Imperial College London
2407848116

AF566643

Hypertension and Cardiovascular Disease

Emmanuel A. Andreadis
Editor

Hypertension and Cardiovascular Disease

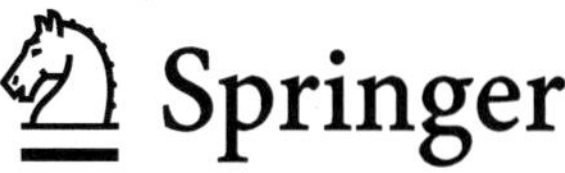

Editor
Emmanuel A. Andreadis
Fourth Internal Medicine Department
Evangelismos State General Hospital
Athens
Greece

ISBN 978-3-319-39597-5 ISBN 978-3-319-39599-9 (eBook)
DOI 10.1007/978-3-319-39599-9

Library of Congress Control Number: 2016952231

Printed on acid-free paper

This Springer imprint is published by Springer Nature
The registered company is Springer International Publishing AG Switzerland

Preface

"*Hypertension And Cardiovascular Disease*" reviews the recent advances in understanding the pathophysiology and the fundamental diagnostic, clinical, and therapeutic aspects of arterial hypertension.

It was with great pleasure that I proceeded in the fulfillment of this venture for two reasons:

First, I felt that despite the considerable bulk of existing literature, the need for such a book is great as knowledge in the field has progressed rapidly over the past years. New large randomized controlled trials and meta-analyses have been published recently providing evidence for a lower blood pressure target for many patients. The impact of these "landmark" studies on hypertension guidelines remains to be seen in the near future. As a hypertension specialist, my ultimate goal is to apply evidence-based medicine to each patient attending the Hypertension Center that I have run at Evangelismos General Hospital for almost two decades and which has been recognized as an Excellence Center by the European Society of Hypertension. Evidence-based practice is not a new concept. It is the integration of best research evidence with clinical expertise and patient values. Personally, I strongly urge my attending and resident physicians to use their clinical skills and past experience to rapidly identify each patient's unique health state and diagnosis, individual risks and benefits of potential treatment strategies, taking into account their patient's personal health status and expectations. Getting the most of each clinical encounter will guide them into making appropriate clinical decisions for their patients.

Second, my vision is to offer to young physicians and other scientists engaged in the clinical cardiovascular field a book that integrates basic medical science knowledge with applied clinical medicine, keeping in mind that physician-scientists are a vital force in transforming clinical observations into testable research hypotheses and translating research findings into medical advances, thus having a substantial effect on people's lives. Therefore, the main goal of this book is to inspire young physicians and urge them to become a critical resource in the future for assuring excellence in medical education and to teach their students that the basis of medicine is science and that scientific rigor should apply to patient care as well as research.

It is clear that this book represents a valuable tool for scientists engaged in the field since it collates and updates knowledge in this area. Each chapter adopts a concise approach to its topic and can therefore be read on its own. As you will find easily, this book focuses on the deleterious consequences that hypertension has on the cardiovascular system, since hypertension often coexists with heart disease, arrhythmia, and dyslipidemia, further increasing total cardiovascular risk. The way we should approach a patient with hypertension and cardiovascular disease is the main objective of this book.

For the completion of this project, I did invite contributors who are widely recognized as global leaders in the field of hypertension. They have worked hard to expertly and concisely review their area of expertise. Each chapter merits multiple reads and can act as a starting point for anyone seeking an up-to-date and scientifically accurate review in the aforementioned areas. I am grateful to the authors who invested their time so generously in this effort. I would like to express my deepest and sincere gratitude for their valuable contribution to the fulfillment of this project. Their outstanding work has given this book the opportunity to succeed as an educational resource for the scientific community and to enhance the clinical skills of practicing physicians.

My sincere thanks to my wonderful wife for her invaluable help, immense support, and infinite patience while I worked on this book and to my beloved daughter for her encouragement in my research and clinical activities and for her understanding. Most importantly, I thank my colleague Charalampia V. Geladari for her enthusiasm, creativity, commitment, and dedication to bringing this book into fruition. She urged me, supported me, and organized every detail in completing this ambitious goal.

I would also like to thank Grant Weston, the Editor of Springer International Publishing, who worked so diligently with us toward the publication of this book.

Last, but not least, this book would have not been published without the decisive contribution of the Professor Vasilios Papadementriou, the peer-reviewer of this book.

Athens, Greece Emmanuel A. Andreadis

Contents

Contributors

Tonje A. Aksnes, M.D., Ph.D. Department of Cardiology, Oslo University Hospital Ullevaal, Oslo, Norway

Emmanuel A. Andreadis, M.D., Ph.D. 4th Department of Internal Medicine, "Evangelismos" State General Hospital, Athens, Greece

Hypertension and Cardiovascular Disease Prevention Outpatient Clinic, "Evangelismos" State General Hospital, Athens, Greece

Nadia Boubouchairopoulou, M.Sc. Hypertension Center STRIDE-7, National and Kapodistrian University of Athens, Third Department of Medicine, Sotiria Hospital, Athens, Greece

Chrysoula Boutari, M.D. 2nd Propedeutic Department of Internal Medicine, Aristotle University, Thessaloniki, Greece

Paola Chrysostomou Department of Veterans Affairs Medical Center, and National Institutes of Health (NIH), Intramural Research Program (IRP), Institute of Clinical Research, Washington, DC, USA

Antonio Coca, M.D., Ph.D. Hypertension and Vascular Risk Unit, Hypertension, Nutrition and Aging Unit, Department of Internal Medicine, Hospital Clinic, IDIBAPS (Institut d´Investigacions Biomèdiques August Pi i Sunyer), University of Barcelona, Barcelona, Spain

Dennis Cokkinos, M.D., Ph.D. Clinical, Experimental Surgery, Translational Research Centre, Biomedical Research Foundation Academy of Athens, Athens, Greece

Amelie F. Constant, Ph.D. Department of Economics, Migration Economics, United Nations University, UNU-MERIT, Maastricht, The Netherlands

Society of Government Economists SGE, Washington, DC, USA

IZA, Bonn, Germany

Temple University, Philadelphia, PA, USA

Giovanni de Simone, M.D., FESC, FACC, FAHA Hypertension Research Center, FEDERICO II University Naples, Naples, Italy

Mónica Domenech, M.D., Ph.D. Hypertension and Vascular Risk Unit, Hypertension, Nutrition and Aging Unit, Department of Internal Medicine, Hospital Clinic, IDIBAPS (Institut d´Investigacions Biomèdiques August Pi i Sunyer), University of Barcelona, Barcelona, Spain

Michael Doumas, M.D., Ph.D. Department of Medicine, Veteran Affairs Medical Center and George Washington University, Washington, DC, USA

2nd Propedeutic Department of Internal Medicine, Aristotle University, Thessaloniki, Greece

Maria Dulak-Lis, Ph.D. Institute of Cardiovascular and Medical Sciences, BHF Glasgow Cardiovascular Research Centre, University of Glasgow, Glasgow, UK

Serap E. Erdine, M.D. Department of Cardiology, Istanbul University Cerrhpa, School of Medicine, Istanbul, Turkey

Charles Faselis, M.D. Cardiology Department, Veterans Affairs Medical Center, Washington, DC, USA

George Washington University School of Medicine, Washington, DC, USA

Ioannis Felekos, M.D. Department of Cardiology, Hippokrateion Hospital, Athens, Greece

Eleni V. Geladari, M.D. Division of Cardiology, Department of Medicine, Beth Israel Deaconess Medical Center, Harvard Medical School, Boston, MA, USA

4th Department of Internal Medicine, "Evangelismos" General Hospital, Athens, Greece

First Internal Medicine Department, Evangelismos General Hospital, Athens, Greece

Charalampia V. Geladari, M.D. Division of Cardiology, Department of Medicine, Beth Israel Deaconess Medical Center, Harvard Medical School, Boston, MA, USA

4th Department of Internal Medicine, Hypertension and Cardiovascular Disease Prevention Outpatient Center, Evangelismos General Hospital, Athens, Greece

Styliani A. Geronikolou, M.Sc., Ph.D. Clinical, Experimental Surgery, Translational Research Centre, Biomedical Research Foundation Academy of Athens, Athens, Greece

Geoffrey A. Head, B.Sc., Ph.D. Baker IDI Heart and Diabetes Institute, Melbourne, VIC, Australia

Janusz Kaczorowski, Ph.D. Department of Family and Emergency Medicine, Université de Montréal and CRCHUM, Montreal, QC, Canada

Yuan-Yuan Kang, Ph.D. Centre for Epidemiological Studies and Clinical Trials, Shanghai Key Laboratory of Hypertension, The Shanghai Institute of Hypertension, Ruijin Hospital, Shanghai Jiaotong University School of Medicine, Shanghai, China

Sverre E. Kjeldsen, M.D., Ph.D., FAHA, FESC Department of Cardiology, Oslo University Hospital Ullevaal, Oslo, Norway

Peter Kokkinos, Ph.D., FACSM, FAHA Cardiology Department, Veterans Affairs Medical Center, Washington, DC, USA

Georgetown University School of Medicine, Washington, DC, USA

Department of Exercise Science, Arnold School of Public Health, University of South Carolina, Columbia, SC, USA

George Washington University School of Medicine, Washington, DC, USA

Maria Irene Kontaridis, Ph.D. Division of Cardiology, Department of Medicine, Beth Israel Deaconess Medical Center, Boston, MA, USA

Department of Biological Chemistry and Molecular Pharmacology, Harvard Medical School, Boston, MA, USA

Division of Cardiology, Department of Medicine, Beth Israel Deaconess Medical Center, Center for Life Sciences, Boston, MA, USA

Athanasios J. Manolis, M.D., FESC, FACC, FAHA Department of Cardiology, Asklepeion General Hospital, Athens, Greece

Augusto C. Montezano, Ph.D. Institute of Cardiovascular and Medical Sciences, BHF Glasgow Cardiovascular Research Centre, University of Glasgow, Glasgow, UK

Carmine Morisco, M.D. Hypertension Research Center, FEDERICO II University Naples, Naples, Italy

Martin G. Myers, M.D., FRCPC Division of Cardiology, Schulich Heart Program, Sunnybrook Health Sciences Centre, Toronto, ON, Canada

Department of Medicine, University of Toronto, Toronto, ON, Canada

Puneet Narayan, M.D. Department of Medicine, Veterans Affairs Medical Center, Washington, DC, USA

Petros Nihoyannopoulos, M.D., FRCP, FESC, FACC, FAHA Department of Cardiology, Imperial College London, London, UK

National Kapodistrian University of Athens, Athens, Greece

Paolo Palatini, M.D. Department of Medicine, University of Padova, Padova, Italy

Vascular Medicine, DIMED, University of Padova, Padova, Italy

Vasilios Papademetriou, M.D. Department of Medicine, Georgetown University, Washington, DC, USA

Division of Hypertension and Vascular Medicine, Veteran Affairs Medical Center, Washington, DC, USA

Theodore G. Papaioannou, Ph.D. Assistant Professor in Biomedical Engineering at the Medical School of National and Kapodistrian University of Athens, Department of Medicine, Athens, Greece

Panagiota Pietri, M.D. Hypertension Unit, Athens Heart Center, Athens Medical Center, Athens, Greece

Andreas Pittaras, M.D. Cardiology Department, Veterans Affairs Medical Center, Washington, DC, USA

Department of Medicine, George Washington University School of Medicine, Washington, DC, USA

Athanasios D. Protogerou Cardiovascular Prevention and Research Unit, Department of Pathophysiology, Medical School, National and Kapodistrian University of Athens, Athens, Greece

Mohammad Shenasa, M.D. Heart and Rhythm Medical Group, Department of Cardiovascular Services, O'Connor Hospital, San Jose, CA, USA

George S. Stergiou, M.D., FRCP Hypertension Center STRIDE-7, National and Kapodistrian University of Athens, Third Department of Medicine, Sotiria Hospital, Athens, Greece

Rhian M. Touyz, M.D., Ph.D. Institute of Cardiovascular and Medical Sciences, BHF Glasgow Cardiovascular Research Centre, University of Glasgow, Glasgow, UK

Bruno Trimarco, M.D. Hypertension Research Center, FEDERICO II University Naples, Naples, Italy

Costas Tsioufis, M.D., Ph.D., FESC, FACC First Cardiology Clinic, Department of Cardiology, University of Athens, Hippokration Hospital, Athens, Greece

Department of Medicine, Georgetown University, Washington, DC, USA

Sofia Tsiropoulou, Ph.D. Institute of Cardiovascular and Medical Sciences, BHF Glasgow Cardiovascular Research Centre, University of Glasgow, Glasgow, UK

Charalambos Vlachopoulos, M.D., FESC First Cardiology Department, Athens University School of Medicine, Hippokration Hospital, Athens, Greece

Dimitrios A. Vrachatis, M.D., M.Sc., Ph.D. Department of Medicine, Medical School, National and Kapodistrian University of Athens, Athens, Greece

Ji-Guang Wang, M.D., Ph.D. Centre for Epidemiological Studies and Clinical Trials, Shanghai Key Laboratory of Hypertension, The Shanghai Institute of Hypertension, Ruijin Hospital, Shanghai Jiaotong University School of Medicine, Shanghai, China

The Shanghai Institute of Hypertension, Shanghai, China

Misbah Zaheer, M.D. Department of Medicine, Georgetown University, Washington, DC, USA

Chapter 1
Hypertension: A Growing Threat

Emmanuel A. Andreadis

Abbreviations

ABP	Ambulatory Blood Pressure
ACC	American College of Cardiology
AF	Atrial Fibrillation
AHA	American Heart Association
AML/ATOR	Amlodipine/Atorvastatin
ARIC	Atherosclerosis Risk in Communities
ASH/ISH	American Society of Hypertension/International Society of Hypertension
BP	Blood Pressure
BPV	Blood Pressure Variability
CAD	Coronary Artery Disease
CDC	Center for Disease Control
CHD	Coronary Heart Disease
CHNS	China Health and Nutrition Survey
CVD	Cardiovascular Disease
DBP	Diastolic Blood Pressure
DM	Diabetes Mellitus
ESH/ESC	European Society of Hypertension/European Society of Cardiology
HHD	Hypertensive Heart Disease
HRT	Hormone Replacement Therapy
HTN	Hypertension
IHD	Ischemic Heart Disease
JNC8	Eighth Joint National Committee
LVH	Left Ventricular Hypertrophy
MH	Masked Hypertension

E.A. Andreadis, M.D., Ph.D.
4th Department of Internal Medicine, "Evangelismos" State General Hospital, AHEPA Building, Room 528 Ipsilantou 45-47, Athens, ATT 13122, Greece

Hypertension and Cardiovascular Disease Prevention Outpatient Clinic, "Evangelismos" State General Hospital, Athens, Greece
e-mail: andreadise@usa.net

E.A. Andreadis (ed.), *Hypertension and Cardiovascular Disease*,
DOI 10.1007/978-3-319-39599-9_1

MI	Myocardial Infarction
NHANES	National Health and Nutrition Examination Survey
PWV	Pulse Wave Velocity
RAAS	Renin Angiotensin System
SBP	Systolic Blood Pressure
SCD	Sudden Cardiac Death
SHR	Spontaneously Hypertensive Rats
TOD	Target Organ Damage
WCE	White Coat Effect
WHD	World Hypertension Day
WHL	World Hypertension League
WHO	World Health Organization

Hypertension Is a Growing Threat Worldwide and a Primary Risk Factor for Cardiovascular Disease

Hypertension (HTN), commonly known as high blood pressure (BP), remains a mounting threat in modern societies despite the implementation of new clinical guidelines and the broad availability of effective pharmaceutical agents. This is due *firstly* to the fact that HTN is considered the major risk factor for cardiovascular disease (CVD), *secondly* to the continued increase of the HTN prevalence and *thirdly* to the inadequate BP control regardless of the remarkable advances in antihypertensive drug therapy [1]. In addition, it has been observed that HTN is associated with a constellation of other risk factors, such as hypercholesterolemia and diabetes mellitus (DM). Fundamentally, the assessment and accurate stratification of global risk in individual patients is critical for the overall CVD risk reduction, and is nowadays regarded as the main determinant for HTN management [2]. Specifically, it has been suggested that in order to prevent CVD complications, a paradigm shift away from the treatment of risk factors in isolation, towards an integrated cardiovascular risk-management approach, is required [3]. According, to the World Health Report 2002, HTN specialists should take firm actions against the major and contributing risk factors associated with HTN and cardiovascular diseases, such as diabetes, cancers and chronic respiratory diseases: tobacco, alcohol, physical inactivity and unhealthy diet [4].

It is known that HTN, is a major modifiable risk factor for cardiovascular and renal diseases, and the single most important risk factor for stroke [5–7]. However, many people have high BP levels that go undetected for months or even years before they are diagnosed as having essential HTN [8]. Franco et al., reported that if HTN remains untreated it shortens life expectancy by 5 years during adulthood. This association is stronger than estimated previously, and affects both sexes similarly [9]. Survey data regarding HTN prevalence based on gender, indicate that systolic blood pressure (SBP) is higher among younger men than women, whereas it becomes higher in women beyond the age of sixty in Canada, and the age of seventy in the US, compared to men [10]. Menopause is considered to play a central role in the higher BP levels observed in middle-aged and elderly women, suggesting that the loss of estrogens may be a critical component of this association. However, hormone replacement therapy (HRT) in most cases does not significantly reduce BP in postmenopausal women, pointing to other co-existing unrevealed mechanisms involved in the higher BP levels observed in women after menopause that are yet to be identified. On the other hand, androgens may decrease only slightly in postmenopausal women, if at all, implying that male sex hormones may also be responsible for increases in BP levels. Several mechanisms by which androgens increase BP have been proposed with the renin-angiotensin-aldosterone system (RAAS) playing a central role in mediating HTN in spontaneously hypertensive rats (SHR) in several animal studies [11].

Furthermore, HTN affects one billion people worldwide and the World Health Organization (WHO) estimates that raised BP levels kill nine million people every year [12] (Figs. 1.1 and 1.2). Interestingly, in a study by Lawes et al., 7.6 million premature deaths, 13.5 % of the global total, were attributed to uncontrolled high BP. People, living in low and middle-income economies, middle-aged individuals (around 45–69 years of age), and patients whose BP level was within the prehypertensive range, were found to represent the most afflicted populations. Indicatively, in the East Asia-Pacific region, up to 66 % of some subtypes of CVD can be attributed to HTN, underscoring the need for a primary healthcare system that will identify high-risk individuals and the importance of implementing new and effective

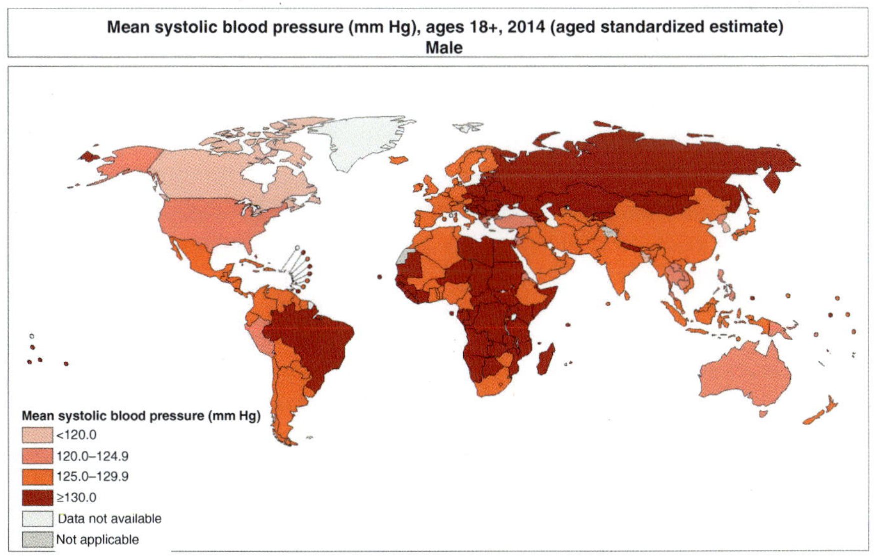

Fig. 1.1 Mean systolic blood pressure (mmHg) in males aged 18+, in 2014, across the continents (Reused with permission from the World Health Organization (WHO))

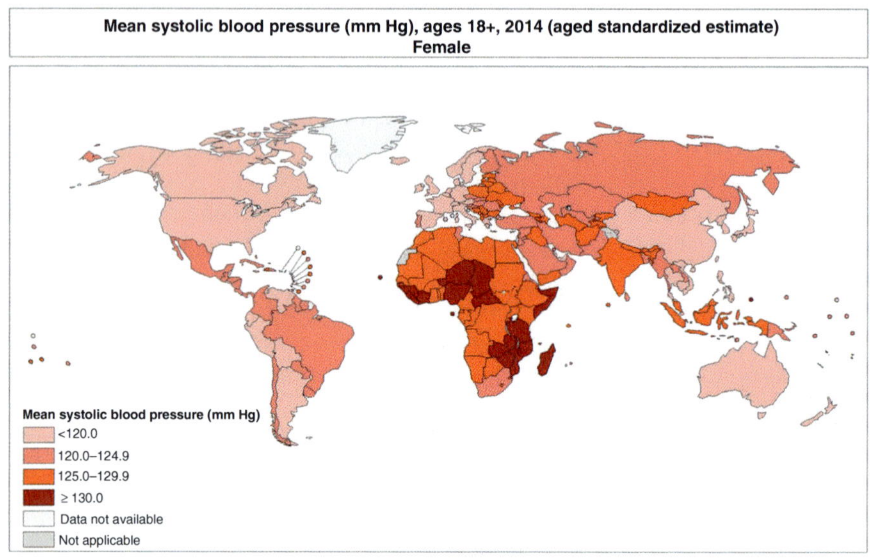

Fig. 1.2 Mean systolic blood pressure (mmHg) in women aged 18+, in 2014, across the continents (Reused with permission from the World Health Organization (WHO))

BP-lowering strategies to prevent fatal complications in these populations [13–15]. Additionally, when the total global impact of known risk factors on the overall burden of the CVD is considered, 54 % of stroke and 47 % of ischemic heart disease (IHD) worldwide, was attributed to HTN [13] (Fig. 1.3). Furthermore, researchers cautioned that even though HTN is not an infectious disease, the risky behaviors associated with it, like smoking rates, patterns of alcohol consumption, and suboptimal physical activity, are spreading fast and seem to be as effectively transmitted as infectious agents [16]. Interestingly, based on available data it is estimated that the number of deaths attributable to HTN over the next 20 years may well substantially exceed the number resulting from HIV/AIDS. This has led epidemiologists to describe HTN using terms such as: "the new HIV epidemic" [16].

Since HTN gives no clear warning signs or symptoms before its diagnosis is fully established, it is referred to as a "silent killer", and thus, both its prevention and management represent one of the greatest challenges in public health care today [12]. CVD is undeniably the number one cause of death worldwide [17]. Data from a survey study suggests that HTN is responsible for an estimated 395,000 cardiovascular deaths annually, making it the leading cause of death in the USA after smoking [18] (Fig. 1.4). It is also an important risk factor for myocardial infarction (MI), since it is associated with the development of atherosclerosis [19, 20]. Links between HTN and MI are clearly established, as high BP poses an increased mechanical stress on blood vessels, thereby contributing to endothelial dysfunction, the progression of atherosclerosis, and plaque rupture [21]. Notably, the Framingham Heart Study has added much to our understanding of the epidemiology of BP and CVD [22]. In 1959, Kagan et al. first recruited men and women from the town of Framingham, Massachusetts, and followed them up over a 6 year period, in order to

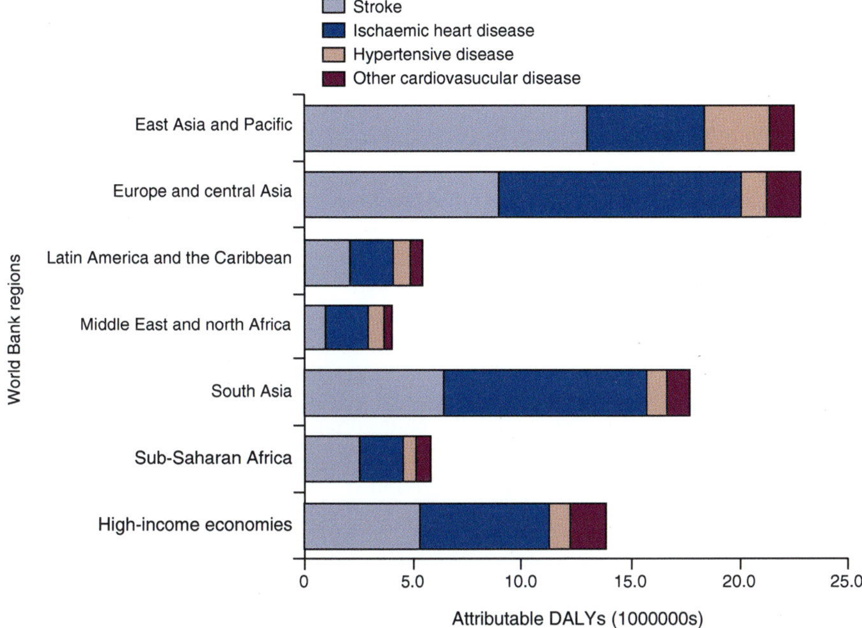

Fig. 1.3 Disability-adjusted life years (DALYs) attributable to high blood pressure by region and endpoint in 2001 (Reused with permission from Lawes et al. [13])

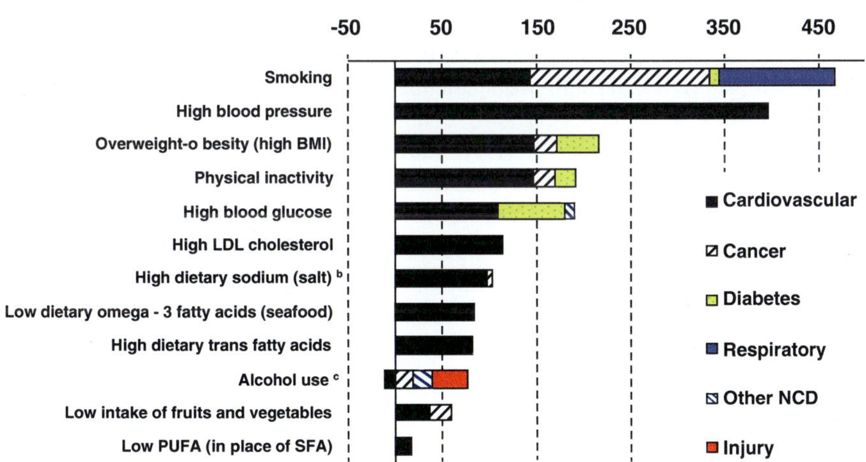

Fig. 1.4 HTN is the leading cause of death in the USA after smoking (Reused with permission from Danaei et al. [18])

assess the relationship between BP and the development of coronary heart disease (CHD). Researchers, concluded that both SBP and diastolic BP (DBP) rise proportionally with increasing age in both men and women [23]. It has also been shown that the increase in BP observed with ageing is mostly associated with structural changes in the arteries and especially with large artery stiffness [24]. Consequently, age-related stiffening of the arteries leads to increased pulse wave velocity (PWV), which is also considered as an independent predictor of cardiovascular morbidity and mortality in hypertensive patients [25]. Several studies have demonstrated that continued rises in BP result in higher CVD risk. This highlights the importance of optimal BP control at early stages of disease, allowing target organ damage (TOD) to be prevented in a timely manner [26].

Blood Pressure Components as Independent Predictors of Cardiovascular Risk

Until 1990, DBP was still considered as a better predictor for CHD and cerebrovascular stroke than SBP, worldwide [27]. Since then, data from a prospective study have shown that mortality from both CHD and stroke increases progressively and linearly from BP levels as low as 115 mmHg systolic and 75 mmHg diastolic upward, and it has been observed that with increments of 20 mmHg systolic or 10 mmHg diastolic pressure, mortality from both IHD and stroke doubles [28]. Moreover, Framingham Heart Study Investigators reported that even high-normal BP (SBP of 130–139 mmHg, DBP of 85–89 mmHg, or both) was associated with an increased risk of CVD as compared to lower BP levels, emphasizing the need to determine whether lowering high-normal BP can reduce the risk of CVD [29]. Apart from SBP and DBP, overwhelming evidence shows that BP variability (BPV) is a key factor in predicting cardiovascular outcomes. Significant BP variations within a 24-h period are associated with increased CVD risk [30]. A study conducted by Parati et al., showed that in diabetic patients, the incidence of CHD is significantly greater in those with increased 24-h systolic BPV [30]. Moreover, it has been observed that nocturnal systolic HTN is an independent risk factor for coronary artery disease (CAD) in patients with diabetic nephropathy [31]. A large meta-analysis of prospective studies from Europe, Asia, and South America, suggested that this non-dipping BP pattern also predicted total mortality and cardiovascular events compared to the normal or extreme dipping pattern, independent of cohort and confounding variables and after adjustment for 24-h BP [32]. Recently, it has been showed that non-dipper sustained hypertensives have a twofold greater risk of developing atrial fibrillation (AF) than dipper ones [33]. This may be due to the fact that nighttime HTN may be a powerful determinant of long-standing left ventricular diastolic dysfunction, which subsequently increases atrial stretch. Furthermore, it has been observed that nighttime hemodynamics, are associated with higher sympathetic and reduced vagal activity, which may trigger AF. Additionally, sympathetic activation is associated with the stimulation of the renin-angiotensin-aldosterone axis, which leads to increased left ventricular diastolic preload, both atrial and ventricular fibrosis, thus exerting direct cellular electrophysiological effects [33]. However, further research is needed to elucidate the role held by hypertensive heart disease (HHD) progression in arrhythmogenesis and sudden cardiac death (SCD).

Furthermore, studies have demonstrated that whereas normal morning BP surge is a physiological phenomenon, an exaggerated morning BP surge is associated with increased CVD risk and mortality [34]. Left ventricular hypertrophy (LVH) and carotid artery atherosclerosis have also been found to be independently associated with increased morning BP surge [35, 36]. On the other hand, Verdecchia et al. suggests that in untreated hypertensive subjects without overt cardiovascular disease an excessive BP surge does not portend an increased risk of events [37]. We anticipate that ongoing research regarding morning BP surge may allow determination of its prognostic importance with respect to other BP components, such as dipping or non-dipping pattern, systolic and/or diastolic HTN.

Hypertension Prevalence Across the Continents

Based on a pooled analysis of available national and regional data, Kearney et al., reported that HTN prevalence continues to increase, worldwide [38]. The overall prevalence of raised BP in adults, aged 25 and over, was around 40 % in 2008. Tu et al., found that the age-and sex-adjusted prevalence of HTN in Ontario, among adults aged 20 years and older increased by 60.0 % from 1995 to 2005, and by 20.9 % from 2000 to 2005 [39]. According to the 2013 WHO global brief update, 9.4 million deaths worldwide every year were attributed to complications of HTN. Furthermore, HTN is accountable for 45 % of deaths owing to heart disease, whereas it is responsible for 51 % of deaths due to stroke [12, 40]. According to WHO the prevalence of high BP was highest in Africa, with a reported rate of 46 % for both sexes combined [3]. HTN in sub-Saharan Africa is a widespread problem, and its prevalence is higher in urban versus rural communities [41], owing to lifestyle changes associated with "civilization" such as heavier body weights (obesity), increased pulse rates as well as increased urinary sodium-potassium ratio [42]. Hypertensive TOD is common in Nigeria, where HTN awareness is rather low, and is often the reason that brings patients to healthcare facilities. HTN is also the major risk factor for stroke in Nigeria, and frequently affects younger age groups [43]. Data from NHANES (National Health and Nutrition Examination Survey), a representative sample of adults in the U.S. indicate that the prevalence has increased from fifty million in the period from 1988 through to 1994–65 million in the period from 1999 through to 2004, an increase from 24.4 to 28.9 % [44]. Interestingly, it has been showed that 28 % of Americans with HTN are unaware that they have the condition, 39 % are receiving no therapy, and 65 % have insufficient BP control [14]. The CARMELA Study, a cross-sectional, epidemiologic study assessing cardiovascular risk factors in seven Latin American cities, concluded that HTN prevalence ranged from 9 % in Quito to 29 % in Buenos Aires, and that the majority of the population had other co-existing cardiovascular risk factors, with only 9.19 % of the participants having HTN as a lone cardiovascular risk factor. Scientists suggested that public health programs are needed in order to target prevention, early diagnosis and guide HTN management in order to decrease global CVD risk in Latin American populations [45].

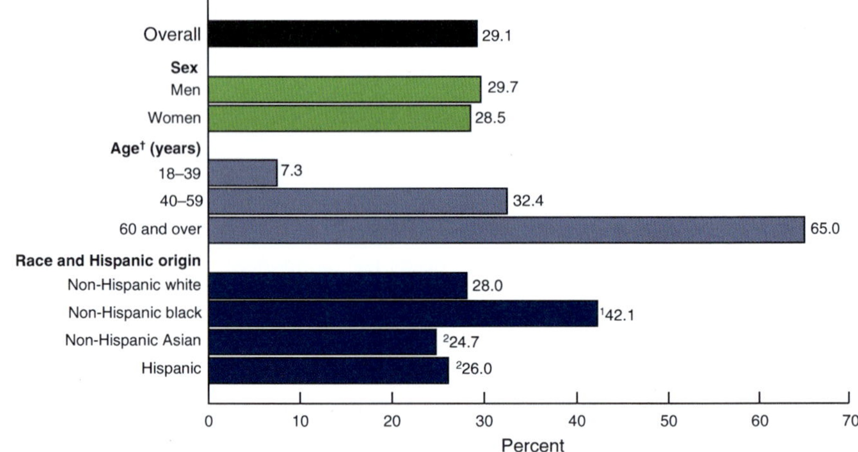

Fig. 1.5 Age-specific and age-adjusted prevalence of hypertension among US adults aged 18 and over, during 2011–2012 (Reused with permission from the National Center for Health Statistics (NCHS) and the Centers for Disease Control and Prevention (CDC))

It has been observed that the prevalence of HTN is higher among blacks than whites or Mexican Americans in both men and women, and increases with age, becoming more predominant among black women [46] (Fig. 1.5). The higher prevalence of HTN reported in blacks has been recognized as the most significant factor for the higher incidence of cardiovascular disease and mortality observed in this population [47]. Moreover, HTN prevalence is higher in blacks living in the USA rather than those living in Africa, a fact that highlights the importance of environmental and behavioural characteristics in this association [48]. Genetic traits, a higher sensitivity to alcohol, as well as a higher renal sodium retention by blacks, have been proposed as the mechanisms for the higher HTN prevalence observed in black Americans versus white Americans [49]. The consequences of aging and the increased prevalence of HTN have been shown in the Framingham Heart Study population in which 90 % of persons who had normal BP at 55 or 65 years of age became hypertensive over the subsequent 20 years. If this residual lifetime risk remains unattenuated, it becomes more than clear that the societal burden of HTN will increase further. This underscores the need for a preventive healthcare system oriented toward primary care [50]. Similarly in the Atherosclerosis Risk In Communities (ARIC) study, which followed up more than 15,000 patients between 45 and 64 years of age for 9 years, the average 5-year age-adjusted increase in systolic BP ranged from 4 to 7 mmHg [51]. Although it has been clearly demonstrated that HTN and atherosclerosis are two distinct disease entities, HTN predisposes to and accelerates atherosclerosis due to the synergistic effect observed between high BP levels and other atherogenic stimuli, both of which induce increased oxidative stress on the arterial wall [52]. It is thus clear that combined antihypertensive and lipid-lowering therapy could further decrease cardiovascular event occurrence and

SCD [53]. In addition, the development of single-pill formulations, such as the single pill amlodipine with atorvastatin (AML/ATOR), is expected to improve patient adherence to treatment and lower costs of therapy [54, 55].

Several factors contributing to the increased prevalence across the USA have been recognized. It has been previously reported that HTN prevalence grows significantly with increasing age. Specifically, pooled data indicate that around 81 % of hypertensive individuals in the USA are older than 45 years of age and obesity, increased body weight, is a crucial factor. The rapid and striking growth of the fast-food industry has meant an increase in consumption of calories, saturated fat, and salt, as well as a reduced intake of fruits, vegetables and complex carbohydrates. High sodium and low potassium intake also contributes to the increased HTN prevalence in the USA. It should be noted that the ratio of dietary sodium to potassium correlates better with BP than the level of either cation alone. Finally, other contributors to the increased prevalence of HTN during lifetime are the excessive alcohol intake, low socioeconomic status, sleep apnea, the use of certain illegal drugs, or the use of over-the-counter medications [6].

The prevalence of HTN in different European countries appears to be 30–45 % of the general population, increasing sharply as the population becomes older [56]. The impact of aging and the accompanying increased prevalence of HTN on stroke mortality in Europe has been analysed using the WHO statistics. Western European countries exhibit a downward trend, in contrast to eastern European countries, which show an increase in death rates from stroke [57]. A review of sample surveys conducted in Europe, indicates that HTN prevalence was highest in Germany (55 %), followed by Finland (49 %), Spain (47 %), England (42 %), Sweden (38 %), and Italy (38 %), whereas on average only 8 % of European hypertensive individuals had their condition controlled compared with 23 % of adults in Canada and the United States [58]. HYPERTENSHELL, a cross-sectional study conducted in 98 Health Centers across Greece, indicated that the level of patient awareness, optimal HTN management and control, is comparable to the best rates of control of HTN given for the problem, with great potentials for further improvements regarding HTN control in the country [59]. At present, with the ongoing global economic crisis and the Depression in Greece, stress perception and HTN prevalence are expected to escalate rapidly. Just how this will affect control rates and patient compliance remains to be seen in years to come.

The prevalence of HTN in China from 2002 to 2012 has increased considerably in both men and women with higher prevalence in north China, as shown in a systematic review and meta-analysis of trends and regional differences [60]. In contrast to African countries, its prevalence in China is higher among younger and rural residents than among urban populations, and patterns are anticipated to rise even further in the future, given the poor status of HTN awareness, treatment, and control. Public health care programs for further improving patient awareness and BP control are still urgently required in this Asian "sleeping giant" [61].

The rise in average life expectancy along with the growing urbanization has led to substantial increases in obesity in all economic regions of the world [62]. Foulds et al. [63], confirmed the well-established relationship between HTN and obesity but found ethnic differences among white, aboriginal, East Asian, and South Asian ethnic background. The higher proportion of HTN and obesity with accompanying high levels of CVD and diabetes were found in aboriginal people as compared to European populations [63]. Available evidence suggests that obesity in hypertensives is associated with an increased risk of renal insufficiency, glucose intolerance and DM. A mix of these three factors may be a potent and dangerous combination and could lead to fatal cardiovascular events [64].

Hypertension Awareness Is Critical for Optimal Blood Pressure Control and Target Organ Damage Prevention

Despite the therapeutic advances in HTN and the acceptance of benefits in lowering BP the number of people with low control of HTN has continued to rise, constituting a major health problem and a growing threat for the communities. Moreover, the increase in obesity and the failure to follow healthy lifestyles, intensifies the need for implementing healthy lifestyles. Discussing the factors responsible for the low control of HTN, Chobanian et al. [6], note: "The failure to adopt healthy lifestyles has been a critical factor in this increase and must be addressed urgently. To make the necessary changes on a broad basis will be difficult, but the benefits will be well worth the effort". The outcome of achieving optimal BP remains disappointing even in randomized controlled trials where patient motivation and physician expertise are ensured [65]. HTN control varies considerably between countries and regions and also by age, sex, ethnicity, socioeconomic status, and education and is especially low in some economically developing countries. The NHANES 1999–2004 database control of BP in the United State was 29 % in 1990–2000 and 37 % in 2003–2004 [66]. In Canada BP control has been achieved only in 16 %. Older hypertensives, those with diabetes type 2 and those with a previous MI had higher rates of treatment and control [67]. In European countries although some improvement in the control rate has subsequently been found in the percentage of the population to attain target BP goals of <140/90 mmHg, it represents a small fraction of the hypertensive population [68]. In the adult English population, control has been achieved in 21.5 % of hypertensive men and 22.8 % of women. An overall control rate of 12 % has been demonstrated in Poland. Furthermore, data from national surveys on HTN treatment and control in Europe have shown the control rate to be 21 % for Sweden, 28 % for Italy, 30 % for Germany and 20.7 % for Turkey [69, 70]. In a large cross-sectional study conducted across 98 Health Centres throughout Greece, involving 11,540 eligible participants and comprising the 0.1 % of the Greek population, the prevalence of HTN was 31.1 % in the overall population and 65.4 % among those older than 65 years of age. In particular, 51.2 % were under treatment and the race of BP control was 32.8 % (men 33.3 %, women 32.3 %) [59]. In the "EPIC" study, another large study of 27,000 patients from several Greek regions, it emerged that the prevalence of HTN was 40 % and the HTN control rate was as low as 15.2 % [71]. Low rates of control have been reported in China Health and Nutrition Survey

(CHNS) in which despite some improvement in the control rate among Chinese adults, the rate from 1991 to 2011 was found to reach 30.1 % [72].

Current population studies are based on clinic BP measurements. If we only use the clinic BP levels, people with masked hypertension (MH) will be regarded as normotensives and those with the white coat effect (WCE) as hypertensives. Pickering realized that when ambulatory blood pressure (ABP) measurements were used, the age-related increase in BP was much smaller than it was indicated by the clinic BP [73]. Specifically, the clinic BP should be higher than ambulatory BP in older adults and this is inclined to happen after the age of 40. On the other hand, in younger individuals, the clinic BP readings tend to underestimate true ABP values leading to the phenomenon of MH. Thus, there is a growing need for people in the prehypertensive range or with MH to be identified who are at highest risk of damage. Such patients could stand to benefit most from early treatment as indicated by meta-analyses of prospective studies reporting the incidence of CVD to be about two times higher than those with normal or optimal BP and similar to the incidence of sustained HTN [74].

It should be made clear that patient knowledge and awareness of HTN are important factors in achieving optimal BP control. Having recognized that more than half of the hypertensive population globally is unaware of their condition, the World Hypertension League (WHL), an umbrella organization of 85 national HTN societies and leagues, initiated an international awareness campaign on HTN in 2005 and established May 17 of each year as World Hypertension Day (WHD). The League supported by an increasing number of national societies conveys the message to the public through several media, such as the Internet and television. The enthusiasm and motivation that every country-member exhibits in this global effort guarantees the success of this program; there is growing confidence that the message will eventually reach all afflicted populations [75]. Moreover, apart from increased patient awareness, several studies have indicated that the educational programs improve patient compliance with antihypertensive therapy, and also control detrimental lifestyle habits of hypertensive patients.

Summarizing proper patient knowledge about HTN early diagnosis, and adherence to treatment along with the new clinical guidelines and innovative therapies, such as polypill formulations, are expected to control the growing threat of this devastating condition worldwide (Fig. 1.6).

Definitions of Hypertension

Clinical practice requires some strict criteria for the definition of HTN in order to determine the need for diagnosis and treatment. More than 35 years ago, Evan and Rose [76] offered an operational definition of HTN; "HTN should be defined in terms of BP level above which investigation and treatment do more good than harm". When scientific societies use numerical definitions of HTN, they rely on the fact that physicians feel more secure when dealing with precise criteria, even if

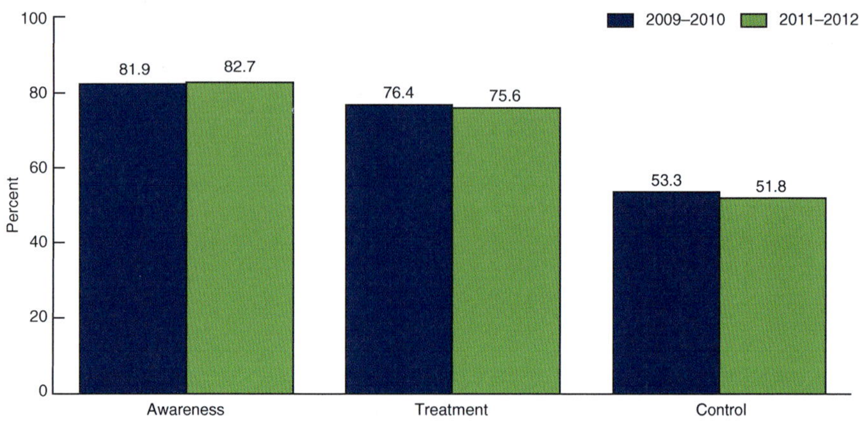

Fig. 1.6 Age-adjusted awareness, treatment, and control of hypertension among US adults with hypertension during 2009–2012 (Reused with permission from the National Center for Health Statistics (NCHS) and the Centers for Disease Control and Prevention (CDC))

these criteria are arbitrary, as Pickering pointed out [77]. Nevertheless, as medical practice requires that some criteria be used to determine the need for treatment, definitions need to be flexible, taken into consideration the benefits and risks and costs of action or inaction.

The European Society of Hypertension/European Society of Cardiology (ESH/ESC) guidelines released in 2013 continue to classify BP <140/90 mmHg into optimal, normal and high normal, recognizing the increased awareness for patients with BP above optimal levels [74]. This classification remains unchanged from the 2003 and 2007 ESH/ESC guidelines. The American Society of Hypertension/International Society of Hypertension (ASH/ISH) clinical practice guidelines tend to use 140/90 mmHg for all adults, up to 80 years of age [78]. The term "prehypertension" has been used when systolic or/and diastolic BP is between 120 and 139 mmHg or/and 80 and 89 mmHg, respectively. Furthermore, there is a discrepancy between ASH/ISH hypertension guidelines and Eighth Joint National Committee (JNC 8) [79]. They both use similar levels for diagnosing HTN but different definition of the elderly. Specifically, JNC 8 guidelines define as elderly those who are 60 years or older whereas ASH/ISH those who are 80 years or older.

In a recent evaluation of the cost-effectiveness of HTN therapy in U.S. adults according to the 2014 JNC 8 guidelines, Moran noted that the implementation of these guidelines would not only prevent about 56,000 cardiovascular events and 13,000 deaths annually, but would also result in cost savings [80]. To amplify the clinical significance of the recent guidelines the American Heart Association (AHA), American College of Cardiology (ACC) and the Center of Disease Control and Prevention (CDC) recommend a dividing line of 139/89 mmHg between normal and high BP goal. Their goal is to help reduce the U.S. death rate from CVD and stroke by 20 % in 2020 [81]. Evidence on the control of HTN seems to play a relatively small role in the decreased mortality from coronary disease in U.S. but a remarkable role in the decreased mortality from CVD. Nevertheless, the benefits of lowering BP reduce the risk of CVD and death as a whole offsetting the side effects from therapy, the required changes in lifestyle and the increase in financial cost. As health care providers should by nature be optimistic, health workers, the academic research community, civil society, the private sector and families and individuals all have a role to play. Only their strenuous effort can connect the testing technology and treatments available to prevent and control HTN and thereby delay or prevent life-threatening complications.

Future Perspectives

HTN has been a major health problem worldwide regardless of the remarkable advances in drug therapy. Furthermore, despite the increased awareness and treatment of BP the outcomes of achieving BP control remain unacceptably low. The discrepancy between improved therapy and more uncontrolled disease guided Chobanian to describe this phenomenon as a "hypertension paradox" [82]. However, we are confident that with proper patient knowledge about HTN, early diagnosis using available innovative BP measuring techniques, and adherence to treatment along with the implementation of new clinical guidelines and novel therapies, we will be able to restrict the escalating cardiovascular risk generated by this "silent killer".

References

1. Antonakoudis G, Poulimenos L, Kifnidis K, Zouras C, Antonakoudis H. Blood pressure control and cardiovascular risk reduction. Hippokratia. 2007;11:114–9.
2. Volpe M, Alderman MH, Furberg CD, Jackson R, Kostis JB, Laragh JH, et al. Beyond hypertension toward guidelines for cardiovascular risk reduction. Am J Hypertens. 2004;17:1068–74.
3. World Health Organization. Integrated management of cardiovascular risk, report of a WHO meeting. Geneva: World Health Organization; 2002.
4. World Health Organization. The World Health Report 2002 'Reducing risks and promoting healthy life'. Geneva, Switzerland: World Health Organization; 2002.
5. Whelton PK. Epidemiology of hypertension. Lancet. 1994;344:101–6.
6. Chobanian AV, Bakris GL, Black HR, Cushman WC, Green LA, Izzo Jr JL, et al. Seventh report of the Joint National Committee on prevention, detection, evaluation, and treatment of high blood pressure. Hypertension. 2003;42:1206–52.
7. Yusuf S, Hawken S, Ounpuu S, Dans T, Avezum A, Lanas F, et al. Effect of potentially modifiable risk factors associated with myocardial infarction in 52 countries (the INTERHEART study): case-control study. Lancet. 2004;364:937–52.
8. Chockalingam A, Campbell NR, Fodor JG. Worldwide epidemic of hypertension. Can J Cardiol. 2006;22:553–5.
9. Franco OH, Peeters A, Bonneux L, de Laet C. Blood pressure in adulthood and life expectancy with cardiovascular disease in men and women: life course analysis. Hypertension. 2005;46:280–6.

10. Joffres M, Falaschetti E, Gillespie C, Robitaille C, Loustalot F, Poulter N, et al. Hypertension prevalence, awareness, treatment and control in national surveys from England, the USA and Canada, and correlation with stroke and ischaemic heart disease mortality: a cross-sectional study. BMJ Open. 2013;3:e003423.
11. Reckelhoff JF. Gender differences in the regulation of blood pressure. Hypertension. 2001;37:1199–208.
12. World Health Organization. A global brief on hypertension. WHO/DCO/WHD/2013.2. 3 Apr 2013. http://apps.who.int/iris/bitstream/10665/79059/1/WHO_DCO_WHD_2013.2_eng.pdf..
13. Lawes CM, Vander Hoorn S, Rodgers A, International Society of Hypertension. Global burden of blood-pressure-related disease. Lancet. 2008;371:1513–8.
14. Martiniuk AL, Lee CM, Lawes CM, Ueshima H, Suh I, Lam TH, et al. Hypertension: its prevalence and population-attributable fraction for mortality from cardiovascular disease in the Asia-Pacific region. J Hypertens. 2007;25:73–9.
15. Ueshima H, Sekikawa A, Miura K, Turin TC, Takashima N, Kita Y, et al. Cardiovascular disease and risk factors in Asia a selected review. Circulation. 2008;118:2702–9.
16. Lloyd-Sherlock P, Ebrahim S, Grosskurth H. Is hypertension the new HIV epidemic? Int J Epidemiol. 2014;43:8–10.
17. Mathers CD, Lopez AD, Murray CJL. The burden of disease and mortality by condition: data, methods, and results for 2001. Glob Burden Dis Risk Factors. 2006;45:88.
18. Danaei G, Ding EL, Mozaffarian D, Taylor B, Rehm J, Murray CJ, et al. The preventable causes of death in the United States: comparative risk assessment of dietary, lifestyle, and metabolic risk factors. PLoS Med. 2009;6:e1000058.
19. Richards AM, Nicholls MG, Troughton RW, Lainchbury JG, Elliott J, Frampton C, et al. Antecedent hypertension and heart failure after myocardial infarction. J Am Coll Cardiol. 2002;39:1182–8.
20. Picariello C, Lazzeri C, Attanà P, Chiostri M, Gensini GF, Valente S. The impact of hypertension on patients with acute coronary syndromes. Int J Hyper. 2011;563:657.
21. Rakugi H, Yu H, Kamitani A, Nakamura Y, Ohishi M, Kamide K, et al. Links between hypertension and myocardial infarction. Am Heart J. 1996;132:213–21.
22. Franklin SS, Wong ND. Hypertension and cardiovascular disease: contributions of the Framingham Heart Study. Glob Heart. 2013;8:49–57.
23. Kagan A, Gordon T, Kannel WB, Dawber TR. Proceedings of the council for high blood pressure research. J Am Heart Assoc. 1959:53–81.
24. Pinto E. Blood pressure and ageing. Postgrad Med J. 2007;83:109–14.
25. Cecelja M, Chowienczyk P. Role of arterial stiffness in cardiovascular disease. JRSM Cardiovasc Dis. 2012;1:11.
26. Carretero OA, Oparil S. Essential hypertension part I: definition and etiology. Circulation. 2000;101:329–35.
27. Collins R, Peto R, MacMahon S, Hebert P, Fiebach NH, Eberlein KA, et al. Blood pressure, stroke, and coronary heart disease: part 2, short-term reductions in blood pressure: overview of randomized drug trials in their epidemiological context. Lancet. 1990;335:827–38.
28. Lewington S, Clarke R, Qizilbash N, Peto R, Collins R, Prospective Studies Collaboration. Age specific relevance of usual blood pressure to vascular mortality: a meta-analysis of individual data for one million adults in 61 prospective studies. Lancet. 2002;360:1903–13.
29. Vasan RS, Larson MG, Leip EP, Evans JC, O'Donnell CJ, Kannel WB, et al. Impact of high-normal blood pressure on the risk of cardiovascular disease. N Engl J Med. 2001;345:1291–7.
30. Parati G, Ochoa JE, Salvi P, Lombardi C, Bilo G. Prognostic value of blood pressure variability and average blood pressure levels in patients with hypertension and diabetes. Diabetes Care. 2013;36:S312–24.
31. Tamura K, Tsurumi Y, Sakai M, Tanaka Y, Okano Y, Yamauchi J, et al. A possible relationship of nocturnal blood pressure variability with coronary artery disease in diabetic nephropathy. Clin Exp Hypertens. 2007;29:31–42.
32. Boggia J, Li Y, Thijs L, Hansen TW, Kikuya M, Björklund-Bodegård K, et al. Prognostic accuracy of day versus night ambulatory blood pressure: a cohort study. Lancet. 2007;370:1219–29.

33. Pierdomenico SD, Lapenna D, Cuccurullo F. Risk of atrial fibrillation in dipper and nondipper sustained hypertensive patients. Blood Press Monit. 2008;13:193–7.
34. Kario K. Morning surge in blood pressure and cardiovascular risk evidence and perspectives. Hypertension. 2010;56:765–73.
35. Kaneda R, Kario K, Hoshide S, Umeda Y, Hoshide Y, Shimada K. Morning blood pressure hyperreactivity is an independent predictor for hypertensive cardiac hypertrophy in a community-dwelling population. Am J Hypertens. 2005;18:1528–33.
36. Yano Y, Hoshide S, Inokuchi T, Kanemaru Y, Shimada K, Kario K. Association between morning blood pressure surge and cardiovascular remodeling in treated elderly hypertensive subjects. Am J Hypertens. 2009;22:1177–82.
37. Verdecchia P, Angeli F, Mazzotta G, Garofoli M, Ramundo E, Gentile G, et al. Day-night dip and early-morning surge in blood pressure in hypertension. Prospective implications. Hypertension. 2012;60:34–42.
38. Kearney PM, Whelton M, Reynolds K, Muntner P, Whelton PK, He J. Global burden of hypertension: analysis of worldwide data. Lancet. 2005;365:217–23.
39. Tu K, Chen Z, Lipscombe LL, Canadian Hypertension Education Program Outcomes Research Taskforce. Prevalence and incidence of hypertension from 1995 to 2005: a population-based study. CMAJ. 2008;178:1429–35.
40. Mendis S. Hypertension: a silent contributor to the global cardiovascular epidemic. Regional Health Forum. 2013;17:6.
41. Opie LH, Seedat YK. Hypertension in sub-Saharan African populations. Circulation. 2005;112:3562–8.
42. Poulter NR, Khaw K, Hopwood BE, Mugambi M, Peart WS, Sever PS. Determinants of blood pressure changes due to urbanization: a longitudinal study. J Hypertens Suppl. 1985;3: S375–7.
43. Ogah OS, Okpechi I, Chukwuonye II, Akinyemi JO, Onwubere BJ, Falase AO, et al. Blood pressure, prevalence of hypertension and hypertension related complications in Nigerian Africans: a review. World J Cardiol. 2012;4:327–40.
44. Cutler JA, Sorlie PD, Wolz M, Thom T, Fields LE, Roccella EJ. Trends in hypertension prevalence, awareness, treatment, and control rates in United States adults between 1988–1994 and 1999–2004. Hypertension. 2008;52:818–27.
45. Hernández-Hernández R, Silva H, Velasco M, Pellegrini F, Macchia A, Escobedo J, et al. Hypertension in seven Latin American cities: the cardiovascular risk factor multiple evaluation in Latin America (CARMELA) study. J Hypertens. 2010;28:24–34.
46. Lloyd-Jones D, Adams R, Carnethon M, De Simone G, Ferguson TB, Flegal K, et al. Heart disease and stroke statistics—2009 update a report from the American Heart Association Statistics Committee and Stroke Statistics Subcommittee. Circulation. 2009;119:e21–181.
47. Lloyd-Jones D, Adams RJ, Brown TM, Carnethon M, Dai S, De Simone G, American Heart Association Statistics Committee and Stroke Statistics Subcommittee, et al. Executive summary: heart disease and stroke statistics–2010 update: a report from the American Heart Association. Circulation. 2010;121:948–54.
48. Cooper RS, Wolf-Maier K, Luke A, Adeyemo A, Banegas JR, Forrester T, et al. An international comparative study of blood pressure in populations of European vs. African descent. BMC Med. 2005;3:2.
49. Fuchs FD. Why do Black Americans have higher prevalence of hypertension? An enigma still unsolved. Hypertension. 2011;57:379–80.
50. Vasan RS, Beiser A, Seshadri S, Larson MG, Kannel WB, D'Agostino RB, et al. Residual lifetime risk for developing hypertension in middle-aged women and men: the Framingham Heart Study. JAMA. 2002;287:1003–10.
51. Diez Roux AV, Chambless L, Merkin SS, Arnett D, Eigenbrodt M, Nieto FJ, et al. Socioeconomic disadvantage and change in blood pressure associated with aging. Circulation. 2002;106:703–10.
52. Alexander RW. Theodore Cooper Memorial Lecture. Hypertension and the pathogenesis of atherosclerosis. Oxidative stress and the mediation of arterial inflammatory response: a new perspective. Hypertension. 1995;25:155–61.

53. Barkas F, Liberopoulos E, Elisaf M. Impact of compliance with antihypertensive and lipid-lowering treatment on cardiovascular risk benefits. Hellenic J Atheroscler. 2013;1:18–25.
54. Patel BV, Leslie RS, Thiebaud P, Nichol MB, Tang SS, Solomon H, et al. Adherence with single-pill amlodipine/atorvastatin vs a two-pill regimen. Vasc Health Risk Manag. 2008;4:673–81.
55. Hussein MA, Chapman RH, Benner JS, Tang SS, Solomon HA, Joyce A, et al. Does a single-pill antihypertensive/lipid-lowering regimen improve adherence in US managed care enrolees? A non-randomized, observational, retrospective study. Am J Cardiovasc Drugs. 2010;10:193–202.
56. Pereira M, Lunet N, Azevedo A, Barros H. Differences in prevalence, awareness, treatment and control of hypertension between developing and developed countries. J Hypertens. 2009;27:963–75.
57. Redon J, Olsen MH, Cooper RS, Zurriaga O, Martinez-Beneito MA, Laurent S, et al. Stroke mortality and trends from 1990 to 2006 in 39 countries from Europe and Central Asia: implications for control of high blood pressure. Eur Heart J. 2011;32:1424–31.
58. Wolf-Maier K, Cooper RS, Banegas JR, Giampaoli S, Hense HW, Joffres M, et al. Hypertension prevalence and blood pressure levels in 6 European countries, Canada, and the United States. JAMA. 2003;289:2363–9.
59. Efstratopoulos AD, Voyaki SM, Baltas AA, Vratsistas FA, Kirlas DE, Kontoyannis JT, et al. Prevalence, awareness, treatment and control of hypertension in Hellas, Greece: the Hypertension Study in General Practice in Hellas (HYPERTENSHELL) National Study. Am J Hypertens. 2006;19:53–60.
60. Wang X, Bots ML, Yang F, Hoes AW, Vaartjes I. Prevalence of hypertension in China: a systematic review and meta-regression analysis of trends and regional differences. J Hypertens. 2014;32:1919–27.
61. Gao Y, Chen G, Tian H, Lin L, Lu J, Weng J, et al. Prevalence of hypertension in China: a cross-sectional study. PLoS One. 2013;8:e65938.
62. Finucane MM, Stevens GA, Cowan MJ, Danaei G, Lin JK, Paciorek CJ, et al. National, regional, and global trends in body-mass index since 1980: systematic analysis of health examination surveys and epidemiological studies with 960 country-years and 9.1 million participants. Lancet. 2011;377:557–67.
63. Foulds HJ, Bredin SS, Warburtona DE. The relationship between hypertension and obesity across different ethnicities. J Hypertens. 2012;30:359–67.
64. Re RN. Obesity-related hypertension. Ochsner J. 2009;9:133–6.
65. Mancia G, Grassi G. Systolic and diastolic blood pressure control in antihypertensive drug trials. J Hypertens. 2002;20:1461–4.
66. Ong KL, Cheung BM, Man YB, Lau CP, Lam KS. Prevalence, awareness, treatment, and control of hypertension among United States adults 1999–2004. Hypertension. 2007;49:69–75.
67. Petrella RJ, Merikle EP, Jones J. Prevalence, treatment, and control of hypertension in primary care: gaps, trends, and opportunities. J Clin Hypertens (Greenwich). 2007;9:28–35.
68. Erdine S, Aran SN. Current status of hypertension control around the world. Clin Exp Hypertens. 2004;26:731–8.
69. Erdine S. How well is hypertension controlled in Europe? J Hypertens. 2000;18:1348–9.
70. Erdine S. European society of hypertension scientific newsletter: update on hypertension management. How well is hypertension controlled in Europe? 2007;8:3
71. Psaltopoulou T, Orfanos P, Naska A, Lenas D, Trichopoulos D, Trichopoulou A. Prevalence, awareness, treatment and control of hypertension in a general population sample of 26,913 adults in the Greek EPIC study. Int J Epidemiol. 2004;33:1345–52.
72. Guo J, Zhu YC, Chen YP, Hu Y, Tang XW, Zhang B. The dynamics of hypertension prevalence, awareness, treatment, control and associated factors in Chinese adults: results from CHNS 1991-2011. J Hypertens. 2015;33:1688–96.
73. Pickering TG. The natural history of hypertension: prehypertension or masked hypertension? J Clin Hypertens (Greenwich). 2007;9:807–10.

74. Mancia G, Fagard R, Narkiewicz K, Redón J, Zanchetti A, Böhm M, et al. 2013 ESH/ESC Guidelines for the management of arterial hypertension. The Task Force for the management of arterial hypertension of the European Society of Hypertension (ESH) and of the European Society of Cardiology (ESC). J Hypertens. 2013;31:1281–357.
75. Chockalingam A. World Hypertension Day and global awareness. Can J Cardiol. 2008;24:441–4.
76. Evans JG, Rose G. Hypertension. Br Med Bull. 1971;27:37–42.
77. Pickering G. Hypertension: definitions, natural histories and consequences. Am J Med. 1972;52:570–83.
78. Weber MA, Schiffrin EL, White WB, Mann S, Lindholm LH, Kenerson JG, et al. Clinical Practice Guidelines for the Management of Hypertension in the Community. A Statement by the American Society of Hypertension and the International Society of Hypertension. J Hypertens. 2014;32:3–15.
79. James P, Oparil S, Carter BL, Cushman WC, Dennison-Himmelfarb C, Handler J, et al. 2014 evidence-based guideline for the management of high blood pressure in adults: report from the panel members appointed to the Eighth Joint National Committee (JNC 8). JAMA. 2014;311:507–20.
80. Moran AE, Odden MC, Thanataveerat A, Tzong KY, Rasmussen PW, Guzman D, et al. Cost-effectiveness of hypertension therapy according to 2014 guidelines. N Engl J Med. 2015;372:447–55.
81. Go AS, Bauman MA, Coleman King SM, Fonarow GC, Lawrence W, Williams KA, et al. An effective approach to high blood pressure control. A science advisory from the American Heart Association, the American College of Cardiology, and the Centers for Disease Control and Prevention. Hypertension. 2014;63:878–85.
82. Chobanian AV. Shattuck Lecture. The hypertension paradox – more uncontrolled disease despite improved therapy. N Engl J Med. 2009;361:878–87.

Chapter 2
Techniques for Measuring Blood Pressure in the Office Setting

Martin G. Myers and Janusz Kaczorowski

Techniques for Measuring Blood Pressure in the Office Setting

This section will describe the current techniques and devices for the measurement of blood pressure (BP) in the office setting. The primary focus will be on electronic, oscillometric sphygmomanometers which are becoming the standard for BP measurement in clinical practice. The reasons for the decline in the use of the mercury sphygmomanometer and the evidence supporting its replacement by electronic devices will be discussed. This section will conclude with a review of the current status of office BP measurement in clinical practice and its future in relationship to home BP and 24-h ambulatory BP monitoring (ABPM).

Manual Blood Pressure Measurement

During the past century, the measurement of BP has been synonymous with the mercury sphygmomanometer. This device had the apparent advantages of having simple mechanical components and being accurate when properly used. Virtually all landmark epidemiologic and treatment studies to establish BP cut-off points for diagnosis and treatment targets used the mercury sphygmomanometer which

M.G. Myers, M.D., FRCPC (✉)
Division of Cardiology, Schulich Heart Program, Sunnybrook Health Sciences Centre, Toronto, ON, Canada

Department of Medicine, University of Toronto, Toronto, ON, Canada
e-mail: martin.myers@sunnybrook.ca

J. Kaczorowski, Ph.D.
Department of Family and Emergency Medicine, Université de Montréal and CRCHUM, Montreal, QC, Canada

E.A. Andreadis (ed.), *Hypertension and Cardiovascular Disease*,
DOI 10.1007/978-3-319-39599-9_2

established its predominant position for use in clinical practice. Developed in 1896 by Riva-Rocci, it has remained virtually unchanged except for auscultation being added by Sergei Korotkoff in 1905. The main alternative has been the aneroid sphygmomanometer which is smaller and more portable than the mercury recorder. However, the mechanical components used to record BP are not as stable and aneroid devices have a tendency to lose accuracy with repeated use. Consequently, periodic re-calibration is recommended, but this is often not performed in clinical practice. Thus, the mercury sphygmomanometer has continued to be the most common device for routine use in the office.

Detailed guidelines were developed over several decades by organizations such as the American Heart Association with recommendations generally focused on how health professionals ought to use the manual sphygmomanometer and how patient-related factors that could influence the accuracy of the readings should be reduced. The guidelines stimulated research into various aspects of the measurement process which could affect the accuracy of the BP readings. For example, the belief that conversation during a BP recording relaxed patients and lowered their BP was not supported by research which showed that talking to the patient actually increased BP [1]. Although manual BP readings using the mercury sphygmomanometer were relatively accurate and reproducible in research studies in which BP was measured in accordance with the guidelines, observational and experimental studies from 'real-life' clinical settings reported that proper technique for recording BP was often not followed [2]. Besides conversation, factors such as not allowing the patient to rest before readings, rapid cuff deflation, digit preference (rounding off readings to zero values) and recording only single readings reduced accuracy and introduced a 'white coat effect' with the office BP being often substantially higher and poorly correlated with the awake ambulatory BP [3].

Despite the apparent limitations of manual BP in routine clinical practice, the guidelines continued to recommend its use with greater emphasis being placed on educating health professionals on the proper technique for BP measurement [4]. However, the success of these efforts was limited and attempts to maintain the use of the mercury sphygmomanometer were further thwarted by concerns about the environmental hazards of mercury. Regulations were enacted in the European Community [5] to eliminate mercury from the workplace, including healthcare settings, and the mercury sphygmomanometer also began disappearing from hospitals and physicians' offices in North America.

As a consequence, manual BP measurement in the office was often left with the aneroid device despite its uncertain accuracy. Non-mercury sphygmomanometers are now also available for manual BP measurement in the office or hospital but, to date, none has achieved widespread use. Examples include the Accoson Greenlight 300, Heine Gama G7, Nissei DM-3000, Rossamax Mandaus and Welch-Allyn Maxi Stabil 3. At the moment, mercury and aneroid sphygmomanometers are still frequently used in the office setting, especially outside of Europe.

Electronic Sphygmomanometers

Numerous clinical outcome studies using electronic 24-h ABPM and, to a lesser extent, home BP monitoring have reported that BP readings recorded outside of the office are significantly better predictors of future cardiovascular risk in relation to BP status [6, 7]. These studies led to ABPM being recommended as the preferred method for diagnosing and managing hypertension with home BP as an alternative when ABPM was not feasible [8–10]. Some recommendations even questioned the usefulness of manually recording BP in the office setting altogether [9]. These developments have contributed to greater use of electronic sphygmomanometers in an attempt to overcome some of the shortcomings of manual office BP.

Whereas manual sphygmomanometers measure BP by recording the Korotkoff sounds in the anti-cubital fossa, most electronic devices now use the oscillometric method for recording BP. This method involves a sensor placed over the brachial or radial artery to detect changes in oscillations of the vessel wall as the BP cuff is deflated. Mathematically derived algorithms translate these oscillometric changes into values for systolic and diastolic BP. Some devices also record the oscillations during inflation of the cuff which allows for a more rapid determination of the BP.

The accuracy of the various electronic sphygmomanometers has been evaluated independent of the manufacturer using recognized procedures such as the International [11], British Hypertension Society [12] and Association for the Advancement of Medical Instrumentation protocols [13]. There has been some concern about the accuracy of electronic sphygmomanometers in patients with atrial fibrillation. A systematic review [14] of the literature did not reveal any specific problems in recording BP in the presence of atrial fibrillation when using oscillometric devices, although a greater variability of readings in the presence of irregular cardiac rhythms was recognized for all types of sphygmomanometers, including manual devices. Any loss of accuracy in the presence of atrial fibrillation can be minimized by averaging multiple manual or electronic BP readings.

Semi-automated Electronic Devices

Semi-automated electronic sphygmomanometers were initially developed for self-measurement of BP by patients in the home. These devices require activation usually by pressing a button in order to obtain a BP reading. Early recorders detected the Korotkoff sounds to measure BP but these were subsequently replaced by oscillometric devices. More recent features of oscillometric home BP recorders include taking multiple readings after initial device activation, electronic memory for storage of readings, capacity to transmit readings remotely via Bluetooth and mobile phone or Wi-Fi (BP telemonitoring) and devices which detect oscillations in the radial artery at the wrist.

In addition to their intended use, some home BP recorders have been adapted for professional use in the office or research setting. For example, the Omron HEM-705 home BP recorder was used to take BP in the ASCOT study [15] and a similar device is currently being used in some physicians' offices in Europe. From a practical perspective, standard home BP devices are generally not suitable for the office use in that they have not been designed for the frequent use and demands of a busy clinical practice. Also, semi-automated electronic sphygmomanometers adapted for professional use generally require the presence of medical personnel to activate the device for each reading.

Automated Office Blood Pressure (AOBP)

Fully automated, electronic sphygmomanometers have now been developed for professional use in the office [3]. These devices record multiple BP readings without any involvement of the patient or medical staff while the patient rests in a quiet place such as in an examining room or alone in a section of the waiting room. Examples include the BpTRU [16], Omron HEM-907 [17] and Microlife Watch BP Office [18]. These sphygmomanometers are capable of automatically taking 3–5 readings at pre-set intervals with only one minute of rest required before the first reading is taken. The net result is a mean office BP which is similar to the awake ambulatory BP and home BP [19, 20]. Initial studies on AOBP required the patient to be resting alone in a quiet examining room. However, more recent studies have reported that AOBP can also be recorded in a quiet place in a community pharmacy [21] or in the waiting room of the doctor's office [22, 23], although, when feasible, an unused examining room is still to be preferred.

AOBP has important advantages over manual BP as recorded in routine clinical practice. Whereas manual BP in primary care settings is on average 15/7 mmHg higher than the mean awake ambulatory BP, AOBP virtually eliminates this white coat effect [3]. AOBP is also more accurate in that its readings are more closely correlated than routine manual office BP with the awake ambulatory BP [20] and AOBP is not affected by digit preference which occurs in about one half of manual BP measurements [24]. AOBP does not require the presence of a health professional in order to record multiple readings since measurements are taken automatically once the device has been activated. A purported disadvantage of AOBP is that this technique takes four to six minutes to record three to five readings, the precise time depending on which recorder and which settings are used. However, the time to obtain the AOBP is no different from manual BP when one takes into consideration the five minutes of rest recommended before the first of two or more manual BP readings are recorded. It is true that when a single manual office BP is recorded without any antecedent rest, less time will be required, but the accuracy of the reading will be compromised.

Alternatives to AOBP

As noted above, home BP recorders are not sufficiently robust for professional use in the office. However, many patients have a home BP recorder which could be used for self-measurement in the office without a health professional being present. This technique has been examined in four studies [19, 25–27] in which patients used semi-automated oscillometric sphygmomanometers which required activation of the device to take multiple readings while they were resting alone in a quiet examining room. The results were somewhat surprising in that the mean BP in each instance was still about 5 mmHg higher than either the awake ambulatory BP, home BP or AOBP. Having a patient involved in the BP measurement process seems to increase the BP reading. This suggests that AOBP recorders ought to be fully automated.

Twenty-four hour ABPM is now recognized as the preferred method for diagnosing hypertension. However, ABPM is expensive and not always available or feasible, especially in lower income countries. In such instances, AOBP can be combined with home BP for the detection and diagnosis of hypertension as well as to follow patients after treatment is initiated.

AOBP and Target Organ Damage

In a study [28] involving 147 hypertensive patients attending the offices of primary care physicians in the community, ambulatory BP but not routine manual office BP correlated with left ventricular mass, an intermediate measure of target organ damage. In contrast, Andreadis et al. [29] reported that both AOBP and the awake ambulatory BP recorded in hypertensive patients attending a university hospital clinic correlated ($r=0.27$) significantly with left ventricular mass whereas a clinic reading showed a poor correlation ($r=0.12$). Other studies have shown that AOBP exhibits a significantly stronger correlation than manual BP with the intima-media thickness of the carotid artery in normotensive volunteers [30]. Also, AOBP and ambulatory BP both correlated significantly with microalbuminuria in hypertensive patients [31].

The cut-point at which AOBP is associated with an increase in cardiovascular events has been examined in 3,627 community-dwelling subjects aged over 65 years [32]. An AOBP reading was recorded at baseline and subjects were followed for a mean of 4.9 years for the development of myocardial infarction, congestive heart failure and stroke. A significant increase in cardiovascular events was seen at an AOBP of 135–144 mmHg systolic and 80–89 mmHg diastolic (Fig. 2.1). These results are consistent with AOBP having a cut-point of 135/85 mmHg for defining hypertension, the same cut-point previously derived using data from studies comparing AOBP with the awake ambulatory BP and home BP (20.21).

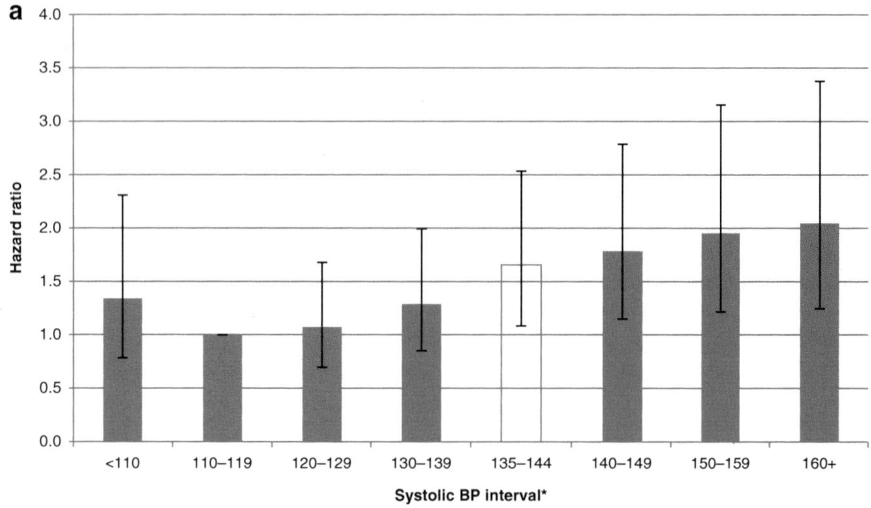

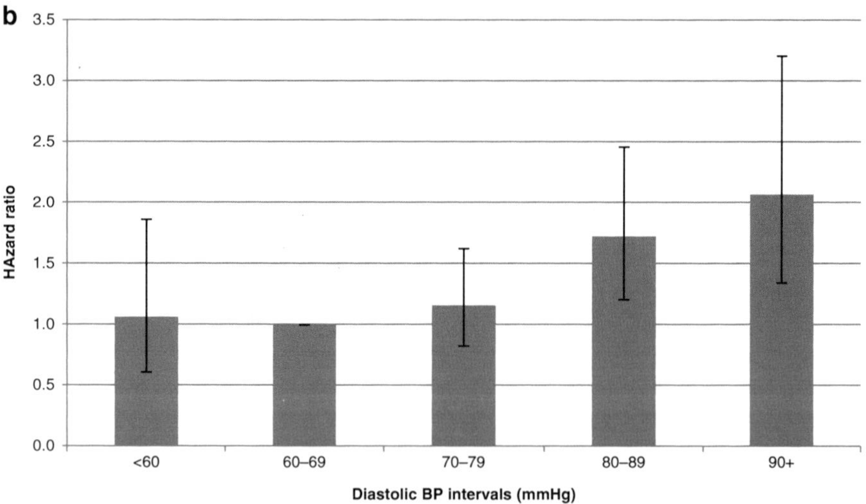

Fig. 2.1 Panels (**a**, **b**). Adjusted hazard ratios with 95 % confidence intervals according to category of systolic and diastolic blood pressure. A cut-point of 135/85 mmHg is based on analysis from a separate Cox regression models that used different categories for SBP [32]

AOBP and the Guidelines

The use of electronic devices for recording home BP and 24-h ambulatory BP was first recommended in the 1999 guidelines of the Canadian Hypertension Society [33]. Although electronic sphygmomanometers such as the Roche Arteriosonde 1216 were used to record clinic BP 40 years ago, only recently has this type of device been recommended for routine clinical practice [34]. The 2014 ASH/ISH guidelines [35] expressed a preference for electronic sphygmomanometers over manual devices for office BP measurement. Other organizations have gone further to include AOBP in their recommendations. The 2013 ESH/ESC guidelines [36] stated that there was no longer any role for the mercury sphygmomanometer in office BP measurement. Semi-automated manual or electronic devices were recommended instead. The guidelines then made a specific recommendation to use AOBP, if feasible, because of its improved reproducibility and closer approximation to the daytime ambulatory BP and home BP. In 2015, the Canadian Hypertension Education Program [37] recommended that manual BP should not be used to diagnose hypertension. Instead, electronic devices should be used with the AOBP being preferred.

The Future of Office BP Measurement

During the past decade, there have been dramatic changes in how hypertension is diagnosed. After an extensive evaluation of the evidence, the 2011 NICE guidelines [9] virtually excluded office BP from making a diagnosis of hypertension, preferring ABPM and home BP. This recommendation was based upon the overwhelming evidence that office BP is a relatively poor technique for evaluating future cardiovascular risk in comparison to ABPM and home BP. Recent guidelines generally agree that ABPM and home BP are preferable but office BP is still considered useful to screen for hypertension and in the management of patients once a diagnosis has been made. Of interest, the only study [38] which has demonstrated that screening for hypertension in the community can lead to a reduction in future cardiovascular events used AOBP readings.

Electronic sphygmomanometers improve the accuracy of office BP readings by reducing human involvement in the measurement process to a minimum. AOBP goes even further, by virtually eliminating human error [39] and bias in BP measurement while reducing the anxiety experienced by some patients when readings are recorded in the presence of a health professional. AOBP also automatically records multiple readings whereas a nurse or physician using a semi-automated electronic device often only takes a single reading.

Devices which record AOBP in both arms are now available [40]. If one arm has a systolic BP 10 mmHg or higher than the other arm, the higher arm should be used for recording AOBP during future office visits. Some devices for AOBP are now able to detect the presence of atrial fibrillation with reasonably good accuracy [41]. This feature is useful for diagnosing atrial fibrillation which is common in the elderly, the same population having an increased prevalence of hypertension. It can also be useful in the management of atrial fibrillation, either to estimate the frequency of paroxysmal episodes or to assess the response to anti-arrhythmic therapy.

The correlation between ABPM, home BP and AOBP is significantly stronger than for manual BP in clinical practice. Even semi-automated electronic devices record significantly higher BP readings under research conditions in the office setting. The present evidence strongly suggests that AOBP is a better technique for evaluating an individual's BP status compared to manual BP. All that is required is the use of a fully automated electronic sphygmomanometer to record multiple BP readings with the patient resting quietly alone. Since it is almost as easy to record AOBP as it is to measure BP using a semi-automated electronic sphygmomanometer, there would seem to be little reason why AOBP should not be the technique of choice for recording BP in the office setting.

References

1. Le Pailleur C, Helft G, Landais P, Montgermont P, Feder JM, Metzger JP, et al. The effects of talking, reading, and silence on the 'white coat' phenomenon in hypertensive patients. Am J Hypertens. 1998;11:203–7.
2. Reeves RA. Does this patient have hypertension – how to measure blood pressure. JAMA. 1995;273:1211–7.
3. Myers MG, Godwin M, Dawes M, Kiss A, Tobe SW, Kaczorowski J. Measurement of blood pressure in the office – recognizing the problem and proposing the solution. Hypertension. 2010;55:195–200.
4. Pickering TG, Hall JE, Appel LJ, Falkner BE, Graves J, Hill MN, et al. Recommendations for blood pressure measurement in humans and experimental animals Part 1: blood pressure measurement in humans a statement for professionals from the subcommittee of Professional and Public Education of the AM Heart Association Council on High Blood Pressure Research. Hypertension. 2005;45:142–61.
5. Scientific Committee on Emerging and Newly Identified Health Risks. Mercury sphygmomanometers in healthcare and the feasibility of alternatives. SCENIHR, 2009. [http://ec.europa.eu/health/ph_risk/committees/04_scenihr/scenihr_opinions_en.htm#2]. Accessed 1 Oct 2015.
6. O'Brien E, Parati G, Stergiou G, Asmar R, Beilin L, Bilo G, et al. European Society of Hypertension position paper on ambulatory blood pressure monitoring. J Hypertens. 2013;31:1731–68.
7. Parati G, Stergiou GS, Asmar R, Bilo G, de Leeuw P, Imai Y, et al. European Society of Hypertension guidelines for blood pressure monitoring at home: a summary report of the Second International Consensus Conference on Home Blood Pressure Monitoring. J Hypertens. 2008;26:1505–26.
8. Myers MG, Tobe SW, McKay DW, Bolli P, Hemmelgarn BR, McAlister FA, On behalf of the Canadian Hypertension Education Program. New algorithm for the diagnosis of hypertension.-Canadian Hypertension Education Program recommendations (2005). Am J Hypertens. 2005;18:1369–74.
9. National Institute for Health and Clinical Excellence: Hypertension NICE Clinical Guidelines 127. National Clinical Guidelines Centre. London, August 2011.
10. Piper M, Evans CV, Burda BU, Margolis KL, O'Connor E, Whitlock EP. Diagnostic and predictive accuracy of blood pressure screening methods with consideration of rescreening intervals: a systematic review for the U.S. Preventative Services Task Force. Ann Intern Med. 2015;162:192–204.
11. O'Brien E, Atkins N, Stergiou G, Karpettas N, Parati G, Asmar R, et al. European Society of Hypertension international protocol revision 2010 for the validation of blood pressure measuring devices in adults. Blood Press Monit. 2010;15:23–38.
12. O'Brien E, Petrie J, Littler W, et al. The British Hypertension Society protocol for the evaluation of blood pressure measuring devices. J Hypertens. 1993;11 Suppl 2:S43–62.

13. Association for the Advancement of Medical Instrumentation. American National Standard. Electronic or automated sphygmomanometers ANSI/AAMI SP10-2002. 3330 Washington Boulevard, Suite 400, Arlington, VA 22201–4598, USA: AAMI; 2003.
14. Myers MG, Stergiou GS. Should oscillometric blood pressure monitors be used in patients with atrial fibrillation? J Clin Hypertens. 2015;17:565–6.
15. Dahlhof B, Sever PS, Poulter NR, Wedel H, Beevers DG, Caulfield M, et al. Prevention of cardiovascular events with an antihypertensive regimen of amlodipine adding perindopril as required versus atenolol, adding bendroflumethazide as required, in the Anglo-Scandinavian Cardiac Outcomes Trial – Blood pressure lowering arm (ASCOT-BPLA): a multicenter randomized controlled trial. Lancet. 2005;366:895–906.
16. Wright JM, Mattu GS, Perry Jr TL, Gelfer ME, Strange KD, Zorn A, Chen Y. Validation of a new algorithm for the BPM-100 electronic oscillometric office blood pressure monitor. Blood Press Monit. 2001;6:161–5.
17. White WG, Anwar YA. Evaluation of the overall efficacy of the Omron office digital blood pressure HEM-907 monitor in adults. Blood Press Monit. 2001;6:107–10.
18. Stergiou GS, Tzamouranis D, Protogerou A, Nasothimiou E, Kapralos C. Validation of the Microlife Watch BP Office professional device for office blood pressure measurement according to the International Protocol. Blood Press Monit. 2008;13:299–303.
19. Myers MG, Valdivieso M, Chessman M, Kiss A. Can sphygmomanometers designed for self-measurement of blood pressure in the home be used in office practice? Blood Press Monit. 2010;15:300–4.
20. Myers MG. The great myth of office blood pressure measurement. J Hypertens. 2012;30:1894–8.
21. Chambers LW, Kaczorowski J, O'Reilly S, Ignagni S, Hearps SJC. Comparison of blood pressure measurements using an automated blood pressure device in community pharmacies and family physicians' offices: a randomized controlled trial. CMAJ Open. 2013;1(1):E37–42. doi:10.9778/cmajo.2013005.
22. Greiver M, White D, Kaplan DM, Katz K, Moineddin R, Doabchian E. Where should automated blood pressure measurements be taken? Blood Press Monit. 2012;17:137–8.
23. Armstrong D, Matangi M, Brouillard D, Myers MG. Automated office blood pressure – being alone and not location is what matters most. Blood Press Monit. 2015;20:204–8.
24. Myers MG, Godwin M, Dawes M, Kiss A, Tobe SW, Grant FC, Kaczorowski J. Conventional versus automated measurement of blood pressure in primary care patients with systolic hypertension: randomized parallel design controlled trial. BMJ. 2011;342:d286.
25. Myers MG, Meglis G, Polemidiotis G. The impact of physician vs automated blood pressure readings on office-induced hypertension. J Hum Hypertens. 1997;11:491–3.
26. Stergiou GS, Efstathiou SP, Alamara CV, Mastorantonakis SE, Roussias LG. Home or self blood pressure measurement? What is the correct term? J Hypertens. 2003;21:2259–64.
27. Al-Karkhi I, Al-Rubaiy R, Rosenqvist U, Falk M, Nystrom FN. Comparisons of automated blood pressures in a primary health care setting with self-measurements at the office and at home using the Omron i-C10 device. Blood Press Monit. 2015;20:98–103.
28. Myers MG, Oh P, Reeves RA, Joyner CD. Prevalence of white coat effect in treated hypertensive patients in the community. Am J Hypertens. 1995;8:591–7.
29. Andreadis EA, Agaliotis GD, Angelopoulos ET, Tsakanikas AP, Chaveles IA, Mousoulis GP. Automated office blood pressure and 24-h ambulatory measurements are equally associated with left ventricular mass index. Am J Hypertens. 2011;24:661–6.
30. Campbell NRC, McKay DW, Conradson H, Lonn E, Title LM, Anderson T. Automated oscillometric blood pressure versus auscultatory blood pressure as a predictor of carotid intima-medial thickness in male fire-fighters. J Hum Hypertens. 2007;21:588–90.
31. Andreadis EA, Agaliotis GD, Angelopolous ET, Tsakanikas AP, Kolyvas GN, Mousoulis GP. Automated office blood pressure is associated with urine albumin excretion in hypertensive subjects. Am J Hypertens. 2012;25:969–73.

32. Myers MG, Kaczorowski J, Paterson JM, Dolovich L, Tu K. Thresholds for diagnosing hypertension based upon automated office blood pressure measurements and cardiovascular risk. Hypertension. 2015;66:489–95.
33. Feldman RD, Campbell N, Larochelle P, Bolli P, Burgess ED, Carruthers SG, et al. 1999 Canadian recommendations for the management of hypertension. CMAJ. 1999;161 Suppl 12:S1–22.
34. Rabi DM, Daskalopoulou SS, Padwal RS, Khan NA, Grover SA, Hackam DG, et al. The 2011 Canadian Hypertension Education Program recommendations for the management of hypertension: blood pressure measurement, diagnosis, assessment of risk and therapy. Can J Cardiol. 2011;27:415–33.
35. Weber ME, Schiffrin EL, White WB, Mann S, Lindholm LH, Kenerson KG, et al. Clinical practice guidelines for the management of hypertension in the community – a statement of the American Society of Hypertension and the International Society of Hypertension. J Hypertens. 2014;32:3–15.
36. Mancia G, Fagard R, Krzysztof N, Redon J, Zanchetti A, Bohm M, et al. 2013 ESH/ESC guidelines for the management of arterial hypertension. J Hypertens. 2013;31:1281–357.
37. Cloutier L, Daskalopoulou DS, Padwal RS, Lamarre-Cliché M, Bolli P, McLean D, et al. A new algorithm for the diagnosis of hypertension in Canada. Can J Cardiol. 2015;31:620–30.
38. Kaczorowski J, Chambers LW, Dolovich L, Paterson JM, Karwalajtys T, Gierman T, et al. Improving cardiovascular health at the population level: 39 community cluster randomized trial of Cardiovascular Health Awareness Program (CHAP). BMJ. 2011;342:d442.
39. Myers MG. Eliminating the human factor in office blood pressure measurement. J Clin Hypertens. 2014;16:83–6.
40. Lohmann FW, Eckert S, Verberk WJ. Interarm differences in blood pressure should be determined by measuring both arms simultaneously with an automated oscillometric device. Blood Press Monit. 2011;16:37–42.
41. Kearley K, Selwood M, Van den Bruel A, Thompson M, Mant D, Hobbs FR, Fitzmaurice D, Heneghan C. Triage tests for identifying atrial fibrillation in primary care: a diagnostic accuracy study comparing single-lead ECG and modified BP monitors. BMJ Open. 2014;4:e004565. doi:10.1136/bmjopen-2013-004565.

Chapter 3
Home Blood Pressure Measurements

Nadia Boubouchairopoulou and George S. Stergiou

Introduction

Despite the fact that conventional measurement of blood pressure (BP) in the office (OBP) is regarded as the gold standard for both the diagnosis and long-term management of hypertension, it is recognized that it may lead to incorrect clinical decisions. The white-coat and the masked hypertension phenomenon are very common with OBP measurements and associated with intermediate cardiovascular risk that lies between that of normotension and hypertension [1, 2]. Furthermore, the small number of BP readings, the unusual setting, and the observer bias further weaken the reliability of OBP in the diagnosis and management of hypertension [3].

In the last decades, self-monitoring of BP by patients at home (HBPM) and 24-h ambulatory BP monitoring (ABPM) have both gained ground compared to OBPM for hypertension management, aiming to overcome the abovementioned drawbacks. Both these BP measurement methods present several similarities, as they provide multiple measurements taken in the individual's usual environment. However, they also important differences, as HBPM is performed only at home and in the sitting posture, whereas ABPM is performed in ambulatory conditions, at work, at home and during sleep [4, 5]. Therefore, it is still debated whether their role in the clinical management of hypertension is interchangeable or complementary [4, 6, 7].

Unlike ABPM, the clinical value of which is strongly supported by evidence from short-term and longitudinal trials, HBPM has been less well investigated. Recently, evidence has accumulated from studies investigating the diagnostic value of HBPM and its association with target organ damage and cardiovascular risk,

N. Boubouchairopoulou, M.Sc. • G.S. Stergiou, M.D., FRCP (✉)
Hypertension Center STRIDE-7, National and Kapodistrian University of Athens, Third Department of Medicine, Sotiria Hospital, 152 Mesogion Avenue, Athens 11527, Greece
e-mail: gstergi@med.uoa.gr

E.A. Andreadis (ed.), *Hypertension and Cardiovascular Disease*,
DOI 10.1007/978-3-319-39599-9_3

aiming to support the utility of this method as an indispensable tool for the initial evaluation of elevated BP, for treatment initiation and adjustment, as well as for long-term follow-up of treated hypertensives [1].

Clinical Value of HBPM

Diagnostic Value

Several studies during the last decade have demonstrated the efficiency of HBPM in diagnosing hypertensive patients and identifying the white-coat and masked hypertension phenomena which remain undetected with OBP measurements, by investigating the sensitivity and specificity of HBPM and considering ABPM as reference method [1].

HBPM appeared to be more efficient in identifying normotensive individuals but less accurate in detecting truly hypertensives, as it was associated with high specificity and negative predictive value (>80 %) but relatively lower sensitivity and positive predictive value (60–70 %) [1, 8]. Nevertheless, these results should be interpreted with caution as ABPM was used as reference method in most of the studies. Thus, these conclusions are based on the assumption that ABPM is perfectly reproducible and reliable, which certainly is not the case. Moreover, the diagnostic disagreement between the two methods in several cases was minimal and clinically irrelevant, and mostly present in subjects whose BP levels were very close to the diagnostic thresholds [1, 9].

As mentioned above, the usefulness of HBPM is manifested through the identification of white-coat and masked hypertension phenomena, which remain undiagnosed and inadequately treated when considering exclusively OBP measurements [4, 10–12]. White-coat hypertension is defined by normal HBPM (<135/85 mmHg) but elevated OBP values (≥140/90 mmHg systolic/diastolic BP, or both), thus not truly reflecting the "true" BP of an individual [1]. These individuals should not be considered as normotensives, as they present an intermediate cardiovascular risk between normotensives and hypertensives and are more likely to develop sustained hypertension within the next years [13]. On the other hand, masked hypertensives have elevated HBPM (≥135/85 mmHg) but normal OBP levels (<140/90 mmHg), and are associated with preclinical target organ damage and cardiovascular risk similar to sustained hypertensives. Masked hypertension is often present in treated patients reflecting the peak effect of morning antihypertensive drug treatment on OBP measurements and trough or plateau effect using morning and evening HBPM respectively. When the diagnosis of these phenomena is confirmed by repeat OBP and HBPM or ABPM measurements, the administration of antihypertensive therapy should be considered, especially in subjects with high total cardiovascular risk [1, 12].

The diagnostic accuracy of HBPM, its good reproducibility, its ability to provide a large number of measurements, its wide availability and the minimum effort required for its application, should lead to its wide implementation as primary diagnostic method for hypertension diagnosis and identification of white-coat and masked hypertension [5].

Treatment Titration

The long-term use of HBPM by patients treated for hypertension is recommended by recent guidelines as it enhances their compliance to therapy, and prevents them from adhering to therapy only before an office visit, a phenomenon known as "white-coat adherence" which is associated with increased cardiovascular risk [4, 10]. Poor compliance is indeed the most common cause of resistant hypertension despite the fact that patients are administered intensive antihypertensive treatment [14]. HBPM not only prevents normotensive individuals from receiving unnecessary medication, but also enables physicians to closely monitor BP of treated hypertensive patients. With HBPM treated hypertensive patients might receive less intensive therapy with equal protection from target organ damage [1, 8, 15]. However, there is incomplete evidence on the possible effects on target organ damage progression with antihypertensive treatment because the studies with long-term therapy and HBPM or ABPM are very few and in cases with contradictory results [16, 17].

HBPM has the unique advantage to enables patients to take multiple measurements not only through a period of time of weeks, but also months and even years and at minimal cost. Thus, it is undeniably more suitable for long-term follow-up of normotensives at high risk and of treated hypertensives compared to ABPM or OBPM [3, 18].

Prediction of Preclinical Organ Damage

The association of HBPM with several indices of preclinical damage, including echocardiographic left ventricular mass and index (LVM and LVMI), urinary albumin excretion rate, glomerular filtration rate, carotid intima-media thickness and pulse wave velocity, has been investigated. In these studies HBPM has been proven to be superior to OBP [1, 4, 15, 18], while when considering the strength of the association with several indices, the results were comparable with those obtained by ABPM and superior to these by OBP [1, 18].

Two meta-analyses have concluded that HBPM is a stronger predictor of LVMI, urinary albumin excretion rate and even silent cerebrovascular disease compared to OBP, with the strongest evidence reported for LVMI and fewer studies with weaker associations for other indices [19, 20]. Systolic BP assessed by both HBPM and ABPM is more closely correlated with LVMI than OBP, demonstrating the advantage of the two out-of-office BP measurement methods, and preliminary evidence suggests that HBPM might be superior even to ABPM [12].

Prognostic Value

The ultimate criterion to identify a useful method for the assessment of a cardiovascular risk factor in clinical practice is its actual ability to predict future cardiovascular events. Two meta-analyses have investigated the evidence sourced from outcome trials assessing the prognostic ability of HBPM compared to OBP measurements [21, 22]. Both were based on data from 8 prospective studies and 17,688 patients followed for 3.2–10.9 years, which resulted in the availability of information based on almost 100,000 person/years of follow-up and showed HPBM to be superior to OBP measurements, with this difference being beyond chance for systolic BP. Moreover in the meta-analysis by Ward et al., even when HBPM was adjusted for OBP, it still retained its prognostic ability, whereas OBP lost its significance after adjustment for HBPM [22]. Thus, the availability of reliable HBPM is likely to make OBP measurements obsolete in terms of cardiovascular events prediction [23].

Nocturnal HBPM

ABPM is considered as the gold standard in assessing nocturnal BP which has been shown to predict cardiovascular events in all populations and appears to be the aspect of the 24 h BP profile that has the strongest prognostic ability. Whether the nocturnal BP dip during sleep or the morning BP surge upon the morning rise contributes more in the cardiovascular risk prediction it is still debatable [24].

New technological advancement of HBPM devices offer the option to evaluate nocturnal BP on repeated days by patients at home [24]. These innovative HBPM devices are usually programmed to take 3 automated hourly BP readings at sleep for 3 consecutive nights, providing thereby a similar number of nocturnal BP readings as the usual 24-h ABPM. Studies have shown that daytime and nighttime BP assessed by these novel HBPM devices has similar levels as those obtained by conventional 24-h ABPM and there is satisfactory agreement between the two methods in identifying non-dippers [25]. Taking also into account that these measurements can be repeated for longer periods than these of ABPM, HBPM can be regarded as an appealing alternative [24, 26, 27].

Advantages and Limitations (Table 3.1)

Advantages

HBPM is widely available in general practice, with a relatively low-cost (in fact patients usually decide to cover themselves the cost of the devices) and is well accepted by patients for long-term use [1], highlighting its potential use as primary method of BP monitoring for both physicians and patients [10, 15, 28].

Table 3.1 Advantages and limitations of home blood pressure monitoring

Advantages	Limitations
Need of minimal training (with automated devices) Large sample of blood pressure readings Absence of placebo effect Absence of observer error and bias (automated devices with memory or PC link) Good reproducibility Detection of white-coat and masked hypertension phenomena Association with preclinical organ damage Prediction of cardiovascular events Wide availability Good acceptance by users Improvement of patients' compliance with drug therapy Improvement of hypertension control rates Cost-effectiveness	Devices often not properly validated Misreporting (over- or under-) of readings by patients Need of user training (minimal with automated devices) and medical supervision May induce anxiety in some patients Some patients may self-modify their drug treatment on the basis of casual BP readings Measurements do not reflect usual daily activities Inability to monitor nocturnal BP (possible with some novel home monitors) Questionable accuracy of oscillometric devices in the presence of arrhythmias

Indeed, from the physicians' point of view HBPM can be considered as superior to OBP and similar to ABPM in terms of reproducibility, which is mainly attributed to the large number of readings obtained [28]. Moreover, as aforementioned, the evaluation of BP in the patients' usual environment enables the accurate diagnosis of hypertension through the identification of the white coat and the masked hypertension phenomena, which both affect almost one third of treated and untreated subjects attending hypertension clinics [28]. Particularly in treated patients, HBPM has been proved to enhance their compliance by involving them in their monitoring, thereby leading to improved hypertension control rates [4, 29].

In line with the above, recent studies have shown HBPM to be highly cost-effective, through the need of fewer clinic visits, more adequate treatment adjustment and avoidance of unnecessary treatment in white coat hypertensives [4, 12, 30]. However, its cost-effectiveness has not been thoroughly investigated and more studies should be performed [3].

Limitations

Despite its many advantages, HBPM inevitably presents some limitations which occasionally restrict its use. Self HBPM may induce anxiety which leads to BP increase and also to excessive monitoring, while sometimes the conditions under which the measurements are taken are not representative (stress, pain, etc.) and providing false evidence and overestimating BP levels [3, 28]. This can induce some patients to perform self-modification of their drug treatment without medical consultation on the basis of casual home BP measurement (high or low) [3, 4].

Patients' usual misreporting of their self-taken BP readings still remains the "Achilles' heel" of HBPM, leading in over- or under treatment, especially in high risk hypertensives or those with high BP variability [4, 12, 31]. There is evidence that less than 70 % of HBPM readings reported by patients to the doctor are usually identical to those recorded by the device. Electronic HBPM devices with automated memory or PC link and home-telemonitoring can all prevent misreporting and ensure an unbiased and reliable HBPM evaluation.

It should be mentioned that even if HBPM is performed under ideal circumstances, it only provides BP readings at home and in the sitting posture, whereas ABPM provides BP data in dynamic conditions, at work, at home, and also during sleep [5]. Nevertheless, even ABPM is not truly ambulatory, since patients have to stay still during each measurement.

Clinical Application (Table 3.2)

The current European and American guidelines recommend HBPM to be used in the long-term follow-up of almost all subjects with treated hypertension and also in untreated subjects for the initial evaluation of elevated BP [32, 33]. However, HBPM should be always applied after adequate training and under close medical supervision.

Devices

HBPM can be performed using auscultatory aneroid devices, or electronic arm, wrist or finger devices. Regular calibration of devices and training of patients are important prerequisites for the use of auscultatory method. Considering the fact that for the wide application of HBPM the aforementioned prerequisites are not feasible

Table 3.2 Practical recommendations for optimal application of home blood pressure monitoring

Device	Automated upper-arm device validated according an established protocol.
Cuff	Bladder size according to individual arm circumference.
Conditions	Relaxed, after 5 min sitting rest.
Monitoring schedule	7-days monitoring before each office visit with duplicate morning (before drug intake) and evening measurements. Not fewer than 3 days (12 readings).
Evaluation	Calculation of average BP of all readings after discarding the first day. Casual readings have little clinical relevance.
Diagnostic thresholds	Normal home BP: <130/80 mmHg; Hypertension: ≥135/85 mmHg; Intermediate levels are considered borderline.
Long-term follow up	1–2 duplicate measurements per week. Too frequent monitoring and self-modification of treatment on the basis of casual measurements to be avoided.

but rather unrealistic, automated electronic devices, especially these using an oscillometric algorithm and having an arm cuff are currently recommended for HBPM. Auscultatory devices might be preferred only in case of arrhythmias, or pre-eclampsia, yet these indications are also debatable. Some wrist devices have passed the internationally accepted validation protocols, however they are regarded as less accurate than upper arm devices, mainly because of anatomical differentiations of the wrist, and of difficulty in following the correct wrist position (at heart level and relaxed) [4, 8, 12]. On the other hand, finger devices are not accurate and have been withdrawn from the market [4, 8, 12].

The accuracy of electronic BP monitors should be tested against conventional mercury sphygmomanometry according to established validation protocols. The US Association for the Advancement of Medical Instrumentation (AAMI) in 1987 [34] and the British Hypertension Society in 1990 [35] have developed the first protocols for devices' validation, and both have been later revised. In 2002 the European Society of Hypertension International Protocol has been developed, requiring considerably smaller sample size and therefore being widely accepted and applied worldwide [36]. However, many of the electronic devices for HBPM available on the market have not been subjected to independent validation or have failed [12]. Updated lists of devices which have passed at least one of the aforementioned validation protocols are available at the British Hypertension Society website (www.bhsoc.org) and the Medaval website for the evaluation of BP monitors (www.medaval.org). The fact that a device has passed a validation protocol does not guarantee that it will provide accurate readings to each individual [12]. Indeed, in some cases, even a BP monitor that has achieved passing grades may present a measurement error of more than 5 or 10 mmHg compared to mercury sphygmomanometer for reasons which remain rather unclear and might be related to the individual's arterial wall properties.

The use of a cuff with inflatable bladder of appropriate size for the arm of each individual is of equal importance as the accuracy of the HBPM device [8]. The length of the inflatable bladder should cover 80–100 % of the arm circumference and the width should be about half of the length. Cuffs which are too small for the arm size tend to overestimate BP (common in obese subjects), whereas cuffs which are too large (in children or lean women) tend to underestimate BP. It is recommended that subjects with arm circumference larger than 32 cm should use a cuff larger than the standard size, while those with arm circumference smaller than 24 cm a smaller cuff than the standard [4].

Methodology

The European Society of Hypertension [37] and the American Heart Association [5] guidelines for HBPM recommend that patients should perform a standard HBPM schedule for the initial evaluation of BP levels (untreated subjects) and before each visit to the physician (for treated hypertensives). The recommended HBPM schedule includes duplicate measurements (with one minute interval) in the morning (before drug intake if treated), and the evening for 7 routine work days (and not less than 3 days), with weekends preferably excluded as the corresponding BP values are usually lower than in workdays [3, 12]. However, for the long-term follow-up of treated hypertensives, HBPM once or twice per week seems to be appropriate to ensure maintenance of adequate BP control [4, 12]. In all cases, individuals should ensure that they are in sitting posture with supported back and arm and uncrossed legs, and that BP measurements are taken after 5 min rest. Moreover, the cuff must be placed on the nondominant arm, at the heart's level and the centre of the bladder should be placed over the brachial artery. Talking during the measurement and coffee or smoking for at least 30 min before the measurement should be discouraged [4].

All HBPM readings should be recorded in a form, or better automatically saved on the device memory or PC [4]. A total of 24 HBPM readings (7 days) should be routinely obtained for clinical decision making and 12 readings seems to be the minimum acceptable sample. The first day HBPM readings should be better discarded particularly when less that the full 7-day schedule has been obtained, as they are typically higher and more variable than the next days [4].

Interpretation

The HBPM interpretation is based on assessing the average BP of 7 days (minimum 3), whereas casual BP readings little clinical value. As mentioned above, the average home BP of all readings is calculated after discarding those of the first day [4].

According to the European and American guidelines, the hypertension threshold for average home BP is 135/85 mmHg, which is the same as for awake ABPM [3, 4, 8]. Levels exceeding this threshold are considered elevated. Home BP levels ranging between 130 and 135 mmHg for systolic and 80–85 mmHg diastolic BP are regarded as borderline (pre-hypertension range), and those <130/80 mmHg as normal [3, 12]. Comparison between the morning and evening home BP values are particularly useful in treated hypertensives for the evaluation of the duration of antihypertensive drug action and the 24 h BP control [12].

References

1. Stergiou GS, Kollias A, Zeniodi M, et al. Home blood pressure monitoring: primary role in hypertension management. Curr Hypertens Rep. 2014;16:462.
2. Stergiou GS, Asayama K, Thijs L, et al. Prognosis of white-coat and masked hypertension: International Database of HOme blood pressure in relation to Cardiovascular Outcome. Hypertension. 2014;63:675–82.
3. Stergiou GS, Kollias A, Nasothimiou E. Home blood pressure monitoring: application in clinical practice. Hipertensión y Riesgo Vascular. 2011;28:149–53.

4. Parati G, Stergiou GS, Asmar R, et al. European Society of Hypertension guidelines for blood pressure monitoring at home: a summary report of the Second International Consensus Conference on Home Blood Pressure Monitoring. J Hypertens. 2008;26:1505–26.
5. Pickering TG, Miller NH, Ogedegbe G, et al. Call to action on use and reimbursement for home blood pressure monitoring: a joint scientific statement from the American Heart Association, American Society of Hypertension, and Preventive Cardiovascular Nurses Association. Hypertension. 2008;52:10–29.
6. Mancia G, Fagard R, Narkiewicz K, et al. ESH/ESC Guidelines for the management of arterial hypertension: the Task Force for the management of arterial hypertension of the European Society of Hypertension (ESH) and of the European Society of Cardiology (ESC). J Hypertens. 2013;31:1281–357.
7. O'Brien E, Parati G, Stergiou G, et al. European Society of Hypertension position paper on ambulatory blood pressure monitoring. J Hypertens. 2013;31:1731–68.
8. Celis H, Den Hond E, Staessen JA. Self-measurement of blood pressure at home in the management of hypertension. Clin Med Res. 2005;3:19–26.
9. Stergiou GS, Salgami EV, Tzamouranis DG, et al. Masked hypertension assessed by ambulatory blood pressure versus home blood pressure monitoring: is it the same phenomenon? Am J Hypertens. 2005;18:772–8.
10. Imai Y, Hosaka M, Elnagar N, et al. Clinical significance of home blood pressure measurements for the prevention and management of high blood pressure. Clin Exp Pharmacol Physiol. 2014;41:37–45.
11. Green BB, Cook AJ, Ralston JD, et al. Effectiveness of home blood pressure monitoring, Web communication, and pharmacist care on hypertension control: a randomized controlled trial. JAMA. 2008;299:2857–67.
12. Mallick S, Kanthety R, Rahman M. Home blood pressure monitoring in clinical practice: a review. Am J Med. 2009;122:803–10.
13. Ohkubo T, Asayama K, Kikuya M, et al. How many times should blood pressure be measured at home for better prediction of stroke risk? Ten-year follow-up results from the Ohasama study. J Hypertens. 2004;22:1099–104.
14. McManus RJ, Mant J, Haque MS, et al. Effect of self-monitoring and medication self-titration on systolic blood pressure in hypertensive patients at high risk of cardiovascular disease: the TASMIN-SR randomized clinical trial. JAMA. 2014;312:799–808.
15. Staessen JA, Den Hond E, Celis H, et al. Antihypertensive treatment based on blood pressure measurement at home or in the physician's office: a randomized controlled trial. JAMA. 2004;291:955–64.
16. Karpettas N, Destounis A, Kollias A, et al. Prediction of treatment-induced changes in target-organ damage using changes in clinic, home and ambulatory blood pressure. Hypertens Res. 2014;37:543–7.
17. Stergiou GS, Karpettas N, Destounis A, et al. Home blood pressure monitoring alone vs. combined clinic and ambulatory measurements in following treatment-induced changes in blood pressure and organ damage. Am J Hypertens. 2014;27:184–92.
18. Verdecchia P, Angeli F, Mazzotta G, et al. Home blood pressure measurements will not replace 24-hour ambulatory blood pressure monitoring. Hypertension. 2009;54:188–95.
19. Fuchs SC, Mello RG, Fuchs FC. Home blood pressure monitoring is better predictor of cardiovascular disease and target organ damage than office blood pressure: a systematic review and meta-analysis. Curr Cardiol Rep. 2013;15:413.
20. Bliziotis IA, Destounis A, Stergiou GS. Home versus ambulatory and office blood pressure in predicting target organ damage in hypertension: a systematic review and meta-analysis. J Hypertens. 2012;30:1289–99.
21. Stergiou GS, Siontis KC, Ioannidis JP. Home blood pressure as a cardiovascular outcome predictor: it's time to take this method seriously. Hypertension. 2010;55:1301–3.
22. Ward AM, Takahashi O, Stevens R, et al. Home measurement of blood pressure and cardiovascular disease: systematic review and meta-analysis of prospective studies. J Hypertens. 2012;30:449–56.

23. Stergiou GS, Parati G. Home blood pressure monitoring may make office measurements obsolete. J Hypertens. 2012;30:463–5.
24. Head GA. The prognostic value of self-assessed nocturnal blood pressure. J Clin Hypertens (Greenwich). 2015;17:349–51.
25. Stergiou GS, Nasothimiou EG, Destounis A, et al. Assessment of the diurnal blood pressure profile and detection of non-dippers based on home or ambulatory monitoring. Am J Hypertens. 2012;25:974–8.
26. Ishikawa J, Hoshide S, Eguchi K, et al. Nighttime home blood pressure and the risk of hypertensive target organ damage. Hypertension. 2012;60(4):921–8.
27. Kario K, Hoshide S, Haimoto H, et al. Sleep blood pressure self-measured at home as a novel determinant of organ damage: Japan Morning Surge Home Blood Pressure (J-HOP) Study. J Clin Hypertens (Greenwich). 2015;17:340–8.
28. McManus RJ, Glasziou P, Hayen A, et al. Blood pressure self monitoring: questions and answers from a national conference. BMJ. 2008;337:a2732.
29. Cappuccio FP, Kerry SM, Forbes L, et al. Blood pressure control by home monitoring: meta-analysis of randomised trials. BMJ. 2004;329:145.
30. Stergiou G, Mengden T, Padfield PL, et al. Self monitoring of blood pressure at home. BMJ. 2004;329:870–1.
31. Myers MG, Stergiou GS. Reporting bias: achilles' heel of home blood pressure monitoring. J Am Soc Hypertens. 2014;8:350–7.
32. ESH/ESC Task Force for the Management of Arterial Hypertension. 2013 Practice guidelines for the management of arterial hypertension of the European Society of Hypertension (ESH) and the European Society of Cardiology (ESC): ESH/ESC Task Force for the Management of Arterial Hypertension. J Hypertens. 2013;31:1925–38.
33. Weber MA, Schiffrin EL, White WB, et al. Clinical practice guidelines for the management of hypertension in the community: a statement by the American Society of Hypertension and the International Society of Hypertension. J Clin Hypertens (Greenwich). 2014;16:14–26.
34. Association for the Advancement of Medical Instrumentation. American National Standard. Electronic or automated sphygmomanometers ANSI/AAMI SP10-1987. 3330 Washington Boulevard, Suite 400, Arlington, VA 22201–4598, USA: AAMI, 1987.
35. O'Brien E, Petrie J, Littler W, et al. The British Hypertension Society Protocol for the evaluation of automated and semi-automated blood pressure measuring devices with special reference to ambulatory systems. J Hypertens. 1990;8:607–19.
36. O'Brien E, Atkins N, Stergiou G, et al. European Society of Hypertension International Protocol revision 2010 for the validation of blood pressure measuring devices in adults. Blood Press Monit. 2010;15:23–38.
37. Parati G, Stergiou GS, Asmar R, et al. European Society of Hypertension practice guidelines for home blood pressure monitoring. J Hum Hypertens. 2010;24:779–85.

Chapter 4
24-hour Ambulatory Blood Pressure Measurements

Geoffrey A. Head

Introduction

Ambulatory Blood Pressure Monitoring (ABPM) is now recognised as the gold standard method for measuring a patient's BP. The process involves wearing a portable BP monitor which inflates an upper arm cuff to determine BP at regular intervals over a complete 24 h period. The value of this measurement is that it provides an estimate of the diurnal changes in BP while the patient undergoes their normal daily activities and importantly measurements are made during sleep. Measurement of BP in the physician's office provide only a small sample of measurement of the patient's BP and can be subject to higher readings due to the presence of the physician which is known as a "white coat effect". Alternatively in some cases BP can be lower than normal in the doctor's office particularly in subjects where normal activities are stressful resulting in hypertension. Such patients are known as "masked" hypertensives. Thus ABPM provides a much more reliable estimate of the patient's true BP and avoids much of the misdiagnosis that can occur in subjects with either "whitecoat hypertension" or "masked hypertension" [33]. Nevertheless clinic BP assessments by the physician will continue to remain as an important screening tool.

The Value of Ambulatory BP Monitoring

ABPM provides the most accurate information for the diagnosis of hypertension and the provision of optimal care such as determining the effectiveness of antihypertensive therapy. The evidence supporting the use of ABPM has reached a point

G.A. Head, B.Sc., Ph.D.
Baker IDI Heart and Diabetes Institute,
75 Commercial Road, Melbourne, VIC 3004, Australia
e-mail: geoff.head@baker.edu.au; http://www.bakerIDI.edu.au

E.A. Andreadis (ed.), *Hypertension and Cardiovascular Disease*,
DOI 10.1007/978-3-319-39599-9_4

where expert groups such as the National Institute for Health and Clinical Excellence in the United Kingdom advocate that every suspected case of hypertension be validated with ambulatory monitoring if tolerated. The latter caveat reflects that not all patients are comfortable wearing a device over 24 h. Nevertheless there is a considerable international movement to increase the use of ABPM for the diagnosis and management of hypertension [16].

The strongest argument for the use of ABPM over other techniques for the measurement of BP has come from the increasing recognition of its superior prognostic value in terms of predicting future cardiovascular events. This may arise in part from the large number of BP measurements that are made within the 24 h period which would be expected to increase the likelihood of estimating the patient's BP. Perhaps more importantly is that the measurements are made during a person's normal daily activities and during sleep where the BP is expected to fall. There are a very large number of prospective studies that have compared the prognostic value of different measurements of BP with the clear consensus that ABPM is a superior predictor of cardiovascular outcomes than clinic BP assessments [3, 4, 6, 7, 10–12, 14, 15, 21, 22, 29, 32, 34, 36, 37]. The outcomes include, myocardial infarction, stroke as well as secondary indices of end organ damage such as left ventricular hypertrophy, microalbuminuria and carotid artery wall thickness. A more recent study compared the prognostic value of ABPM, home BP measurement and Clinic BP in predicting cardiovascular mortality, myocardial infarction, stroke, heart failure hospitalization and coronary intervention with a 16 year follow up period. Using a sophisticated multivariate adjusted Cox model only systolic and diastolic ambulatory BP was a predictor which suggests that ABPM is prognostically superior to office and home measurements [30]. These studies support the view that end organ damage is a surrogate for the long term level of BP of the individual patient which ABPM may be better at estimating than other techniques.

When Should ABPM Be Used?

The principal use of ABPM is to confirm the diagnosis of hypertension, masked hypertension or suspected white coat hypertension. ABPM is particularly useful for determining suspected nocturnal hypertension or a lack of the normal night-time reduction in BP. Patients whose reduction in BP is less than 10 % during sleep have been termed "non-dippers" and are at considerably more cardiovascular risk. Importantly ABPM can also be used to determine the effectiveness or not of antihypertensive treatment. Indeed ABPM is essential for defining patients with resistant hypertension which has been defined as BP remaining above a defined target of 140/90 mmHg despite at least three different classes of antihypertensive agent including a diuretic.

ABPM is appropriate and accurate for a wide range of age groups and conditions including children, adolescents, elderly and obese subjects. ABPM can be useful in detecting hypertension, particularly white coat hypertension early in pregnancy which is important as it can avoid inappropriate pharmacological treatment of pregnant women. However, ABPM should not be used in an individual pregnant woman to assess the risk of pre-eclampsia or progression from gestation hypertension to pre-eclampsia [5].

ABPM is not necessary and indeed contraindicated if it will delay antihypertensive treatment in patients with high cardiovascular risk such as those with grade 3 hypertension (BP ≥ 180/110 mmHg) [20]. For such patients antihypertensive therapy should be commenced as soon as practical. For most patients ABPM is appropriate being safe and not usually associated with complications. The newer ABPM devices are light, quiet and comfortable to wear but some patients report that inflation of the cuff can cause some transient discomfort, particularly in people with hypertension due to the pressure required to reach systolic pressure or when multiple repetitions of the reading are triggered due to errors in measurement. To minimise this issue, some devices adjust the inflation maximum pressure according to what is required and will reinflate if the maximum has not been reached. ABPM may not be accurate when there is irregular heart rate due to arrhythmias [20].

How Is ABPM Performed?

ABPM should be performed by an appropriately trained person who is familiar with instructing the patient and fitting the device correctly. The battery operated monitor which includes a pressure pump is worn on a belt connected to a cuff on the upper arm and uses an oscillometric technique to detect systolic, diastolic and mean BP as well as heart rate [27]. Only validated devices should be used that have been approved by one of the authorities such as the European society of hypertension (ESH-IP:2010, [31]) or the Association for the Advancement of Medical Instrumentation (AAMI/ANSI/ISO, ISO 81060–2:2013). ABP monitors measure the arm cuff pressure oscillations during deflation and defines the maximal amplitude of the oscillation as the mean arterial BP and then uses an algorithm on the ascending and descending slope of the oscillation amplitude to calculate systolic and diastolic BP [1]. The algorithms are a closely guarded commercial secret and cannot be independently validated but it is recognised that ABPM devices differ slightly from the manual method using Korotkoff sounds.

One of the most important aspects for accurate assessment of ambulatory BP is to use the correct cuff size for the particular patient. This is particularly important if the patient has a very large or conical shaped upper arm as the use of a smaller cuff will over read quite considerably. Furthermore it is important to use only the cuffs supplied by the manufacturer with each device. Measure BP in both arms and if the difference in systolic is less than 10 mmHg, use the non-dominant arm. If the difference in systolic BP is greater than 10 mmHg, use the arm with the higher pressure.

ABPM devices are usually programmed to take readings at set intervals of 15–30 min during the day and every 30–60 min at night, in order to avoid interfering with activity or sleep. It is important to fully inform the patients usually with a written set of instructions including phone numbers in case of emergency as well is a verbal description of what to expect, what to do and what not to do. They need to be clear that the device will automatically inflate periodically over the 24 h period and that when the cuff starts to inflate the patient should stop moving, talking and keep the arm still and relaxed while breathing normally. The day chosen to perform the ABPM should be as close to the normal activities as possible rather than a rest day or holiday. Obviously patients need to be informed to avoid vigorous activities that may interfere with the accurate assessment of BP and it is highly desirable to keep a diary of events during the 24 h period particularly those related to sleep, activities, medication and any symptoms that may be related to postural BP such as dizziness. In some cases ABPM during the night time period may interfere with normal sleep and give higher values or suggest a lack of nocturnal dipping. If this is the case the monitoring should be repeated provided the patient is willing.

When the recording period is complete the patient should return to the clinic and return the device where it is connected to a computer for analysis. The computer calculates the average 24 h, day time, night time as well as sleep and awake (if recorded) average systolic and diastolic BP and heart rate.

Interpreting ABPM Recordings

Most ABPM analysis software will display a graph of individual data points over the recording period and give the averages for 24 h, daytime and night time (Figs. 4.1 and 4.2). Measurements obtained from ABPM must be interpreted carefully with reference to diary information and timing of medicines. Recordings are considered

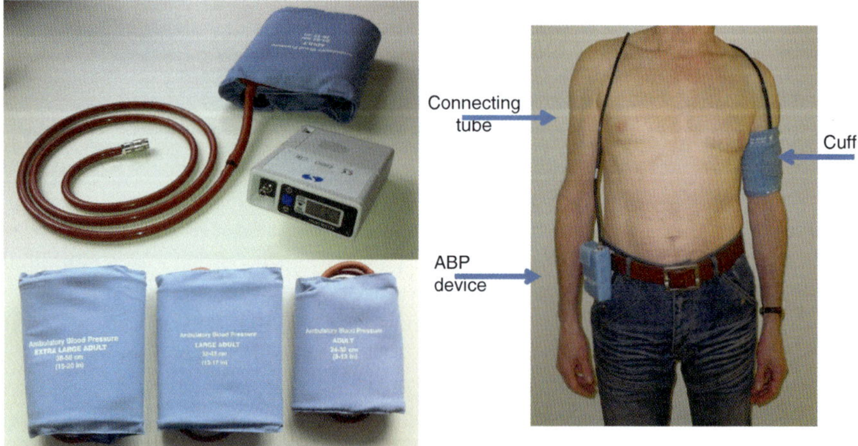

Fig. 4.1 Example of an ambulatory blood pressure monitor (*upper left*), multiple cuff sizes (*lower left*) and the device when fitted to a patient (*right*) (Reproduced with permission from [19])

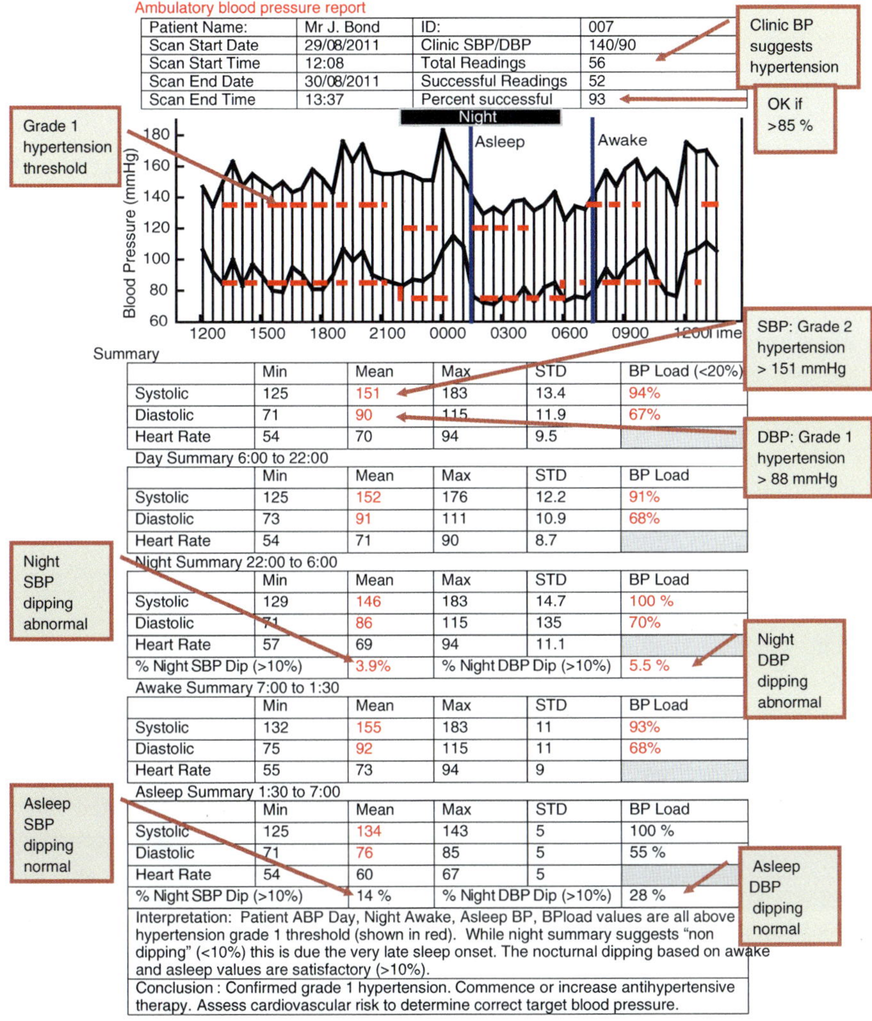

Ambulatory blood pressure report

Patient Name:	Mr J. Bond	ID:	007
Scan Start Date	29/08/2011	Clinic SBP/DBP	140/90
Scan Start Time	12:08	Total Readings	56
Scan End Date	30/08/2011	Successful Readings	52
Scan End Time	13:37	Percent successful	93

Summary

	Min	Mean	Max	STD	BP Load (<20%)
Systolic	125	151	183	13.4	94%
Diastolic	71	90	115	11.9	67%
Heart Rate	54	70	94	9.5	

Day Summary 6:00 to 22:00

	Min	Mean	Max	STD	BP Load
Systolic	125	152	176	12.2	91%
Diastolic	73	91	111	10.9	68%
Heart Rate	54	71	90	8.7	

Night Summary 22:00 to 6:00

	Min	Mean	Max	STD	BP Load
Systolic	129	146	183	14.7	100 %
Diastolic	71	86	115	135	70%
Heart Rate	57	69	94	11.1	
% Night SBP Dip (>10%)		3.9%	% Night DBP Dip (>10%)		5.5 %

Awake Summary 7:00 to 1:30

	Min	Mean	Max	STD	BP Load
Systolic	132	155	183	11	93%
Diastolic	75	92	115	11	68%
Heart Rate	55	73	94	9	

Asleep Summary 1:30 to 7:00

	Min	Mean	Max	STD	BP Load
Systolic	125	134	143	5	100 %
Diastolic	71	76	85	5	55 %
Heart Rate	54	60	67	5	
% Night SBP Dip (>10%)		14 %	% Night DBP Dip (>10%)		28 %

Interpretation: Patient ABP Day, Night Awake, Asleep BP, BPload values are all above hypertension grade 1 threshold (shown in red). While night summary suggests "non dipping" (<10%) this is due the very late sleep onset. The nocturnal dipping based on awake and asleep values are satisfactory (>10%).

Conclusion : Confirmed grade 1 hypertension. Commence or increase antihypertensive therapy. Assess cardiovascular risk to determine correct target blood pressure.

Fig. 4.2 An example of an ABPM report (Reproduced with permission from [19])

to be valid when there is a minimum of 20 daytime measurements and at least seven measurements at night [33]. Reference and threshold values of systolic BP/diastolic BP for hypertension categories are shown in Table 4.1 [17, 18] with the threshold equivalent for grade 1 or moderate hypertension of clinic 140/90 mmHg being 135/85 mmHg (daytime value). The night time threshold for hypertension is 137/76 mmHg and normal BP is considered as 120/80 mmHg in the day and 105/65 mmHg at night. ABPM values above these normal values but below the hypertension threshold are classed as 'high-normal' (Table 4.1). Treatment targets based on ABPM are generally lower than for clinic BP readings but the two values

Table 4.1 Classification of hypertension thresholds and treatment targets in adults

		ABP predicted from clinic BP (mmHg)		
Classification	Clinic BP	24-h	Night	Day
Grade 3 hypertension	180/110	163/101	157/93	168/105
Grade 2 hypertension	160/100	148/93	139/84	152/96
Grade 1 hypertension	140/90	133/84	121/76	136/87
Uncomplicated hypertension	140/90	133/84	121/76	136/87
High cardiovascular risk	130/80	125/76	112/67	128/78
Hypertension and proteinuria	125/75	121/71	107/63	124/74
Normal	120/80	115/75	105/65	120/80

Adapted from Head et al. [17, 18, 20]

converge when BP is lower and the difference is greater when BP is very high. Night-time (sleeping) average systolic and diastolic BP should both be at least 10 % lower than daytime (awake) average [27]. The example shown in Fig. 4.2 highlights the different conclusions that can be reached about nocturnal dipping when considering fixed clock times or sleep times. Based on clock times, the subject would be considered a non-dipper (5.5 %) while by sleep times the patient dipped (28 %) adequately. An often quoted measure called BP load which is the percentage time during which BP readings exceed hypertension threshold over 24 h should be less than 20 %. The example in Fig. 4.2 shows the patient has a BP load value of 98 % for systolic and 67 % for diastolic.

"White Coat Hypertension" or isolated office hypertension as it is otherwise known, is defined as untreated individuals with 24-h ambulatory BP less than 130/80 mmHg, awake ambulatory BP less than 135/85 mmHg but elevated clinic measurements above the hypertension threshold [33]. These patients are generally at low cardiovascular risk but are at greater risk of developing true hypertension and require continued assessment of absolute cardiovascular risk and continued monitoring with clinic and home BP measurements. The diagnosis should be confirmed by repeating the ambulatory assessment or using home BP monitoring. ABPM should be repeated every 1–2 years depending on the patient's individual total cardiovascular risk.

"Masked uncontrolled hypertension" is a condition found in approximately 15 % of patients where clinic measurements of BP are below hypertension threshold but ABPM assessments are above threshold [33]. Suspicion of masked hypertension can arise from the presence of unexplained left ventricular hypertrophy. Masked uncontrolled hypertension can be caused by a lack of nocturnal BP reduction or even nocturnal hypertension possibly associated with sleep apnoea.

One of the important issues is whether ABPM can be used to manage antihypertensive therapy. Surprisingly there have been relatively few studies directly comparing the outcome with treatment of patients randomly assigned to either standard clinical decision-making or using ABPM thresholds. One of the few studies showed that using ABPM instead of clinic BP lead to less intensive drug treatment with the preservation of BP control and reduction in left ventricular hypertrophy [35].

A standard ABPM device will not give any relevant information as to the occurrence of cardiac arrhythmias and may be less accurate in determining BP where there is an irregular cardiac rhythm such as in atrial fibrillation. However, there are newer devices that have an embedded algorithm to detect arrhythmias during the inflation and deflation of the cuff [24]. Nevertheless, the standard ABPM devices remain appropriate under these conditions [33]. ABPM is not designed to detect postural hypotension as the measurements occur at a fixed interval and devices do not contain inclinometers which would be required to record a patient's position. However, ABPM can be used to assess whether there is high variability of BP which is often associated with orthostatic hypotension [9].

Novel ABPM Related Indices

There has been considerable interest in other measures that can be derived from ABPM apart from the standard measurements described above. Short-term BP variability has been a major interest as it is thought to reflect contributions from the autonomic nervous system. There are a host of indices related to standard deviation which have been suggested as independent risk factors over and above the absolute level of BP. New indices which reflect short term BP variability more precisely our "Average Real Variability" [28] and "Time Rate of variation" [38]. Both of these reflect the reading to reading changes in BP with the latter adjusted for the length of time between measurements.

An index which is determined from the relationship between systolic and diastolic BP over the 24 h has been called the ambulatory arterial stiffness index (AASI). This index which is correlated with vascular compliance is a predictor of cardiovascular mortality [2, 8] and associated with subclinical target organ damage in hypertensive subjects [13].

With the realisation that most cardiovascular events occur in the morning period, there has been great interest in determining the contribution of the morning surge in BP to these events and also targeting therapy to be most effective during this period. The morning BP surge defined by the difference between the minimum BP during the night and 2 h post waking has been associated with greater risk independently of ambulatory BP or nocturnal BP [23]. A mathematical construct combining the rate and amplitude of the morning surge in BP known as the morning BP Power is elevated in true and white coat hypertensive patients compared to normotensive subjects [17, 18] and is associated with the reactivity of the sympathetic nervous system [25]. Importantly this measure has been shown to be an independent risk factor for cardiovascular events and stroke [26].

Acknowledgements The current article was in part adapted from [19] with permission.

References

1. Babbs CF. Oscillometric measurement of systolic and diastolic blood pressures validated in a physiologic mathematical model. Biomed Eng Online. 2012;11:56.
2. Ben-Dov IZ, Gavish B, Kark JD, Mekler J, Bursztyn M. A modified ambulatory arterial stiffness index is independently associated with all-cause mortality. J Hum Hypertens. 2008;22(11):761–6.
3. Bjorklund K, Lind L, Zethelius B, Berglund L, Lithell H. Prognostic significance of 24-h ambulatory blood pressure characteristics for cardiovascular morbidity in a population of elderly men. J Hypertens. 2004;22(9):1691–7.
4. Clement DL, De Buyzere ML, De Bacquer DA, de Leeuw PW, Duprez DA, Fagard RH, et al. Prognostic value of ambulatory blood-pressure recordings in patients with treated hypertension. N Engl J Med. 2003;348(24):2407–15.
5. Davis GK, Mackenzie C, Brown MA, Homer CS, Holt J, McHugh L, et al. Predicting transformation from gestational hypertension to preeclampsia in clinical practice: a possible role for 24 hour ambulatory blood pressure monitoring. Hypertens Pregnancy. 2007;26(1):77–87.
6. Dawes MG, Coats AJ, Juszczak E. Daytime ambulatory systolic blood pressure is more effective at predicting mortality than clinic blood pressure. Blood Press Monit. 2006;11(3):111–8.
7. Dolan E, Stanton A, Thijs L, Hinedi K, Atkins N, McClory S, et al. Superiority of ambulatory over clinic blood pressure measurement in predicting mortality: The dublin outcome study. Hypertension. 2005;46(1):156–61.
8. Dolan E, Thijs L, Li Y, Atkins N, McCormack P, McClory S, et al. Ambulatory arterial stiffness index as a predictor of cardiovascular mortality in the dublin outcome study. Hypertension. 2006;47(3):365–70.
9. Ejaz AA, Kazory A, Heinig ME. 24-hour blood pressure monitoring in the evaluation of supine hypertension and orthostatic hypotension. J Clin Hypertens. 2007;9(12):952–5.
10. Elliott HL. 24-hour blood pressure control: Its relevance to cardiovascular outcomes and the importance of long-acting antihypertensive drugs. J Hum Hypertens. 2004;18(8):539–43.
11. Fagard RH, Thijs L, Staessen JA, Clement DL, De Buyzere ML, De Bacquer DA. Prognostic significance of ambulatory blood pressure in hypertensive patients with history of cardiovascular disease. Blood Press Monit. 2008;13(6):325–32.
12. Fan HQ, Li Y, Thijs L, Hansen TW, Boggia J, Kikuya M, et al. Prognostic value of isolated nocturnal hypertension on ambulatory measurement in 8711 individuals from 10 populations. J Hypertens. 2010;28(10):2036–45.
13. Garcia-Garcia A, Gomez-Marcos MA, Recio-Rodriguez JI, Gonzalez-Elena LJ, Parra-Sanchez J, Fe Munoz-Moreno M, et al. Relationship between ambulatory arterial stiffness index and subclinical target organ damage in hypertensive patients. Hypertens Res. 2010;34(2):180–6.
14. Hansen TW, Jeppesen J, Rasmussen S, Ibsen H, Torp-Pedersen C. Ambulatory blood pressure and mortality: a population-based study. Hypertension. 2005;45(4):499–504.
15. Hansen TW, Kikuya M, Thijs L, Bjorklund-Bodegard K, Kuznetsova T, Ohkubo T, et al. Prognostic superiority of daytime ambulatory over conventional blood pressure in four populations: a meta-analysis of 7,030 individuals. J Hypertens. 2007;25(8):1554–64.
16. Head GA. Ambulatory bp monitoring is ready to replace clinic bp in the diagnosis of hypertension: pro side of the argument. Hypertension. 2014;64(6):1175–81.
17. Head GA, Chatzivlastou K, Lukoshkova EV, Jennings GL, Reid CM. A novel measure of the power of the morning blood pressure surge from ambulatory blood pressure recordings. Am J Hypertens. 2010;23(10):1074–81.
18. Head GA, Mihailidou AS, Duggan KA, Beilin LJ, Berry N, Brown MA, et al. Definition of ambulatory blood pressure targets for diagnosis and treatment of hypertension in relation to clinic blood pressure: prospective cohort study. BMJ. 2010;340:c1104.
19. Head GA, McGrath BP, Mihailidou AS, Nelson MR, Schlaich MP, Stowasser M, et al. Ambulatory blood pressure monitoring. Aust Fam Physician. 2011;40(11):877–80.

20. Head GA, McGrath BP, Mihailidou AS, Nelson MR, Schlaich MP, Stowasser M, et al. Ambulatory blood pressure monitoring in Australia: 2011 consensus position statement. J Hypertens. 2012;30(2):253–66.
21. Imai Y. Prognostic significance of ambulatory blood pressure. Blood Press Monit. 1999;4(5):249–56.
22. Ingelsson E, Bjorklund-Bodegard K, Lind L, Arnlov J, Sundstrom J. Diurnal blood pressure pattern and risk of congestive heart failure. JAMA. 2006;295(24):2859–66.
23. Kario K, Pickering TG, Umeda Y, Hoshide S, Hoshide Y, Morinari M, et al. Morning surge in blood pressure as a predictor of silent and clinical cerebrovascular disease in elderly hypertensives: a prospective study. Circulation. 2003;107(10):1401–6.
24. Kollias A, Stergiou GS. Automated measurement of office, home and ambulatory blood pressure in atrial fibrillation. Clin Exp Pharmacol Physiol. 2014;41(1):9–15.
25. Lambert E, Chatzivlastou K, Schlaich M, Lambert G, Head G. Morning surge in blood pressure is associated with reactivity of the sympathetic nervous system. Am J Hypertens. 2014;27(6):783–92.
26. Luo Y, Wang Y-L, WU Y-B, Liang Y-L, Head GA, McGrath B, et al. Association between the rate of the morning surge in blood pressure and cardiovascular events and stroke. Chin Med J. 2013;126(3):510–4.
27. McGrath BP. Ambulatory blood pressure monitoring. Med J Aust. 2002;176(12):588–92.
28. Mena L, Pintos S, Queipo NV, Aizpurua JA, Maestre G, Sulbaran T. A reliable index for the prognostic significance of blood pressure variability. J Hypertens. 2005;23(3):505–11.
29. Mesquita-Bastos J, Bertoquini S, Polonia J. Cardiovascular prognostic value of ambulatory blood pressure monitoring in a portuguese hypertensive population followed up for 8.2 years. Blood Press Monit. 2010;15(5):240–6.
30. Niiranen TJ, Maki J, Puukka P, Karanko H, Jula AM. Office, home, and ambulatory blood pressures as predictors of cardiovascular risk. Hypertension. 2014;64:218–86.
31. O'Brien E, Atkins N, Stergiou G, Karpettas N, Parati G, Asmar R, et al. European society of hypertension international protocol revision 2010 for the validation of blood pressure measuring devices in adults. Blood Press Monit. 2010;15(1):23–38.
32. Ohkubo T, Imai Y, Tsuji I, Nagai K, Watanabe N, Minami N, et al. Prediction of mortality by ambulatory blood pressure monitoring versus screening blood pressure measurements: a pilot study in ohasama. J Hypertens. 1997;15(4):357–64.
33. Parati G, Stergiou G, O'Brien E, Asmar R, Beilin L, Bilo G, et al. European society of hypertension practice guidelines for ambulatory blood pressure monitoring. J Hypertens. 2014;32(7):1359–66.
34. Perloff D, Sokolow M, Cowan R. The prognostic value of ambulatory blood pressures. JAMA. 1983;249(20):2792–8.
35. Staessen JA, Byttebier G, Buntinx F, Celis H, O'Brien ET, Fagard R. Antihypertensive treatment based on conventional or ambulatory blood pressure measurement. A randomized controlled trial. Ambulatory blood pressure monitoring and treatment of hypertension investigators. JAMA. 1997;278(13):1065–72.
36. Staessen JA, Thijs L, Fagard R, O'Brien ET, Clement D, de Leeuw PW, et al. Predicting cardiovascular risk using conventional vs ambulatory blood pressure in older patients with systolic hypertension. Systolic hypertension in europe trial investigators. JAMA. 1999;282(6):539–46.
37. Verdecchia P, Porcellati C, Schillaci G, Borgioni C, Ciucci A, Battistelli M, et al. Ambulatory blood pressure. An independent predictor of prognosis in essential hypertension. Hypertension. 1994;24(6):793–801.
38. Zakopoulos NA, Tsivgoulis G, Barlas G, Papamichael C, Spengos K, Manios E, et al. Time rate of blood pressure variation is associated with increased common carotid artery intima-media thickness. Hypertension. 2005;45(4):505–12.

Chapter 5
Central Blood Pressure Measurement

Dimitrios A. Vrachatis, Theodore G. Papaioannou, and Athanasios D. Protogerou

Introduction

Peripheral (p) arterial blood pressure (BP) has monopolized clinical interest in arterial hypertension for more than a century. Although it is quite inaccurately measured with the available non-invasive methods, when compared to the intra-arterial pBP, it has been rightfully established as vital part of routine clinical examination. Upon recognition of the BP amplification phenomenon, researchers have also shed light on central BP (cBP) and its magnitude beyond pBP. In brief, BP amplification may be described as a rise of systolic BP (SBP) (and pulse pressure; PP) throughout the arterial tree, as moving apart from the aortic valve [1]. On the contrary, mean arterial pressure (MAP) and diastolic BP (DBP) remain almost unchanged (i.e. brachial SBP may be greater by ~20 mmHg than cSBP, while DBP and MAP only differ by ~1–2 mmHg from center to periphery) [1]. From an energy point of view, this phenomenon should be regarded as a distortion, rather than amplification phenomenon of the central pressure waveform as it travels towards the peripheral arteries. This observation was initially based on invasive data, which however are still limited to very small and disease specific populations. Therefore more invasive data are needed to quantify the actual amplification phenomenon between different arterial sites, especially in healthy subjects.

D.A. Vrachatis, M.D., M.Sc., Ph.D.
Department of Medicine, Medical School, National and Kapodistrian University, Athens, Greece
e-mail: dvrachatis@gmail.com

T.G. Papaioannou, Ph.D.
Assistant Professor in Biomedical Engineering at the Medical School of National and Kapodistrian University of Athens, Department of Medicine, Athens, Greece
e-mail: thepap@med.uoa.gr

A.D. Protogerou (✉)
Cardiovascular Prevention and Research Unit, Department of Pathophysiology, Medical School, National and Kapodistrian University of Athens,
75, Mikras Asias Street (Building 16 - 3rd floor), Athens 115 27, Greece
e-mail: aprotog@med.uoa.gr

E.A. Andreadis (ed.), *Hypertension and Cardiovascular Disease*,
DOI 10.1007/978-3-319-39599-9_5

This phenomenon is largely considered to be generated by (i) pressure wave reflections (amplitude and timing/travel distance before merging with the forward travelling pressure waves), (ii) heart rate, (iii) stiffness and diameter gradient, and thus it is greatly depending on age, gender and height [2]. Although its complex pathophysiology has not been fully elucidated, numerous invasive [3] and non-invasive studies [4] have illustrated that blood pressure lowering drugs do have different effects on aortic SBP compared to brachial (b) SBP and that cBP might have a better predictive ability when compared to brBP for future CV events and all-cause mortality in several, but not all, populations [5].

While the potential superiority of central blood pressure versus brachial blood pressure in the management of arterial hypertension is under intensive investigation [6], in parallel various of methods for direct or indirect estimation of cBP have been developed, mainly for research purposes. It should be noted that, traditionally, both aortic and carotid BP are referred as cBP. However, carotid BP is mainly used as a surrogate of aortic BP, assuming that BP amplification is negligible between these two points of interest. This assumption is, though, vaguely proven and supported by invasive data in the literature, whereas data on other central haemodynamics -like pressure wave reflections- provide only indirect information [7].

Following we will deal with the available methods for measurement of cBP (summarized in Table 5.1) and attempt to describe clearly the potential advantages as well as their limitations. However, it must be stated that no consensus has been reached so far for multiple issues that affect the methodology of cBP measurement. It must be also underlined that direct measurement of cBP may only be conducted invasively, while non-invasive approaches provide an indirect estimation of the actual central pressures. Of note, this is also true for the methods used during the previous decades to non-invasively "measure" the bBP with automated oscillometric devices. These devices measure mean arterial bBP and then derive systolic and diastolic BP with the application of proprietary algorithms. For these reason, and although we acknowledge the essential difference between measurement and estimation in the text, we use the term "measurement" instead of "estimation" for both the bBP and cBP.

Invasive Central Pressure Measurement

Invasive is considered the "gold-standard" method to accurately measure cBP. It may be conducted either with (a) fluid-filled catheter-manometer system or (b) with special pressure wire systems. From a historical viewpoint, Hales R.S. is appraised as a pioneer in cBP assessment since, in 1733, he was the first to cannulate a horse's carotid artery using a long glass tube and subsequently observe the pumping equilibrium of blood into the tube [8]. Undoubtedly, the interventional nature of direct cBP measurement – accompanied by the potential complications – constitutes its major disadvantage.

Table 5.1 Advantages and disadvantages of methods and techniques for non-invasive central blood pressure assessment

Method	Waveform acquisition	Calibration pressure derived at the	Calibration pressures	Calibration vs. waveform acquisition	Advantages	Disadvantages
Tonometry	Common carotid arery	Brachial artery	DBP/MAP	Asynchronous	Proximity to aorta SBP is not used for calibration, potentially minimizing the brachial cuff measurement error	Aortic to carotid amplification may not be negligible[a] Assumption that MAP/DBP are constant in the arterial tree Operator dependent
	Radial artery	Brachial artery	SBP/DBP or MAP/DBP	Asynchronous	Easier than carotid tonometry May be less operator independent if special equipment is used May be used for ambulatory BP monitoring	Brachial to radial amplification may not be negligible
Ultrasound	Common carotid arery	Brachial artery	DBP/MAP	Asynchronous	Proximity to aorta	Aortic to carotid amplification may not be negligible[a] Assumption that MAP/DBP are constant in the arterial tree Operator dependent
Oscillometry	Brachial artery	Brachial artery	SBP/DBP or MAP/DBP	Synchronous	Operator independent Waveform and BP acquisition in the same artery May be used for ambulatory BP monitoring	Waveform disparity depending on cuff inflation pressure

DBP diastolic blood pressure, *MAP* mean arterial pressure, *SBP* systolic blood pressure
[a]When carotid SBP considered as surrogate of aortic SBP

Fluid Filled Catheters

This approach requires catheterization of a peripheral artery and advancement of a catheter that incorporates an infusion system into the point of interest (i.e. above the aortic valve). The catheter (usually filled with normal saline) is connected to an external pressure transducer (hydraulic coupling) that provides a dynamic monitoring of arterial pressure waveform and calculates its' levels. Calibration (zeroing) of the system is achieved through exposure to atmospheric air. Zeroing process is affected by patient positioning (hydrostatic level) and proper removal of air bubbles from the catheter and its' connectors. More, it is recommended that it should be conducted immediately prior to its use. A limitation of such systems is that they provide over-filtered pressure signals and present a relatively low frequency response. Their greatest advantage is their considerable low cost compared to high fidelity pressure wires or micro-tipped catheters that will be discussed in the next paragraph.

Pressure Wires

Utilization of high-fidelity catheter micro-tip pressure transducers is considered to be the actual "gold-standard" against which the accuracy of all other approaches is assessed. They provide high-fidelity pressure waveforms and are characterized by a higher frequency response (depending on their analog/digital converter) than fluid-filled systems; therefore they are more suitable for pulse wave analysis and the derivation of more complex haemodynamic indices, such as augmentation index. We should emphasize the clear discrimination between "true" pressure wires that incorporate a pressure catheter tip and those that require initial calibration with a fluid-filled system. Currently evidence on the direct comparison between the two systems is not available and the magnitude of the potential error introduced by the fluid-filled system is not known. Major limitation of pressure wires is their high cost.

Non-invasive Central Pressure Estimation

The Main Method and the Related Techniques

The currently prevailing method to non-invasively measure cBP requires the following three steps: (1) acquisition of a physiologically relevant to the peripheral BP waveform signal e.g. either direct pressure wave, distention wave or other; (2) BP calibration of the peripheral waveform; (3) transformation of the peripheral BP to aortic BP waveform.

Techniques for the Acquisition of the Peripheral Waveform

Applanation Tonometry

Applanation tonometry utilizes Newton's third law of motion ("for every action, there is an equal and opposite reaction") in order to estimate arteries' internal pressure. Special (mechanical or electrical) transducers (tonometers), comprising of single-element or multi-array sensors, are employed in order to compress a superficial artery against a (relatively) solid surface. This set-up allows the tonometer to sense forces or displacement of the compressed vessel.

In order to achieve optimal recording both positioning and pressure of the tonometer shall be steady, as "noise" may easily be introduced in the recorded signal. The following features have been proposed to characterize an acceptable waveform recording: (i) Highest possible pulse amplitude, (ii) Sharp upstroke of the recorded pulse from the minimum diastolic value, (iii) Sharp inflection (incisura) indicative of aortic valve closure, (iv) Near exponential decline in diastolic pressures, especially at end-diastole, (v) Lowest possible length variation of the diastolic part of the sequential recorded pressure waves.

Radial artery tonometry, has been introduced in the early 90s for pBP waveform recording [9]. This approach tackles the aforementioned practical prerequisites, as the artery may be applanated against a hard bony surface. Moreover, the patient may easily be instructed to keep his/her forearm steady, while housings in which the tonometer is mounted and placed over the wrist have been developed. In such systems, the force applied by the tonometer may be electronically controlled. Still, we underline that there is missing standardization regarding patient positioning (sitting or supine) during examination, a fact that is often overlooked [10].

Oscillometry

Oscillometry in the brachial artery is utilized the last few years to measure cBP. The physiological signals in this approach are collected by a inflatable cuff (at different BP levels from diastolic to suprasystolic depending on the device used, which is positioned around the upper arm at the level of brachial artery, the same way as conventionally done for brachial BP measurement [11]. This method is operator-independent, provides simultaneously brachial and aortic BP readings and it may also be utilized for ambulatory patient monitoring [12]. It represents the most promising method so far for measuring cBP, facilitating the application of cBP assessment in the large population studies and clinical trials.

Peripheral (Pressure) Waveform Calibration

Pressure waveforms derived from the aforementioned techniques are not already calibrated in mmHg, so such a process is required in order to extract cBP. For this purpose, BP – as measured conventially by standard validated oscillometric devices or the mercury sphygmomanometer – at the level of brachial artery is utilized. MAP & DBP or alternatively SBP & DBP are used for calibration purposes. However, the physiologic signal (pressure or other) waveform acquisition is not always measured at the same level as brachial BP. Although the aforementioned oscillometric technique provides the brachial waveform, on the contrary tonometry is usually conducted at the radial artery. Therefore, a series of assumptions, that may introduce systematic errors, are required: (i) in general the DBP and MAP are considered similar throughout the arterial tree, however very small errors, potentially below 0.5 mmHg might be introduced; (ii) brachial to radial SBP amplification is considered to be negligible, however non-invasive data suggest that the brachial to radial amplification may reach 5 mmHg [13]. Actually, recent data underline the role of waveform calibration on the predictive role of the estimated central pressures on clinical events [14] as well as regarding the association with organ damage [15]. In these studies [14, 15] calibration with MAP and DBP provided better results than calibration with SBP and DBP; however these findings cannot be generalized and may be device and setting dependent.

Transformation of the Peripheral BP Waveform to Aortic BP (or Waveform)

Transformation of the peripherally acquired waveform to its aortic "ancestor" has been a point of debate as different approaches have been utilized in order to overcome the inherent limitations of the acquisition techniques. These approaches involve mainly transfer functions of the peripheral waveform [8]. In brief, transfer functions are derived by combination of advanced mathematical techniques (e.g. time or frequency domain analysis). Different transfer functions have been developed by different research groups and vary accordingly in the commercially available devices [9, 16–18]. The detailed presentation of all these models is beyond the scope of this chapter, however it must be noted that the final error of each algorithm ranges from a few to several (1–2 to 10–20) mmHg but depends mainly on the method of calibration (MAP & DBP versus SBP & DBP) rather than the mathematical models per se.

Alternative Method Based on Direct Carotid Waveforms Acquisition and Related Techniques

Because the carotid artery is anatomically close to the aorta, the carotid waveforms have been considered as surrogates of the actual aortic waveforms. The carotid waveforms are not calibrated in mmHg, so such a process is required. Given the fact that MAP and DBP are considered to be constant throughout the arterial tree the carotid waveform can be calibrated by the brachial derived MAP and DBP – as measured conventially by standard validated oscillometric devices or the mercury sphygmomanometer – in order to get carotid (central) SBP.

Direct Acquisition of the Carotid (Central) Pressure Waveform by Applanation Tonometry at the Carotid Artery

Whilst applanation tonometry is mainly utilized at the level of the radial artery (see previous section for technical details), application of this approach in the carotid artery is also feasible. However as already discussed, to the best of our knowledge, data regarding head-to-head evaluation of carotid (by tonometry) vs. aortic BP are scarce [7]. Nevertheless, the limited, non-randomized, available studies suggest that the clinical performance of carotid BP to associate with organ damage or to predict the incidence of mortality is rather comparable to that of aortic BP [19, 20].

Moreover, the left or right common carotid tonometry has been "accused" of a range of methodological drawbacks [8]. First, there is absence of a solid anatomic surface in the cervical region against which the carotid artery may be compressed. Second, it is strenuous for the patient to keep his/her neck totally motionless during the examination; this also applies for the operator who manually handles the tonometer. Potential activation of baroreceptors, displacement of carotid plaques, relative hypo-perfusion are also included in the potential – although hardly seen or proven – disadvantages of this approach.

Direct Acquisition of the Carotid (Central) Distention Waveform by Ultrasound at the Carotid Artery

Alternatively to the applanation technique, acquisition of an arterial wall distension waveform utilizing ultrasounds (echo-tracking) is technically feasible, though highly operator-dependent. This approach may be theoretically applied in any superficial artery, but available data regarding cBP practically refer to the carotid artery only [21] and scarcely to the femoral artery [20]. In brief, a high-precision echo-tracking device coupled with a Doppler system is used- the transducer of which is placed (manually or by a stereotaxic arm) perpendicular to the longitudinal axis of the carotid artery. Subsequently, the corresponding signals from the anterior and posterior artery walls is recorded and analyzed. Main limitation of this approach is that it is based on the assumption that intra-arterial blood pressure variation is analogous to arterial distension. Indeed, this may be only partially confirmed as the pressure/diameter relationship is not linear [22]. In fact the arterial wall does not behave as a pure elastic material thus introducing an hysteris loop that could mislead cBP waveform estimation.

Further Non-invasive Approaches

Derivation of the central BP through peripheral waveform utilizing the, linear, correlation between the two pressures has also been proposed [23, 24]. However, BP amplification may vary under a series of circumstances (e.g. age, heart rate, vasoactive substances). This could introducing systematic errors as the relationship between central and peripheral BP may not always be linear. Such an approach is useful for large epidemiological studies but not for clinical use.

The final approach refers to "graphical" estimation of central BP based upon inspection of the peripheral waveform [25]. In particular, it has been shown that in patients in whom the second systolic peak of the radial artery pressure wave can be detected, this peak is linearly associated with the maximal aortic systolic pressure [26].

Perspective – Conclusions

Central haemodynamics have been a rapidly evolving field of clinical research in arterial hypertension. Although consensus has yet to be achieved regarding the optimal method and technique for non-invasive measurement of cBP, undoubtedly significant progress has been accomplished during the last decades. A recently developed method, which is based on brachial cuff oscillometry and the use of mathematical transformations to derive the aortic BP, seems at the moment the most promising and suitable way in order to massively apply cBP measurement in clinical research, and potentially in future clinical practice. The potential superiority of cBP compared to pBP in the clinical management of arterial hypertension will be essentially tested (proven or negated) only when devices able to measure non-invasively and accurately cBP, pBP and BP amplification, will become available. To this end, the so far neglected, but huge, inaccuracies in pBP assessment are equally important and should be addressed together with the innovation in central haemodynamics.

Conflicts of Interest ADP has received equipment for research and an unrestricted research grant from IEM (Stolberg, Germany), a manufacturer of central blood pressure measuring device; TGP has received equipment for research purposes from IEM (Stolberg, Germany) and he serves as consultant for Microsoft (Microsoft Research, Redmond, USA)

References

1. Kroeker EJ, Wood EH. Comparison of simultaneously recorded central and peripheral arterial pressure pulses during rest, exercise and tilted position in man. Circ Res. 1955;3(6):623–32.
2. Protogerou AD, Papaioannou TG, Blacher J, Papamichael CM, Lekakis JP, Safar ME. Central blood pressures: do we need them in the management of cardiovascular disease? Is it a feasible therapeutic target? J Hypertens. 2007;25(2):265–72.
3. Chirinos JA, Zambrano JP, Chakko S, Veerani A, Schob A, Perez G, et al. Relation between ascending aortic pressures and outcomes in patients with angiographically demonstrated coronary artery disease. Am J Cardiol. 2005;96(5):645–8.
4. Safar ME, Blacher J, Pannier B, Guerin AP, Marchais SJ, Guyonvarc'h PM, et al. Central pulse pressure and mortality in end-stage renal disease. Hypertension. 2002;39(3):735–8.

5. Agabiti-Rosei E, Mancia G, O'Rourke MF, Roman MJ, Safar ME, Smulyan H, et al. Central blood pressure measurements and antihypertensive therapy: a consensus document. Hypertension. 2007;50(1):154–60.
6. Sharman JE, Marwick TH, Gilroy D, Otahal P, Abhayaratna WP, Stowasser M, et al. Randomized trial of guiding hypertension management using central aortic blood pressure compared with best-practice care: principal findings of the BP GUIDE study. Hypertension. 2013;62(6):1138–45.
7. Chen CH, Ting CT, Nussbacher A, Nevo E, Kass DA, Pak P, et al. Validation of carotid artery tonometry as a means of estimating augmentation index of ascending aortic pressure. Hypertension. 1996;27(2):168–75.
8. Papaioannou TG, Protogerou AD, Stamatelopoulos KS, Vavuranakis M, Stefanadis C. Non-invasive methods and techniques for central blood pressure estimation: procedures, validation, reproducibility and limitations. Curr Pharm Des. 2009;15(3):245–53.
9. Karamanoglu M, O'Rourke MF, Avolio AP, Kelly RP. An analysis of the relationship between central aortic and peripheral upper limb pressure waves in man. Eur Heart J. 1993;14(2):160–7.
10. Vrachatis D, Papaioannou TG, Konstantopoulou A, Nasothimiou EG, Millasseau S, Blacher J, et al. Effect of supine versus sitting position on noninvasive assessment of aortic pressure waveform: a randomized cross-over study. J Hum Hypertens. 2014;28(4):236–41.
11. Alpert BS, Quinn D, Gallick D. Oscillometric blood pressure: a review for clinicians. J Am Soc Hypertens. 2014;8(12):930–8.
12. Protogerou AD, Argyris A, Nasothimiou E, Vrachatis D, Papaioannou TG, Tzamouranis D, et al. Feasibility and reproducibility of noninvasive 24-h ambulatory aortic blood pressure monitoring with a brachial cuff-based oscillometric device. Am J Hypertens. 2012;25(8): 876–82.
13. Segers P, Mahieu D, Kips J, Rietzschel E, De Buyzere M, De Bacquer D, et al. Amplification of the pressure pulse in the upper limb in healthy, middle-aged men and women. Hypertension. 2009;54(2):414–20.
14. Wassertheurer S, Baumann M. Assessment of systolic aortic pressure and its association to all cause mortality critically depends on waveform calibration. J Hypertens. 2015;33(9):1884–9.
15. Protogerou AD, Argyris AA, Papaioannou TG, Kollias GE, Konstantonis GD, Nasothimiou E, et al. Left-ventricular hypertrophy is associated better with 24-h aortic pressure than 24-h brachial pressure in hypertensive patients: the SAFAR study. J Hypertens. 2014;32(9):1805–14.
16. Chen CH, Nevo E, Fetics B, Pak PH, Yin FC, Maughan WL, et al. Estimation of central aortic pressure waveform by mathematical transformation of radial tonometry pressure. Validation of generalized transfer function. Circulation. 1997;95(7):1827–36.
17. Fetics B, Nevo E, Chen CH, Kass DA. Parametric model derivation of transfer function for noninvasive estimation of aortic pressure by radial tonometry. IEEE Trans Biomed Eng. 1999;46(6):698–706.
18. Hope SA, Tay DB, Meredith IT, Cameron JD. Comparison of generalized and gender-specific transfer functions for the derivation of aortic waveforms. Am J Physiol Heart Circ Physiol. 2002;283(3):H1150–6.
19. Asmar RG, London GM, O'Rourke ME, Safar ME, Coordinators RP. Investigators. Improvement in blood pressure, arterial stiffness and wave reflections with a very-low-dose perindopril/indapamide combination in hypertensive patient: a comparison with atenolol. Hypertension. 2001;38(4):922–6.
20. Protogerou AD, van Sloten TT, Henry RMA, Dekker JM, Nijpels G, Stehouwer CDA. Pulse pressure measured at the level of the femoral artery, but not at the level of the aorta, carotid and brachial arteries, is associated with the incidence of coronary heart disease events in a population with a high prevalence of type 2 diabetes and impaired glucose metabolism – The Hoorn study. Artery Res. 2015;9:19–26.
21. Van Bortel LM, Balkestein EJ, van der Heijden-Spek JJ, Vanmolkot FH, Staessen JA, Kragten JA, et al. Non-invasive assessment of local arterial pulse pressure: comparison of applanation tonometry and echo-tracking. J Hypertens. 2001;19(6):1037–44.

22. London GM, Pannier B. Arterial functions: how to interpret the complex physiology. Nephrol Dial Transplant. 2010;25(12):3815–23.
23. Borow KM, Newburger JW. Noninvasive estimation of central aortic pressure using the oscillometric method for analyzing systemic artery pulsatile blood flow: comparative study of indirect systolic, diastolic, and mean brachial artery pressure with simultaneous direct ascending aortic pressure measurements. Am Heart J. 1982;103(5):879–86.
24. Davies JI, Band MM, Pringle S, Ogston S, Struthers AD. Peripheral blood pressure measurement is as good as applanation tonometry at predicting ascending aortic blood pressure. J Hypertens. 2003;21(3):571–6.
25. Adji A, O'Rourke MF. Determination of central aortic systolic and pulse pressure from the radial artery pressure waveform. Blood Press Monit. 2004;9(3):115–21.
26. Pauca AL, Kon ND, O'Rourke MF. The second peak of the radial artery pressure wave represents aortic systolic pressure in hypertensive and elderly patients. Br J Anaesth. 2004;92(5):651–7.

Chapter 6
The Progression of Hypertensive Heart Disease to Left Ventricular Hypertrophy and Heart Failure

Styliani A. Geronikolou and Dennis Cokkinos

Epidemiology of Hypertension

Although statistics of cardiovascular disease (CVD) change over time, hypertension (HTN) remains a leading cause of cardiac morbidity and mortality. Many recent reviews stress its etiologic correlation with heart failure (HF). Thus, Roger [67] describing the HF epidemic stresses that 4.9 million Americans carry this diagnosis with survival estimates of 50 % at 5 years. She mentions that the attributable risk of hypertension varies between 10 and 13 % in various studies [67].

According to the date of Olmsted County, hypertension is responsible for the largest proportion of new HF (HF) population cases; actually the incidence attributable risk of this increased from 15 % in 1979–1984 to 29 % in 1979–2002 [22].

Khatibzadeh [43] found that, worldwide, HTN as a risk factor for HF varied widely from 7 to 65 % [43]. For Greece they report a prevalence of 55 %. Cheng [9] reported that HTN was the most prevalent risk factor for incident CVD over the years (population attributable 0.25 between 1987 to 1989 and 0.29 between 1996 to 1998 [9].

In the elderly, HTN is the most prevalent HF risk factor. Butler found a continuous positive association between systolic blood pressure and HF risk [8].

De Goma [11] re-emphasized the importance of both 24-h ambulatory and standard office-based blood pressure as risk factors for cardiovascular mortality with Hazard Ratios (HR) for various increases of systolic blood pressure up to 1.4 [11].

S.A. Geronikolou • D. Cokkinos (✉)
Clinical, Experimental Surgery, Translational Research Centre,
Biomedical Research Foundation Academy of Athens, Athens, Greece
e-mail: dcokkinos@bioacademy.gr

E.A. Andreadis (ed.), *Hypertension and Cardiovascular Disease*,
DOI 10.1007/978-3-319-39599-9_6

Hypertension and Cardiac Hypertrophy

Hypertension is strongly linked to left ventricular hypertrophy (LVH). In many studies it is recognized that LVH itself is associated with increased mortality, independently of age, gender and the levels of blood pressure itself [13, 28].

LVH itself is a risk factor, with a mortality rate at 16 %, as compared to 2 % in its absence according to Devereux [13]. He stresses that this increase of adverse events of LVH is dependent on age, gender, the levels of blood pressure, lipid levels, smoking and even the angiographically determined presence of coronary artery disease (CAD). Mortality increases as the concentric pattern of remodeling (REM) is associated to an increase in LV mass. Moreover, in patients whose LVH increased during the study, subsequent events increased substantially [16]. Many of the aforementioned studies are older. However, in 2011, Katholi and Couri stress that LVH is a strong factor for atrial fibrillation, congestive HF and sudden death in women [42].

It should not be forgotten that even electrocardiographically (ECG)-diagnosed LVH which obviously can be applied in much larger populations, is associated with a three-fold increased risk for CHD, and a 1.4–2.9 increased risk for HF. Interestingly, in various studies by echocardiography (Echo), the increase in HF risk was roughly similar: 1.6–3.7 [8, 22]

Great discussion still exists whether the simpler technique, electrocardiography is adequate in comparison to (Echo) for population and epidemiologic purposes. An older study had showed that it failed to detect LVH in 50 % of cases [15]. There is a general consensus that ECG has good specificity but low sensitivity. Moreover, many of the more sensitive techniques, such as the Cornell index are sometimes difficult to calculate. In consequence, a clinician interested in the welfare and the future of his patients would advice Echo to be performed in every newly diagnosed case of HTN. The examination should include cardiac structure, including concentric and eccentric REM, LVH by standard criteria, left atrial dilatation, contractility (fractional, shortening is simple and more accurate than calculating ejection fraction), and diastolic function. During the examination the carotids and ascending and abdominal aorta should also be examined. Here, it must be stressed that a variety of definitions of LVH exist. Ducimetiere and Richard [21] correlated cardiac insufficiency and LVH in general population, in two cities: Goeteborg and Framingham. In clinical HF cases, they found arterial HTN in 24 % and 37 % respectively [21].

Many of the above studies have been performed by Echo. However, in the MESA study MRI was employed. With this technique CVD events were correlated to LV mass. Interestingly, as regards the emergence of HF events, a strong correlation was seen with LV mass and volume, but not with their ratio, when it was adjusted for risk factors such as age, gender, race, smoking, HDL, BP, diabetes and anti-hypertensive and hypolipidemic therapy [5]. The same authors concluded that association between LVH with heart and coronary heart disease can be mediated through concentric LV, REM, whereas HF is more closely associated to LV mass. Probably, the most widely accepted is that of Devereux who found that hypertensives with LVH had a LVMI (left ventricular mass index 140 ± 15 g/m^2, while normals had 9 ± 26 g/m^2

and hypertensives without LVH 97 ± 15 g/m^2 [17]. Ang [2] angiographically defined LVH cutoff as g/m^2 > 105 in men and > 95 in women [2].

It must also be re-iterated that while very strong correlations exist between LVH and cardiovascular morbidity-mortality, the favorable effects of LVH regression have not been studied to a similar extent [17]. This will be further discussed.

Clinical Correlations

Clinical correlations of LVH with simple clinical factors should be given. Thus, according to Devereux [17] who cites various studies, 60 % of the variability of LV mass can be attributed to systolic BP, body height and mass, male gender and diabetes mellitus. Interestingly, Ang repeated that 75 % of patients with stable angina have LVH, even in the presence of normal ambulatory blood pressure (45 %) [2]. Chronic uremia is commonly associated with LVH [53, 56].

Tissue Cardiac Correlates

A very large number of studies have addressed the histological, anosohistochemical and molecular changes underlying LVH. van Berlo gave a very detailed review, 2 years ago [79]. These authors stress that LVH is the result of myocyte growth in a cross sectional area (myocyte hypertrophy). They re-iterate the different types of LVH, i.e. eccentric or dilative growth response in which the chamber effectively dilates with wall thinning through a predominate lengthening of individual myocytes.

In an old but very pertinent study, Grossman [34] hypothesize that increased systolic tension development results in fiber thickening to normalize wall stress, while diastolic tension results into cardiac lengthening, which improves ventricular mechanical efficiency but does not normalize diastolic wall stress. The importance of the latter mechanism will be addressed further on [34].

van Berlo describe how the hypertrophic response of the myocardium is initiated by many diverse signal transduction pathways. They also stress that the transition from pure hypertrophy to HF is accompanied by an eccentric growth, with chamber dilation wall thinning and predominant myocyte lengthening [79]. There exists a very intense discussion as to what differentiates between "physiological" or "compensatory" LVH to the "pathological" or maladaptive state. Here, it should be stressed that two nature-proved paradigms are pregnancy and regular exercise. The hypertrophy of the Burmese python, during a large meal, has necessarily been studied very sparsely. Most authors give a simple statement that functional assessment of cardiac growth; normal or even hyperkinetic function is essential to define the "compensated" state, although intrinsic cardiomyocyte function may already be depressed [19]

Tardiff again stresses that cardiac HF can be adaptive or maladaptive. Cardiovascular function is a simple differentiating factor, stressing that early β-adrenergic receptor (β-ARs) dysfunction drives the pathogenic hypertensive phenotype [72].

Dorn [20] also stress the relevant cellular features of LVH. They emphasize that myocyte H is accompanied by increased sarcomerogenesis and increased expression of ANP and BNP. The role of hyperplasia is not adequately known, even with more recent studies of a possible contribution of cell regeneration and hyperplasia [20]

Hunter and Chien [39] additionally point out that in physiological hearts the CMCs grow evenly in length and width, while they become wider during pressure and longer during volume overload respectively. According to the authors, this abnormal morphological evaluation can disrupt sarcomere alignment and cardiac dysfunction [39]. So far, contractile dysfunction has been mainly discussed. However, echocardiography has made an entity of diastolic dysfunction widely known. In fact, in most individuals over 65 years, "diastolic dysfunction" is diagnosed. Vogel [82] studied the natural history of pre-clinical diastolic dysfunction in 388 individuals of mean age 67 ± 12 years (75 % females over 3 years) in Olmsted County, Minessota. At this time interval 11.6 % developed symptomatic HF, 14.5 % atrial fibrillation and 10 % died [82].

Molecular Markers

Inevitably, we come to the molecular cardiac markers. One aspect which is derived from rat and mice studies is the expression of the "hypertrophic" gene program which mostly co-exists with the "fetal" gene program. This is mostly characterized by a shift from the fast "α" isoform of the myosin heavy chain to the slow "β" isoform- representative of the fetal myocardium. MCs overexpressing αMHC demonstrate faster contraction but are more sensitive to hypoxia. Importantly, adult mice or rats have an approximately 90 % αMHC expression while in the rabbit they are about equally expressed. In the human ventricles, αMHC is represented in only 3-10 %; atria express αMHC much more abundantly. Many noxious processes cause a shift from αMHC to βMHC, i.e. diabetes, HF, hypothyroidism [33]. Actually, genetic over-expression of SERCA 2α in mice prevents the transition from hypertrophy to early HF [40], while a characteristic of the heart with HF is a decrease in SERCA-Z. However, at which stage from "compensated" to "decompensated" LVH this occurs is difficult to assess [3]. With this opportunity it should be stressed that the question of cut-off of molecular changes of "physiological" or "pathological" H is very difficult to outline. A former review by Swynghedauw [70] is still very pertinent as to which genes are re-expressed or blunted during REM. Thus, β-MHC, the less efficient A3, Na^+, K^+, ATPase subunit, atrial natriuretic peptide, myocyte lengthening gene are re-expressed while calcium ATPase of SERCA2, the adrenergic receptor β1, the muscarinic receptors M2 and myoglobin are blunted [70].

Here, a very intriguing finding by Pandya [62] should be mentioned. They reiterate that the re-expression of the fetally expressed β-myosin heavy chain (β-MHC) is a principal marker of pathological LVH. However, they argue that it is a marker of fibrosis rather than cellular hypertrophy [62].

Another preferential feature of "H" or "F" phenotype is the shift from fatty acid to glucose oxidation. However, it is not widely appreciated that this shift is not completely compensatory; thus, energy deprivation or impairment occurs, with a decrease in tissue high energy phosphate levels, expressed by a decrease of ATP, P(r) and the P(r)/ATP and ATP/ADP ratio [60]. Van Bilsen [80] outlines the suggested causative role of genomic alterations in the chain of events from hypertrophy to HF (Fig. 6.1): Reductions in PGC1α and Nrf1/2 (left side of Fig. 6.1) impair mitochondrial replication and the gene expression constituting respiratory chain complexes, whereas, the PPARs expression/activity (right side of Fig. 6.1) reduce leads to diminished expression of fatty acid oxidation (FAO) genes. Consequently, a preferred therapeutic approach would stimulate glucose oxidation rather than to normalize substrate metabolism by stimulating fatty acid utilization [80].

Izumiya [41] showed that the vascular endothelial growth factor (VEGF) is essential for maintaining capillaries density; disruption of this compensatory reaction by VEGF blockade promotes the transition from compensatory H to HF [41].

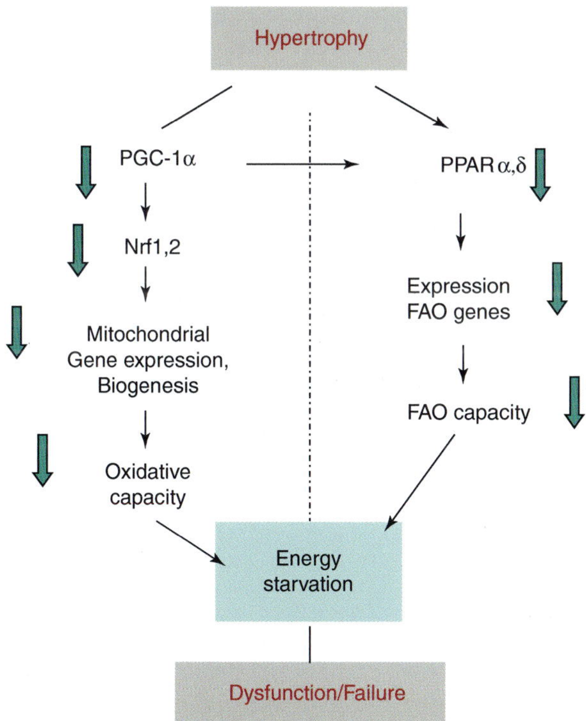

Fig. 6.1 Causative factors chain of events from HPT to HF hypothesis (Reproduced by van Bilsen [80]. Licence No 3727530217090)

Another factor-very recently described- attenuating this transition is Canopy 2. This is pro-angiogenic and is induced by hypoxia and the HIF-1α (hypoxia-inducible factor) [35].

ROS production is a main aspect of H and REM. Takimoto and Kass [71] point out that free oxygen radicals produce: hypertrophy apoptosis, MMP activation, fibrosis, contractile dysfunction and ultimately pathologic REM [71]. The polyphenolic compound quercetin (QCN) included in antioxidative diets prevents maladaptive myocardial remodeling as suggested in an experiment on hyperlipidemic mice [77].

Fanelli and Zatz [23] point out that oxidative stress induces HTN through activation of the RAAS [23]. Not only does Angio-II induce oxidative stress, but these two entities interact to promote exaggerated H. Also, they both activate NFKb –a key inflammatory agent. Discussion still exists whether Angiotensin –II is a direct mediator of LVH. This brings into focus the question, whether drugs produce LVH regression through blood pressure reduction. Animal studies have given significant insights. Thus, Mazzolai [52] found marked right and left ventricular H in transgenic mice overexpressing Angio-II in the heart [52]. Mellor [55] have shown that "ageig-related cardiomyocyte functional decline is gender and angiotensin II dependent" [55].

Once contractile insufficiency with a reduction of cardiac output occurs, another vicious cycle sets in: that of enhanced neuro-hormonal response, mainly represented by:

(a) Enhanced release of adrenergic amines. This causes down- regulation and desensitization of cardiac adrenergic receptors.
(b) Enhanced release of angiotensin and aldosterone : this causes peripheral vasoconstriction which together with retention of salt and water causes increases in pre- and after load. The end results of "α" and "β" are in contractility deterioration and hemodynamic overload.

This last occurrence sets in motion a hitherto little recognized mechanism, mechanoreceptor activation, which elicits growth stimuli. Mechanotransduction activation can lead to apoptosis and increase of extracellular matrix leading to fibrosis [38]. Here it should be stated that many cells can sense mechanical forces. Though mechanotransduction, the mechanical signal is converted into a biochemichal or biophysical signal. A family of proteins –the polycystins- physically interact with most of the mechanosensing proteins regulating this phenomenon [66].

Mann [49] describes how stretch induces signal transduction in the heart is effected by two parallel mechanisms: Directly through activation of integrins, stretch –activated ion channels, the Na^+/H^+ exchanger (NHE) heterotrimetric G proteins of the Gq and Gi class, and possibly angiotensin II, cytokines of the IL-β family, IGF-1 and possibly endothelin-1 [49].

Here, a little discussed factor should be described, inflammation through innate immunity activation. Pressure overload by itself sets into motion a cascade of pro-inflammatory factors, i.e. nuclear factor kB activation, interleukin 1β, up-regulation and eventually toll-like receptor-2, which by itself mediates adaptive hypertrophy [36]. Additionally, the toll-interacting protein (Tollip) diminishes pressure overload hypertrophy in mice [47].

Signaling Effectors

Van Berlo et al. [79] and Frey and Olson [27] describe how the above mentioned factors mediate H in a molecular basis [27, 79]. The former reviewers outline how β-adrenergic receptors (β-ARs) act through hypertrophic kinases: the β-ARs activate adenyl cyclase and induce CAMP elevation. CAMP increases activate PKA which regulates cardiac contractility by phosphorylating Ca^{++} handling and contractile proteins. Importantly, prolonged β-ARs activation ultimately leads to their desensitization, with loss to catecholamine contractile response. This sets into motion a vicious cycle of further sympathetic neuro-hormonal activation. PKCa protects the myocardium by increasing the sarcoplasmic reticulum Ca^{++} levels and Ca^{++} cycling efficiency. Also, PKCa inhibition can blunt the hypertrophic control by the following mechanisms [6]:

- By augmenting contractile function, the need for enhanced neuroendocrine level is diminished.
- Ca^{++}/calmodulin –dependent kinase II (CaMK II) signaling is a regulator of cardiac demand. HF according to Anderson [1]. As suggested by the name, CaMK II isozymes are activated by Ca^{++}/calmodulin. This kinase is also activated by ROS. CaMK II also regulates intracellular Ca^{++} handling. As will be described in the therapy section, an inhibitor of CaMK II would decrease cardiac H and REM. Phosphodisterase -5 inhibition with sildenafil has an antihypertrophic effect, independent of blood pressure reduction [58]. Sildenafil, has mild inotropic effects, which, in the case of PKCa inhibition interrupts the vicious neurohormonal catecholamine cycle [84]

The MAPK signaling cascade consists of three main branches, which are all potentiated in pathological H. Of these, JNKs and p38 kinases serve as transducers of stress or injury responses. ERK1/2 activation produces concentric cardiac H, which however, does not progress to HF nor produces cell death [7].

In the mouse heart chronic transverse aortic constriction increases p38 MAP activities, together with an increase in apoptosis [83].

Another anti-hypertrophic agent is NO [64]. The endothelial NO synthase enhancer (eNOS) diminishes REM after an experimental infarction [26].

Histone deacetylases (**HDACs**) act in diverse ways: IIα HDACs suppress cardiac hypertrophy according to Zhang [85]. However, inhibition of class I HDACs reduces pressure overload hypertrophy [31]. Proto-oncogenes participate in normal cell proliferation and in cell transformation. After cardiac myocytes terminal differentiation, they cannot further divide except in the fetal period. Komuro [46] examined eight oncogenes in rat hearts in order to determine the role of cellular oncogenes in the growth of the heart. Pressure overload increased the levels of cellular c-fos, c-myc, and c-Ha-ras in stage specific manner. Although oncogenes were reported experiment suggests that oncogenes may be expressed in cardiomyocytes [46].

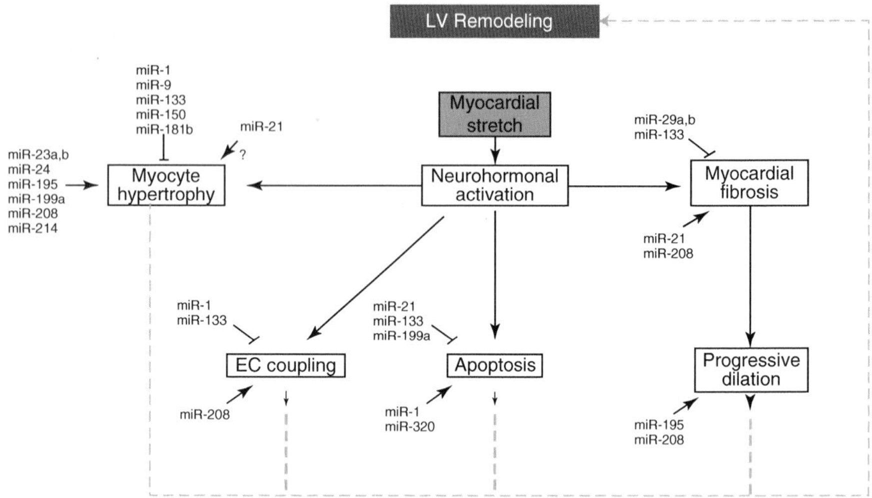

Fig. 6.2 The role of miRs in LV REM (Reproduced by Topkara and Mann [75]. Licence No 3727520931190)

Major players in cardiac structure and function are **micro-RNAs**. Very recently, Feng [24] signaled microRNA profiles in the development of cardiac hypertrophy [24]. They found that with transverse aortic constriction producing LVH, many microRNAs were up- and down-regulated. In the former group, they placed miR-331, 339b, 3557p, 221, 34c, while in the latter miR-194-451, 352, 98.

In the flow chart of Fig. 6.2, Topkara and Mann [74] outline the role of the suggested miRNAs in LV remodeling: more specifically, they regulate the gene expression, leading to "HF phenotype". Their role, though, is not causative but synergistic. Thus, miRNAs hold promise as biomarkers in disease progression as well as future therapeutic targets in HF management [74, 75].

Forms of Hypertrophy in Humans

Significant efforts have been dedicated in differentiating physiologic versus pathological hypertrophy in the human. Katholi and Couri point out that in the athlete, mostly representing physiologic LVH cardiac function, both systolic and diastolic is normal, while LV wall thickness is not greater than 12 mm, an increased wall thickness between 13 and 15 mm represents a grey area. Cardiovascular magnetic resonance imaging can be very helpful [65].

Pathological hypertrophy which subsequently leads to HF is characterized by a decrease in the utilization of fatty acids and the increase of glucose oxidation. However, this results into an energy depletion, resulting into a diminution of high energy phosphates. Thus, initially ATP levels are maintained while the energy

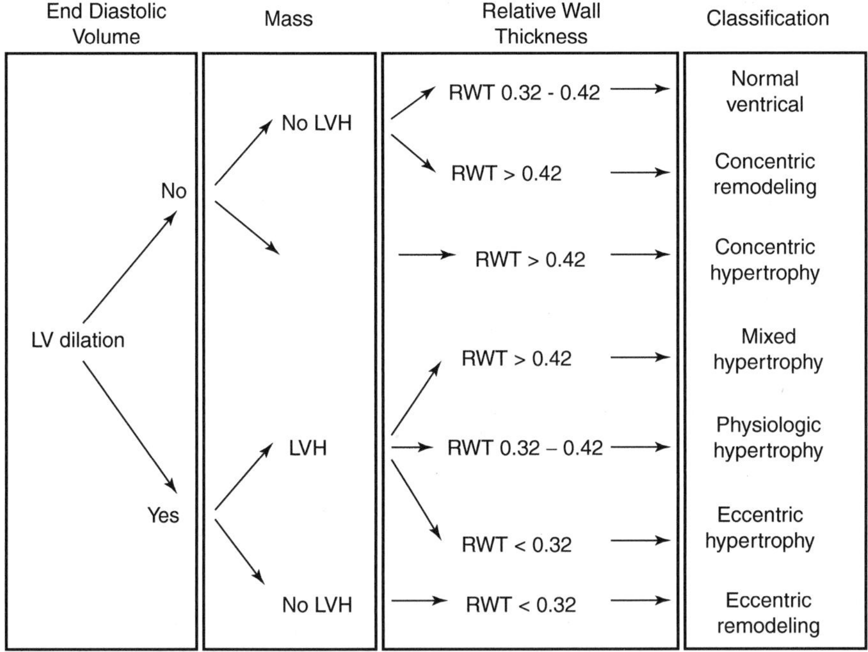

Fig. 6.3 Patterns of LV remodeling based on EDV, Wall Mass, and RWT (Reproduced by Gaasch and Zile [30]. Licence No 3727520332373)

reserve compound phosphocreatine is diminished; consequently, the PCr/ATP ratio is the first to be decreased [45, 59].

The patterns of LV remodeling based on EDV, Wall Mass, and RWT are reviewed by Gaash [30] and represented in Fig. 6.3. This LV remodeling pattern is determined by the type of overload: a systolic pressure overload is caused by concentric geometry/hypertrophy, whereas, a volume overload leads to eccentric geometry/hyper-trophy. The differential effects of pressure and volume overload biological mechanisms underlying such LV remodeling are prominent research targets [30].

The Impact of LVH and Its Regression

As already mentioned, LVH has a very adverse prognosis. Apart from the already measured techniques of assessing, the ECG and ECHO and to a much narrower scale CMR, plasma biomarkers have been used to determine prognosis [12]. Thus, Zile [86] found that the following markers predicted LVH [86]: MMP-7, MMP-9, TIMP-1, PiiiNP and NT-proBNP predicted LVH with an area under the curve (AVC) of 0.8, while MMP-2, TIMP-4, PiiiNP and the decreased MMP-8 predicted the presence of diastolic HF with an AUC of 0.79. The panel performed better than a single, N-proBNP alone and better than clinical co-variates alone. Many studies suggest that LVH regression is beneficial.

An important paper by the LIFE study showed that electrocardiographic LVH regression by the Cornell product and Sokolow-Lyon criteria was associated with a reduction of 14–17 % of cardiovascular death, non fatal myocardial infarction or stroke [61].

In a similar sub-study of the LIFE study, Devereux included 941 patients with initially ECG-diagnosed LVH followed for 4.8 years for cardiovascular events. They found that a lower-in- treatment LV mass index was associated with reduction of the composite events, HR 0.78, specifically cardiovascular mortality 0.62, stroke (HR 0.76), myocardial infarction (HR 0.85), and all cause mortality 0.72, independently of systolic blood pressure and assigned treatment [18].

The results of another group are interesting Verdecchia studied 880 initially untreated patients, followed for a median of 3.5 years. They found that the risk of celebrovascular events was 2.8 times higher in patients with no regression of development of new LVH [81].

Shillaci [68], reviewing many of the already reported studies, stress another point- that LVH regression induced by antihypertensive treatment decreases all major events such as stroke, myocardial infarctions, sudden cardiac death, cardiovascular death in general, atrial fibrillation, HF and importantly new-onset diabetes mellitus [61, 68].

Nadour and Biedeman review the importance of LVH regression. They stress that in most studies a poor correlation of blood pressure reduction and LV mass regression is found [57]. They believe that in most studies a poor correlation of blood pressure reduction and LV mass exists, and that a reduction of 15 % should be aimed at, in order to achieve the best improvement in prognosis..

How well can LVH regression be achieved? Interestingly, antihypertensive drugs have different effects on LVH regression. Dahlof [10] undertook an analysis of 109 treatment studies comprising 2357 patients. They found only modest results: 11.9 % reduction of LV mass in parallel to a reduction of mean arterial pressure of 14.9 %. They found that angiotensin converting enzyme inhibitor reduced LV mass by 15 %, β-blockers by 8 %, calcium antagonists by 8.5 %, and diuretics by 11.3 %. Interestingly, diuretics predominantly reduced cavity diameter, while the other drugs affected wall thickness [10] The results of the study of Dahlof showed that angiotensin converting enzyme inhibitors as compared to placebo achieved a 15 % LV mass regression against 8–11.3 % of all other drug families [10, 69].

Devereux in 2000 reviewed more recent clinical studies [13]. Valsartan was found to have a twice as large reduction of LV mass than atenolol at 8 months [73].

In a more recent study, Fereira [25] reviewed 694 manuscripts examining the relationship between anti-hypertensive drugs and cardiac hypertrophy regression. They mentioned that ACE inhibitor and Angiotensin receptor blockers achieved a 13 % LV mass regression, while beta-blockers and diuretics a 5–8 % reduction. They also noted that most studies showed that LVH regression is associated with a decrease in cardiovascular morbidity and mortality [25]. Some important more recent studies should be mentioned. In the 4E trial, E*plerenone* was as effective as

Enalarpil over 9 months, while combination of the two was superior [63]. According to Galzerano [32] *Telmisartan* reduced LV mass more than *Carvedilol* (11 % vs 9 %) [32]. Finally, in a more recent meta-analysis of 80 trials LV mass decreased by 13 % with ARBs, 10 % with ACEIs, 11 % with calcium antagonists, 8 % with diuretics and 6 % with beta-blockers [44, 51]. Mayet [51] found that regression of LVH after blood pressure decrease with *Ramipril* with addition of *Felodipine* and *Bendrofluazide* at 6 months improved midwall shortening to normal levels.

In the PRESERVE trial *Enalarpil* and *Nifedipine* had similar effects on LVH regression at 1 year [14]. In the LIFE study McKinsey and Kass address additional novel drug targets for LVH [54]. Their proposals are based on the already described mechanisms which induce pathological LVH. Thus, drug families discussed are the following:

- Rho kinase inhibition. Fasudil is such a drug.
- Statins have pleiotropic actions but clinical evidence is still scant although in patients treated for diastolic HF they showed a survival benefit [29].
- Rapamycin which is am mTOR inhibitor
- Anti-Akt therapy
- Antioxidant agents
- PDE5 inhibition
- Calcineurin inhibition
- Inhibition of Transient Receptor Potential (TRPC) channels which are mechanosensitive [50]
- Calmodulin dependent protein kinase inhibition
- Protein kinase C inhibition
- HDACs inhibition [76]

Hou and Kang [37] propose some more targets to effect regression of pathological cardiac hypertrophy [37]:

- Promotion of cardiovascular angiogenesis (stimulation of VEGFR-1).
- Activation of PKG-1 pathway, which inhibits hypertrophic growth
- Activation of the HIF-1 transcriptional activity. HIF-1 is critical for maturation of newly formed vessels.

In their aforementioned review Frey and Olsen [27] propose some additional targets:

- GP130/STAT 3 signaling (Gp130 is a receptor for several cytokines, which promote LVH) [78].
- Lipid metabolism modulation

Thus, they propose that peroxisome proliferator-activated receptor- agonists (PPARγ) namely pioglitazone can blunt pressure overload LVH in mice [4].

MMP/TNF inhibition

- CHAMP (cardiac helicase activated by MEF2 protein) activation [48]
- Na^+/H^+ exchanger inhibition, specifically cariporide.

Conclusions

From the above data one can make the following conclusions:

HTN is a major cause of HF. HF is the consequence of LVH. Hypertrophy induced by increased blood pressure is maladaptive and pathological. Thus, the co-existence of LVH in HTN is an adverse prognostic sign. Many and diverse signaling pathways are involved in the process towards LVH. A distinction is made between signaling pathways leading to physiological or pathological hypertrophy. Therapy by various drugs cause regression of H in different degrees. This regression is accompanied by better prognosis but is modest up to 11–12 %. Thus, additional and novel agents towards this goal are being continually introduced and tested.

References

1. Andersen DC, Ganesalingam S, Jensen CH, Sheikh SP. Do neonatal mouse hearts regenerate following heart apex resection? Stem Cell Rep. 2014;2:406–13.
2. Ang DS, Pringle SD, Struthers AD. The cardiovascular risk factor, left ventricular hypertrophy, is highly prevalent in stable, treated angina pectoris. Am J Hypertens. 2007;20:1029–35.
3. Arai M, Matsui H, Periasamy M. Sarcoplasmic reticulum gene expression in cardiac hypertrophy and heart failure. Circ Res. 1994;74:555–64.
4. Asakawa M, Takano H, Nagai T, Uozumi H, Hasegawa H, Kubota N, Saito T, Masuda Y, Kadowaki T, Komuro I. Peroxisome proliferator-activated receptor gamma plays a critical role in inhibition of cardiac hypertrophy in vitro and in vivo. Circulation. 2002;105:1240–6.
5. Bluemke DA, Kronmal RA, Lima JA, Liu K, Olson J, Burke GL, Folsom AR. The relationship of left ventricular mass and geometry to incident cardiovascular events: the MESA (Multi-Ethnic Study of Atherosclerosis) study. J Am Coll Cardiol. 2008;52:2148–55.
6. Braz JC, Gregory K, Pathak A, Zhao W, Sahin B, Klevitsky R, Kimball TF, Lorenz JN, Nairn AC, Liggett SB, Bodi I, Wang S, Schwartz A, Lakatta EG, Depaoli-Roach AA, Robbins J, Hewett TE, Bibb JA, Westfall MV, Kranias EG, Molkentin JD. PKC-alpha regulates cardiac contractility and propensity toward heart failure. Nat Med. 2004;10:248–54.
7. Bueno OF, DE Windt LJ, Tymitz KM, Witt SA, Kimball TR, Klevitsky R, Hewett TE, Jones SP, Lefer DJ, Peng CF, Kitsis RN, Molkentin JD. The MEK1-ERK1/2 signaling pathway promotes compensated cardiac hypertrophy in transgenic mice. Embo J. 2000;19:6341–50.
8. Butler J, Kalogeropoulos AP, Georgiopoulou VV, Bibbins-Domingo K, Najjar SS, Sutton-Tyrrell KC, Harris TB, Kritchevsky SB, Lloyd-Jones DM, Newman AB, Psaty BM. Systolic blood pressure and incident heart failure in the elderly. The cardiovascular health study and the health, ageing and body composition study. Heart. 2011;97:1304–11.
9. Cheng S, Claggett B, Correia AW, Shah AM, Gupta DK, Skali H, NI H, Rosamond WD, heiss G, Folsom AR, Coresh J, Solomon SD. Temporal trends in the population attributable risk for cardiovascular disease: the atherosclerosis risk in communities study. Circulation. 2014;130:820–8.
10. Dahlof B, Pennert K, Hansson L. Reversal of left ventricular hypertrophy in hypertensive patients. A metaanalysis of 109 treatment studies. Am J Hypertens. 1992;5:95–110.
11. Degoma EM, Knowles JW, Angeli F, Budoff MJ, Rader DJ. The evolution and refinement of traditional risk factors for cardiovascular disease. Cardiol Rev. 2012;20:118–29.
12. Desai CS, Ning H, Lloyd-Jones DM. Competing cardiovascular outcomes associated with electrocardiographic left ventricular hypertrophy: the atherosclerosis risk in communities study. Heart. 2012;98:330–4.

13. Devereux RB. Therapeutic options in minimizing left ventricular hypertrophy. Am Heart J. 2000;139:S9–14.
14. Devereux RB, Dahlof B, Levy D, Pfeffer MA. Comparison of enalapril versus nifedipine to decrease left ventricular hypertrophy in systemic hypertension (the PRESERVE trial). Am J Cardiol. 1996;78:61–5.
15. Devereux RB, Koren MJ, De Simone G, Okin PM, Kligfield P. Methods for detection of left ventricular hypertrophy: application to hypertensive heart disease. Eur Heart J. 1993;14(Suppl D):8–15.
16. Devereux RB, Okin PM, Roman MJ. Pre-clinical cardiovascular disease and surrogate endpoints in hypertension: does race influence target organ damage independent of blood pressure? Ethn Dis. 1998;8:138–48.
17. Devereux RB, Pickering TG, Harshfield GA, Kleinert HD, Denby L, Clark L, Pregibon D, Jason M, Kleiner B, Borer JS, Laragh JH. Left ventricular hypertrophy in patients with hypertension: importance of blood pressure response to regularly recurring stress. Circulation. 1983;68:470–6.
18. Devereux RB, Wachtell K, Gerdts E, Boman K, Nieminen MS, Papademetriou V, Rokkedal J, Harris K, Aurup P, Dahlof B. Prognostic significance of left ventricular mass change during treatment of hypertension. JAMA. 2004;292:2350–6.
19. Dorn 2nd GW, Robbins J, Ball N, Walsh RA. Myosin heavy chain regulation and myocyte contractile depression after LV hypertrophy in aortic-banded mice. Am J Physiol. 1994;267:H400–5.
20. Dorn 2nd GW, Robbins J, Sugden PH. Phenotyping hypertrophy: eschew obfuscation. Circ Res. 2003;92:1171–5.
21. Ducimetiere P, Richard JL. Cardiac insufficiency and left ventricular hypertrophy in the general population. In: Swynghedauw B, editor. Research in cardiac hypertrophy and future. John Libbey: Eurotext; 1990. pp. 3–8.
22. Dunlay SM, Weston SA, Jacobsen SJ, Roger VL. Risk factors for heart failure: a population-based case-control study. Am J Med. 2009;122:1023–8.
23. Fanelli C, Zatz R. Linking oxidative stress, the renin-angiotensin system, and hypertension. Hypertension. 2011;57:373–4.
24. Feng HJ, Ouyang W, Liu JH, Sun YG, Hu R, Huang LH, Xian JL, Jing CF, Zhou MJ. Global microRNA profiles and signaling pathways in the development of cardiac hypertrophy. Braz J Med Biol Res. 2014;47:361–8.
25. Ferreira Filho C, Abreu LC, Valenti VE, Ferreira M, Meneghini A, Silveira JA, Riera AR, Colombari E, Murad N, Santos-Silva PR, Silva LJ, Vanderlei LC, Carvalho TD, Ferreira C. Anti-hypertensive drugs have different effects on ventricular hypertrophy regression. Clinics (Sao Paulo). 2010;65:723–8.
26. Fraccarollo D, Widder JD, Galuppo P, Thum T, Tsikas D, Hoffmann M, Ruetten H, Ertl G, Bauersachs J. Improvement in left ventricular remodeling by the endothelial nitric oxide synthase enhancer AVE9488 after experimental myocardial infarction. Circulation. 2008;118:818–27.
27. Frey N, Olson EN. Cardiac hypertrophy: the good, the bad, and the ugly. Annu Rev Physiol. 2003;65:45–79.
28. Frohlich ED, Apstein C, Chobanian AV, Devereux RB, Dustan HP, DZAU V, Fauad-Tarazi F, Horan MJ, Marcus M, Massie B, et al. The heart in hypertension. N Engl J Med. 1992;327:998–1008.
29. Fukuta H, Sane DC, Brucks S, Little WC. Statin therapy may be associated with lower mortality in patients with diastolic heart failure: a preliminary report. Circulation. 2005;112:357–63.
30. Gaasch WH, Zile MR. Left ventricular structural remodeling in health and disease: with special emphasis on volume, mass, and geometry. J Am Coll Cardiol. 2011;58:1733–40.
31. Gallo P, Latronico MV, Gallo P, Grimaldi S, Borgia F, Todaro M, Jones P, Gallinari P, DE Francesco R, Ciliberto G, Steinkuhler C, Esposito G, Condorelli G. Inhibition of class I histone deacetylase with an apicidin derivative prevents cardiac hypertrophy and failure. Cardiovasc Res. 2008;80:416–24.

32. Galzerano D, Tammaro P, Del Viscovo L, Lama D, Galzerano A, Breglio R, Tuccillo B, Paolisso G, Capogrosso P. Three-dimensional echocardiographic and magnetic resonance assessment of the effect of telmisartan compared with carvedilol on left ventricular mass a multicenter, randomized, longitudinal study. Am J Hypertens. 2005;18:1563–9.
33. Giordano FJ, He H, Mcdonough P, Meyer M, Sayen MR, Dillmann WH. Adenovirus-mediated gene transfer reconstitutes depressed sarcoplasmic reticulum Ca2+-ATPase levels and shortens prolonged cardiac myocyte Ca2+ transients. Circulation. 1997;96:400–3.
34. Grossman W, Jones D, Mclauren L. Wall stress and patterns of hypertrophy in the human left ventricle. J Clin Invest. 1975;56:56–64.
35. Guo J, Mihic A, WU J, Zhang Y, Singh K, Dhingra S, Weisel RD, LI RK. Canopy 2 attenuates the transition from compensatory hypertrophy to dilated heart failure in hypertrophic cardiomyopathy. Eur Heart J. 2015;36:2530–40.
36. Higashikuni Y, Tanaka K, Kato M, Nureki O, Hirata Y, Nagai R, Komuro I, Sata M. Toll-like receptor-2 mediates adaptive cardiac hypertrophy in response to pressure overload through interleukin-1beta upregulation via nuclear factor kappaB activation. J Am Heart Assoc. 2013;2, e000267.
37. Hou J, Kang YJ. Regression of pathological cardiac hypertrophy: signaling pathways and therapeutic targets. Pharmacol Ther. 2012;135:337–54.
38. Humphrey JD, Dufresne ER, Schwartz MA. Mechanotransduction and extracellular matrix homeostasis. Nat Rev Mol Cell Biol. 2014;15:802–12.
39. Hunter JJ, Chien KR. Signaling pathways for cardiac hypertrophy and failure. N Engl J Med. 1999;341:1276–83.
40. Ito K, Yan X, Feng X, Manning WJ, Dillmann WH, Lorell BH. Transgenic expression of sarcoplasmic reticulum Ca(2+) atpase modifies the transition from hypertrophy to early heart failure. Circ Res. 2001;89:422–9.
41. Izumiya Y, Shiojima I, Sato K, Sawyer DB, Colucci WS, Walsh K. Vascular endothelial growth factor blockade promotes the transition from compensatory cardiac hypertrophy to failure in response to pressure overload. Hypertension. 2006;47:887–93.
42. Katholi RE, Couri DM. Left ventricular hypertrophy: major risk factor in patients with hypertension: update and practical clinical applications. Int J Hypertens. 2011;2011:495349.
43. Khatibzadeh S, Farzadfar F, Oliver J, Ezzati M, Moran A. Worldwide risk factors for heart failure: a systematic review and pooled analysis. Int J Cardiol. 2013;168:1186–94.
44. Klingbeil AU, Schneider M, Martus P, Messerli FH, Schmieder RE. A meta-analysis of the effects of treatment on left ventricular mass in essential hypertension. Am J Med. 2003;115:41–6.
45. Kolwicz Jr SC, Purohit S, Tian R. Cardiac metabolism and its interactions with contraction, growth, and survival of cardiomyocytes. Circ Res. 2013;113:603–16.
46. Komuro I, Kurabayashi M, Takaku F, Yazaki Y. Expression of cellular oncogenes in the myocardium during the developmental stage and pressure-overloaded hypertrophy of the rat heart. Circ Res. 1988;62:1075–9.
47. Liu Y, Jiang XL, Liu Y, Jiang DS, Zhang Y, Zhang R, Chen Y, Yang Q, Zhang XD, Fan GC, LI H. Toll-interacting protein (Tollip) negatively regulates pressure overload-induced ventricular hypertrophy in mice. Cardiovasc Res. 2014;101:87–96.
48. Liu ZP, Olson EN. Suppression of proliferation and cardiomyocyte hypertrophy by CHAMP, a cardiac-specific RNA helicase. Proc Natl Acad Sci U S A. 2002;99:2043–8.
49. Mann DL. Left ventricular size and shape: determinants of mechanical signal transduction pathways. Heart Fail Rev. 2005;10:95–100.
50. Maroto R, Raso A, Wood TG, Kurosky A, Martinac B, Hamill OP. TRPC1 forms the stretch-activated cation channel in vertebrate cells. Nat Cell Biol. 2005;7:179–85.
51. Mayet J, Ariff B, Wasan B, Chapman N, Shahi M, Poulter NR, Sever PS, Foale RA, Thom SA. Improvement in midwall myocardial shortening with regression of left ventricular hypertrophy. Hypertension. 2000;36:755–9.

52. Mazzolai L, Nussberger J, Aubert JF, Brunner DB, Gabbiani G, Brunner HR, Pedrazzini T. Blood pressure-independent cardiac hypertrophy induced by locally activated renin-angiotensin system. Hypertension. 1998;31:1324–30.
53. McClellan WM. Epidemiology and risk factors for chronic kidney disease. Med Clin North Am. 2005;89:419–45.
54. Mckinsey TA, Kass DA. Small-molecule therapies for cardiac hypertrophy: moving beneath the cell surface. Nat Rev Drug Discov. 2007;6:617–35.
55. Mellor KM, Curl CL, Chandramouli C, Pedrazzini T, Wendt IR, Delbridge LM. Ageing-related cardiomyocyte functional decline is sex and angiotensin II dependent. Age (Dordr). 2014;36:9630.
56. Michea L, Villagran A, Urzua A, Kuntsmann S, Venegas P, Carrasco L, Gonzalez M, Marusic ET. Mineralocorticoid receptor antagonism attenuates cardiac hypertrophy and prevents oxidative stress in uremic rats. Hypertension. 2008;52:295–300.
57. Nadour W, Biederman RW. Is left ventricular hypertrophy regression important? Does the tool used to detect it matter? J Clin Hypertens (Greenwich). 2009;11:441–7.
58. Nagayama T, Hsu S, Zhang M, Koitabashi N, Bedja D, Gabrielson KL, Takimoto E, Kass DA. Sildenafil stops progressive chamber, cellular, and molecular remodeling and improves calcium handling and function in hearts with pre-existing advanced hypertrophy caused by pressure overload. J Am Coll Cardiol. 2009;53:207–15.
59. Neubauer S. The failing heart—an engine out of fuel. N Engl J Med. 2007;356:1140–51.
60. Neubauer S, Krahe T, Schindler R, Horn M, Hillenbrand H, Entzeroth C, Mader H, Kromer EP, Riegger GA, Lackner K, et al. 31P magnetic resonance spectroscopy in dilated cardiomyopathy and coronary artery disease. Altered cardiac high-energy phosphate metabolism in heart failure. Circulation. 1992;86:1810–8.
61. Okin PM, Devereux RB, Jern S, Kjeldsen SE, Julius S, Nieminen MS, Snapinn S, Harris KE, Aurup P, Edelman JM, Wedel H, Lindholm LH, Dahlof B. Regression of electrocardiographic left ventricular hypertrophy during antihypertensive treatment and the prediction of major cardiovascular events. JAMA. 2004;292:2343–9.
62. Pandya K, Kim HS, Smithies O. Fibrosis, not cell size, delineates beta-myosin heavy chain reexpression during cardiac hypertrophy and normal aging in vivo. Proc Natl Acad Sci U S A. 2006;103:16864–9.
63. Pelliccia F, Patti G, Rosano G, Greco C, Gaudio C. Efficacy and safety of eplerenone in the management of mild to moderate arterial hypertension: systematic review and meta-analysis. Int J Cardiol. 2014;177:219–28.
64. Prabhu SD. Nitric oxide protects against pathological ventricular remodeling: reconsideration of the role of NO in the failing heart. Circ Res. 2004;94:1155–7.
65. Puntmann VO, Jahnke C, Gebker R, Schnackenburg B, Fox KF, Fleck E, Paetsch I. Usefulness of magnetic resonance imaging to distinguish hypertensive and hypertrophic cardiomyopathy. Am J Cardiol. 2010;106:1016–22.
66. Retailleau K, Duprat F. Polycystins and partners: proposed role in mechanosensitivity. J Physiol. 2014;592:2453–71.
67. Roger VL. The heart failure epidemic. Int J Environ Res Public Health. 2010;7:1807–30.
68. Schillaci G, Pirro M, Mannarino E. Left ventricular hypertrophy reversal and prevention of diabetes: two birds with one stone? Hypertension. 2007;50:851–3.
69. Schmieder RE, Martus P, Klingbeil A. Reversal of left ventricular hypertrophy in essential hypertension. A meta-analysis of randomized double-blind studies. JAMA. 1996;275:1507–13.
70. Swynghedauw B. Molecular mechanisms of myocardial remodeling. Physiol Rev. 1999;79:215–62.
71. Takimoto E, Kass DA. Role of oxidative stress in cardiac hypertrophy and remodeling. Hypertension. 2007;49:241–8.
72. Tardiff JC. Cardiac hypertrophy: stressing out the heart. J Clin Invest. 2006;116:1467–70.

73. Thurmann PA, Kenedi P, Schmidt A, Harder S, Rietbrock N. Influence of the angiotensin II antagonist valsartan on left ventricular hypertrophy in patients with essential hypertension. Circulation. 1998;98:2037–42.
74. Topkara VK, Mann DL. Clinical applications of miRNAs in cardiac remodeling and heart failure. Per Med. 2010;7:531–48.
75. Topkara VK, Mann DL. Role of microRNAs in cardiac remodeling and heart failure. Cardiovasc Drugs Ther. 2011;25:171–82.
76. Trivedi CM, Luo Y, Yin Z, Zhang M, Zhu W, Wang T, Floss T, Goettlicher M, Noppinger PR, Wurst W, Ferrari VA, Abrams CS, Gruber PJ, Epstein JA. Hdac2 regulates the cardiac hypertrophic response by modulating Gsk3 beta activity. Nat Med. 2007;13:324–31.
77. Ulasova E, Perez J, Hill BG, Bradley WE, Garber DW, Landar A, Barnes S, Prasain J, Parks DA, Dell'Italia LJ, Darley-Usmar VM. Quercetin prevents left ventricular hypertrophy in the Apo E knockout mouse. Redox Biol. 2013;1:381–6.
78. Uozumi H, Hiroi Y, Zou Y, Takimoto E, Toko H, Niu P, Shimoyama M, Yazaki Y, Nagai R, Komuro I. gp130 plays a critical role in pressure overload-induced cardiac hypertrophy. J Biol Chem. 2001;276:23115–9.
79. Van Berlo JH, Maillet M, Molkentin JD. Signaling effectors underlying pathologic growth and remodeling of the heart. J Clin Invest. 2013;123:37–45.
80. Van Bilsen M, Van Nieuwenhoven FA, Van Der Vusse GJ. Metabolic remodelling of the failing heart: beneficial or detrimental? Cardiovasc Res. 2009;81:420–8.
81. Verdecchia P, Angeli F, Gattobigio R, Sardone M, Pede S, Reboldi GP. Regression of left ventricular hypertrophy and prevention of stroke in hypertensive subjects. Am J Hypertens. 2006;19:493–9.
82. Vogel MW, Slusser JP, Hodge DO, Chen HH. The natural history of preclinical diastolic dysfunction: a population-based study. Circ Heart Fail. 2012;5:144–51.
83. Wang Y, Huang S, Sah VP, Ross Jr J, Brown JH, Han J, Chien KR. Cardiac muscle cell hypertrophy and apoptosis induced by distinct members of the p38 mitogen-activated protein kinase family. J Biol Chem. 1998;273:2161–8.
84. Westermann D, Becher PM, Lindner D, Savvatis K, Xia Y, Frohlich M, Hoffmann S, Schultheiss HP, Tschope C. Selective PDE5A inhibition with sildenafil rescues left ventricular dysfunction, inflammatory immune response and cardiac remodeling in angiotensin II-induced heart failure in vivo. Basic Res Cardiol. 2012;107:308.
85. Zhang CL, Mckinsey TA, Chang S, Antos CL, Hill JA, Olson EN. Class II histone deacetylases act as signal-responsive repressors of cardiac hypertrophy. Cell. 2002;110:479–88.
86. Zile MR, Desantis SM, Baicu CF, Stroud RE, Thompson SB, Mcclure CD, Mehurg SM, Spinale FG. Plasma biomarkers that reflect determinants of matrix composition identify the presence of left ventricular hypertrophy and diastolic heart failure. Circ Heart Fail. 2011;4(3):246–56.

Chapter 7
Systemic Hemodynamics in Hypertension

Paolo Palatini

Introduction

Several lines of research have documented an association between increased sympathetic nervous system activity and hypertension in the young. A widespread autonomic nervous system abnormality, clinically manifested as a hyperkinetic circulation characterized by elevations in heart rate, cardiac output, and plasma norepinephrine levels has been repeatedly demonstrated in the early phases of hypertension [1–6]. The co-distribution of blood pressure and cardiac index was investigated in two large Michigan populations using the mixture analysis method [7]. Distinct subgroups of individuals with elevated blood pressure and cardiac index were identified in both populations, with a prevalence of 17–24 %. Among the subjects in Tecumseh, Michigan, with borderline hypertension (mean age 32 years), 37 % showed a hyperdynamic circulation and other signs of sympathetic overactivity [4]. Sympathetic overactivity may be detected many years before the blood pressure increases to hypertensive levels suggesting that sympathetic activation is a primary event and not a mere consequence of some other aberration [4]. Plasma norepinephrine and epinephrine levels, as well as norepinephrine turnover and platelet norepinephrine content, are elevated in hypertensive subjects [8, 9]. Excessive sympathetic activity in hypertensives has been demonstrated also using spectral analysis of heart rate variability. About 30 % of the young subjects from the Tecumseh Offspring Study had sympathetic predominance at spectral analysis of heart rate variability [10]. In a sample of young adults with stage 1 hypertension from the HARVEST Study, over one third of subjects had sympathetic

P. Palatini, M.D. (✉)
Department of Medicine, University of Padova, Padova, Italy

Vascular Medicine, DIMED, University of Padova, via Giustiniani, 2, Padova 35128, Italy
e-mail: palatini@ux1.unipd.it

E.A. Andreadis (ed.), *Hypertension and Cardiovascular Disease*,
DOI 10.1007/978-3-319-39599-9_7

predominance and reduced heart rate variability [11]. During a 6-year follow-up, subjects with sympathetic predominance developed sustained hypertension requiring antihypertensive treatment three times more frequently than subjects with normal autonomic tone. In addition, at the end of follow-up subjects with sympathetic predominance showed an increase in total cholesterol and body weight and an impairment of large artery compliance. According to some investigators, even normotensive individuals with a positive family history of hypertension may have an increased ratio of sympathetic to parasympathetic activity at the cardiac level [12]. An abnormal autonomic cardiac regulation has been found to be present also in subjects with white-coat hypertension [13, 14]. Fagard et al. found a low-frequency to high-frequency ratio of 1.11 in a group of white-coat hypertensives that was significantly higher than in a group of normotensive subjects of control (0.81) [14]. The impact of enhanced sympathetic activity in hypertension has been confirmed by studies performed with microneurographic assessment of sympathetic nerve traffic to skeletal muscle. A marked increase in muscle sympathetic nervous activity was found in subjects with both borderline and established hypertension [8, 15]. In addition, a number of prospective studies have shown that increased cardiovascular reactivity to stressful stimuli is predictive of future hypertension and that it may contribute to the development of cardiovascular disease [16, 17]. Japanese investigators [18] have shown that increases in baseline plasma norepinephrine are predictive of future blood pressure elevation in normotensive or borderline hypertensive subjects. Julius et al. demonstrated that both sympathetic and parasympathetic blockade were needed to normalize cardiac output in borderline hypertension and that enhanced sympathetic activity was associated with decreased parasympathetic cardiac activity [2]. The above findings strongly suggest that the stimuli for the altered hemodynamic state in the early stage of hypertension emanate from the medulla oblongata, where sympathetic and parasympathetic activities are integrated in a reciprocal fashion. In conclusion, the data from the literature indicate that sympathetic predominance starts early in life and is present in a sizable portion of the hypertensive population. Exaggerated sympathetic activity in hypertension has detrimental effects on target organs and may favor the development of cardiovascular complications. In fact, in addition to its effect on blood pressure, alteration of autonomic nervous system activity may lead to an increase in other cardiovascular risk factors, producing tachycardia, lipid abnormalities, insulin resistance and obesity [19] (Fig. 7.1).

Systemic Hemodynamics in Hypertension

The sympathetic predominance present in the early stage of hypertension has important influences on systemic hemodynamics. Studies in hypertensive subjects have demonstrated elevated resting cardiac output with normal total peripheral resistance in young, mildly hypertensive individuals [1, 4, 7–9]. However, this hemodynamic picture tends to change with aging. Low levels of cardiac output

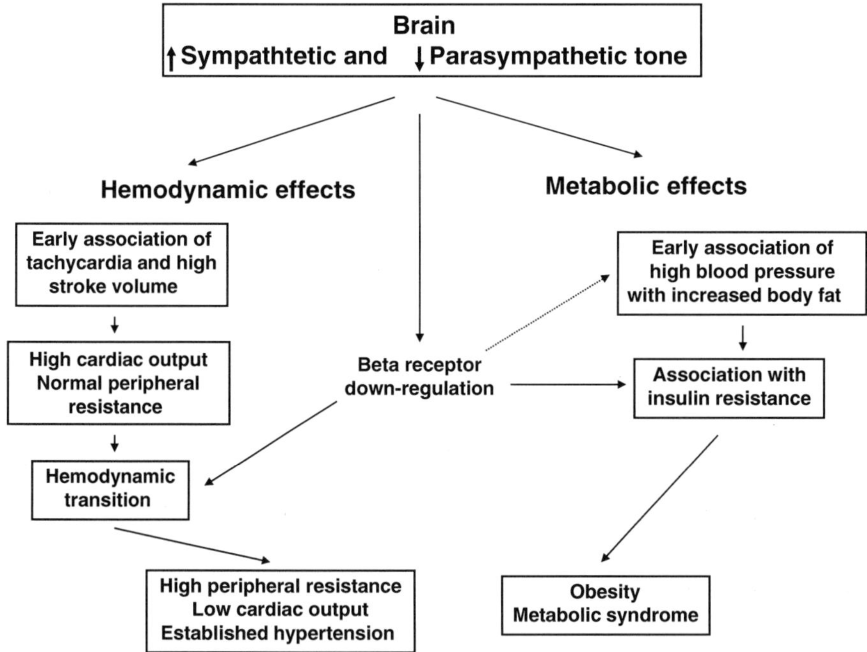

Fig. 7.1 The sketch illustrates the mechanisms through which increased sympathetic tone and reduced vagal activity lead to changes in hemodynamic and metabolic variables in hypertension. Beta-receptor down-regulation is a key factor in the process that leads to the hemodynamic transition from a high cardiac output-normal peripheral resistance to a normal cardiac output-high peripheral resistance state and favors the development of obesity and metabolic abnormalities

and high peripheral resistance have been reported in older and more severely hypertensive individuals [20–22]. When overt left ventricular hypertrophy develops in the course of hypertension, left ventricular ejection fraction starts to decline and coronary flow reserve is significantly depressed [21]. This, together with the prevalent evidence of resting and stress-induced ischemia, indicates that myocardial ischemia unrelated to coronary atherosclerosis can occur in patients with severe hypertension and left ventricular hypertrophy. Data from available longitudinal studies [4, 20, 23] suggest that progression from mild to moderate to severe hypertension is paralleled by evolution of the hemodynamic profile. From the increased cardiac index with normal peripheral resistance state present in the early stage the hemodynamic picture progressively changes to a normal or even reduced cardiac index with increased resistance state (Fig. 7.1). Pioneer studies by S Julius and P Lund-Johansen have shown that sympathetic overactivity is associated with high cardiac output and rapid heart rate early in the course of hypertension, but later cardiac output decreases and vascular resistance increases due to a downregulation of adrenoreceptors [4, 20, 23]. However, at variance with the above data some authors using echocardiographic measurement, did not find an evolution of cardiac output and peripheral resistance with aging [24]. The hemodynamic transition from a phase of high cardiac output to a high-resistance phase of hypertension has been actually documented by Lund-Johansen in his unique long-term longitudinal hemodynamic study [20]. The mechanism of this hemodynamic transition has been explained by Julius through a series of pathogenetic studies. Cardiac output returns from elevated to normal values as beta-adrenergic receptors are downregulated and stroke volume decreases because of decreased left ventricular compliance [25, 26]. The high blood pressure induces vascular hypertrophy, which in turn leads to increased vascular resistance at baseline and excessive vascular reactivity to vasoconstrictor stimuli. Paralleling the hemodynamic transition is a resetting of the sympathetic tone in the course of hypertension [27]. According to Julius, the mechanism of the change of sympathetic tone from elevated in borderline hypertension to apparently normal in established hypertension can be explained within the conceptual framework of the "BP-seeking" properties of the brain [21]. In the initial phases of hypertension, the central nervous system seeks to maintain systemic blood pressure at a high level. As hypertension advances and vascular hypertrophy develops, arterioles become hyperresponsive to vasoconstrictor stimuli. At this point, less sympathetic drive is needed to maintain pressure-elevating vasoconstriction, and the central sympathetic drive is downregulated. Sympathetic stimulation may directly promote the development of left ventricular hypertrophy and large-artery stiffness. The effect of sympathetic activity on the heart was shown by Julius et al. [28] in a dog model in which repeated episodes of increased blood pressure and norepinephrine levels failed to induce permanent hypertension but caused left ventricular hypertrophy. An association of cardiac hypertrophy with increased plasma catecholamine values has also been described in human studies [29]. This relationship was found only in men, which can explain why sympathetic overactivity is more deleterious in men than in women. As mentioned above, in the HARVEST study, hypertensive participants with sympathetic predominance exhibited impaired large-artery distensibility indices when compared with those with normal autonomic nervous system activity in spite of their young age [11]. These results are consistent with a previous report that showed an association between enhanced sympathetic activity, white-coat effect, and reduced arterial distensibility in a group of 50-year-old patients with hypertension [30]. The HARVEST Study extended those observations by showing that the detrimental effect of sympathetic activity on large-vessel distensibility also occurs in early life [11]. Longitudinal studies have demonstrated that plasma norepinephrine concentrations predict both future blood pressure elevation and weight gain in lean normotensives [18, 31], indicating that sympathetic overactivity may be the linchpin connecting future blood pressure elevation and increase in body weight. Japanese investigators followed a cohort of healthy individuals for up to 10 years and found that those whose blood pressure and body weight increased with time initially had elevated heart rate and plasma norepinephrine values [18]. In our laboratory, we have shown decreased beta-adrenergic responsiveness to infusion of beta agonists in hypertension and have speculated that this downregulation may play a role in weight gain during the long term [26, 31].

Structural and Functional Cardiac Changes in Hypertension

Although reduced cardiac output and dysfunction of left ventricular chamber occur commonly in hypertension, it is not clear at what stage of the disease these changes develop. It is known that left ventricular structure and function at rest are normal or even supernormal in the early stage of hypertension [32, 33]. However, initial abnormalities of left ventricular function can be detected during strenuous exercise [34, 35]. Exercise hemodynamics during traditional ergometric tests do not generally differ between young normotensive and stage 1 hypertensive subjects. However, a lower efficiency of the left ventricle in young hypertensive subjects without cardiac abnormalities has been found during long lasting exercise [36]. In our laboratory we compared intraarterial blood pressure changes during a long-distance run with those during traditional bicycle ergometry in a group of normotensive and a group of hypertensive joggers by means of ambulatory intra-arterial monitoring [37]. In both groups the traditional ergometric test to exhaustion caused parallel changes in systolic and diastolic blood pressure. A different blood pressure pattern was observed during long distance track running. In all individuals a sharp rise in systolic blood pressure reaching maximum values 2–4 min after the start was recorded followed by a progressive decline throughout the run and an increase only during a final sprint. A poor relationship was observed between the blood pressure values at peak exercise and baseline levels as the normotensives showed a significantly higher blood pressure response than the hypertensives. These results showed that the blood pressure increase with strenuous effort is reduced in hypertensive individuals, probably because of latent impairment of cardiac performance.

To investigate whether the abnormal blood pressure trend observed in hypertensive subjects during prolonged exercise is actually due to impaired left ventricular function, in a later experiment we measured left ventricular function by means of M-mode echocardiography during prolonged in-door exercise (1 h) performed in the semi-recumbent position in 13 physically trained, young, mild hypertensives and 12 trained normotensives with similar working capacity [36]. Blood pressure changes during the first 20 min of exercise were similar in the two groups, but thereafter the between-group blood pressure difference tended to decline progressively in keeping with the results previously obtained during long-distance running, and after 1 h the difference between the two groups was no longer significant. Two parameters of left ventricular systolic performance, systolic blood pressure/end-systolic volume (ESV) and end-systolic stress/ESV at rest were greater in the hypertensives ($P<0.0001$ and $P=0.034$), while left ventricular diastoling filling was impaired ($p=0.05$). Left ventricular ejection fraction ($P=0.018$), systolic blood pressure/ESV ($P<0.0001$) and stress/ESV ($P=0.027$) remained greater in the hypertensives than the normotensives throughout the test documenting the existence of an increased ejective performance in the former. Indexes of ejective performance in the hypertensives were greater also when normalized for left ventricular wall thickness. Stroke volume increased to a lower extent in the hypertensives, even though the between-group difference was not statistically significant. These data indicate that left ventricular ejective performance is increased in the early stage of hypertension not only at rest but also during vigorous exercise. However, in spite of increased pump function the hypertensive subjects were unable to increase their blood pressure to the same extent as the normotensives during strenuous exercise. This suggests that left ventricular contractility may be impaired in the early stage of hypertension. Indeed, whether the myocardium preserves a normal contractile performance in arterial hypertension has been a matter of dispute. In agreement with our previous results, some investigators [32, 38–40] who used endocardial indexes to measure left ventricular systolic function found increased ejective systolic performance in subjects with hypertension. However, it should be born in mind that left ventricular contractility may be overestimated by the measurement of fractional shortening at the endocardium [41]. Using midwall fractional shortening to evaluate left ventricular performance, some investigators demonstrated that in hypertensive subjects left ventricular contractility was actually depressed [42, 43] (Fig. 7.2). This suggests that supranormal left ventricular performance found by earlier studies in hypertensive subjects [38–40] was an artefact due to estimation of left ventricular muscle shortening from the motion of the endocardial surface. Data by Palmon et al. [44] obtained in subjects with left ventricular concentric remodelling demonstrated that circumferential myocardial shortening is uniformly reduced across the left ventricular wall and that ejective performance may be normal in the presence of depressed myocardial contractility. At variance with those results, some authors found enhanced left ventricular systolic function in young subjects with mild hypertension when it was assessed either at the endocardium or the midwall [45].

Several studies have shown that in mild to moderate hypertensive patients left ventricular chamber performance is usually preserved at rest, but may be abnormal when evaluated during exercise [46–48]. Thus, in a further experiment using the same ergometric protocol as described above we measured left ventricular fractional

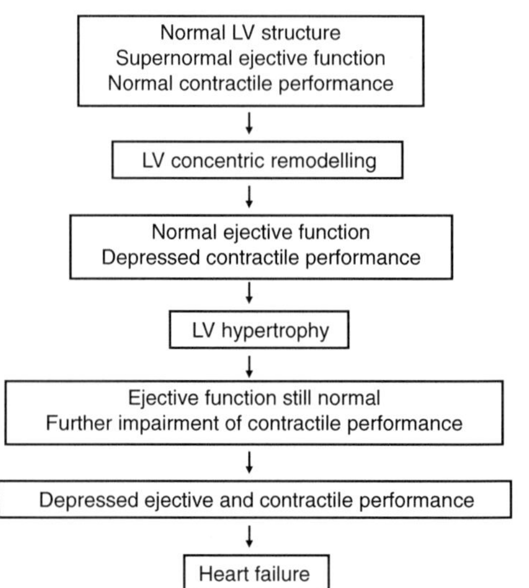

Fig. 7.2 Evolution of structural and functional left ventricular (*LV*) characteristics in hypertension. In the early stage of hypertension LV ejective function is often supernormal with a normal LV contractility. Structural adaptations of the LV walls can preserve a normal cardiac output for long but they eventually lead to depressed LV contractility with ominous consequences for the left ventricle

shortening both at the endocardium and at the midwall during long-lasting exercise in a group of young hypertensive subjects and a group of normotensive controls [49]. In agreement with our previous results [36] we found increased indexes of left ventricular ejective performance in the hypertensives during exercise. Indeed, the hypertensives increased their stroke volume and cardiac output adequately during bicycle ergometry through an increase in left ventricular ejective performance. A new finding of this study was that in the hypertensive subjects the endocardial fractional shortening, predicted on the basis of the shortening/stress relationship in the normotensive controls, overestimated midwall fractional shortening throughout rest ($P = 0.04$) and exercise ($P = 0.004$). In addition, among the hypertensive subjects we could identify two different subgroups, one with left ventricular geometry similar to that of the normotensive controls and one with increased relative wall thickness. Thickening of the left ventricular wall allowed the subjects of the latter group to increase their ejective performance adequately during highly demanding effort. However, left ventricular concentric remodelling is the key factor in the process that leads to impaired left ventricular contractility. De Simone et al. [43] using midwall fractional shortening/meridional end-systolic stress relation in a population of 474 hypertensive subjects identified a subgroup of patients with abnormal left ventricular myocardial function who had concentric left ventricular hypertrophy. In a population of 635 mild hypertensives we found that relative wall thickness was the strongest predictor of the difference between left ventricular performance measured at midwall and at the endocardium and that subjects with left ventricular remodelling had a depressed left ventricular contractility [50]. Thus, even though left ventricular wall hypertrophy appears as a valid compensatory mechanism to increase pump function both at rest and during exercise, it is likely that in the long run this mechanism leads to left ventricular contractile dysfunction.

This issue was further explored within the frame of the HARVEST study in young to middle age subjects with stage 1 hypertension [51]. In 722 participants we evaluated whether and how frequently left ventricular systolic performance was depressed by examining the relation between impairment in left ventricular performance measured at the endocardium (ejective function) and myocardial function assessed at the midwall (contractile function). This analysis confirmed that myocardial contractility may often be depressed in young patients with borderline to mild hypertension. In fact, 8.9 % of our subjects had an abnormal midwall fractional shortening-stress relation. Left ventricular ejective performance was abnormal less often because the endocardial fractional shortening-stress relation was depressed in 5.7 % of the subjects. The group of patients with decreased left ventricular contractility exhibited cardiac structural and hemodynamic features associated with increased cardiovascular risk, including increased ventricular septum, posterior wall, and relative wall thicknesses, impaired diastolic filling, and reduced stroke volume and cardiac output. However, among the subjects with depressed left ventricular contractility, 55 % had lower than normal ejective performance, whereas the other 45 % had an ejective function still within the normal range. The latter group had greater wall thickness than the former and a clearer tendency to left ventricular concentric remodelling. Patients with increased relative wall thickness are known to have abnormal systolic pump performance, characterized by low stroke volume and low cardiac output [52]. To prevent an excessive decrease in stroke volume, these subjects have to empty their ventricles more completely at end-systole to compensate for the lower diastolic volume. In our group with depressed contractility and normal ejective performance this could be achieved thanks to an augmented sympathetic activity, as documented by a 50 % increase in the level of urinary norepinephrine. Signs of increased sympathetic activity have been reported also by Lehman and Keul [53] in subjects with established hypertension and initial left ventricular dysfunction and by Yasuda et al. [54] in hypertensive subjects with left ventricular hypertrophy, which contributed to maintaining left ventricular systolic function within the normal range. However, sympathetic overactivity also favors the left ventricular hypertrophic process, starting a vicious cycle with deleterious effects on the left ventricular chamber structure and function which in the long run may lead to left ventricular failure. Indeed, in a 7-year follow-up of the HARVEST participants we found that the discrepancy between the ejective and contractile left ventricular performance was a significant predictor of worsening of the hypertensive condition [55]. This series of studies allowed us to conclude that increased left ventricular ejective performance on a background of depressed left ventricular contractility can temporarily preserve cardiac output but leads to an unfavorable structural left ventricular pattern with ominous consequences for the left ventricle. Detection of depressed left ventricular contractility at echocardiography irrespective of whether left ventricular endocardial performance is normal should prompt early antihypertensive treatment in stage 1 hypertension. Attention should be focused especially on subjects with autonomic nervous system abnormalities, clinically manifested as a hyperkinetic circulation characterized by elevations in heart rate, blood pressure, catecholamine levels and cardiac output, a condition that has been repeatedly demonstrated in hypertension of the young [56, 57]. Physical training, through its favorable modulation of the autonomic nervous system activity should be particularly beneficial in this clinical setting [58, 59].

Pathogenetic Mechanisms

The above data stress the importance of the increase in left ventricular wall thickness and of left ventricular concentric remodelling in the process that leads to left ventricular systolic dysfunction in hypertension. Several determinants of left ventricular mass have been identified, including growth factors such as catecholamines, insulin, the renin-angiotensin-aldosterone system, sodium intake etc [10, 29, 60]. However, studies within populations have variously demonstrated positive, absent or even negative associations between left ventricular mass and these putative factors [10, 29, 60]. A relationship between sympathetic stimulation and cardiac hypertrophy has been shown in several experimental studies [10]. The growth of cultured embryonal cardiac cells is stimulated by norepinephrine through an alpha-effect [61, 62]. As mentioned above, in animal models, repeated pressor episodes coupled to norepinephrine increase determined left ventricular hypertrophy without causing chronic hypertension [28]. Theoretically, the interrelationship between sympathetic activity and the renin-angiotensin system can reinforce the tendency to develop left ventricular hypertrophy as both norepinephrine and angiotensin are known to have trophic properties [62]. A direct association between markers of sympathetic activity and left ventricular hypertrophy has been demonstrated in some studies. A study in 111 adolescents and young adults from the Tecumseh Offspring Study can help clarify this controversial point [10] (Fig. 7.3). Among these subjects we could identify two different groups according to the low frequency and the high frequency components of heart rate variability, which are well known markers of the autonomic tone balance. Thirty-eight subjects showed signs of sympathetic overactivity, and had higher heart rate, blood pressure, waist/hip ratio, and cholesterol than the rest of the group. In the subjects with sympathetic overactivity, insulin emerged as the strongest univariate correlate of interventricular septum and posterior wall thicknesses, and of left ventricular mass. Cholesterol and triglycerides were other correlates of echocardiographic variables. On the contrary, the marginal univariate relationship with diastolic blood pressure did not remain significant in multivariate analysis. In the subjects with normal sympathetic activity, blood pressure was strongly correlated with left ventricular wall thicknesses and mass both in univariate and multivariate analyses while insulin and lipids were not. The interactive effect of sympathetic activity and insulin on echocardiographic data was confirmed when the multivariate analyses were performed in all subjects taken together. In this analysis, markers of sympathetic activity alone did not show an independent association with left ventricular size and structure. However, when the interaction term between sympathetic activity and insulin was incorporated in the model this term was a potent explanatory variable of echocardiographic data. These results show that higher insulin against a background of increased sympathetic activity is a major determinant of the left ventricular wall growth and remodelling during adolescence. In contrast, in subjects with normal autonomic tone and no metabolic abnormalities the main determinant of left ventricular wall thickness and mass is the hemodynamic load while insulin has only a negligible effect. In summary, these data

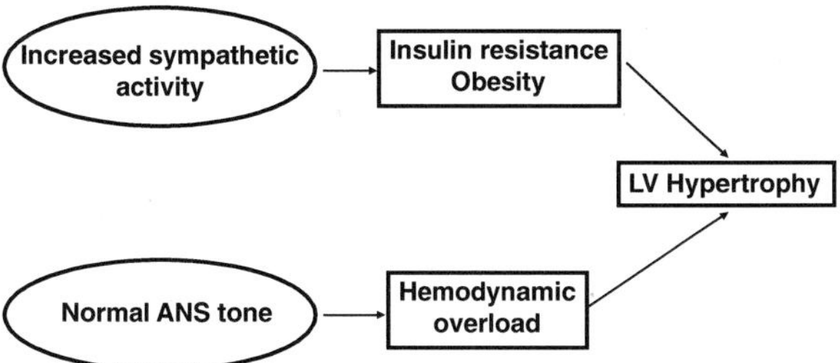

Fig. 7.3 Factors promoting left ventricular hypertrophy in hypertension. In patients with sympathetic predominance obesity and insulin resistance play a major role whereas in subjects with normal autonomic nervous system tone the hemodynamic load is the main determinant of the left ventricular wall growth. LV indicates left ventricular

indicate that in subjects with an elevated sympathetic tone insulin and the degree of overweight contribute to left ventricular structure whereas in subjects with normal sympathetic tone the hemodynamic factors are major contributors (Fig. 7.3). A practical consequence of these findings is that metabolic disturbances in hypertension can increase the overall cardiovascular risk also by favoring the development of left ventricular hypertrophy.

Effect of Regular Exercise Training on Cardiac Structure in Hypertension

Regular endurance exercise causes a reduction of the sympathetic tone and an increase of vagal activity with beneficial effects on heart rate, blood pressure and other components of the metabolic syndrome [63, 64] (Fig. 7.4). In addition, aerobic fitness has been found to be associated with reduction in cardiovascular responsiveness to psychophysiological stressors [65]. A reduction of blood pressure reactivity to stressors has been described in physically active individuals [66], which may be involved with the blood pressure lowering effect of regular exercise. In a homogeneous cohort of young to middle age subjects screened for stage 1 hypertension, we demonstrated that subjects who performed regular physical activity had a smaller blood pressure and heart rate reaction to public speaking and a lower risk of developing hypertension than sedentary subjects [67]. The reason why regular aerobic exercise decreases reactivity to stressors is unclear. Similarities between central and peripheral cardiovascular responses to exercise and psychosocial stressors have lead to the theory of 'cross-stressor adaptation'. According to this view, adaptations to repeated bouts of exercise can lead also to adaptations to daily life stressors [59]. Though not all studies have been positive, regular physical activity can result in

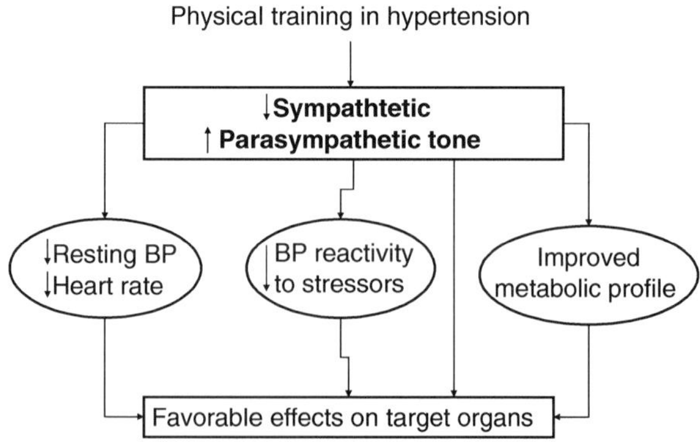

Fig. 7.4 Effects of regular physical activity in hypertension. Through modulation of sympathetic and vagal activity physical training improves the hemodynamic and metabolic profile of the hypertensive patient with favorable consequences on cardiac and vascular structure and function

decreased cardiac-sympathetic drive, in part by enhancing baroreceptor sensitivity [68]. A study of untreated hypertensive patients demonstrated that even a short period of moderate intensity aerobic exercise training significantly reduced muscle sympathetic discharge in subjects with increased central sympathetic activation and increased arterial baroreflex regulation [69]. Central autonomic adaptations in response to exercise would thus be responsible for the reduced blood pressure responsiveness to psychological stress and might also represent a mechanistic pathway for the decreased tendency to develop hypertension in physically active subjects [17]. Insulin resistance in hypertension is frequently associated with activation of the sympathetic nervous system [70] and improved insulin sensitivity has been observed after exercise training [71]. Elevated sympathetic activity has been associated with increases in arterial wall thickening and left ventricular mass [72]. Thus, to retard or even prevent hypertensive complications, atherosclerosis and cardiovascular morbidity, in young hypertensive subjects with signs of sympathetic predominance and/or increased reactivity to stressors a program of physical activity may be beneficial. The favorable effects of regular physical activity on the heart have been demonstrated by several studies [73, 74]. In the HARVEST study [75], during a median follow-up of 8.3 years, 10.3 % of the sedentary subjects and only 1.7 % of the active subjects developed left ventricular hypertrophy ($P<0.001$). In a logistic regression, after controlling for sex, age, family history for hypertension, hypertension duration, body mass, blood pressure, baseline left ventricular mass, lifestyle factors, and follow-up length, the odds ratio of left ventricular hypertrophy for the active subjects was 0.24 (95 % CI, 0.07–0.85). Exercise-related beneficial effects in the same cohort have been found also for arterial elasticity [76] and carotid intima-media thickness [77].

Isolated Systolic Hypertension of the Young

Isolated systolic hypertension is the dominant form of hypertension after the sixth decade of life [78–80]. In the elderly, high pulse pressure is related to progression of large artery atherosclerosis and the consequent loss of distensibility [80]. The mechanisms underlying elevated pulse pressure in younger age groups are not well known and the clinical significance of isolated systolic hypertension in young and middle-age subjects is still controversial. Traditionally, systolic hypertension in the young has been considered as the result of increased cardiac output and hyperkinetic circulation [81, 82]. However, in the Enigma study [83], systolic hypertension appeared to result from both increased cardiac output and large artery stiffness, suggesting that systolic hypertension in young individuals may not be innocuous. According to some studies [84], young people with systolic hypertension have initial target organ damage but according to others [81, 82] systolic hypertension of the young is the mere consequence of exaggerated pulse pressure amplification from the aorta to the brachial artery and has been considered as spurious hypertension. In an analysis of the HARVEST study, we observed that in subjects with systolic hypertension at enrollment, the risk of developing hypertension needing treatment during 6 years of follow-up was intermediate between the normotensive and the systolic-diastolic hypertensive participants [85]. The study was made in 1141 participants aged 18–45 years and 101 nonhypertensive subjects of control. At baseline, 13.8 % of the subjects had isolated systolic hypertension, 24.8 % had isolated diastolic hypertension, and 61.4 % had systolic-diastolic hypertension. The risk of developing hypertension needing treatment was higher in all hypertensive groups than in the nonhypertensive subjects (Fig. 7.5). However, within the hypertensive participants the risk was higher among the systolic-diastolic hypertensives (odds ratio 5.2, 95 % CI 2.9–9.2), and the diastolic hypertensives (odds ratio 2.6, 95 % CI 1.5–4.5) than the systolic hypertensives (odds ratio 2.2, 95 % CI 1.2–4.5). Similar results were obtained when the definition of hypertension was based on ambulatory blood pressure (Fig. 7.5). The odds ratios were 5.1 (95 % CI 3.1–8.2), 5.6 (95 % CI 3.2–9.8), and 3.3 (95 % CI 1.7–6.3), respectively. In a later study, using central blood pressure measurement we could identify two distinct systolic hypertension subgroups with different arterial elasticity characteristics. Subjects with isolated systolic hypertension and high central blood pressure had reduced large artery compliance, as assessed from arterial pulse waveform analysis, in comparison with systolic hypertension subjects with low central systolic blood pressure attesting to increased large artery stiffness [86]. In addition, patients with high central blood pressure exhibited impaired small artery compliance and increased total peripheral resistance a condition which favors central pressure augmentation [87]. In stiffer

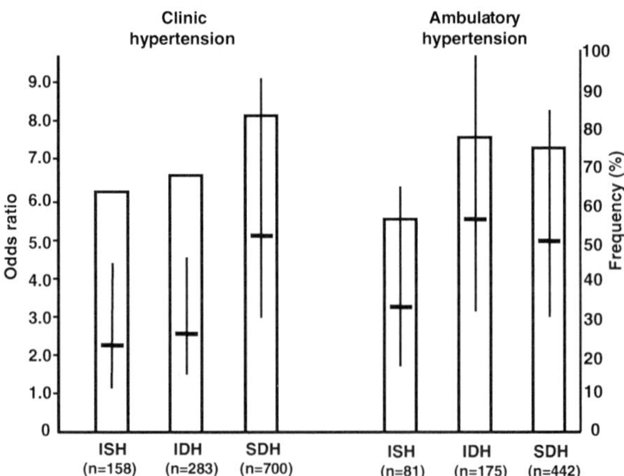

Fig. 7.5 Odds ratios and 95 % confidence intervals for development of hypertension needing treatment and frequency of incident clinic and ambulatory hypertension during 6 years of follow-up in 1,141 participants from the HARVEST study. At baseline, 13.8 % of the subjects had isolated systolic hypertension, 24.8 % had isolated diastolic hypertension, and 61.4 % had systolic-diastolic hypertension. The risk of developing hypertension needing treatment was increased in all hypertensive groups but was higher among the systolic-diastolic or the diastolic hypertensives than among the systolic hypertensives. The risk in 101 nonhypertensive subjects of control was used as a reference (Adapted from Ref. [85])

arteries the reflected wave merges with the incident wave in systole and augments aortic systolic blood pressure thereby reducing systolic blood pressure amplification. This may explain why our subjects with high central systolic blood pressure had an increased likelihood of developing more severe hypertension during the follow-up. Trained individuals may have a high pulse pressure with normal diastolic blood pressure due to high stroke volume and cardiac output. Indeed, isolated systolic hypertension has been found to be more common in physically trained individuals than in sedentary subjects [88]. Thus, spurious systolic hypertension is common in young sports persons and this is thought to be the consequence of the progressive decrease in arterial diameter from the heart to the arm and the corresponding increase in arterial impedance [81, 82]. This is why central systolic pressure has been found to be much lower than brachial systolic pressure in these subjects. Central blood pressure is a more important determinant of target organ damage such as vascular hypertrophy or left ventricular hypertrophy than is brachial blood pressure [89]. In addition, central systolic blood pressure has been found to be an independent predictor of cardiovascular morbidity and mortality [90]. Thus, peripheral systolic hypertension in physically active people may be an innocent clinical condition and assessment of central systolic blood pressure can distinguish between truly hypertensive subjects and subjects with spurious hypertension. The HARVEST study has shown that mean blood pressure was a significant precursor of sustained hypertension in the young age whereas pulse pressure had even a negative association with this outcome [85]. In contrast, systolic hypertension in the elderly results from increased elastic artery stiffness, which increases pulse-wave velocity and wave reflection amplitude [87]. Therefore, high pulse pressure is considered as an ominous haemodynamic parameter in the old age as it proved to be a strong precursor of cardiovascular disease [78, 79].

High Resting Heart Rate in Hypertension

A relationship between sinus tachycardia and adverse cardiovascular outcome was shown for the first time by Levy et al. [91], who found that cardiovascular mortality was higher among subjects with high resting heart rate at baseline evaluation than among those with normal heart rate. Starting from the eighties a large number of studies have confirmed this association showing that fast heart rate is a strong predictor of cardiovascular events and mortality [92, 93]. The correlation with sudden death was a particularly close one [93]. In the Framingham Study, as well as in other studies the relationship between heart rate and cardiovascular mortality was stronger among males than among females and was maintained even after excluding individuals who died in the first 2 years after baseline evaluation [92]. In the last 15 years, numerous new studies that used refined statistical analyses confirmed the findings of the above cited pioneering studies. In the Copenhagen Male study, Jensen and colleagues [94] assessed whether a raised resting heart rate was a robust predictor of cardiovascular mortality independent of inflammation. In that study, after adjusting for both C-reactive protein and fibrinogen, as well as other conventional risk factors, a 10 bpm increase in heart rate was still associated with increased risk of cardiovascular mortality. An association between heart rate and death from cardiovascular disease was also found in a large Norwegian cohort of 180,353 men and 199,490 women aged 40–45 years without cardiovascular history or diabetes [95]. Recent results from the MESA (Multi-Ethnic Study of Atherosclerosis) study [96] showed that elevated resting heart rate was also associated with increased risk for incident heart failure. The relationship between heart rate and adverse outcome persists into old age as shown by the Jerusalem Longitudinal Cohort study, a prospective longitudinal study of a representative cohort born in 1920–21 [97]. This study showed that heart rate declines in the old, and that a greater decline is associated with greater longevity.

The relationship between high heart rate and cardiovascular outcomes might be explained by tachycardia merely reflecting poor physical fitness. To establish whether elevated resting heart rate is an independent risk factor for mortality or a mere marker of physical fitness both variables were included in the FINRISK Study [98] a large cohort of 10,519 men and 11,334 women. After adjusting also for age, gender, total cholesterol, blood pressure, body mass index, and high-density lipoprotein cholesterol, each 15 bpm increase in heart rate was associated with an adjusted hazard ratio of 1.24 (95 % CI, 1.11–1.40) in men. A similar association was observed among the women (HR 1.32, 95 % CI, 1.08–1.60). In keeping with the FINRISK study, results obtained within the frame of the Cooper Clinic Study [99] showed a protective role of low resting heart rate on all-cause and cardiovascular disease mortality in 53,322 subjects. Patients with high heart rate were at greater risk for cardiovascular and all-cause mortality compared with those with bradycardia irrespective of degree of physical fitness. Among the unfit individuals, those with tachycardia had the greatest risk of cardiovascular and all cause mortality whereas those with bradycardia had a similar risk as the fit individuals with high heart rate. This study clearly demonstrated that heart rate and cardiorespiratory fitness independently contribute to the risk of mortality. The vast majority of epidemiologic studies in general populations have found a linear relationship between heart rate and major outcomes. In a recent analysis of the Framingham Heart Study, the authors examined the association of baseline heart rate with both fatal and nonfatal outcomes fitting restricted cubic splines with 3 knots at 25th, 50th, and 75th percentiles [100]. Baseline heart rate was associated with incident cardiovascular disease (hazard ratio 1.15 per 1 SD increase in heart rate; 95 % CI, 1.07–1.24) in a linear fashion starting from very low heart rate levels. The association was particularly strong with heart failure (HR 1.32, 95 % CI 1.18–1.48).

A number of studies performed in hypertensive populations have shown that the heart rate-mortality association is particularly strong in hypertension. A positive association with adverse outcome has been found in 6 cohort studies and 6 clinical trials [19]. The first study to analyze the relation between heart rate and mortality in patients with hypertension was the Framingham Study [101]. In this cohort of patients followed for 36 years, the relative risk of cardiovascular death adjusted for age and blood pressure was 1.68 among men and 1.70 among women for an increase in heart rate of 40 bpm. The odds ratios for sudden death were 1.93 and 1.37, respectively. To exclude the possibility that the excess mortality observed among persons with tachycardia were due to a chronic underlying disease, serial analyses were carried out excluding the events that occurred during the first 6 years after baseline assessment. These analyses confirmed the predictive value of heart rate for mortality, making it unlikely that this association was due to an underlying chronic disease. A study by Benetos et al. analyzed the relation between mortality and tachycardia in a cohort of 12,123 men and 7263 women from a French population between the ages of 40 and 69 [102]. Among the men, all-cause and cardiovascular mortality steadily increased with higher heart rates in both normotensive and hypertensive individuals whereas these relationships were weaker among the women. In the Glasgow Blood Pressure Clinic Study [103] hypertensive patients with a heart rate persistently >80 bpm had an increased risk of all-cause and cardiovascular mortality. The highest risk of all-cause mortality was found for a final heart rate of 81–90 bpm, and the lowest risk for a final heart rate of 61–70 bpm. In the hypertensive patients of the Cooper Clinic study [99], people with high resting heart rate (≥80 bpm) were found to be at greater risk for cardiovascular and all-cause mortality compared with those with hypertension and lower heart rate (<60 bpm). An association between heart rate and mortality was found also in people with pre-hypertension from the ARIC study [104].

Similar results were obtained in the patients enrolled in the 6 clinical trials. In the Systolic Hypertension in Europe (Syst-Eur) trial, elderly patients with heart rate >79 bpm had a 1.89 greater risk of all-cause mortality and a 1.60 greater risk of cardiovascular mortality than subjects with heart rate below that level [105]. In the LIFE study a 10 bpm increament in heart rate was associated with a 25 % increased risk of cardiovascular mortality and a 27 % greater risk of all-cause death [106]. Persistence or development of a heart rate ≥84 bpm was associated with an 89 % greater risk of cardiovascular death and a 97 % increased risk of all-cause mortality with a significant interaction between baseline and follow-up heart rate. In the INternational VErapamil-SR/trandolapril STudy (INVEST) study [107], a 5-bpm increment in resting heart rate was associated with a 6 % excess risk in the primary composite outcome (all-cause death, non-fatal myocardial infarction, or non-fatal stroke). Of particular interest are the results obtained in the VALUE study [108]. Also in this study, both baseline and in-trial heart rates were powerful predictors of the composite cardiovascular outcome after adjustment for other risk factors (Fig. 7.6). The VALUE study also showed that the risk of cardiovascular events remained elevated in the patients who had a blood pressure well controlled by treatment if their heart rate was elevated. The lowest risk was found in the group of patients with well controlled blood pressure and low heart rate. Thus, the main message of this study is that the risk of hypertensive patients can be lowered only marginally by antihypertensive treatment if their heart rate remains elevated. In an analysis of the ONTARGET and TRANSCEND studies which included mainly patients with hypertension, the risk of cardiovascular mortality increased by 41–58 % among the patients with a heart rate >70 bpm and by 77 % in those with heart rate >78 bpm [109].

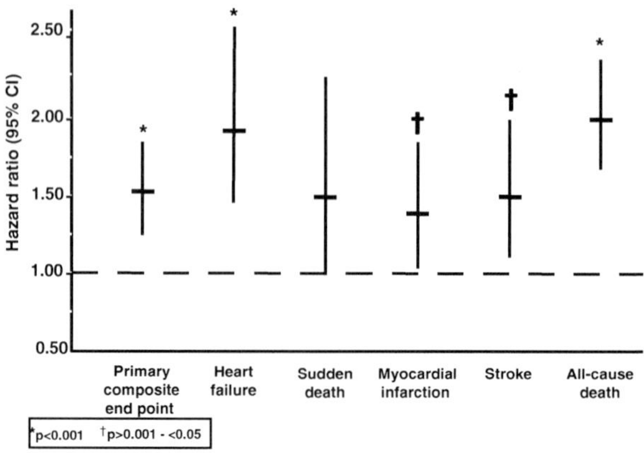

Fig. 7.6 Hazard ratios and 95 % confidence intervals for outcome events from multivariate Cox regression models by in-trial heart rate (recorded at year 1) in the VALUE study. Hazard ratios reflect risk in the top heart rate quintile versus bottom heart rate quintile (Adapted from Ref. [108].

Recent research has shown that the relationship between heart rate and CV events in hypertension is particularly strong for ambulatory heart rate recorded over the 24 h. Within the frame of the ABP-International study, we investigated the association of heart rate measured with intermittent ambulatory recording with cardiovascular outcomes in 7600 hypertensive patients from Italy, U.S.A., Japan, and Australia [110]. All were untreated at baseline examination and were followed for 5 years. In a multivariable Cox model, night-time heart rate emerged as the strongest predictor of fatal combined with nonfatal events with a hazard ratio of 1.13 (95 % CI, 1.04–1.22) for a 10-bpm increment of the night-time heart rate. This relationship remained significant when subjects taking beta-blockers during the follow-up or subjects who had an event within 5 years after enrolment were excluded from analysis.

The prognostic significance of heart rate has also been evaluated in resistant hypertension, in which a U-shaped relationship between heart rate and cardiovascular outcome was found, particularly for heart rate measured with ambulatory monitoring [111].

In conclusion, the data from the literature consistently demonstrated that heart rate is a potent risk factor for mortality and/or cardiovascular disease in hypertension. In all of the studies in which patients who died within the initial years of follow-up were excluded from analysis the association between elevated heart rate and risk of cardiovascular events or mortality remained significant excluding the possibility of reverse causality [112].

Conclusions

Hypertension is a self-accelerating condition and if left untreated the blood pressure increases progressively. In the young age the acceleration is usually slow but at a certain point during the lifetime the increase of blood pressure becomes exponential. This process occurs because of restructuring of the arterioles whose wall when exposed to excessive pressure thickens because of smooth muscle hypertrophy and arteriolar remodelling. Reduction in arteriolar lumen causes an increase of vascular resistance and the blood pressure increases to maintain adequate capillary blood flow. At some time point in the acceleration curve target organ damage starts to develop leading with time to cardiovascular, cerebral and renal damage. At that "point of no return" antihypertensive treatment can still reduce the occurrence of morbid events but the underlying cardiac and arterial abnormalities cannot be reverted. It follows that detection of early target organ damage is crucial for preventing later cardiovascular complications. With modern antihypertensive treatment only a strict minority of hypertensive patients develop left ventricular hypertrophy and the related hemodynamic and left ventricular functional changes. However, subtle abnormalities of cardiac function can occur early in the course of the disease and detecting those alterations would allow the clinician to start antihypertensive treatment on due time. For example, in the Tecumseh study, the blood pressure amplification in the prehypertension group happened between 21 and 31 years of age [4]. Thus our attention should be focused especially on young subjects with prehypertension or stage 1 hypertension. Our echocardiographic studies have shown that the discrepancy between the ejective and contractile left ventricular performance is related to the concentric remodelling of the left ventricle and that it is a significant predictor of worsening of the hypertensive condition [49–51]. Left ventricular ejective performance on a background of depressed left ventricular contractility can temporarily preserve cardiac output but leads to an unfavorable structural left ventricular pattern with ominous consequences for the left ventricle. Detection of depressed left ventricular contractility at echocardiography irrespective of whether left ventricular endocardial performance is normal should thus prompt early antihypertensive treatment in stage 1 hypertension. Attention should be focused especially on subjects with autonomic nervous system abnormalities, clinically manifested as a hyperkinetic circulation characterized by elevations in heart rate, blood pressure, cardiac output, and catecholamine levels a condition that has been repeatedly demonstrated in hypertension of the young [56, 57]. Physical training, through its favorable modulation of the autonomic nervous system activity should be particularly beneficial in this clinical setting [63, 66–69] and may defer the necessity for antihypertensive drug treatment.

References

1. Julius S, Conway J. Hemodynamic studies in patients with borderline blood pressure elevation. Circulation. 1968;38:282–8.
2. Julius S, Pascual AV, London R. Role of parasympathetic inhibition in the hyperkinetic type of borderline hypertension. Circulation. 1971;44:413–8.
3. Goldstein DS. Plasma catecholamines and essential hypertension: an analytical review. Hypertension. 1983;5:86–99.
4. Julius S, Krause L, Schork N, et al. Hyperkinetic borderline hypertension in Tecumseh, Michigan. J Hypertens. 1991;9:77–84.

5. Palatini P, Vriz O, Nesbitt S, et al. Parental hyperdynamic circulation predicts insulin resistance in offspring: the Tecumseh Offspring Study. Hypertension. 1999;33:769–74.
6. Grassi G. Role of the sympathetic nervous system in human hypertension. J Hypertens. 1998;16:1979–87.
7. Schork NJ, Weder AB, Schork MA, et al. Disease entities, mixed multi-normal distributions, and the role of the hyperkinetic state in the pathogenesis of hypertension. Stat Med. 1990;9:301–14.
8. Jennings GL. Noradrenaline spillover and microneurography measurements in patients with primary hypertension. J Hypertens. 1998;16(Suppl):S35–8.
9. Kjeldsen SE, Zweifler AJ, Petrin J, et al. Sympathetic nervous system involvement in essential hypertension: increased platelet noradrenaline coincides with decreased ß-adrenoreceptor responsiveness. Blood Press. 1994;3:164–71.
10. Palatini P, Majahalme S, Amerena J, et al. Determinants of left ventricular structure and mass in young subjects with sympathetic over-activity. The Tecumseh Offspring Study. J Hypertens. 2000;18:769–75.
11. Palatini P, Longo D, Zaetta V, et al. Evolution of blood pressure and cholesterol in stage 1 hypertension: role of autonomic nervous system activity. J Hypertens. 2006;24:1375–81.
12. Maver J, Strucl M, Accetto R. Autonomic nervous system activity in normotensive subjects with a family history of hypertension. Clin Auton Res. 2004;14:358–9.
13. Neumann SA, Jennings JR, Muldoon MF, Manuck SB. White-coat hypertension and autonomic nervous system dysregulation. Am J Hypertens. 2005;18:584–8.
14. Fagard RH, Stolarz K, Kuznetsova T, Kawecka-Jaszcz K. Sympathetic activity, assessed by power spectral analysis of HR variability, in white-coat, masked and sustained hypertension versus true normotension. J Hypertens. 2007;25:2280–5.
15. Calhoun DA, Mutinga ML, Wyss JM, Oparil S. Muscle sympathetic nervous system activity in black and Caucasian hypertensive subjects. J Hypertens. 1994;12:1291–6.
16. Matthews KA, Katholi CR, McCreath H, et al. Blood pressure reactivity to psychological stress predicts hypertension in the CARDIA study. Circulation. 2004;110:74–8.
17. Steptoe A. Psychophysiological stress reactivity and hypertension. Hypertension. 2008;52:220–1.
18. Masuo K, Kawaguchi H, Mikami H, et al. Serum uric acid and plasma norepinephrine concentrations predict subsequent weight gain and blood pressure elevation. Hypertension. 2003;42:474–80.
19. Palatini P. Role of elevated heart rate in the development of cardiovascular disease in hypertension. Hypertension. 2011;58:745–50.
20. Lund-Johansen P. Newer thinking on the hemodynamics of hypertension. Curr Opin Cardiol. 1994;9:505–11.
21. Julius S. The blood pressure seeking properties of the central nervous system. J Hypertens. 1988;6:177–85.
22. Palatini P, Julius S. Heart rate and the cardiovascular risk. J Hypertens. 1997;15:3–17.
23. Julius S, Jamerson K, Mejia A, et al. The association of borderline hypertension with target organ changes and higher coronary risk. Tecumseh Blood Pressure Study. JAMA. 1990;264:354–8.
24. Slotwiner DJ, Devereux RB, Schwartz JE, et al. Relation of age to left ventricular function and systemic hemodynamics in uncomplicated mild hypertension. Hypertension. 2001;37:1404–9.
25. Stein CM, Nelson R, Deegan R, et al. Forearm beta adrenergic receptor-mediated vasodilation is impaired, without alteration of forearm norepinephrine spillover, in borderline hypertension. J Clin Invest. 1995;96:579–85.
26. Valentini M, Julius S, Palatini P, et al. Attenuation of haemodynamic, metabolic and energy expenditure responses to isoproterenol in patients with hypertension. J Hypertens. 2004;22:1999–2006.
27. Julius S, Nesbitt S. Sympathetic overactivity in hypertension A moving target. Am J Hypertens. 1996;9:113s–20.

28. Julius S, Li Y, Brant D, et al. Neurogenic pressor episodes fail to cause hypertension, but do induce cardiac hypertrophy. Hypertension. 1989;13:422–9.
29. Hartford M, Wikstrand J, Wallentin I, et al. Left ventricular mass in middle-aged men. Relationship to blood pressure, sympathetic nervous activity, hormonal and metabolic factors. Clin Exper Hypertens. 1983;5:1429–51.
30. Lantelme P, Milon H, Gharib C, et al. White coat effect and reactivity to stress: cardiovascular and autonomic nervous system responses. Hypertension. 1998;31:1021–9.
31. Julius S, Valentini M, Palatini P. Overweight and hypertension: a 2-way street? Hypertension. 2000;35:807–13.
32. Hartford M, Wikstrand JCM, Wallentin I, Ljungman SMJ. Left ventricular wall stress and systolic function in untreated primary hypertension. Hypertension. 1985;7:97–104.
33. Palatini P, Mormino P, Santonastaso M, et al. Target organ damage in stage I hypertensive subjects with white coat and sustained hypertension: results from the HARVEST study. Hypertension. 2004;31:57–63.
34. Seals DR, Rogers MA, Hagberg JM, et al. Left ventricular dysfunction after prolonged exercise in healthy subjects. Am J Cardiol. 1988;61:875–9.
35. Vanoverschelde JL, Younis LT, Melin JA, et al. Prolonged exercise induces left ventricular dysfunction in healthy subjects. J Appl Physiol. 1991;70:1356–63.
36. Palatini P, Bongiovì S, Mario L, et al. Above normal left ventricular performance is present during exercise in young subjects with mild hypertension. Eur Heart J. 1995;16:232–42.
37. Palatini P, Mos L, Mormino P, et al. Intra-arterial blood pressure monitoring in the evaluation of the hypertensive athlete. Eur Heart J. 1990;11:348–54.
38. De Simone G, Di Lorenzo L, Moccia D, et al. Hemodynamic hypertrophied left ventricular patterns in systemic hypertension. Am J Cardiol. 1987;60:1317–21.
39. Lutas EM, Devereux RB, Reis G, et al. Increased cardiac performance in mild essential hypertension: left ventricular mechanics. Hypertension. 1985;7:979–88.
40. De Simone G, Di Lorenzo L, Costantino G, et al. Supernormal contractility in primary hypertension without left ventricular hypertrophy. Hypertension. 1988;11:457–63.
41. Aurigemma GP, Silver KH, Priest MA, Gaash WH. Geometric changes allow normal ejection fraction despite depressed myocardial shortening in hypertensive left ventricular hypertrophy. J Am Coll Cardiol. 1995;26:195–202.
42. Shimizu G, Hirota Y, Kita Y, et al. Left ventricular midwall mechanics in systemic arterial hypertension: myocardial function is depressed in pressure-overload hypertrophy. Circulation. 1991;83:1676–84.
43. De Simone G, Devereux RB, Roman MJ, et al. Assessment of left ventricular function by the midwall fractional shortening-systolic stress relation in human hypertension. J Am Coll Cardiol. 1994;23:1444–51.
44. Palmon LC, Reichek N, Yeon SB, et al. Intramural myocardial shortening in hypertensive left ventricular hypertrophy with normal pump function. Circulation. 1994;89:122–31.
45. Hinderliter AL, Light KC, Willis IV PW. Patients with borderline elevated blood pressure have enhanced left ventricular contractility. Am J Hypertens. 1995;8:1040–5.
46. Blaufox ME, Wexler JP, Sherman RA, et al. Left ventricular ejection fraction and its response to therapy in essential hypertension. Nephron. 1981;28:112–7.
47. Melin JA, Wijns W, Pouler H, et al. Ejection fraction response to upright exercise in hypertension: relation to loading conditions and to contractility. Int J Cardiol. 1987;17:37–49.
48. Miller DD, Ruddy TD, Zusman RM, et al. Left ventricular ejection fraction response during exercise in asymptomatic systemic hypertension. Am J Cardiol. 1987;59:409–13.
49. Palatini P, Frigo G, Visentin P, et al. Left ventricular contractile performance in the early stage of hypertension in humans. Eur J Appl Physiol. 2001;85:118–24.
50. Palatini P, Visentin P, Nicolosi G, et al. Endocardial versus midwall measurement of left ventricular function in mild hypertension: an insight from the Harvest Study. J Hypertens. 1996;14:1011–7.
51. Palatini P, Visentin PA, Mormino P, et al. Left ventricular performance in the early stages of systemic hypertension. Am J Cardiol. 1998;81:418–23.

52. Aurigemma GP, Gaash WH, McLaughlin M, et al. Reduced left ventricular systolic pump performance and depressed myocardial contractile function in patients > 65 years of age with normal ejection fraction and a high relative wall thickness. Am J Cardiol. 1995;76:702–5.
53. Lehmann M, Keul J. Korrelationen zwischen hamodynamischen Grossen und Plasmakatecholaminen bei Normo-und Hypertonikern in Ruhe und wahrend Korperarbeit. Klin Wochenschr. 1983;61:403–11.
54. Yasuda M, Nishikimi T, Akioka K, et al. Relationship between cardiac function and the sympathetic nervous system during exercise in patients with essential hypertension. Jpn Circ J. 1988;52:1121–31.
55. Saladini F, Zaetta V, Visentin P, et al. Left ventricular systolic dysfunction in the early stage of hypertension. Proceedings of the 18th scientific meeting of the European Society of Hypertension, Berlin. 2008.
56. Mancia G, Grassi G, Giannattasio C, Seravalle G. Sympathetic activation in the pathogenesis of hypertension and progression of organ damage. Hypertension. 1999;34:724–8.
57. Palatini P, Julius S. The role of cardiac autonomic function in hypertension and cardiovascular disease. Curr Ther Rep. 2009;11:199–205.
58. Hull EM, Young SH, Ziegler MG. Aerobic fitness affects cardiovascular and catecholamine responses to stressors. Psychophysiol. 1984;21:353–60.
59. Salmon P. Effects of physical exercise on anxiety, depression, and sensitivity to stress: a unifying theory. Clin Psychol Rev. 2001;21:33–61.
60. Frohlich ED. The heart in hypertension. Clin Nephrol. 1991;36:160–5.
61. Kamide K, Rakugi H, Higaki J, et al. The renin-angiotensin and adrenergic nervous system in cardiac hypertrophy in fructose-fed rats. Am J Hypertens. 2002;15(1 Pt 1):66–71.
62. Malmqvist K, Ohman KP, Lind L, et al. Relationships between left ventricular mass and the renin-angiotensin system, catecholamines, insulin and leptin. J Intern Med. 2002;252:430–9.
63. Fagard RH. Exercise therapy in hypertensive cardiovascular disease. Prog Cardiovasc Dis. 2011;53:404–11.
64. Thompson PD, Buchner D, Piña IL, et al. AHA Scientific Statement. Exercise and physical activity in the prevention and treatment of atherosclerotic cardiovascular disease. Circulation. 2003;107:3109–16.
65. Crews DJ, Landers DM. A meta-analytic review of aerobic fitness and reactivity to psychosocial stressors. Med Sci Sports Exe. 1987;19:S114–20.
66. Rimmele U, Zellweger BC, Marti B, et al. Trained men show lower cortisol, heart rate and psychological responses to psychosocial stress compared with untrained men. Psychoneuroendocrinology. 2007;32:627–35.
67. Palatini P, Bratti P, Palomba D, et al. Regular physical activity attenuates the BP response to public speaking and delays the development of hypertension. J Hypertens. 2010;28:1186–93.
68. O'Sullivan SE, Bell C. The effects of exercise and training on human cardiovascular reflex control. J Autonom Nerv Syst. 2000;81:16–24.
69. Laterza MC, de Matos LD, Trombetta IC, et al. Exercise training restores baroreflex sensitivity in never-treated hypertensive patients. Hypertension. 2007;49:1298–306.
70. Julius S. The hemodynamic link between insulin resistance and hypertension. J Hypertens. 1991;9:983–6.
71. Kohno KH, Matsuoka K, Takenaka K, et al. Depressor effect by exercise training is associated with amelioration of hyperinsulinemia and sympathetic overactivity. Intern Med. 2000;39:1013–9.
72. Dinenno FA, Jones PP, Seals DR, Tanaka H. Age-associated arterial wall thickening is related to elevations in sympathetic activity in healthy humans. Am J Physiol Heart Circ Physiol. 2000;278:H1205–10.
73. Baglivo HP, Fabregues G, Burrieza H, et al. Effect of moderate physical training on left ventricular mass in mild hypertensive persons. Hypertension. 1990;15 Suppl 1:I-153–6.
74. Zanettini R, Bettega D, Agostoni O, et al. Exercise training in mild hypertension: effects on blood pressure, left ventricular mass and coagulation factor VII and fibrinogen. Cardiology. 1997;88:468–73.

75. Palatini P, Visentin P, Dorigatti F, Mos L. Regular physical activity prevents development of left ventricular hypertrophy in hypertension. Eur Heart J. 2009;30:225–32.
76. Saladini F, Benetti E, Mos L, et al. Regular physical activity is associated with improved small artery distensibility in young to middle-age stage 1 hypertensives. Vasc Med. 2014;19:458–64.
77. Palatini P, Puato M, Rattazzi M, Pauletto P. Effect of regular physical activity on carotid intima-media thickness. Results from a 6-year prospective study in the early stage of hypertension. Blood Press. 2011;20:37–44.
78. Staessen J, Amery A, Fagard R. Isolated systolic hypertension in the elderly. J Hypertens. 1990;8:393–405.
79. Kannel WB, Dawber TR, McGee DL. Perspectives on systolic hypertension. The Framingham Study. Circulation. 1980;61:1179–82.
80. Grebla RG, Rodriguez CJ, Borrell LN, Pickering TG. Prevalence and determinants of isolated systolic hypertension among young adults: the 1999–2004 US National Health and Nutrition Examination Survey. J Hypertens. 2010;28:15–23.
81. Hulsen HT, Nijdam ME, Bos WJ, et al. Spurious systolic hypertension in young adults; prevalence of high brachial systolic blood pressure and low central pressure and its determinants. J Hypertens. 2006;24:1027–32.
82. O'Rourke MF, Vlachopoulos C, Graham RM. Spurious systolic hypertension in youth. Vasc Med. 2000;5:141–5.
83. Mc Eniery CM, Yasmin, Wallace S, et al. Increased stroke volume and aortic stiffness contribute to isolated systolic hypertension in young adults. Hypertension. 2005;46:221–6.
84. Sorof JM, Alexandrov AV, Garami AZ, et al. Carotid ultrasonography for detection of vascular abnormalities in hypertensive children. Pediatr Nephrol. 2003;18:1020–4.
85. Saladini F, Dorigatti F, Santonastaso M, et al. Natural history of hypertension subtypes in young and middle-age adults. Am J Hypertens. 2009;22:531–7.
86. Saladini F, Santonastaso M, Mos L, et al. Isolated systolic hypertension of young to middle-age individuals implies a relatively low risk of developing hypertension needing treatment when central blood pressure is low. J Hypertens. 2011;29:1311–9.
87. Nichols WW. Clinical measurement of arterial stiffness obtained from noninvasive pressure waveforms. Am J Hypertens. 2005;18:3S–10.
88. Mahmud A, Feely J. Spurious systolic hypertension of youth: fit young men with elastic arteries. Am J Hypertens. 2003;16:229–32.
89. Roman MJ, Okin PM, Kizer JR, et al. Relation of central and brachial blood pressure to left ventricular hypertrophy and geometry: the Strong Heart Study. J Hypertens. 2010;28:384–8.
90. Wang KL, Cheng HM, Chuang SY, et al. Central or peripheral systolic or pulse pressure: which best relates to target organs and future mortality? J Hypertens. 2009;27:461–7.
91. Levy RL, White PD, Stroud WD, et al. Transient tachycardia: prognostic significance alone and in association with transient hypertension. JAMA. 1945;129:585–8.
92. Kannel WB, Kannel C, Paffenbarger Jr RS, et al. Heart rate and cardio-vascular mortality: The Framingham Study. Am Heart J. 1987;113:1489–94.
93. Jouven X, Desnos M, Guerot C, et al. Predicting sudden death in the population: the Paris Prospective Study 1. Circulation. 1999;99:1978–83.
94. Jensen MT, Marott JL, Allin KH, et al. Resting heart rate is associated with cardiovascular and all-cause mortality after adjusting for inflammatory markers: the Copenhagen City Heart Study. Eur J Prev Cardiol. 2012;19:102–8.
95. Tverdal A, Hjellvik V, Selmer R. Heart rate and mortality from cardiovascular causes: a 12 year follow-up study of 379,843 men and women aged 40–45 years. Eur Heart J. 2008;29:2772–81.
96. Opdahl A, Ambale Venkatesh B, et al. Resting heart rate as predictor for left ventricular dysfunction and heart failure: MESA (Multi-Ethnic Study of Atherosclerosis). J Am Coll Cardiol. 2014;63:1182–9.
97. Stessman J, Jacobs JM, Stessman-Lande I, et al. Aging, resting pulse rate, and longevity. J Am Geriatr Soc. 2013;61:40–5.

98. Cooney MT, Vartiainen E, Laatikainen T, et al. Elevated resting heart rate is an independent risk factor for cardiovascular disease in healthy men and women. Am Heart J. 2010;159:612–9. e3.
99. Saxena A, Minton D, Lee DC, et al. Protective role of resting heart rate on all-cause and cardiovascular disease mortality. Mayo Clin Proc. 2013;88:1420–6.
100. Ho JE, Larson MG, Ghorbani A, et al. Long-term cardiovascular risks associated with an elevated heart rate: the Framingham Heart Study. J Am Heart Assoc. 2014;3, e000668.
101. Gillman MW, Kannel WB, Belanger A, D'Agostino RB. Influence of heart rate on mortality among persons with hypertension: The Framingham study. Am Heart J. 1993;125:1148–54.
102. Benetos A, Rudnichi A, Thomas F, et al. Influence of heart rate on mortality in a French population. Role of age, gender, and blood pressure. Hypertension. 1999;33:44–52.
103. Paul L, Hastie CE, Li WS, et al. Resting heart rate pattern during follow-up and mortality in hypertensive patients. Hypertension. 2010;55:567–74.
104. King DE, Everett CJ, Mainous AG, et al. Long-term prognostic value of resting heart rate in subjects with prehypertension. Am J Hypertens. 2006;19:796–800.
105. Palatini P, Thijs L, Staessen J, et al. Predictive value of clinic and ambulatory heart rate for mortality in elderly subjects with systolic hypertension. Arch Int Med. 2002;162:2313–21.
106. Okin PM, Kjeldsen SE, Julius S, et al. All-cause and cardiovascular mortality in relation to changing heart rate during treatment of hypertensive patients with electrocardiographic left ventricular hypertrophy. Eur Heart J. 2010;31:2271–9.
107. Kolloch R, Legler UF, Champion A, et al. Impact of resting heart rate on outcomes in hypertensive patients with coronary artery disease: findings from the INternational VErapamil-SR/trandolapril STudy (INVEST). Eur Heart J. 2008;29:1327–34.
108. Julius S, Palatini P, Kjeldsen S, et al. Usefulness of heart rate to predict cardiac events in treated patients with high-risk systemic hypertension. Am J Cardiol. 2012;109:685–92.
109. Rambihar S, Gao P, Teo K, et al. Heart rate is associated with increased risk of major cardiovascular events cardiovascular and All-cause death in patients with stable chronic cardiovascular disease – an analysis of ONTARGET/TRANSCEND. Circulation. 2010;122:A12667.
110. Palatini P, Reboldi G, Beilin LJ, et al. Predictive value of night-time heart rate for cardiovascular events in hypertension. The ABP-International study. Int J Cardiol. 2013;168:1490–5.
111. Salles GF, Cardoso CR, Fonseca LL, et al. Prognostic significance of baseline heart rate and its interaction with beta-blocker use in resistant hypertension: a cohort study. Am J Hypertens. 2013;26:218–26.
112. Palatini P, Benetos A, Grassi G, et al. Identification and management of the hypertensive patient with elevated heart rate: statement of a European Society of Hypertension Consensus Meeting. J Hypertens. 2006;24:603–10.

Chapter 8
Structural Alterations in the Hypertensive Heart Disease Result in Intercalated Disc Remodeling and Arrhythmias

Maria Irene Kontaridis, Eleni V. Geladari, and Charalampia V. Geladari

Abbreviations

ACEI	Angiotensin converting enzyme inhibitor
ACM	Arrhythmogenic cardiomyopathy
AF	Atrial fibrillation
AJ	Adherens junction
APC	Adenomatous polyposis coli
ARB	Angiotensin receptor blocker
ARVC	Arrhythmogenic right ventricular cardiomyopathy
αT-catenin	Alpha T-catenin
BB	Beta-blocker

M.I. Kontaridis, Ph.D. (✉)
Division of Cardiology, Department of Medicine, Beth Israel Deaconess Medical Center, Center for Life Sciences, Room 908, 3 Blackfan Circle, Boston, MA 02115, USA

Department of Biological Chemistry and Molecular Pharmacology, Harvard Medical School, Boston, MA, USA
e-mail: mkontari@bidmc.harvard.edu

E.V. Geladari, M.D.
4th Department of Internal Medicine, "Evangelismos" General Hospital, Athens, Greece

First Internal Medicine Department, Evangelismos General Hospital, Athens, Greece

Division of Cardiology, Department of Medicine, Beth Israel Deaconess Medical Center, Harvard Medical School, Boston, MA, USA

C.V. Geladari, M.D.
Division of Cardiology, Department of Medicine, Beth Israel Deaconess Medical Center, Harvard Medical School, Boston, MA, USA

4th Department of Internal Medicine, Hypertension and Cardiovascular Disease Prevention Outpatient Center, "Evangelismos" General Hospital, Athens, Greece

E.A. Andreadis (ed.), *Hypertension and Cardiovascular Disease*,
DOI 10.1007/978-3-319-39599-9_8

β-catenin	Beta catenin
BP	Blood pressure
Ca^{2+}	Calcium ions
CaMKII	Calcium/calmodulin kinase II
CaN	Calcineurin A
CCB	Calcium channel blocker
CCS	Cardiac conduction system
CK1	Casein kinase-1
CM	Cardiomyocyte
Cx	Connexin
DCM	Dilated cardiomyopathy
DKO	Double knockout
Dvl	Dishevelled
EC	Excitation-contraction
ECM	Extracellular cell matrix
GJ	Gap junction
GSK	Glycogen synthase kinase
HCM	Hypertrophic cardiomyopathy
HF	Heart failure
HHD	Hypertensive heart disease
HTN	Hypertension
ICM	Ischemic cardiomyopathy
ID	Intercalated disc
IDC	Idiopathic dilated cardiomyopathy
K_v	Voltage-gated calcium channel
LA	Left atrium
LRP	Lipoprotein receptor-related protein
LTCC	Long-type calcium channel
LV	Left ventricle
LVH	Left ventricular hypertrophy
LVM	Left ventricular mass
MI	Myocardial infarction
MCT	Monocrotaline
MMP	Matrix metaloproteinase
Na^+	Sodium
N-Cad CKO	N-cadherin knockout mice
NCX	Na^+-Ca^{2+} exchanger pump
PG	Plakoglobin
PKP2	Plakophilin-2
RA	Right atrium
RAAS	Renin angiotensin aldosterone system
RV	Right ventricle

RyR	Ryanodine receptor
SCD	Sudden cardiac death
SERCA	Sarco-endoplasmic reticulum ATP-ase
SHR	Spontaneously hypertensive rats
SR	Sarcoplasmic reticulum
TCF/LEF	T-cell factor/lymphoid enhancer factor
TGF-β1	Transforming growth factor
TIMP	Tissue inhibitor of metalloproteinase
+TIP	Microtubule plus-end-tracking protein
T-tubule	Transverse tubule
VF	Ventricular fibrillation
VT	Ventricular tachycardia
WT	Wild type

Hypertension Is a Major Contributor to the Onset of Cardiovascular Disease

Hypertension (HTN) is the leading cause of cardiovascular disease and the single most important risk factor for cerebrovascular stroke [1, 2]. Adequate control of high blood pressure (BP) is critical to the prevention of HTN. However, despite the introduction of antihypertensive medications and the implementation of new therapies in recent years, HTN remains a major worldwide public health concern, with 26.4 % of the world's adult population having been diagnosed with HTN by the year 2000 [3]. More troubling still is the fact that the prevalence of HTN is only expected to rise, to approximately 1.56 billion, by the year 2025, particularly in rapidly developing countries with limited early routine screening protocols [4, 5]. Moreover, most hypertensives that are not diagnosed early present with substantial complications by the time they receive their first treatment [6], adding to a growing international clinical and economic burden associated with the disease. Therefore, additional educational and medical resources will be needed to prevent and treat HTN and its associated complications [7, 8].

In particular, cardiac arrhythmias are the most common comorbidity that influences hypertensive patients [9–11]. Groundbreaking research highlighting the underlying mechanisms linking HTN to arrhythmias, including left ventricular hypertrophy (LVH), myocardial ischemia, impaired left ventricular function and left atrial enlargement, has been in the spotlight in recent years [12]. The structural and functional alterations that take place in hypertensive heart disease and the pathophysiological disturbances in the composition of the intercalated disc (ID) leading to cardiomyopathies and arrhythmias will be of notable interest in our discussion here.

Cardiac Function

The heart is a vital, multi-chambered organ that pumps blood through the circulatory system to maintain proper oxygenation of the body's tissues. The human heart is made up of four chambers, the left atria (LA), left ventricle (LV), right atria (RA), and right ventricle (RV), and through electrical signals, each pumps (contracts) or relaxes (dilates) to allow blood to pass through. Briefly, de-oxygenated blood returning from the body through the inferior and superior vena cava enters the heart through the RA and is then pumped to the RV. Subsequently, blood from the RV is propelled into the lungs through the pulmonary arteries, where it is enriched with oxygen [13]. Pulmonary veins return oxygenated blood to the LA, which contracts and fills the LV, the main pumping chamber of the heart, where it can be ejected through the aorta into the major circulatory network of the body and the process can begin again [13]. The contraction of the ventricles is referred to as systole, whereas diastole is the term used to describe the relaxation, or dilation, of the heart muscle [14].

Cardiomyocytes (CMs), the muscle cells responsible for generating the contractile force in the heart are critical regulators of cardiac function. CMs are connected and joined to each other by intercalated discs (IDs), which allow rapid transmission of electrical impulses that enable the heart to function in syncytium [15] (Fig. 8.1). Specifically, IDs permit sodium, potassium and calcium ions to easily diffuse from cell to cell, allowing for depolarization and repolarization of the myocardium in a process termed excitation-contraction (EC) coupling, triggering myocyte contraction [16, 17]. EC coupling is initiated by the entry of sodium ions (Na^+) across the sarcolemma through the activation or opening of voltage-dependent Na^+ channels. As the muscle impulse spreads from the sarcolemma to the transverse tubule (T-tubule), calcium ions (Ca^{2+}) are released into the sarcoplasm. In addition, cardiomyocyte depolarization causes Ca^{2+} ions to enter into the sarcoplasm of the heart muscle cells via voltage-sensitive Long (L)-type Ca^{2+} channels (LTCC), triggering the release of Ca^{2+} from the sarcoplasmic reticulum (SR) via ryanodine receptors (RyR), raising the Ca^{2+} concentration into the cardiomyocyte sarcoplasm [18]. Ca^{2+} ions then bind to the protein troponin C on the actin filament, allowing myofibril shortening and actin-myosin "cross-bridge" formation, a process which regulates the normal, rhythmic contraction of cardiac muscle cells [19, 20]. However, the rapid removal of free Ca^{2+} from the sarcoplasm is also critical, since it is not only necessary for the relaxation of the myocardium, but also for the overall health of the CM itself. Relaxation is achieved by removing the Ca^{2+} from the cytosol, either by re-sequestering it in the SR via the sarco-endoplasmic reticulum ATP-ase (SERCA), or extruding it into the extracellular space through the Na^+-Ca^{2+} exchanger (NCX) or Ca^{2+} ATPase pump [15] (Fig. 8.2).

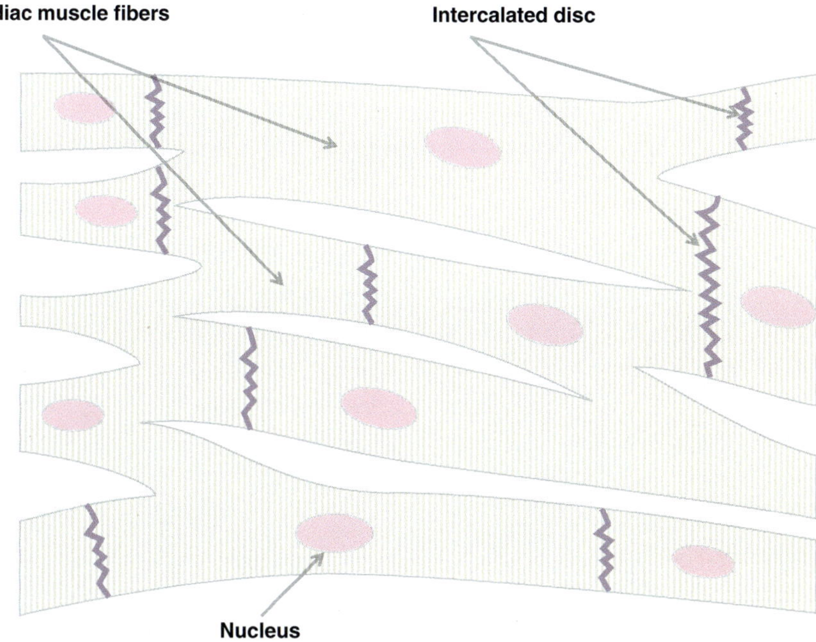

Fig. 8.1 Illustration of a cardiomyocyte. Cardiomyocytes (CMs) are specialized heart muscle cells that together form cardiac muscle fibers that are critical regulators of the contractile motion of the heart. They are often branched and contain only one nucleus. The intercalated discs (IDs) are highly specialized structures at the termini of adjacent CMs. These disks allow for muscle impulses to spread across the cells, and thereby allow for synchronization of the cardiac muscle contractions

Intercalated Discs Are Comprised of Multiple Junctional Complexes

Mechanical and electrical coupling of the CMs play a critical role in the maintenance of the physical and functional integrity of the heart. IDs are electron dense, highly organized structures that join the ends of adjacent CMs to support synchronized contraction of the heart muscle [15]. Therefore, during cardiac contractions, the ID both transmits and coordinates essential signaling events needed for mechanical strength and electrical and chemical communication across the membranes of neighboring cells [21, 22]. In this regard, scientists have recently identified multiple junctional complexes that comprise the ID, including adherens junctions (AJs), desmosomes, and gap junctions (GJs), which together enable the heart to function in this syncytium [23] (Table 8.1).

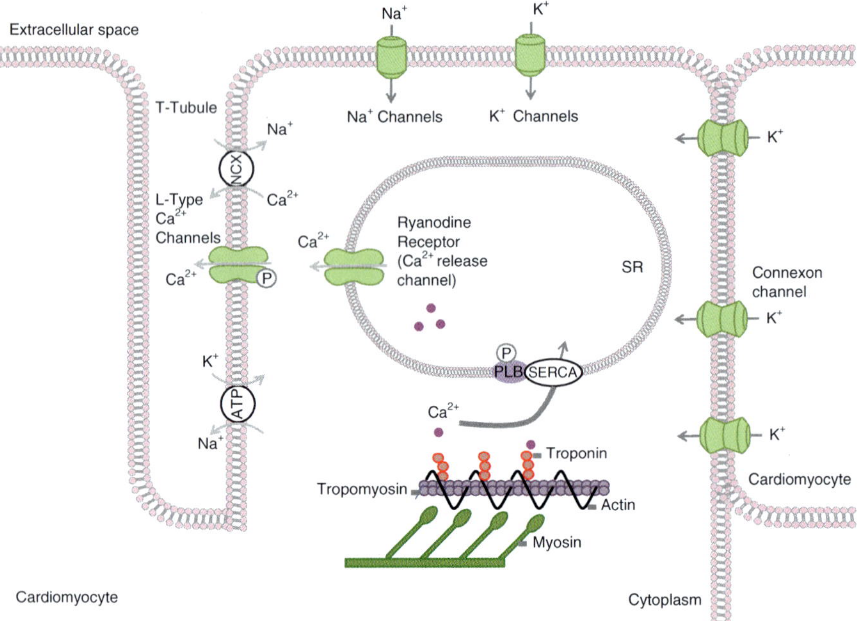

Fig. 8.2 Excitation-contraction coupling in cardiac muscle. The initial event in the cardiac cycle is membrane depolarization, which occurs with ion entry through connexon channels from a neighboring cardiomyocyte (*right*) followed by opening of voltage-gated Na^+ channels and Na^+ entry (*top*). The resultant rapid depolarization of the membrane inactivates Na^+ channels and opens both K^+ channels and Ca^{2+} channels. Entry of Ca^{2+} into the cell triggers the release of Ca^{2+} from the sarcoplasmic reticulum through the ryanodine receptor. Ca^{2+} then binds to the troponin complex and activates the contractile apparatus (*bottom*). Cellular relaxation occurs on removal of Ca^{2+} from the sarcoplasm by the Ca^{2+}-uptake pumps of the sarcoplasmic reticulum, activated when phospholamban becomes phosphorylated and dissociated from the sarco/endoplasmic reticulum calcium ATPase (SERCA) complex (*center*) and by Na^+/Ca^{2+} exchange with the extracellular fluid (*left*). Intracellular Na^+ homeostasis is achieved by the Na^+/K^+ pump (*left*)

Table 8.1 Junctional complexes located at the intercalated disc

1. Adherens Junction (AJ)
2. Desmosome
3. Gap Junction (GJ)
4. Area composita
5. Transitional junction

AJs and desmosomes provide mechanical coupling of CMs, ensuring intercellular communication that allows proper cardiac function. Specifically, AJs hold cardiac muscle cells tightly together as the heart expands and contracts, facilitating the transmission of contractile force from one cell to the next. Therefore, they are crucial in maintaining mechanical strength uniformly across the heart [24]. AJs are

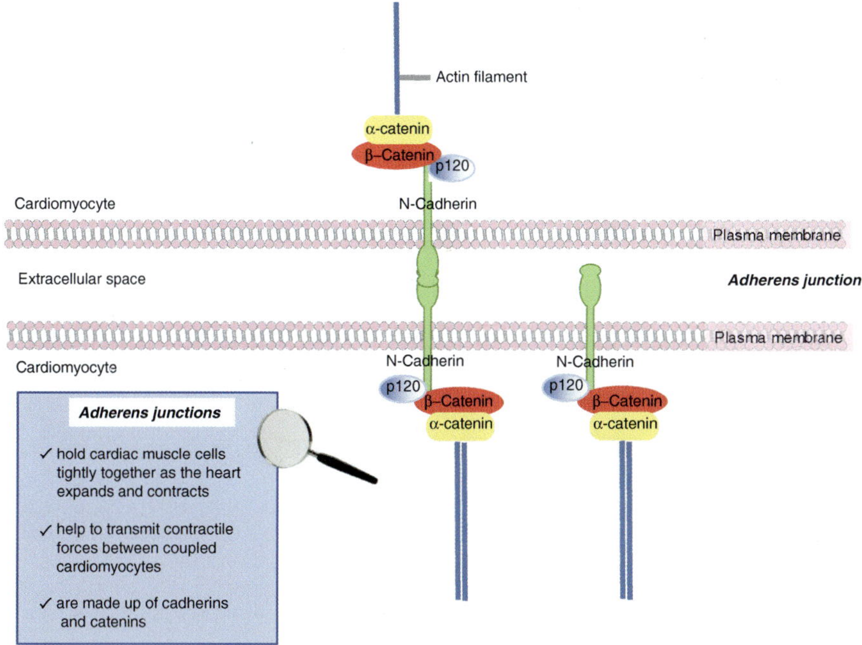

Fig. 8.3 Adherens junctions. Adherens Junctions (AJs) are responsible for mechanically coupling cardiomyocytes (CMs) in the heart. They are made up of N-Cadherin and its cytoplasmic binding proteins, α-catenin and β-catenin. N-Cadherin is a membrane-associated glycoprotein that links the actin microfilaments at the cytoplasmic end with cadherins from the extracellular end of an adjacent CM

made up of N-cadherin and the sarcoplasmic binding proteins catenin and actinin. N-cadherin is a membrane-associated glycoprotein that links actin microfilaments at the sarcoplasmic end of one CM with cadherins on the extracellular end of a neighboring cell [25] (Fig. 8.3).

Desmosomes are comprised of cell adhesion proteins and linking proteins that attach the cell surface adhesion proteins to intracellular cytoskeletal filaments, allowing for mechanical integration of cells within heart muscle and resistance of mechanical stress [26]. Desmoglein and desmocollin are desmosomal proteins that interact with linker proteins, plakoglobin (PG) and desmoplakin, and are a subfamily of the cadherin superfamily that mediate Ca^{2+}-dependent cell-cell adhesion [27] (Fig. 8.4).

GJs, constructed from connexins (Cx), constitute the primary structure of the ID required for intercellular current flow, enabling coordinated action potential propagation and contraction of the heart [28]. Specifically, GJs form channels between adjacent cells. The core proteins in these channels are Cxs, of which 20 members have been identified in humans [29]. Six Cxs form one connexon, and each transverses the plasma membrane of one CM to dock with a connexon of a neighboring cell, creating an extracellular gap [29, 30] (Fig. 8.5). Cx43 is the major GJ protein

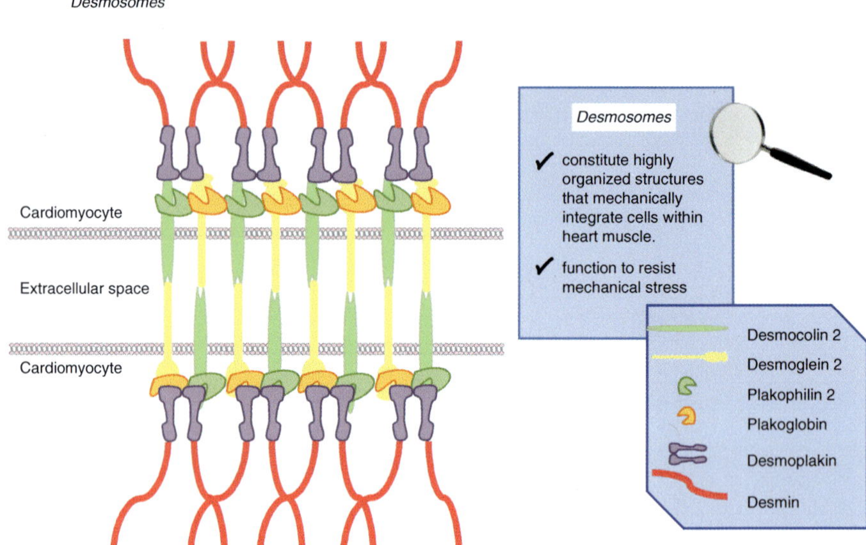

Fig. 8.4 Desmosomes. Desmosomes are intercellular junctions of cardiac muscle that resist mechanical stress and hold adjacent cardiac muscle fibers together. They are made up of several desmosomal proteins. Desmocolin 2 and desmoglein 2 are a subfamily of the cadherin superfamily and interact with linker proteins, such as plakoglobin (PG), desmin, plakophilin 2, and desmoplakin

in working human ventricular CMs [30], with much less Cx45 and Cx40 expressed here [31]. For the most part, Cx45 is strictly localized to the atrioventricular node and adjoining His bundles, and Cx40 is expressed mainly in the atria and the fast connecting tissue of the His-Purkinje system [31].

Recently, an additional junctional complex was identified. This new junction contains molecular components of both desmosomes (plakophilin-2, desmoplakin, desmoglein-2, desmocollin-2) and AJs (N- cadherin, β-catenin) and is localized to the lateralized regions of the CMs [32]. As this highly specialized area is largely devoid of GJs, it was termed "hybrid adherens junction" or "area composita." [32] (Fig. 8.6). Furthermore, it has been suggested that alpha T-catenin (αT-catenin) might mediate the molecular crosstalk between the different junctional complexes of the area composita, due to its unique interaction with the desmosomal protein plakophilin-2 (PKP2) [33]. Alpha (α)–catenins also play a key role in the maintenance of the tissue morphogenesis; they interact with cadherin-binding partners, β-catenin and γ-catenin, as well as with the actin cytoskeleton [34, 35]. In addition, it was recently demonstrated that siRNA-mediated reduction of PKP2 in CMs, but not of some other major plaque components such as desmoplakin, results in progressive disintegration (and loss) of area composita junctional structures, leading destabilization of the ID [36].

Even more recently, in 2006, another unrecognized functional subcellular domain at the ID was identified [21]. This new junctional complex is localized to the

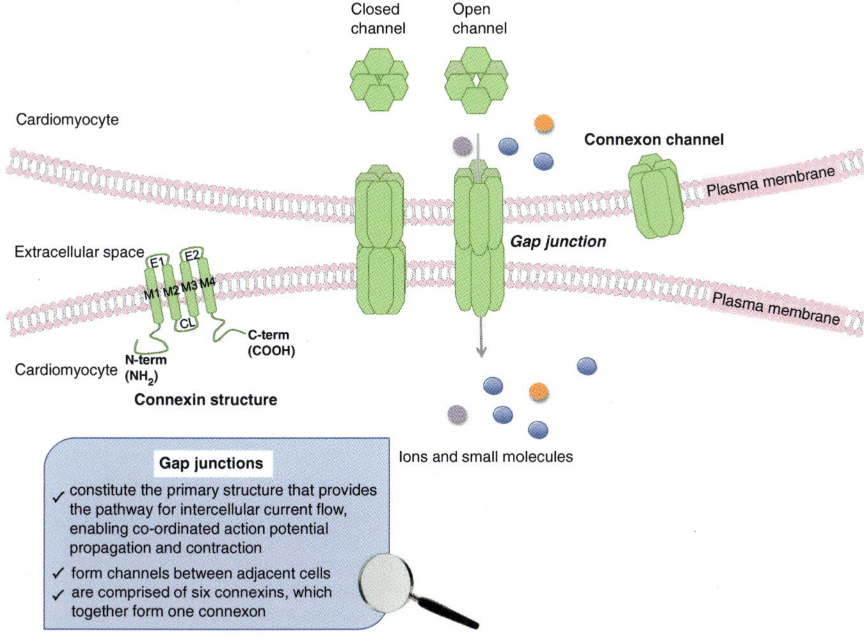

Fig. 8.5 Gap junctions. Gap junction channels constitute the primary structure required for intercellular current flow, enabling coordinated action potential propagation and contraction of the heart. Specifically, GJs form channels between adjacent cells; the core proteins in these channels are connexins (Cxs) (left). Six Cxs form one connexon (right), which transverses the plasma membrane of one cardiomyocyte (CM) and docks with a connexon of a neighboring CM, creating an extracellular gap

interfibrillary region of the CM, between the myofibrillar thin filaments, and is found to be rich in spectrin, a membrane-bound protein that binds to filamentous actin (α-actinin, titin, and ZASP) and produces a robust force-resistant network between cells [21]. This new junction is now known as the "transitional junction" of the ID [21, 37].

Structural Abnormalities in Components of the Intercalated Disc May Play a Role in Cardiac Disease Propagation and Arrhythmogenesis

Growing evidence suggests that anchoring cell-cell junctional components in cardiomyocytes play a key role in the cardiac conduction system (CCS). Moreover, conduction system-related arrhythmias can be found in humans and mouse models of cardiomyopathies harboring defects and/or mutations in key anchoring cell-cell junction proteins [22]. Interestingly, ID remodeling was recently found to play an

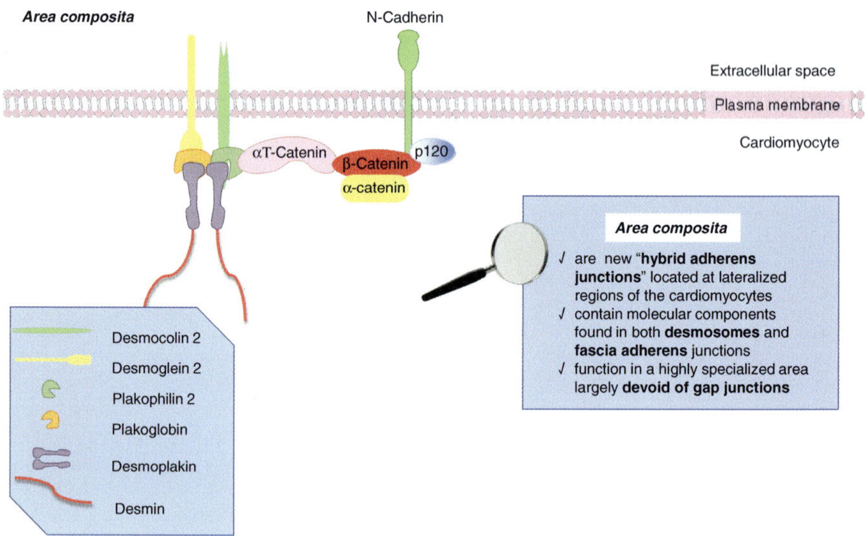

Fig. 8.6 Area composita. Area composita, a newly recognized junction at the intercalated disc (ID), contains molecular components of both desmosomes and adherens junctions (AJs). It is largely devoid of gap junctions (GJs). αT-catenin is thought to mediate the molecular crosstalk between the different junctional complexes of the area composita, due to its unique interaction with the desmosomal protein plakophilin-2 (PKP2)

essential role in ventricular arrhythmogenesis directly, at least in UM-X7.1 cardiomyopathic hamsters, where animals exhibited left ventricular hypertrophy between 10 and 15 weeks of age, had moderate compensated left ventricular contractile dysfunction by 20 weeks, and developed serious decompensated heart failure (HF) at ages beyond 24 weeks [38]. Specifically, at 10–15 weeks of age, these cardiomyopathic hamsters had a remarkable reduction in β-catenin expression in both cellular and nuclear fractions, but not in IDs [38]. Intriguingly, the decrease of total cellular β-catenin preceded Cx43 GJ remodeling, suggesting IDs play an essential role in the pathogenesis of ventricular arrhythmias and HF. Treatment of these mice with olmesartan, an angiotensin II receptor blocker of ID remodeling, attenuated the decrease in cellular and nuclear β-catenin expression and decreased the incidence of ventricular tachycardia (VT) and ventricular fibrillation (VF), improving the survival rate of UM-X7.1 hamsters [38]. This is not attributed to the attenuation of fibrosis, however; rather, decreased incidence of disease was due to the modulation of qualitative (eg. phosphorylation) and/or quantitative Cx43 expression [38]. Thus, angiotensin receptor blockers (ARBs) and/or angiotensin converting enzyme inhibitors (ACEIs) might be a useful therapy for treatment of arrhythmias, through their ability to modulate remodeling of IDs [38].

Interestingly, cardiac-specific deletion of N-Cadherin also leads to a significant decrease in the GJ proteins Cx43 and Cx40, resulting in a decreased ventricular conduction velocity [39]. As such, perturbation of the N-cadherin/β-catenin complex in the heart destabilizes GJs located at the ID, leading to the electrical uncoupling of ventricular myocytes and to the subsequent development of conduction abnormalities, arrhythmogenesis, and sudden cardiac death (SCD) in mice [39]. To investigate whether electrical uncoupling promotes regional ion channel remodeling in N-cadherin conditional knock-out (N-cad CKO) mouse hearts, cardiac excitability and voltage-gated potassium channel (Kv), as well as inwardly rectifying K^+ channel remodeling were measured [40]. These hearts showed slower electrical conduction and significant remodeling of the major outward potassium currents [40]. Specifically, decreased Kv1.5/Kcne2 expression was observed, which correlated with disruption of the actin cytoskeleton and with reduced cortactin levels at the sarcolemma, suggesting a mechanism that tied all these proteins together in promoting electrical heterogeneity and arrhythmogenesis [40].

Multiple clinical and genetic studies have revealed a close relationship between ID protein mutations and the development of cardiomyopathies. Arrhythmic right ventricular cardiomyopathy (ARVC), a rare autosomal recessive condition also called Naxos disease, is characterized by ventricular arrhythmias(predominantly found in the right ventricle) and with SCD [41]. While mutations in PKP2 appear to be the most common in ARVC, additional desmosomal protein mutations are found in patients with this disorder [42]. Indeed, mutations in the gene encoding PG, also known as junction PG or gamma (γ)-catenin, have also been reported [43]. Notably, PG was the first component of the desmosome to be implicated in the pathogenesis of Naxos disease [43], and cardiac-specific loss of PG leads to arrhythmogenic cardiomyopathy and activation of β-catenin/Wnt signaling in the heart [43].

It has been postulated that myocardial canonical Wnt signaling is an important regulator of atrioventricular canal maturation and electric programming [44]. Specifically, in the absence of Wnt-signals, β-catenin is targeted for ubiquitination and proteasomal degradation through the β-TrCP pathway, a consequence of its phosphorylation by casein kinase 1 (CK1) and the APC/Axin/GSK-3β-complex [45] (Fig. 8.7). In the presence of Wnt ligand, however, the co-receptor lipoprotein receptor-related protein (LRP) is brought in complex with Wnt-bound Frizzled, leading to activation of Dishevelled (Dvl) by sequential phosphorylation, polyubiquitination, and polymerization, and displacement of glycogen synthase kinase 3β (GSK-3β) from the axin/adenomatous polyposis coli (APC) complex through an unclear mechanism that may involve substrate trapping and/or endosome sequestration [45]. Stabilized β-catenin is then translocated to the nucleus via Rac1, where it binds to T-cell factor (TCF)/lymphoid enhancer factor (LEF), displacing co-repressors and recruiting additional co-activators to Wnt target genes [44–46] (Fig. 8.8).

PG also has the capacity to modulate Wnt-β-catenin signaling; it competes with β-catenin for binding to transcriptional co-activators TCF/LEF [47, 48]. Upon loss of PG gene expression, β-catenin is translocated to the nucleus where it can interact with TCF/LEF transcription factors and activate target genes [49]. Conversely, increased association between Cx43 and β-catenin is observed at the ID in PG-deficient hearts, and despite GJ remodeling, the PG CKO mice do not exhibit increased rates of ventricular arrhythmias or SCD [49]. Presumably, β-catenin enhances the function of the remaining GJs, thereby protecting PG CKO mice from

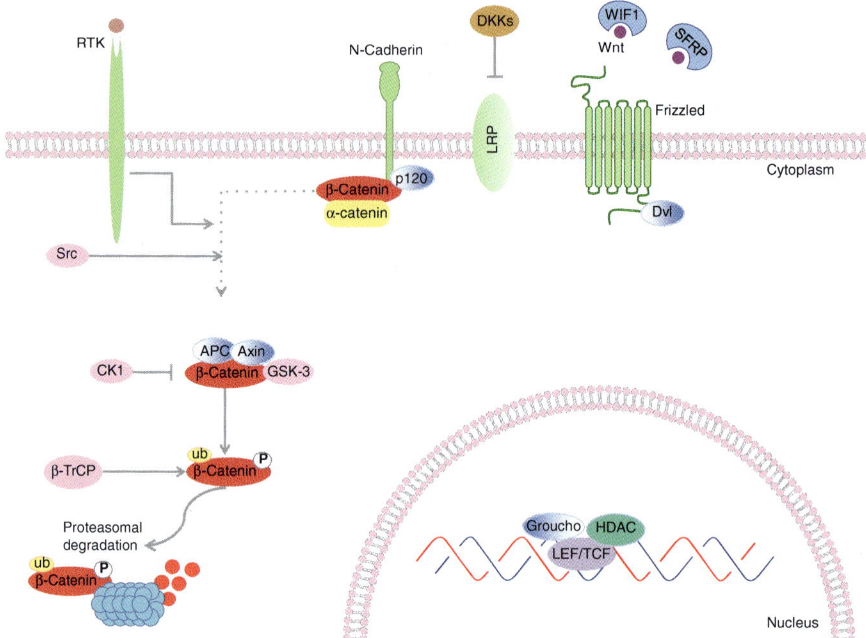

Fig. 8.7 Inhibition of Wnt signaling. In the absence of Wnt ligand, β-catenin is excluded from entering the nucleus, thereby preventing it from activating transcriptional genes required for Wnt signaling. Instead, it becomes targeted for ubiquitination and proteasomal degradation through the β-TrCP pathway. Here, β-catenin becomes phosphorylated by casein kinase 1 (CK1) and the APC/Axin/GSK-3β-complex, targeting it for ubiquitination and destruction by the proteasome

SCD. As previously mentioned, both PG and β-catenin constitute N-Cadherin binding proteins, which link the latter to the actin cytoskeleton and form a "cell adhesion zipper" [50]. To determine whether β-catenin compensates for PG loss in the heart and protects the heart from developing arrhythmias, double knockout mice (DKO) lacking both PG and beta-catenin were generated [51]. While loss of either β-catenin [52] or PG [49] alone in the adult mouse hearts was found to be insufficient to induce conduction abnormalities, deletion of both sarcoplasmic linker proteins caused disassembly of the cardiac ID and generation of lethal arrhythmias [51].

Along with alterations in AJs and desmosomes, remodeling of GJs are also implicated in arrhythmogenic cardiomyopathies [53]. Several laboratory techniques, such as immunofluorescence, immunoblotting, as well as electron microscopy, confirm the presence of markedly decreased Cx43, the major ventricular GJ protein, at the ID of CMs in patients with ARVC [53]. Since spatial heterogeneity in Cx expression is implicated in arrhythmogenesis, the degree of heterogeneity in Cx43 expression and disturbances in electric propagation were analyzed. Heterogeneous ablation of Cx43, where tissue strands are composed of <50 % wild-type (WT) Cx43 expressing cells, led to a marked decrease in propagation velocity and marked dissociation of excitation at the cellular level [53]. However, the small

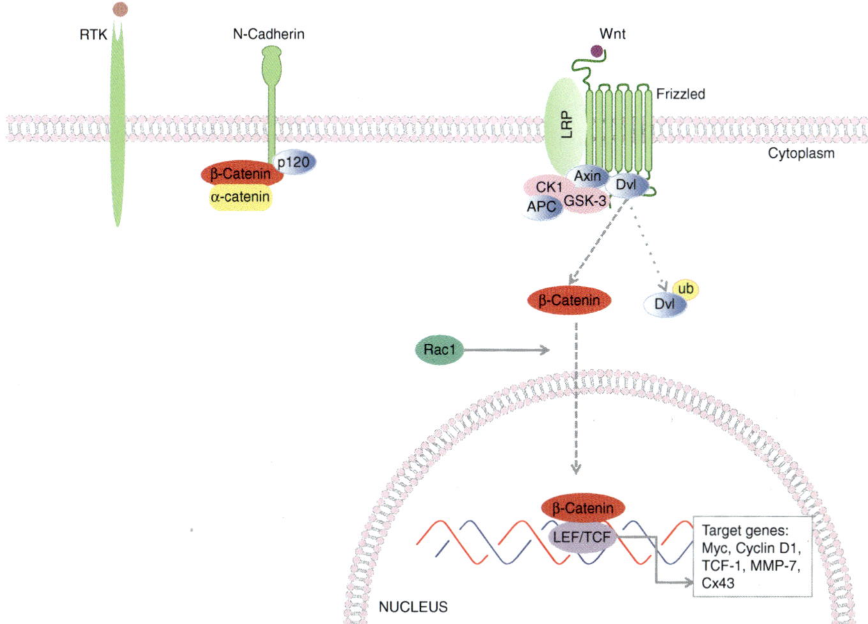

Fig. 8.8 Activation of Wnt signaling. When the Wnt ligand binds to a Frizzled family receptor and a coreceptor of the lipoprotein receptor-related protein (LRP) family, leading to activation of Dishevelled (Dvl) by sequential phosphorylation, poly-ubiquitination, and polymerization, and displacement of glycogen synthase kinase 3β (GSK-3β) from the CK1/axin/adenomatous polyposis coli (APC) complex. This leads to the stabilization of β-catenin and its translocation to the nucleus where it interacts with T-cell factor (TCF)/lymphoid enhancer factor (LEF). β-catenin binding to TCF/LEF proteins provides a transcription activation domain that mediates target gene expression activation

residual electrical conductance in WT Cx43-expressing myocytes was enough to induce excitation of the Cx43 deleted cells [53], suggesting that spatially heterogeneous downregulation of Cx43 expression did not affect overall contractility [54]. Taken together, these data suggest that, while alterations in GJs and Cxs are found in many pro-arrhythmic forms of heart disease, the mechanism(s) by which these alterations occur remain poorly understood and have yet to be determined [55, 56].

It is known that Cx43 interacts with microtubules by binding directly to tubulin [57]. Indeed, Cx-based hemi-channels are directly targeted to cell-cell borders through a pathway that is dependent on microtubules, AJ proteins (N-cadherin and β-catenin), microtubule plus-end-tracking protein (+TIP) EB1, and protein p150-Glued-, its interacting protein [58]. In addition, upon the presence of oxidative stress or ischemia-reperfusion injury, EB1-mediated connexon forward trafficking becomes limited, due to EB1 displacement, and leads to limited microtubule interaction with AJs at the ID and to reduced GJ delivery and coupling to the cell surface [59]. Moreover, a point mutation in EB1 conferring decreased affinity for tubulin also reproduced the effects of EB1 displacement and diminished connexon delivery at cell-cell junctions [59], highlighting the role of EB1 displacement in reducing cell-cell coupling. Thus, protection of the microtubule-based forward delivery of connexons may be useful in improving CM electrical coupling in order to reduce ischemia-related cardiac arrhythmias [59].

Finally, alterations in αT-catenin, which serves as a molecular integrator between AJs and desmosomes in the area composita, can also lead to hybrid adhering junction disorganization, dilated cardiomyopathy and ventricular arrhythmia following acute ischemia [60]. Specifically, deletion of αT-catenin in mouse hearts leads to a reduction of PKP2 expression at the area composita, as well as to decreased Cx43 localization at the ID of adjacent CMs and its proper localization with N-cadherin [60].

In summary, AJ and GJ remodeling play crucial roles in the maintenance of the structural and functional integrity of the myocardium. Therefore, perturbations and/or mutations in the genes encoding junctional proteins may be integral in promoting arrhythmias and SCD through their fostering of mechanical and electrical uncoupling between the adjacent CMs in the heart [22].

Structural Alterations in Hypertensive Heart Disease Results in Intercalated Disc Remodeling and Promotion of Fatal Arrhythmias

Hypertensive heart disease (HHD) is a constellation of functional and structural abnormalities that progress gradually to manifest as arrhythmias and symptomatic HF [61, 62]. In hypertensive patients, left ventricular mass (LVM) can increase either from wall thickening or chamber dilation; wall thickening occurs more commonly in response to pressure overload, and chamber dilation occurs more commonly in response to volume overload, leading to concentric and eccentric hypertrophy, respectively [63] (Fig. 8.9). Several studies indicate that the anatomical changes in the heart that occur as a consequence of HTN are responsible for the increased incidence of ventricular and supraventricular arrhythmias. Patients with HHD exhibit significant LVH, increased myocardial mass, as well as proliferation of fibrous tissue and decreased intercellular coupling, generating arrhythmogenesis [64]. About 96% of hypertensive patients suffer from arrhythmias, which is 10 times higher than the incidence observed in normotensives. Indeed, LVH, impaired left ventricular function with enlarged end-diastolic and systolic volumes, as well as late potentials, can be used to predict the incidence of complex arrhythmias, and pharmacological regression of LVH decreases its incidence [65]. Moreover, there is a significant correlation between HTN and arrhythmias, likely because LVH, systolic and diastolic dysfunction, and increased left atrial size all contribute to maladaptive GJ remodeling. Therefore, it is imperative to control high BP levels through pharmacological regression of LVH in order to improve cardiovascular morbidity and mortality [66].

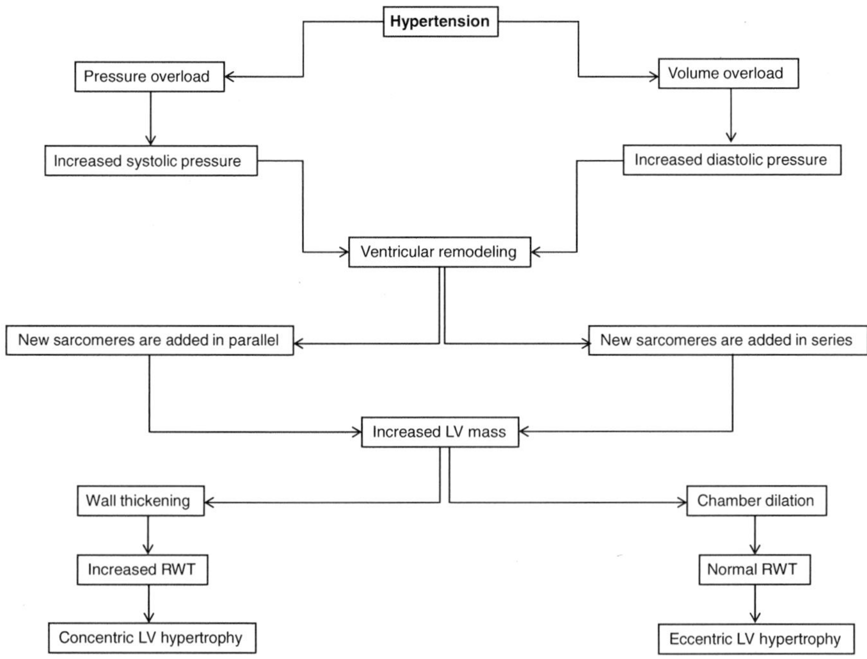

Fig. 8.9 Schematic diagram of the development of concentric and eccentric hypertrophy in hypertension. Hypertension evokes both pressure and volume overload, resulting in increased systolic and diastolic pressures, respectively. Both types of overload lead to ventricular remodeling, but pressure overload leads to the addition of sarcomeres in parallel, whereas volume overload leads to addition of sarcomeres in series. Left ventricular mass (LVM) is increased in both patterns of hypertrophy, but pressure overload leads to wall thickening and concentric left ventricular (LV) hypertrophy, whereas volume overload leads to chamber dilation and eccentric LV hypertrophy. *RWT* relative wall thickness

With increasing prevalence of HTN globally, HHD will soon be the most common cause of HF worldwide. In addition, even if patients with HHD present with LVH, they maintain a normal-sized left ventricular chamber and have preserved systolic function with an ejection fraction greater than 50 % [67]. This is in contrast to other causes of HF, such as ischemic heart disease associated with prior myocardial infarction(s) (MI), and idiopathic dilated cardiomyopathy (IDC), where an enlarged, dilated left ventricular chamber and/or right ventricular enlargement are frequently observed [67, 68]. The main pathological feature of a failing heart is cardiomyocyte hypertrophy and apoptosis along with tissue fibrosis and scarring. However, the fibrotic state is highly prevalent in HHD compared to other causes of HF, since it is found throughout the heart, including the anterior, posterior, and lateral walls of the left ventricle (LV), the interventricular septum, and even the right ventricle (RV). Fibrosis disrupts the coordination of myocardial excitation-contraction coupling in both systole and diastole by altering the composition of the major components of the cardiac extracellular matrix (ECM) (type I and type III fibrillar collagens) [69].

Along with ECM structural changes, myocardial apoptosis and changes in calcium handling associated with impaired relaxation are also observed in HHD. Importantly, there are also substantial changes in the peripheral vasculature (especially resistance vessels) that impair cardiac function [70]. Initially, it would be reasonable to think of LVH as a compensatory mechanism to allow the heart to withstand the hemodynamic strain associated with increased arterial pressure. However, the continued presence of LVH leads to cardiac dysfunction manifested as a reduction of coronary flow reserve, tissue ischemia, development of arrhythmias, heart failure, and sudden death [71]. Transition from compensated LVH to HF is associated with ECM degradation. Since the ECM network ensures tissue strength and allows cell-cell contact between neighboring cells, changes in the collagen network present in HHD impair both systolic and diastolic function [71].

Interestingly, the transition of cardiac fibroblasts to myofibroblasts is an early event that takes place in HHD [72, 73]. Recently, fibrotic state in HHD was shown to be marked by changes in the balance between matrix metalloproteinases (MMPs) and their inhibitors, which alter the composition of the ECM and impair cardiomyocyte function [74]. Specifically, myofibroblasts produce a different ECM than fibroblasts and modify the balance of MMPs and their inhibitors (tissue inhibitors of metalloproteinases [TIMPs]) to promote fibrosis [74]. Altered ECM composition modifies the signals that cardiac myocytes receive from their scaffolding environment, resulting in changes in gene expression associated with hypertrophy and contractile dysfunction. Finally, smooth muscle cells, monocytes, and fibroblasts are recruited by the activated renin-angiotensin-aldosterone system (RAAS) and increased levels of activated transforming growth factor (TGF)-β1 to stimulate a genetic program of wound repair and ECM deposition, leading to perivascular fibrosis and amplification of the profibrotic state [74]. Consequently, therapies targeting the expression, synthesis, or activation of the enzymes responsible for ECM homeostasis might represent novel opportunities to modify the natural progression of HHD.

The changes in cardiac tissue architecture observed in HHD such as LVH, cardiac fiber disarray, increased cardiomyocyte size and fibrosis, constitute what is known as passive ventricular remodeling, which also includes molecular remodeling of GJs [75]. As the heart is a rather heterogeneous organ, all alterations also appear heterogeneously. Thus, GJs composed of Cx43 proteins, found primarily in cardiac ventricles, are particularly affected, as are the Na^+ channels that modify cardiac depolarization [76]. The result of these changes is abnormal electrical and mechanical coupling throughout the heart in terms of irregularity and heterogeneity [76]. HHD progresses and deteriorates HF symptoms, and the heart becomes predisposed to reentry arrhythmias that can prove to be fatal [77–79]. In both animal and human studies, LVH was found to be associated with accentuated conduction delay and altered repolarization during myocardial ischemia, accompanied also by increased vulnerability to arrhythmias and sudden death [31, 80]. Moreover, the increased cell size observed in hypertrophic cardiomyopathy (HCM) seems to be the predominant factor that affects conduction velocity of the electrical impulse [31]. Importantly, in a rat model with monocrotaline (MCT)-induced right ventricular failure, the LV exhibited electrophysiologic remodeling with longer action potentials (at 90 % repolarization), prolonged effective refractory period, and slowing of the longitudinal conduction velocity [81]. As mentioned, the main feature of HHD is the interstitial (in between the individual cells) and diffused fibrosis, which apart from the phenotypical switch from fibroblasts to myofibroblasts, can also be caused by mutations, changes in gene expression, as well as aging [82]. The increased interstitial collagen reduces compliance and leads to irregular electrical coupling, predisposing the patient to arrhythmias and HF [72, 83]. Even though diffuse and patch fibrosis have been shown to be comparable, the short collagen strands associated with the former only marginally affect conduction curves, and is thus thought to be less arrhythmogenic [84].

Increased interstitial fibrosis has been reported in patients with HCM, as well as in mice suffering from hypertrophy induced by chronic pressure-overload [85–87]. Moreover, myocardial disarray is one of the hallmarks of HCM [88]. Passive ventricular remodeling has been described in all forms of heart disease; HCM, DCM, Ischemic Cardiomyopathy (ICM), and Arrhythmogenic Cardiomyopathy (ACM), where a reduction in ventricular Cx43, localized at the ID has been found [89, 90]. Interestingly, an increase in Cx43 expression together with lateralization is observed at the initial stages of HCM, whereas the same protein is found decreased and heterogeneously distributed in later stages [91]. Other studies describe altered Cx43 gene expression without lateralization, and vice versa [92, 93]. Similarly, animal models confirmed some of the observed changes in human heart [38, 94, 95].

Ca^{2+} calmodulin kinase II (CaMKII) expression is also increased in HF. Altered Na^+ channel gating is linked to and may promote VTs in HF. Calmodulin regulates Na^+ channel gating, in part perhaps via phosphorylation by CaMKII, which is associated with a delayed inactivation of the current [96, 97]. This can lead to prolonged repolarization, increased action potential duration and propensity to arrhythmias [97]. Furthermore, it has been shown that in mice with cardiac hypertrophy mediated by calcineurin-A (CaN), reduced Nav1.5 protein expression could be found at the ID [98]. To our knowledge, chronic RAAS inhibition, by eplerenone (an aldosterone antagonist) and losartan (an ARB), limit aging-related interstitial fibrosis, resulting in lower arrhythmogenicity of treated mice. This directly correlates with reduced amounts of patchy fibrosis, the abundance of which induces arrhythmias [99].

In addition, spontaneously hypertensive rats (SHR) or hypertension induced 12-week-old Wistar rats also have abnormal electrical coupling at the GJs that precedes the development of fatal arrhythmias [100]. Permanent changes in GJ distribution (remodeling of GJs) usually results from chronic pathophysiological stimuli such as HTN, diabetes mellitus and ischemia, whereas temporary alterations are usually driven by acute pathophysiological conditions, such as hypokalemia and ischemia/reperfusion injury [100]. Electrical uncoupling can thus lead to malignant arrhythmias through a reentry mechanism. There is no doubt that alterations in GJs can be implicated in the development of fatal arrhythmias and as such, might be promising targets to prevent or attenuate the incidence of lethal events in patients with HHD and hypertrophy [100].

Treatment Options for Hypertensives with Cardiac Disease

Both atrial and ventricular arrhythmias are a common comorbidity in hypertensive patients, and LVH, myocardial ischemia, left atrial enlargement and impaired left ventricular function are considered to be some of the main mechanisms involved in this association. However, ventricular arrhythmias are more common and, when occur, can be lethal (Fig. 8.10). Clinicians have thus suggested a variety of treatment options based on the type of arrhythmia that the hypertensive patient exhibits [101]. Importantly, a strong association between atrial fibrillation (AF), the most common type of arrhythmia, and HTN has been found. Therefore, prevention of AF in patients with HTN is highly dependent on strict BP control in order to reduce the risk of developing hypertensive cardiomyopathy. LVH and atrial enlargement can be reversed by the use of antihypertensive medications, particularly ACE inhibitors and ARBs, which may directly reduce the recurrence of AF [102, 103].

Sudden death in HTN is attributed to increased incidence of ventricular arrhythmias [104]. Beta-blockers (BBs) and amiodarone (class III antiarrhythmic) are

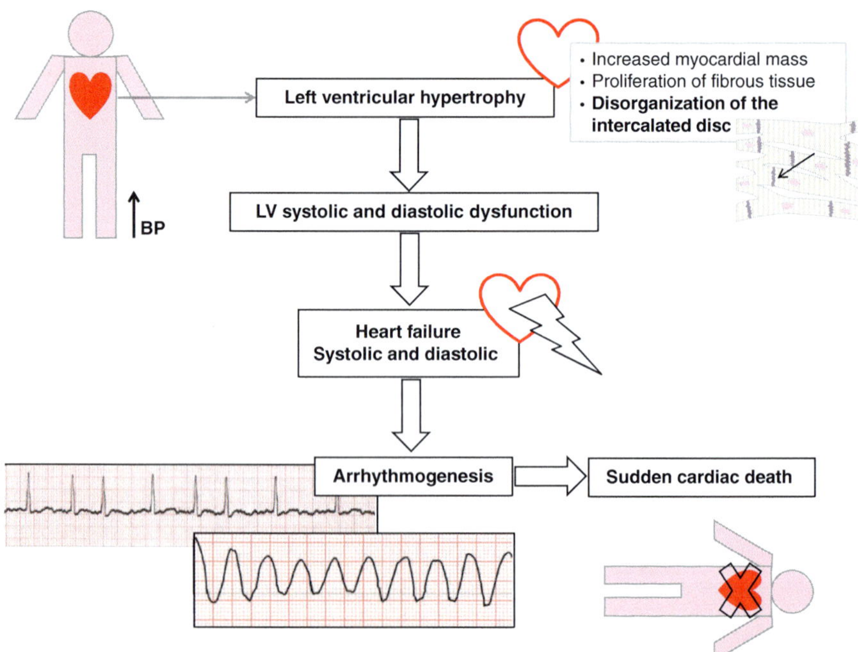

Fig. 8.10 Schematic diagram for the progression of hypertension to arrhythmogenesis and sudden cardiac death. Spontaneous arrhythmogenesis induced by left ventricular hypertrophy (LVH) and structural changes in myocardial architecture that take place in the hypertensive heart may lead to sudden death

considered to be the drugs of choice in ventricular arrhythmia. In addition, calcium channel blockers (CCBs) and ACEI$_s$ have been shown to be effective in the management of ventricular arrhythmias due to their action against LVH [105, 106]. Spironolactone may also be prescribed in hypertensive patients with ventricular arrhythmias first line therapy, because of its ability to reverse hypokalemia and secondly, due to its antifibrotic action in the ventricular myocardium [107]. Ultimately, in severe ventricular arrhythmias refractory to antihypertensive medications, an automatic implantable cardioverter defibrillator should be considered [101].

Finally, several non-invasive electrocardiographic parameters have been defined and widely investigated to identify the hypertensive patient at risk for the development of arrhythmias. A relationship between p wave duration and p wave dispersion and supraventricular arrhythmias has been suggested, and p-wave dispersion may now serve as a new marker for the prediction of AF [12]. In contrast, QT interval dispersion, QT interval dynamicity, late potentials, heart rate variability, T wave morphology analysis (T wave duration/angle), and T wave alternans, have been associated with the occurrence of ventricular arrhythmias [12]. The development of LVH in hypertensive patients appears to be the main link between HTN and the development of ventricular arrhythmias, and in addition to the degree of hypertrophy, may be more important than its presence in arrhythmogenesis in hypertensive patients [108, 109]. The use of antiarrhythmic medications is unclear in the setting of HTN, due to side effect profiles and anti-arrhythmic properties which may worsen patient life expectancies. Indeed, use of appropriate antihypertensive drugs offers optimal control of high BP and, at the same time, proves effective in controlling arrhythmias. Decreased atrial and ventricular ectopy may play a critical role in this association, conferring concurrently less side effects compared to antiarrhythmic therapy [109].

Summary

Taken together, it is clear that further research is needed to unravel the relationships between the various ID structural alterations, the remodeling of the heart, and the onset of arrhythmias. It is now clear, however, that progression of HHD to LVH and HF increases the propensity of arrhythmias due to maladaptive ID remodeling and increased fibrosis, causing impairment of the electrical impulses needed for normal cardiomyocyte function. This pathological process may be reversed by use of antihypertensive therapy and strict control of BP levels. However, further research is needed to highlight important concepts regarding the signaling cascades involved and to bring to light more promising and novel therapeutic molecular targets.

References

1. Lawes CM, Vander Hoorn S, Law MR, Elliott P, MacMahon S, Rodgers A. Blood pressure and the global burden of disease 2000. Part I: Estimates of blood pressure levels. J Hypertens. 2006;24:413–22.
2. Lawes CM, Vander Hoorn S, Law MR, Elliott P, MacMahon S, Rodgers A. Blood pressure and the global burden of disease 2000. Part II: Estimates of attributable burden. J Hypertens. 2006;24:423–30.
3. Kearney PM, Whelton M, Reynolds K, Whelton PK, He J. Global burden of hypertension: analysis of worldwide data. Lancet. 2005;365:217–23.
4. Tibazarwa KB, et al. Hypertension in developing countries. Can J Cardiol. 2014;30(5):527–33.
5. Antikainen RL, Moltchanov VA, Chukwuma Sr C, et al. WHO MONICA Project. Trends in the prevalence, awareness, treatment and control of hypertension: The WHO MONICA Project. Eur J Cardiovasc Prev Rehabil. 2006;13:13–29.
6. Le Heuzey JY, Guize L. Cardiac prognosis in hypertensive patients. Am J Med. 1988;84(Suppl 1B):65–8.
7. Go AS, Mozaffarian D, Roger VL, Benjamin EJ, Berry JD, Blaha MJ, American Heart Association Statistics Committee and Stroke Statistics Subcommittee, et al. Heart disease and stroke statistics—2014 update: a report from the American Heart Association. Circulation. 2014;129(3):e28–292.
8. Chockalingam A, Campbell NR, Fodor JG. Worldwide epidemic of hypertension. Can J Cardiol. 2006;22(7):553–5.
9. Almendral J, Villacastin JP, Arenal A, Tercedor L, Merino JL, Delcan JL. Evidence favoring the hypothesis that ventricular arrhythmias have prognostic significance in left ventricular hypertrophy secondary to systemic hypertension. Am J Cardiol. 1995;76:60D–3.
10. Messerli FH, Grodzicki T. Hypertension, left ventricular hypertrophy, ventricular arrhythmias and sudden death. Eur Heart J. 1992;13(Suppl D):66–9.
11. Ormaetxe JM, Alday JDM, Beobide MA, Iriarte M. Prognostic significance of ventricular arrhythmias in the presence of pathological left ventricular hypertrophy. Eur Heart J. 1993;14(Suppl J):73–5.
12. Yildirir A, Batur MK, Oto A. Hypertension and arrhythmia: blood pressure control and beyond. Europace. 2002;4(2):175–82.
13. Cabin HS, Henry S. The heart and circulation. Yale University School of Medicine heart book. New York: Hearst Books; 1992. p. 5.
14. Fukuta H, Little WC. The cardiac cycle and the physiologic basis of left ventricular contraction, ejection, relaxation, and filling. Heart Fail Clin. 2008;4(1):1–11.
15. Sheikh F, Ross RS, Chen J. Cell-cell connection to cardiac disease. Trends Cardiovasc Med. 2009;19:182–90.
16. Rapila R, Korhonen T, Tavi P. Excitation-contraction coupling of the mouse embryonic cardiomyocyte. J Gen Physiol. 2008;132(4):397–405.
17. Greenstein JL, Winslow RL. Integrative systems models of cardiac excitation-contraction coupling. Circ Res. 2011;108(1):70–84.
18. Bootman MD, et al. Calcium signalling during excitation-contraction coupling in mammalian atrial myocytes. J Cell Sci. 2006;119(Pt 19):3915–25.
19. McDowell SA, et al. Phosphoinositide 3-kinase regulates excitation-contraction coupling in neonatal cardiomyocytes. Am J Physiol Heart Circ Physiol. 2004;286(2):H796–805.
20. Kontaridis MI, Geladari EV, Geladari CV. Role of the SHP2 Protein Tyrosine Phosphatase in Cardiac Metabolism. In: Bence KK, editor. Protein tyrosine phosphatase control of metabolism. New York: Springer; 2013. p. 147–67.
21. Bennett PM, et al. The transitional junction: a new functional subcellular domain at the intercalated disc. Mol Biol Cell. 2006;17:2091–100.
22. Mezzano V, Sheikh F. Cell–cell junction remodeling in the heart: possible role in cardiac conduction system function and arrhythmias? Life Sci. 2012;90(9–10):313–21. doi:10.1016/j.lfs.2011.12.009.

23. Ackermann MA, Kontrogianni-Konstantopoulos A, Li-Yen R Hu. Intercellular connections in the heart: the intercalated disc. INTECH Open Access Publisher. 2012.
24. Gutstein David E, et al. The organization of adherens junctions and desmosomes at the cardiac intercalated disc is independent of gap junctions. J Cell Sci. 2003;116(5):875–85.
25. Franke WW, Borrmann CM, Grund C, Pieperhoff S. The area composita of adhering junctions connecting heart muscle cells of vertebrates. I. Molecular definition in inter- calated disks of cardiomyocytes by immunoelectron microscopy of desmosomal proteins. Eur J Cell Biol. 2006;85:69–82.
26. Saito M, Tucker DK, Kohlhorst D, Niessen CM, Kowalczyk AP. Classical and desmosomal cadherins at a glance. J Cell Sci. 2012;125(11):2547–52.
27. Thomason HA, Scothern A, McHarg S, Garrod DR. Desmosomes: adhesive strength and signalling in health and disease. Biochem J. 2010;429(3):419–33.
28. Willecke K, Eiberger J, Degen J, et al. Structural and functional diversity of connexin genes in the mouse and human genome. Biol Chem. 2002;383:725–37.
29. Bruzzone R, White TW, Paul DL. Connections with connexins: the molecular basis of direct intercellular signaling. Eur J Biochem. 1996;238:1–27.
30. Giepmans BNG. Gap junctions and connexin-interacting proteins. Cardiovasc Res. 2004;62(2):233–45.
31. Spach MS, Heidlage JF, Dolber PC, Barr RC. Electrophysiological effects of remodeling cardiac gap junctions and cell size: experimental and model studies of normal cardiac growth. Circ Res. 2000;86:302–11.
32. Pieperhoff S, Borrmann C, Grund C, Barth M, Rizzo S, Franke WW. The area composita of adhering junctions connecting heart muscle cells of vertebrates. VII. The different types of lateral junctions between the special cardiomyocytes of the conduction system of ovine and bovine hearts. Eur J Cell Biol. 2010;89(5):365–78.
33. Goossens S, et al. A unique and specific interaction between αT-catenin and plakophilin-2 in the area composita, the mixed-type junctional structure of cardiac intercalated discs. J Cell Sci. 2007;120(12):2126–36.
34. Drees F, et al. α-catenin is a molecular switch that binds E-cadherin-β-catenin and regulates actin-filament assembly. Cell. 2005;123(5):903–15.
35. Yamada S, et al. Deconstructing the cadherin-catenin-actin complex. Cell. 2005;123(5): 889–901.
36. Pieperhoff S, Schumacher H, Franke WW. The area composita of adhering junctions connecting heart muscle cells of vertebrates. V. The importance of plakophilin-2 demonstrated by small interference RNA-mediated knockdown in cultured rat cardiomyocytes. Eur J Cell Biol. 2008;87:399–411.
37. Bennett PM. From myofibril to membrane; the transitional junction at the intercalated disc. Front biosci (Landmark ed). 2011;17:1035–50.
38. Yoshida M, et al. Alterations in adhesion junction precede gap junction remodelling during the development of heart failure in cardiomyopathic hamsters. Cardiovasc Res. 2011;92(1):95–105.
39. Li J, et al. Cardiac-specific loss of N-cadherin leads to alteration in connexins with conduction slowing and arrhythmogenesis. Circ Res. 2005;97(5):474–81.
40. Cheng L, et al. Cortactin is required for N-cadherin regulation of Kv1. 5 channel function. J Biol Chem. 2011;286(23):20478–89.
41. Saffitz JE. The pathobiology of arrhythmogenic cardiomyopathy. Annu Rev Pathol. 2011;6:299–321.
42. Saffitz JE. Desmosome mutations in arrhythmogenic right ventricular cardiomyopathy important insight but only part of the picture. Circ Cardiovasc Genet. 2009;2(5):415–7.
43. Protonotarios N, et al. Cardiac abnormalities in familial palmoplantar keratosis. Br Heart J. 1986;56(4):321–6.
44. Gillers BS, et al. Canonical wnt signaling regulates atrioventricular junction programming and electrophysiological properties. Circ Res. 2015;116:398–406.
45. Komiya Y, Habas R. Wnt signal transduction pathways. Organogenesis. 2008;4:68–75.
46. MacDonald BT, Tamai K, He X. Wnt/β-catenin signaling: components, mechanisms, and diseases. Dev Cell. 2009;17:9–26.

47. Garcia-Gras E, et al. Suppression of canonical Wnt/β-catenin signaling by nuclear plakoglobin recapitulates phenotype of arrhythmogenic right ventricular cardiomyopathy. J Clin Invest. 2006;116(7):2012.
48. Lombardi R, et al. Genetic fate mapping identifies second heart field progenitor cells as a source of adipocytes in arrhythmogenic right ventricular cardiomyopathy. Circ Res. 2009;104(9):1076–84.
49. Li J, et al. Cardiac tissue-restricted deletion of plakoglobin results in progressive cardiomyopathy and activation of β-catenin signaling. Mol Cell Biol. 2011;31(6):1134–44.
50. Shapiro L, et al. Structural basis of cell-cell adhesion by cadherins. Nature. 1995;374:327–37.
51. Swope D, et al. Loss of cadherin-binding proteins β-catenin and plakoglobin in the heart leads to gap junction remodeling and arrhythmogenesis. Mol Cell Biol. 2012;32(6):1056–67.
52. Zhou J, et al. Upregulation of gamma-catenin compensates for the loss of beta-catenin in adult cardiomyocytes. Am J Physiol Heart Circ Physiol. 2007;292:H270–6.
53. Asimaki A, Saffitz JE. Gap junctions and arrhythmogenic cardiomyopathy. Heart Rhythm. 2012;9(6):992–5.
54. Beauchamp P, et al. Electrical coupling and propagation in engineered ventricular myocardium with heterogeneous expression of connexin43. Circ Res. 2012;110(11):1445–53.
55. Severs NJ, et al. Remodelling of gap junctions and connexin expression in heart disease. Biochim Biophys Acta (BBA)-Biomembranes. 2004;1662(1):138–48.
56. Severs NJ, et al. Gap junction alterations in human cardiac disease. Cardiovasc Res. 2004;62(2):368–77.
57. Giepmans BNG, et al. Gap junction protein connexin-43 interacts directly with microtubules. Curr Biol. 2001;11(17):1364–8.
58. Shaw RM, et al. Microtubule plus-end-tracking proteins target gap junctions directly from the cell interior to adherens junctions. Cell. 2007;128(3):547–60.
59. Smyth JW, et al. Limited forward trafficking of connexin 43 reduces cell-cell coupling in stressed human and mouse myocardium. J Clin Invest. 2010;120(1):266.
60. Li J, et al. Loss of αT-catenin alters the hybrid adhering junctions in the heart and leads to dilated cardiomyopathy and ventricular arrhythmia following acute ischemia. J Cell Sci. 2012;125(4):1058–67.
61. Pavlopoulos H, Nihoyannopoulos P. The constellation of hypertensive heart disease. Hellenic J Cardiol. 2008;49(2):92–9.
62. Drazner MH. The progression of hypertensive heart disease. Circulation. 2011;123(3):327–34.
63. Ganau A, et al. Patterns of left ventricular hypertrophy and geometric remodeling in essential hypertension. J Am Coll Cardiol. 1992;19(7):1550–8.
64. Aidietis A, Laucevicius A, Marinskis G. Hypertension and cardiac arrhythmias. Curr Pharm Des. 2007;13:2545–55.
65. Perings C, Hennersdorf M, Vester EG, Strauer BE. Arrhythmia risk in left ventricular hypertrophy. Z Kardiol. 2000;89 Suppl 3:36–43.
66. Sultana R, et al. Cardiac arrhythmias and left ventricular hypertrophy in systemic hypertension. J Ayub Med Coll Abbottabad. 2010;22(4):155–8.
67. Zile MR, Brutsaert DL. New concepts in diastolic dysfunction and diastolic heart failure: part II: causal mechanisms and treatment. Circulation. 2002;105:1503–8.
68. Zile MR, Brutsaert DL. New concepts in diastolic dysfunction and diastolic heart failure: part I: diagnosis, prognosis, and measurements of diastolic function. Circulation. 2002;105:1387–93.
69. Shirwany A, Weber KT. Extracellular matrix remodeling in hypertensive heart disease. J Am Coll Cardiol. 2006;48:97–8.
70. Gandhi SK, et al. The pathogenesis of acute pulmonary edema associated with hypertension. N Engl J Med. 2001;344:17–22.
71. Diez J, Lopez B, Gonzalez A, Querejeta R. Clinical aspects of hypertensive myocardial fibrosis. Curr Opin Cardiol. 2001;16:328–35.
72. Janicki JS, Brower GL. The role of myocardial fibrillar collagen in ventricular remodeling and function. J Card Fail. 2002;8 Suppl 6:S319–25.

73. Davis J, Molketin JD. Myofibroblasts: trust your heart and let fate decide. J Mol Cell Cardiol. 2013;70:9–18.
74. Berk BC, Fujiwara K, Lehoux S. ECM remodeling in hypertensive heart disease. J Clin Invest. 2007;117(3):568.
75. Kessler EL, et al. Passive ventricular remodeling in cardiac disease: focus on heterogeneity. Front physiol. 2014;5:482.
76. Kleber AG, Rudy Y. Basic mechanisms of cardiac impulse propagation and associated arrhythmias. Physiol Rev. 2004;84:431–88.
77. Bowers SL, Borg TK, Baudino TA. The dynamics of fibroblast- myocyte-capillary interactions in the heart. Ann N Y Acad Sci. 2010;1188:143–52.
78. van Rijen HV, van Veen TA, Gros D, Wilders R, de Bakker JM. Connexins and cardiac arrhythmias. Adv Cardiol. 2006;42:150–60.
79. Winterton SJ, Turner MA, O'Gorman DJ, Flores NA, Sheridan DJ. Hypertrophy causes delayed conduction in human and guinea pig myocardium: accentuation during ischaemic perfusion. Cardiovasc Res. 1994;28:47–54.
80. Meyerburg RJ, Kessler KM, Castellanos A. Sudden cardiac death. Structure, function, and time-dependence of risk. Circulation. 1992;85(1 Suppl):I2–10.
81. Hardziyenka M, Campian ME, Verkerk AO, Surie S, van Ginneken AC, Hakim S, et al. Electrophysiologic remodeling of the left ventricle in pressure overload-induced right ventricular failure. J Am Coll Cardiol. 2012;59:2193–202.
82. Biernacka A, Frangogiannis NG. Aging and cardiac fibrosis. Aging Dis. 2011;2:158–73.
83. Rohr S. Myofibroblasts in diseased hearts: new players in cardiac arrhythmias. Heart Rhythm. 2009;6:848–56.
84. Kawara T, Derksen R, de Groot JR, Coronel R, Tasseron S, Linnenbank AC, et al. Activation delay after premature stimulation in chronically diseased human myocardium relates to the architecture of interstitial fibrosis. Circulation. 2001;104:3069–75.
85. Swynghedauw B. Molecular mechanisms of myocardial remodeling. Physiol Rev. 1999;79:215–62.
86. Boulaksil M, Noorman M, Engelen MA, van Veen TA, Vos MA, de Bakker JM, et al. Longitudinal arrhythmogenic remodelling in a mouse model of longstanding pressure overload. Neth Heart J. 2010;18:509–15.
87. Xia Y, Lee K, Li N, Corbett D, Mendoza L, Frangogiannis NG. Characterization of the inflammatory and fibrotic response in a mouse model of cardiac pressure overload. Histochem Cell Biol. 2009;131:471–81.
88. Hughes SE. The pathology of hypertrophic cardiomyopathy. Histopathology. 2004;44:412–27.
89. DuPont E, Matsushita T, Kaba RA, Vozzi C, Coppen SR, Khan N, et al. Altered connexin expression in human congestive heart failure. J Mol Cell Cardiol. 2001;33:359–71.
90. Kaplan SR, Gard JJ, Protonotarios N, Tsatsopoulou A, Spiliopoulou C, Anastasakis A, et al. Remodeling of myocyte gap junctions in arrhythmogenic right ventricular cardiomyopathy due to a deletion in plakoglobin (Naxos disease). Heart Rhythm. 2004;1:3–11.
91. Kostin S, Rieger M, Dammer S, Hein S, Richter M, Klövekorn WP, et al. Gap junction remodeling and altered connexin43 expression in the failing human heart. Mol Cell Biochem. 2003;242:135–44.
92. Peters NS, Green CR, Poole-Wilson PA, Severs NJ. Reduced content of connexin43 gap junctions in ventricular myocardium from hypertrophied and ischemic human hearts. Circulation. 1993;88:864–75.
93. Sepp R, Severs NJ, Gourdie RG. Altered patterns of cardiac intercellular junction distribution in hypertrophic cardiomyopathy. Heart. 1996;76:412–7.
94. Ambra R, Di Nardo P, Fantini C, Minieri M, Canali R, Natella F, et al. Selective changes in DNA binding activity of transcription factors in UM- X7.1 cardiomyopathic hamsters. Life Sci. 2002;71:2369–81.
95. Sato PY, Ohkusa T, Honjo H, Suzuki S, Yoshida MA, Ishiguro YS, et al. Altered expression of connexin43 contributes to the arrhyth-mogenic substrate during the development of heart failure in cardiomyopatic hamster. Am J Physiol Heart Circ. 2008;294:H1164–73.

96. Wagner S, Dybkova N, Rasenack EC, Jacobshagen C, Fabritz L, Kirchhof P, et al. Ca2+/calmodulin-dependent protein kinase II regulates cardiac Na^+ channels. J Clin Invest. 2006;116:3127–38.
97. Coppini R, Ferrantini C, Yao L, Fan P, Del Lungo M, Stillitano F, et al. Late sodium current inhibition reverses electromechanical dysfunction in human hypertrophic cardiomyopathy. Circulation. 2013;127:575–84.
98. Bierhuizen MF, Boulaksil M, van Stuijvenberg L, van der Nagel R, Jansen AT, Mutsaers NA, et al. In calcineurin-induced cardiac hypertrophy expression of Nav1.5, Cx40 and Cx43 is reduced by different mechanisms. J Mol Cell Cardiol. 2008;45:373–84.
99. Stein M, Boulaksil M, Jansen JA, Herold E, Noorman M, Joles JA, et al. Reduction of fibrosis-related arrhythmias by chronic renin-angiotensin- aldosterone system inhibitors in an aged mouse model. Am J Physiol Heart Circ Physiol. 2010;299:310–21.
100. Fialová M, et al. Adaptation of the heart to hypertension is associated with maladaptive gap junction connexin-43 remodeling. Physiol Res. 2008;57(1):7.
101. Bagueta J-P, Erdineb S, Malliona J-M. Hypertension and arrhythmia. ESH Update Hypertens manag. 2005;6:24.
102. Schmieder RE, Schlaich MP, Klingbeil AU, Martus P. Update on reversal of left ventricular hypertrophy in essential hypertension (a meta-analysis of all randomized double-blind studies until December 1996). Nephrol Dial Transplant. 1998;13:564–9.
103. Gottdiener JS, Reda DJ, Williams DW, Materson BJ, Cushman W, Anderson RJ. Effect of single-drug therapy on reduction of left atrial size in mild to moderate hypertension: comparison of six antihypertensive agents. Circulation. 1998;98:140–8.
104. Bayès de Luna A, Coumel PH, Leclercq JE. Ambulatory sudden death: mechanisms of production of fatal arrhythmias on the basis of data from 157 cases. Am Heart J. 1989;117:154–9.
105. Malerba M, Muiesan ML, Zulli R, Rizzoni D, Calebich S, Agabiti-Rosei E. Ventricular arrhythmias and changes in blood pressure and left ventricular mass induced by antihypertensive treatment in hypertensive patients. J Hypertens. 1991;9 suppl 6:S162–3.
106. Messerli FH, Nunez BD, Nunez MM, Caravaglia GE. Hypertension and sudden death. Disparate effects of calcium entry blocker and diuretic therapy on cardiac dysrhythmias. Arch Intern Med. 1989;149:1263–7.
107. Aytemir K, Ozer N, Atalar E, et al. P wave dispersion on 12-lead electrocardiogram in patients with paroxysmal atrial fibrillation. Pacing Clin Electrophysiol. 2000;23:1109–12.
108. Ghali JK, Kadakia S, Cooper RS, Liano YL. Impact of left ventricular hypertrophy on ventricular arrhythmias in the absence of coronary artery disease. J Am Coll Cardiol. 1991;17:1277–82.
109. Dunn FG, Oigman W, Sungaard-Riise K, et al. Racial differences in cardiac adaptation to essential hypertension determined by echocardiographic indexes. J Am Coll Cardiol. 1983;1:1348–51.

Chapter 9
Prevention and Treatment of Atrial Fibrillation in Patients with Hypertension

Sverre E. Kjeldsen, Tonje A. Aksnes, Serap E. Erdine, and Athanasios J. Manolis

Introduction

Hypertension is the most common cardiovascular disorder affecting up to 50 % of the adult population [1] with a prevalence rising steeply after the age of 50. Atrial fibrillation (AF) is the most common cardiac arrhythmia with a prevalence of 1–2 %, estimated to at least double in the next 50 years as the population ages [2]. We aimed to describe in more detail the pathophysiological rationale for the coexistence of hypertension and AF and review the effect of various drugs for antihypertensive treatment.

Epidemiology

There are many risk factors for AF, some modifiable and some not (Fig. 9.1). Hypertension increases the risk of AF by about twofold [3], but due to the high prevalence of hypertension in the population, hypertension accounts for more cases of AF than any other risk factor. Hypertension and AF increase the risk of cardiovascular disease, and hypertension commonly coexists with many conditions

---

S.E. Kjeldsen, M.D., Ph.D., FAHA, FESC (✉) • T.A. Aksnes, M.D., Ph.D.
Department of Cardiology, Oslo University Hospital Ullevaal,
Kirkeveien 166, Oslo N-0407, Norway
e-mail: sverrkj@online.no; s.e.kjeldsen@medisin.uio.no; tonjeaksnes@hotmail.com

S.E. Erdine, M.D.
Department of Cardiology, Istanbul University Cerrhpa, School of Medicine, Istanbul, Turkey
e-mail: serap.erdine@gmail.com

A.J. Manolis, M.D., FESC, FACC, FAHA
Department of Cardiology, Asklepeion General Hospital, Athens, Greece
e-mail: ajmanol@otenet.gr

E.A. Andreadis (ed.), *Hypertension and Cardiovascular Disease*,
DOI 10.1007/978-3-319-39599-9_9

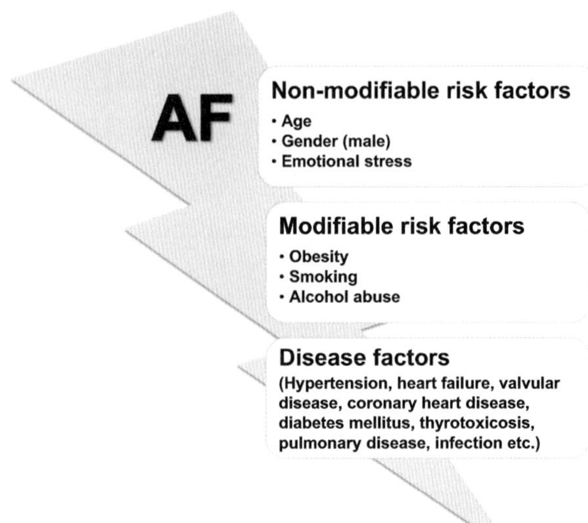

Fig. 9.1 Risk factors for atrial fibrillation

Fig. 9.2 Hypertension (*BT*) and atrial fibrillation (*AF*) are both risk factors for cardiovascular disease (*CVD*)

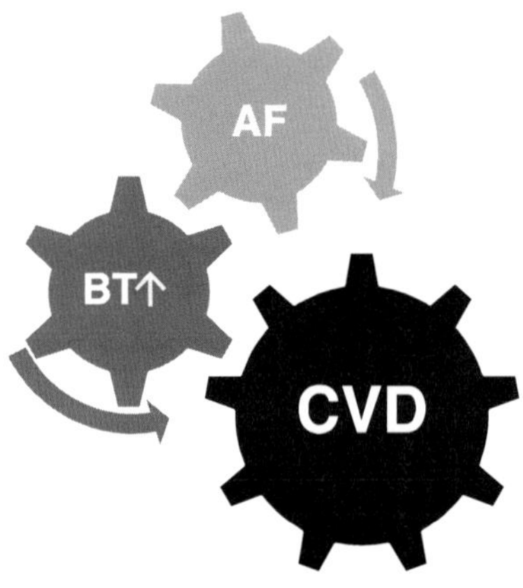

associated with AF, namely in 60–80 % of patients with stroke, chronic kidney disease, diabetes, coronary artery disease, heart failure, and metabolic syndrome [4] (Fig. 9.2). Long-standing hypertension leads to left ventricular hypertrophy, structural changes and enlargement of the left atrium, heterogeneity of atrial conduction, and fibrosis [5], all of which may contribute to the development of AF [6–9] and these conditions accelerate if hypertension is poorly controlled.

Hypertension was reported in up to 90 % of patients with AF who participated in major clinical trials [10]. Further, progression of renal dysfunction is a powerful predictor of new-onset AF in hypertensive patients, independently of left ventricular hypertrophy and left atrial dilatation [11].

In the early stages the presence of multiple risk factors like hypertension, diabetes and obesity predispose patients to AF [12, 13]. However, the development of subclinical and clinical organ damage not only predisposes patients to AF, but the presence of AF may in turn increase the risk of cardiovascular disease. In a subanalysis from the Action in Diabetes and Vascular Disease (ADVANCE) study, in which 75 % were taking antihypertensive treatment with 4.3 years of follow-up, patients with diabetes and AF were at 61 % increased risk for all-cause mortality and had similarly higher risks for cardiovascular death, stroke and heart failure compared to patients who did not have AF [14].

AF is the most common arrhythmia in patients with heart failure and it worsens prognosis in NYHA classes III-IV patients [15], and all-cause mortality [16] and in-hospital mortality are increased in patients with new-onset AF compared with no AF or those with prior documented AF [17]. AF accounts for approximately one third of hospitalizations for heart rhythm disturbances [18], which have increased in recent years by two to three times [19]. In the Valsartan Antihypertensive Long-term Use Evaluation (VALUE) Trial of high-risk hypertensive people incident heart failure was a component of the primary endpoint and most of the patients who developed heart failure also had incident AF [20].

Pathophysiology

In the presence of left ventricular hypertrophy, left ventricular compliance is reduced, left ventricular stiffness and filling pressure increase, coronary flow reserve is decreased, wall stress is increased and there is activation of the sympathetic nervous system and of the renin-angiotensin-aldosterone system (Fig. 9.3). In the atria, proliferation and differentiation of fibroblasts into myofibroblasts and enhanced connective tissue deposition and fibrosis are the hallmarks of this process. Structural remodeling results in electrical dissociation between muscle bundles and in local conduction heterogeneities facilitating the initiation and perpetuation of AF. This electro-anatomical substrate permits multiple small re-entrant circuits that can stabilize the arrhythmia. Over time tissue remodeling promotes and maintains AF by changing the fundamental properties of the atria. Atrial remodeling consists of three components:

1. Electrical remodeling: where at rapid atrial rates, such as those observed during fibrillation paroxysms, intracellular changes in calcium handling lead to a reduction in the action potential duration. Even in the case of prolonged AF, electrical remodeling reverses quickly and completely once sinus rhythm is restored.
2. Contractile remodeling: occurs rapidly. The abnormal calcium handling at the high rates of contraction seen in AF may be responsible for loss of contractility. The contractile remodeling induced by AF may be responsible for its most devastating consequence, which is stroke. Impaired atrial contraction leading to stasis of blood, primarily in the left atrial appendage, is thought to be the major contributor to the development of blood clots, thus promoting thromboembolic events.

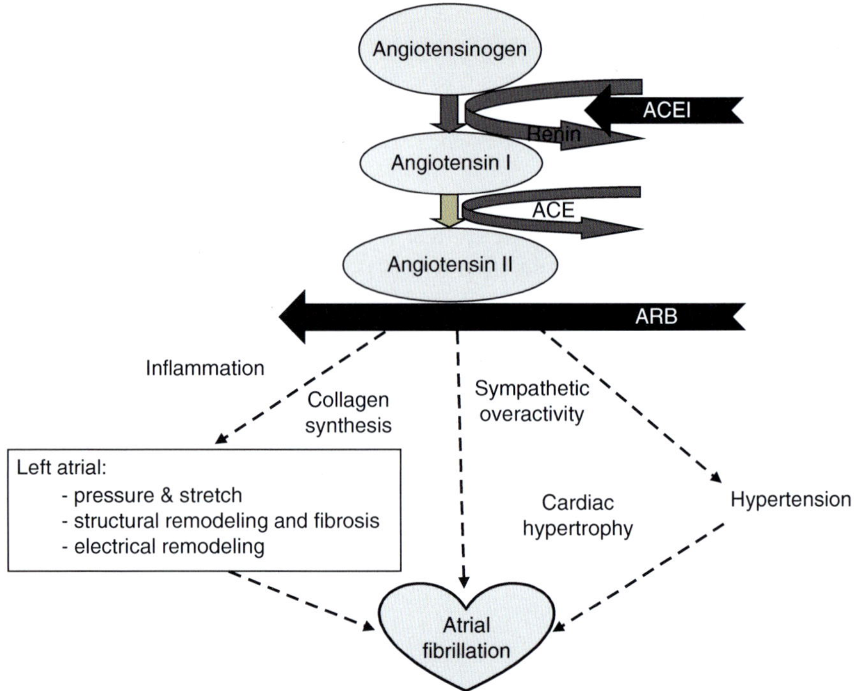

Fig. 9.3 Mechanisms by which ACE-inhibitors and ARBs may prevent atrial fibrillation

3. Structural tissue remodeling: occurs after periods of weeks or months and in this case we have macro- and microscopic changes in the myocardium, which contribute to contractile dysfunction and decreased cardiac output [21].

The levels of systolic blood pressure and duration of hypertension are predictive of adverse left atrial remodeling [22], while a wide pulse pressure [23, 24] and increase in left atrial volume [25] are associated with increased incidence of AF. Both obesity and hypertension were independent predictors of left atrial enlargement, but the co-existence of hypertension with obesity was associated with higher left atrial enlargement [26]. hs-CRP and P-wave dispersion in hypertensive patients are interrelated and associated with AF, suggesting an active role of inflammation in the atrial electrophysiological remodeling predisposing to AF [27].

Consequences of Atrial Fibrillation

Compared to people with normal sinus rhythm, those with AF have a 50–90% higher risk of overall mortality [28]. AF is responsible for 15–20% of all ischemic strokes [29], increases the risk of stroke four- to fivefold [30], and is an independent risk factor for ischemic stroke severity and recurrence [31]. Other consequences of AF include worsening of cognitive function, increased risk of hospitalization and cost, and impaired quality of life. In the Losartan Intervention For Endpoint Reduction in Hypertension Study (LIFE) patients with new-onset AF had approximately twofold increased risk of cardiovascular events, about threefold higher risk of fatal and non-fatal stroke, and fivefold increased rate of hospitalization for heart failure [9]. In the VALUE trial patients with new-onset AF had equally poor cardiovascular prognosis at the end of the follow-up period as those with AF at baseline [32], and new-onset AF was present in many patients who were hospitalized for heart failure whether they had concomitant diabetes or not [20]. In the Antihypertensive and Lipid-Lowering treatment to prevent Heart Attack Trial (ALLHAT), baseline AF or atrial flutter also increased cardiac morbidity and mortality [33].

Prior stroke or transient ischemic attack, increasing age, history of hypertension, diabetes mellitus, structural heart disease and obesity are independent risk factors for stroke [34]. The risks of stroke are doubled (10.4 %) in patients with AF associated with hypertension or diabetes or prior stroke compared to those without these comorbidities (4.3 %). In patients with AF and history of hypertension there was a threefold increase in the annual incidence of stroke compared to those without a history of hypertension [35]. And in at least 33 % of AF patients, the arrhythmia can be asymptomatic [36]. Holter registration and trans-telephonic monitoring studies have demonstrated that asymptomatic episodes of paroxysmal AF are 10–12 times more frequent than symptomatic episodes [37, 38], but the consequences are the same. Patients with history of hypertension but no history of AF who received a pacemaker or ICD, had over 36 % device-detected atrial arrhythmia. Patients who had one episode within the first 3 months had more than doubled the risk of stroke or systemic embolism [39]. Patients with paroxysmal AF have impaired quality of life similar to patients with heart failure, myocardial infarction and patients that have undergone angioplasty [40–42]. AF is independently associated with all forms of dementia and with an increased risk for Alzheimer's disease [43].

Diagnostic Approach and Risk Stratification for Atrial Fibrillation

Among general practitioners and nurse practitioners from 49 practices in central UK, the majority of primary care providers were not able to reliably diagnose the presence or absence of AF on ECG; 20 % of cases of AF were missed and the probability that a diagnosis of AF was correct only in 41 % [44]. A silent AF may be discovered from an AF-related complication as first manifestation or may be diagnosed by an opportunistic ECG [45] (Fig. 9.4). Hypertension increases the risk for AF in men and women by 1.5- and 1.4-fold, respectively, and is the most common underlying risk factor for the development of AF [3]. By multivariate analyses age, sex, body mass index, systolic blood pressure, treatment of hypertension, PR interval, and heart failure accounted for up to 64 % of the risk of new AF within 10 years [46].

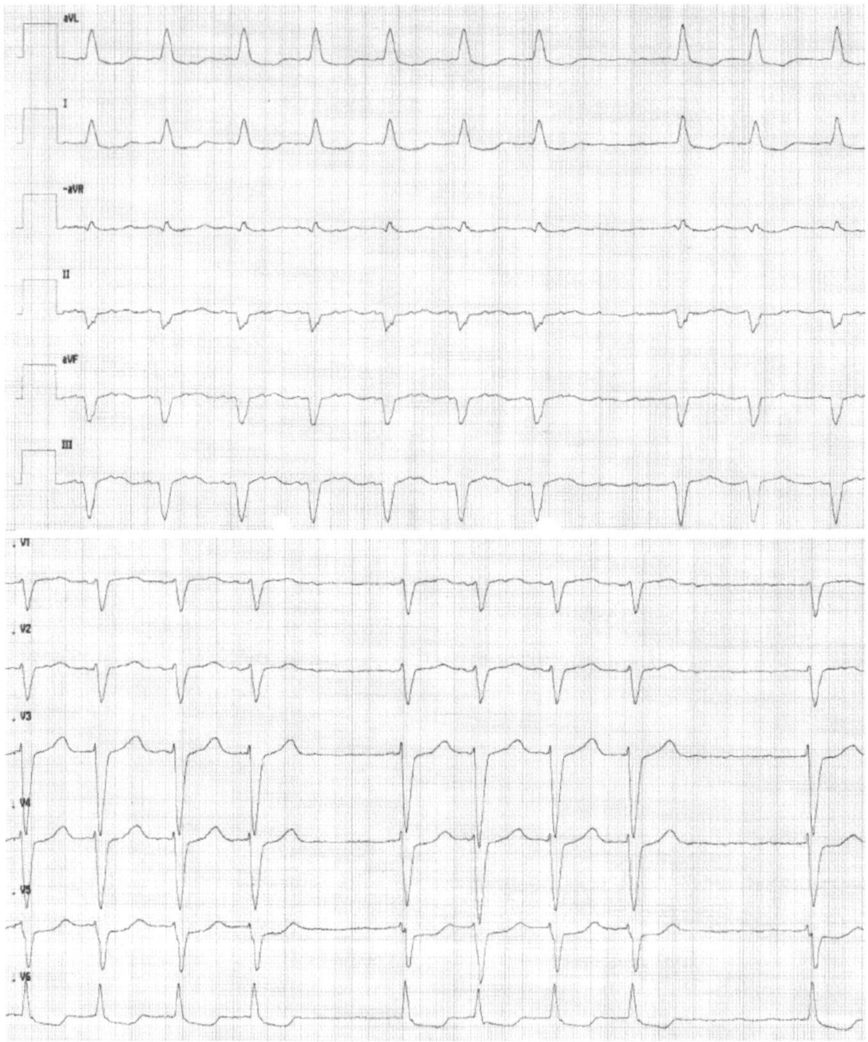

Fig. 9.4 Twelve lead ECG taken at 50 mm/s showing atrial fibrillation in a middle-aged patient with hypertension and left ventricular hypertrophy according to Cornell Product criteria

Risk Stratification and Prevention of Thromboembolism from Atrial Fibrillation

Due to its simplicity and ease of use, the $CHADS_2$ and CHA_2DS_2-VASc score have become the most commonly used predictive rule in clinical practice [47]. The $CHADS_2$ (Congestive heart failure, Hypertension, Age, Diabetes, Stroke) index assigns 1 point each for a history of heart failure, hypertension, age >75 years, and diabetes, and 2 points for a history of stroke or transient ischemic attack. Based on their score, patients can be classified as having low risk (score 0), moderate risk (score 1), or moderate/high risk (score 2 or greater) for stroke. For patients with $CHADS_2$ score ≥2 anticoagulation with new oral anticoagulants (NOAC) or warfarin with an international normalized ratio (INR) of 2.0–3.0 (target 2.5) is recommended unless contraindicated. A refined version known as the CHA_2DS_2-VASc score [48] has been validated in several independent cohorts. The CHA_2DS_2-VASc score outperformed the $CHADS_2$ score in identifying 'truly low risk' individuals who do not need antithrombotic therapy, whilst those with ≥1 stroke risk factors should be considered for oral anticoagulation therapy, whether this is undertaken with well-controlled warfarin or one of NOACs that do not require INR monitoring.

Atrial Fibrillation and Antihypertensive Treatment

Rate and rhythm control plus ablation in patients with AF are discussed elsewhere [45].

Antihypertensive drugs reduce the risk for AF mainly by lowering high blood pressure (Fig. 9.5). However, some antihypertensive drugs may also reduce the risk for AF through other mechanisms and are recommended by the most recent guidelines (Fig. 9.6).

RAS-Blockers (ACEIs and ARBs)

In early meta-analysis of randomised, controlled clinical trials [50, 51], it appeared that renin-angiotensin system (RAS) blockers significantly reduced the relative risk of new-onset AF by 28 % (15–40 %), but this benefit was limited to patients with systolic left ventricular dysfunction or left ventricular hypertrophy. In another meta-analysis [52], the use of an angiotensin-converting enzyme inhibitor (ACEI) or an angiotensin receptor blocker (ARB) was associated with an average 49 % (35–72 %) relative reduction in new-onset AF, a 53 % (24–92 %) lower failure rate of electrical cardioversion of AF, and a 61 % (20–75 %) lower rate of recurrence of AF after electrical cardioversion. A more recent meta-analysis [53] of the effects of RAS-blockade for the prevention of AF comprised 23 randomised studies with a total of 87,048 patients, including 6 hypertension trials, 2 post-myocardial infarction trials, 3 heart failure trials (primary prevention), 8 studies after cardioversion and 4 on medical prevention of paroxysmal AF (secondary prevention). RAS-blockade reduced the odds ratio for AF by 32 %, with similar effects of ACEIs and ARBs. In primary prevention RAS-blockade was most effective in patients with left ventricular hypertrophy and/or heart failure. In secondary prevention, RAS-blockade reduced the odds for AF recurrence after cardio-version by 45 % and on medical therapy by 63 %. However, no effect was found in those with the most refractory AF.

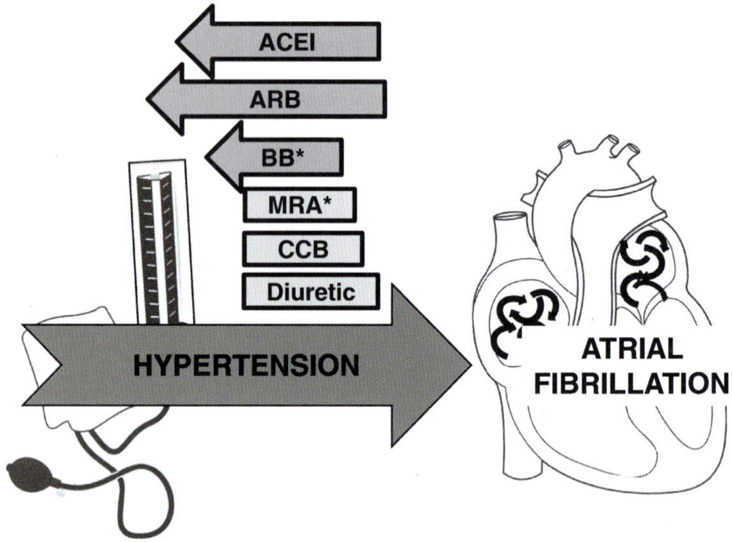

Fig. 9.5 Antihypertensive treatment may reduce the risk of developing atrial fibrillation in hypertensives

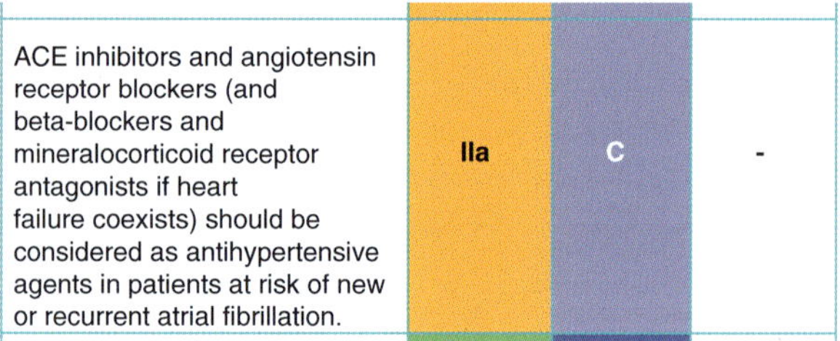

ACE inhibitors and angiotensin receptor blockers (and beta-blockers and mineralocorticoid receptor antagonists if heart failure coexists) should be considered as antihypertensive agents in patients at risk of new or recurrent atrial fibrillation.	IIa	C	-

Fig. 9.6 The 2013 ESH/ESC Hypertension Guidelines [49] state IIa indication for inhibitors of the renin-angiotensin-aldosterone system (ACE-inhibitors, ARBs, aldosterone antagonists and beta-blockers) in people with high risk of developing atrial fibrillation

However, most of the trials included in these meta-analyses were not designed to investigate AF. A pre-specified analysis of the VALUE trial was conducted to compare the effects of the ARB valsartan with the calcium channel blocker amlodipine on new-onset AF in >13,000 patients with hypertension at high cardiovascular risk [32]. Over the course of follow-up, the use of valsartan (vs. amlodipine) was associated with a 16 % reduction ($p<0.0455$) in the incidence of at least 1 documented occurrence of new-onset AF and reduced the incidence of persistent AF by 32 % ($p<0.0046$). Similar findings showing the benefit of ARBs in reducing the incidence of new-onset AF were also documented in pre-specified analysis of data from the LIFE study, in which the incidence of new-onset AF was compared between patients treated with losartan vs. the beta-blocker, atenolol [9]. In the ALLHAT study 42,418 participants were randomized to 4 antihypertensive treatment arms comparing the ability of an ACEI (lisinopril), a dihydropyridine calcium channel blocker (amlodipine), an alpha-adrenoreceptor blocker (doxazosin) relative to a thiazide-like diuretic (chlorthalidone) [33]. New-onset AF or atrial flutter occurred in 641 participants (2.0 %) and, excluding doxazosin (due to the early termination of doxazosin-arm in the year 2000 and shorter follow-up time in these patients; mean 3.2 years vs. mean 4.9 years), did not differ by antihypertensive treatment group. The 2007 ESH/ESC hypertension guidelines [54] summarized evidence from *post hoc* analyses of heart failure and hypertension trials showing a lower evidence of new-onset AF in patients receiving an ARB (in one trial an ACE inhibitor). While warning against the possible bias of *post hoc* analyses, nonetheless the guidelines suggested ARBs and ACE inhibitors as preferred drugs in hypertensive patients at risk of developing AF. A plausible explanation for this was the association between atrial enlargement and LVH, the favourable effects of blockers of the RAS on both cardiac alterations, and the relationship between LVH regression and reduction in new-onset AF [55, 56] (Fig. 9.3).

However, data accumulated since then do not consistently support in all of them this recommendation. Since then, new studies such as ONTARGET, TRANSCEND, PRoFESS and I-PRESERVE were published. In ONTARGET [57] new AF was just slightly less frequent with the ARB (telmisartan) than with the ACE inhibitor (ramipril) treatment, indicating no difference between these two types of RAS-blockade. The placebo comparisons in the TRANSCEND [58] and the PRoFESS [59] trials, could not confirm a protective effect of ARBs against onset of AF, though the absolute numbers were low and the detection power of the analysis may have been insufficient. The HOPE study included patients with high cardiovascular risk without heart failure and left ventricular systolic dysfunction and randomized the patients to treatment with an ACE inhibitor (ramipril) or placebo [60]. No statistically significant difference in the proportion of patients who developed AF was found between the ACE inhibitor and placebo. In TRANSCEND [58], patients intolerant to ACE inhibitors with cardiovascular disease or diabetes with end-organ damage, were randomized to treatment with an ARB (telmisartan) or placebo, and no significant effect on new-onset AF was found: 182 (6.4 %) patients treated with the ARB compared with 180 (6.3 %) patients treated with placebo, developed new AF. However, there are some limitations for the above trials. HOPE and TRANSCEND are not "pure" hypertension trials, although they included a large numbers of hypertensives (≈50 % in HOPE, ≈76 % in TRANSCEND), and were well treated for their blood pressure which may explain why these trials failed to detect a beneficial effect of RAS-blockade. Several relatively small prospective randomized controlled trials have demonstrated that therapy with ACE inhibitors or ARBs conferred an additional benefit on risk of recurrent AF after cardioversion when co-administered with antiarrhythmic drug therapy, usually amiodarone, compared with an antiarrhythmic drug alone [61, 62]. Meta-analyses driven by these studies have reported a significant 45–50 % reduction in RR of recurrent AF [63, 64]. Conversely, a double-blind, placebo-controlled study – Candesartan in the Prevention of Relapsing AF (CAPRAF) – failed to demonstrate any benefit of therapy with candesartan for preservation of sinus rhythm after cardioversion in patients who did not receive antiarrhythmic drug therapy [65]. The largest secondary prevention study, Gruppo Italiano per lo Studio della Sopravvivenza nell'Insufficienza cardiaca AF (GISSI-AF), in 1442 patients with cardiovascular risk factors (mainly hypertension, 85 %) and paroxysmal or recently cardioverted persistent AF, demonstrated no effect of valsartan added on top of optimal medical therapy (including antiarrhythmic drugs and ACE inhibitors) on the primary endpoint of time to first AF recurrence or the number of patients with more than one AF recurrence (26.9 % vs. 27.9 %) compared with placebo at 1-year follow-up [66]. The differences in outcomes showing greater benefit in primary prevention may relate to the fact that inhibitors of the RAS prevent, but do not reverse the development of the structural and electrical remodelling that provides the substrate for AF [66]. There are different mechanisms explaining the beneficial effects of RAS blockers in hypertensive patients with AF (Fig. 9.3). Blockade of the RAS may prevent left atrial dilatation, atrial fibrosis, dysfunction and slowing of conduction velocity, with some studies also indicating direct anti-arrhythmic properties. Favourable effects of RAS-blockers on cardiac alterations like atrial enlargement and left ventricular hypertrophy may also explain the reduction in new-onset AF [55, 56].

Beta-Blockers

Beta-blockers are effective in AF rate-control during AF and possibly in maintaining sinus rhythm, especially in heart failure and in cardiac postoperative settings [67, 68]. In a systematic review including almost 12,000 patients with systolic heart failure (about 90 % received RAS-blockade) and therefore at high risk of AF, the incidence of new-onset AF was significantly lower in the patients treated with beta-blockers compared with those assigned to placebo with a relative risk reduction of 27 % [68]. A history of AF and systolic heart failure may be a specific indication for using beta-blockers. Treatment with sotalol, a non-selective beta-blocker with class III anti-arrhythmic activity, is effective in maintaining sinus rhythm after cardioversion, but has pro-arrhythmic effects and is not recommended as antihypertensive treatment. In hypertension trials like the LIFE study, the ARB-based therapy (losartan) was superior to beta-blocker (atenolol) in reducing the risk of new and recurrent AF.

However, it is also difficult to draw conclusions from the results of trials comparing two or more active antihypertensive treatment regimens, due to uncertainty as to whether the observed effects may represent a detrimental effect of one regimen or a beneficial effect of the other. In the United Kingdom-based General Practice Research Database, with approximately 5 million patient records, it was found that ACE inhibitors, ARBs and beta-blockers were more effective than calcium channel blockers in reducing the risk of AF [69]. Possible mechanisms of action of beta-blockers to this effect may be prevention of adverse remodelling and ischemia, reduced sympathetic drive or counteraction of the beta-adrenergic shortening of action potential which otherwise could contribute to perpetuation of AF [67, 68]. However, recurrence rate of AF is known to be high, even under beta-blocker prophylaxis.

Calcium Channel Blockers

Calcium channel blockers (CCBs) are a heterogeneous group of drugs with antihypertensive properties. Non-dihydropyridines like diltiazem and verapamil are used to slow the ventricular response in AF, and verapamil has also been investigated for its effectiveness in maintaining sinus rhythm after cardioversion. Calcium lowering drugs could hypothetically attenuate the calcium-overload in tachycardia-induced electrical remodelling of the atria [70]. Additional treatment with verapamil significantly reduced the recurrence of AF within 3 months compared with propafenone alone [71]. However, other studies have shown more disappointing results [72, 73]. In the VALUE Trial the ARB valsartan was more effective than the CCB amlodipine in preventing new-onset AF [32].

In a retrospective study using a national integrated medical and pharmacy claims database in the US, almost 5500 patients treated for hypertension with an ACE inhibitor were compared to an equal number of matched patients treated with a CCB. At about 4 years of follow-up the incidence of new AF was significantly lower in the ACE inhibitor-treated patients [73]. In a nested case–control analysis from the United Kingdom-based General Practice Research Database, similar results were found [69]. 4661 patients with AF and 18641 matched controls from a hypertension population were compared and it was found that treatments with ACE inhibitors, ARBs or beta-blockers were associated with a lower risk for AF than treatment with CCBs. However, in such observational studies, bias in treatment cannot be excluded and blood pressure control and changes cannot be evaluated.

Diuretics

Diuretics are often included in antihypertensive treatment regimens, but the effect on new-onset AF has to our knowledge not been thoroughly investigated. Caution to electrolyte balance changes during chronic anti-hypertensive therapy with K+ wasting diuretics such as thiazides, chlorthalidone and indapamide, is recommended.

Mineralocorticoid Receptor Antagonists (MRAs) or Aldosterone Antagonists

Patients with primary hyperaldosteronism have a 12-fold higher risk of developing AF than their matched counterparts with essential hypertension. Increased aldosterone levels have been reported in patients with AF. Pre-treatment with spironolactone in a dog AF model reduced the amount of atrial fibrosis and inducibility of AF. Treatment with spironolactone and eplerenone [74] may prevent AF in patients with heart failure though large studies have not been done in people with hypertension.

Conclusions and Antithrombotic Treatment

Patients with hypertension suffer from an increased risk of AF, and hypertension is the most common disorder in AF trials. Awareness of the increased risk of AF in hypertensive patients may require closer follow-up as AF has a significant effect on cardiovascular outcome. AF is usually a progressive disease that often worsens over time ("AF begets AF") and this worsening is driven by electrical, contractile and structural changes in the atria, known as atrial remodelling. AF leads to reduced cardiac function, and increased risk of thromboembolism. Prevention and new treatment regimens of AF are needed, considering the increasing elderly population, the high percentage of uncontrolled hypertension, the risk of stroke and the worsening of other co-morbidities in the presence of AF. Management of AF includes antihypertensive, antiarrhythmic and antithrombotic drugs. Prevention of AF with antihypertensive drugs such as ACE inhibitors, ARBs, and beta-blockers has been shown to be more effective than other classes mainly in post myocardial infarction and heart failure trials and in other high risk hypertensive patients including those with left ventricular hypertrophy by ECG. Antithrombotic treatment is very effective in the prevention of stroke and new oral antithrombotics that do not require INR monitoring seem to be particularly promising drugs according to recently published trials and guidelines.

References

1. Kearney PM, Whelton M, Reynolds K, Whelton PK, He J. Worldwide prevalence of hypertension: a systematic review. J Hypertens. 2004;22:11–9.
2. Kannel WB, Wolf PA, Benjamin EJ, Levy D. Prevalence, incidence, prognosis, and predisposing conditions for atrial fibrillation: population-based estimates. Am J Cardiol. 1998;82:2N–9.
3. Benjamin EJ, Levy D, Vaziri SM, D'Agostino RB, Belanger AJ, Wolf PA. Independent risk factors for atrial fibrillation in a population-based cohort. The Framingham Heart Study. JAMA. 1994;271:840–4.
4. Wong ND, Lopez VA, L'Italien G, Chen R, Kline SE, Franklin SS. Inadequate control of hypertension in US adults with cardiovascular disease comorbidities in 2003–2004. Arch Intern Med. 2007;167:2431–6.
5. Moser M, Hebert PR. Prevention of disease progression, left ventricular hypertrophy and congestive heart failure in hypertension treatment trials. J Am Coll Cardiol. 1996;27:1214–8.
6. Verdecchia P, Reboldi G, Gattobigio R, Bentivoglio M, Borgioni C, Angeli F, et al. Atrial fibrillation in hypertension: predictors and outcome. Hypertension. 2003;41:218–23.
7. Ciaroni S, Cuenoud L, Bloch A. Clinical study to investigate the predictive parameters for the onset of atrial fibrillation in patients with essential hypertension. Am Heart J. 2000;139:814–9.
8. Krahn AD, Manfreda J, Tate RB, Mathewson FA, Cuddy TE. The natural history of atrial fibrillation: incidence, risk factors, and prognosis in the Manitoba Follow-Up Study. Am J Med. 1995;98:476–84.
9. Wachtell K, Lehto M, Gerdts E, Olsen MH, Hornestam B, Dahlof B, et al. Angiotensin II receptor blockade reduces new-onset atrial fibrillation and subsequent stroke compared to

atenolol: the Losartan Intervention For End Point Reduction in Hypertension (LIFE) study. J Am Coll Cardiol. 2005;45:712–9.
10. Manolis AJ, Agabiti Rosei E, Coca A, Cifkova R, Erdine SE, Kjeldsen S, et al. Hypertension and atrial fibrillation: diagnostic approach, prevention and treatment. Position paper of the WG "hypertension arrhythmias and thrombosis" of the European Society of Hypertension. J Hypertens. 2012;30:239–52.
11. Sciarretta S, Pontremoli R, Rosei EA, Ambrosioni E, Costa V, Leonetti G, et al. Independent association of ECG abnormalities with microalbuminuria and renal damage in hypertensive patients without overt cardiovascular disease: data from Italy-Developing Education and awareness on MicroAlbuminuria in patients with hypertensive Disease study. J Hypertens. 2009;27:410–7.
12. Grundvold I, Skretteberg PT, Liestøl K, Erikssen G, Kjeldsen SE, Arnesen H, et al. Upper normal blood pressures predict incident atrial fibrillation in healthy middle-aged men. A 35-year follow-up study. Hypertension. 2012;59:198–204.
13. Grundvold I, Skretteberg PG, Liestøl K, Gjesdal K, Erikssen G, Kjeldsen SE, et al. Importance of physical fitness on predictive effect of body mass index and weight gain on incident atrial fibrillation in healthy middle-aged men. Am J Cardiol. 2012;110:425–32.
14. Du X, Ninomiya T, de Galan B, Abadir E, Chalmers J, Pillai A, for the ADVANCE Collaborative Group, et al. Risks of cardiovascular events and effects of routine blood pressure lowering among patients with type 2 diabetes and atrial fibrillation: results of the ADVANCE study. Eur Heart J. 2009;30:1128–35.
15. Vardas P, Marakis H. Atrial fibrillation and heart failure. Hellenic J Cardiol. 2004;45:277–81.
16. Mamas MA, Caldwell JC, Chacko S, Garratt CJ, Fath-Ordoubadi F, Neyses L. A meta-analysis of the prognostic significance of atrial fibrillation in chronic heart failure. Eur J Heart Fail. 2009;11:676–83.
17. Rivero-Ayerza M, Scholte Op Reimer W, Lenzen M, Theuns DA, Jordaens L, Komajda M, et al. New-onset atrial fibrillation is an independent predictor of in-hospital mortality in hospitalized heart failure patients: results of the EuroHeart Failure Survey. Eur Heart J. 2008;29:1618–24.
18. Go AS, Hylek EM, Phillips KA, Chang Y, Henault LE, Selby JV, Singer DE. Prevalence of diagnosed atrial fibrillation in adults: national implications for rhythm management and stroke prevention: the AnTicoagulation and Risk Factors in Atrial Fibrillation (ATRIA) Study. JAMA. 2001;285:2370–5.
19. Wattigney WA, Mensah GA, Croft JB. Increasing trends in hospitalization for atrial fibrillation in the United States, 1985 through 1999: implications for primary prevention. Circulation. 2003;108:711–6.
20. Aksnes TA, Schmieder RE, Kjeldsen SE, Ghani S, Hua T, Julius S. Impact of new-onset DM on atrial fibrillation and heart failure development in high risk hypertension (from the VALUE trial). Am J Cardiol. 2008;101:634–8.
21. Van Gelder IC, Hemels ME. The progressive nature of atrial fibrillation: a rationale for early restoration and maintenance of sinus rhythm. Europace. 2006;8:943–9.
22. Vaziri SM, Larson MG, Lauer MS, Benjamin EJ, Levy D. Influence of blood pressure on left atrial size. The Framingham Heart Study. Hypertension. 1995;25:1155–60.
23. Mitchell GF, Vasan RS, Keyes MJ, Parise H, Wang TJ, Larson MG, et al. Pulse pressure and risk of new-onset atrial fibrillation. JAMA. 2007;297:709–15.
24. Larstorp ACK, Ariansen I, Gjesdal K, Olsen MH, Ibsen H, Devereux RB, et al. Association of pulse pressure with new-onset atrial fibrillation in hypertensive patients with left ventricular hypertrophy: the LIFE Study. Hypertension. 2012;60:347–53.
25. Tsang TS, Barnes ME, Bailey KR, Leibson CL, Montgomery SC, Takemoto Y, et al. Left atrial volume: important risk marker of incident atrial fibrillation in 1655 older men and women. Mayo Clin Proc. 2001;76:467–75.
26. Stritzke J, Markus MR, Duderstadt S, Lieb W, Luchner A, Doring A, for the MONIKA/KORA Investigators, et al. The aging process of the heart: obesity is the main risk factor for left atrial

enlargement during aging the MONICA/KORA (monitoring of trends and determinations in cardiovascular disease/cooperative research in the region of Augsburg) study. J Am Coll Cardiol. 2009;54:1982–9.
27. Tsioufis C, Syrseloudis D, Hatziyianni A, Tzamou V, Andrikou I, Tolis P, et al. Relationships of CRP and P wave dispersion with atrial fibrillation in hypertensive subjects. Am J Hypertens. 2010;23:202–7.
28. Benjamin EJ, Wolf PA, D'Agostino RB, Silbershatz H, Kannel WB, Levy D. Impact of atrial fibrillation on the risk of death: the Framingham Heart Study. Circulation. 1998;98:946–52.
29. Go AS. The epidemiology of atrial fibrillation in elderly persons: the tip of the iceberg. Am J Geriatr Cardiol. 2005;14:56–61.
30. Wolf PA, Abbott RD, Kannel WB. Atrial fibrillation as an independent risk factor for stroke: the Framingham Study. Stroke. 1991;22:983–8.
31. Penado S, Cano M, Acha O, Hernández JL, Riancho JA. Atrial fibrillation as a risk factor for stroke recurrence. Am J Med. 2003;114:206–10.
32. Schmieder RE, Kjeldsen SE, Julius S, McInnes GT, Zanchetti A, Hua TA, for the VALUE Trial Group. Reduced incidence of new-onset atrial fibrillation with angiotensin II receptor blockade: the VALUE trial. J Hypertens. 2008;26:403–11.
33. Haywood LJ, Ford CE, Crow RS, Davis BR, Massie BM, Einhorn PT, Williard A, for the ALLHAT Collaborative Research Group. Atrial fibrillation at baseline and during follow-up in ALLHAT (Antihypertensive and Lipid-Lowering Treatment to Prevent Heart Attack Trial). J Am Coll Cardiol. 2009;54:2023–31.
34. Stroke Risk in Atrial Fibrillation Working Group. Independent predictors of stroke in patients with atrial fibrillation: a systematic review. Neurology. 2007;69:546–54.
35. Atrial fibrillation Investigators. Risk factors for stroke and efficacy of antithrombotic therapy in atrial fibrillation. Analysis of pooled data from five randomized controlled trials. Arch Intern Med. 1994;154:1449–57.
36. Savelieva I, Camm AJ. Silent atrial fibrillation—another Pandora's box. Pacing Clin Electrophysiol. 2000;23:145–8.
37. Page RL, Tilsch TW, Connolly SJ, Schnell DJ, Marcello SR, Wilkinson WE, Pritchett EL, for the Azimilide Supraventricular Arrhythmia Program (ASAP) Investigators. Asymptomatic or "silent" atrial fibrillation: frequency in untreated patients and patients receiving azimilide. Circulation. 2003;107:1141–5.
38. Defaye P, Dournaux F, Mouton E. Prevalence of supraventricular arrhythmias from the automated analysis of data stored in the DDD pacemakers of 617 patients: the AIDA study. The AIDA Multicenter Study Group. Automatic Interpretation for Diagnosis Assistance. Pacing Clin Electrophysiol. 1998;21:250–5.
39. Kaufman ES, Israel CW, Nair GM, Armaganijan L, Divakaramenon S, Mairesse GH, et al. Positive predictive value of device-detected atrial high-rate episodes at different rates and durations: an analysis from ASSERT. Heart Rhythm. 2012;9:1241–6.
40. van den Berg MP, Ranchor AV, van Sonderen FL, van Gelder IC, van Veldhuisen DJ. Paroxysmal atrial fibrillation, quality of life and neuroticism. Neth J Med. 2005;63:170–4.
41. Hammer ME, Blumenthal JA, McCarthy EA, Phillips BG, Pritchett EL. Quality-of-life assessment in patients with paroxysmal atrial fibrillation or paroxysmal supraventricular tachycardia. Am J Cardiol. 1994;74:826–9.
42. Dorian P, Jung W, Newman D, Paquette M, Wood K, Ayers GM, et al. The impairment of health-related quality of life in patients with intermittent atrial fibrillation: implications for the assessment of investigational therapy. J Am Coll Cardiol. 2000;36:1303–9.
43. Bunch TJ, Weiss JP, Crandall BG, May HT, Bair TL, Osborn JS, et al. Atrial fibrillation is independently associated with senile, vascular, and Alzheimer's dementia. Heart Rhythm. 2010;7:433–7.
44. Mant J, Fitzmaurice DA, Hobbs FD, Jowett S, Murray ET, Holder R, et al. Accuracy of diagnosing atrial fibrillation on electrocardiogram by primary care practitioners and interpretative diagnostic software: analysis of data from screening for atrial fibrillation in the elderly (SAFE) trial. BMJ. 2007;335:380.

45. Camm AJ, Kirchhof P, Lip GY, Schotten U, Savelieva I, Ernst S, et al. Guidelines for the management of atrial fibrillation: the Task Force for the Management of Atrial Fibrillation of the European Society of Cardiology (ESC). Eur Heart J. 2010;31:2369–429.
46. Schnabel RB, Aspelund T, Li G, Sullivan LM, Suchy-Dicey A, Harris TB, et al. Validation of an atrial fibrillation risk algorithm in whites and African Americans. Arch Intern Med. 2010;170:1909–17.
47. Gage BF, Shannon W, Waterman AD, Boechler M, Rich MW, Radford MJ. Validation of clinical classification schemes for predicting stroke: results from the National Registry of Atrial Fibrillation. JAMA. 2001;285:2864–70.
48. Marinigh R, Lip GY, Fiotti N, Giansante C, Lane DA. Age as a risk factor for stroke in atrial fibrillation patients: Implications for thromboprophylaxis. J Am Coll Cardiol. 2010;56:827–37.
49. The Task Force for the Management of Arterial Hypertension of the European Society of Hypertension (ESH) and of the European Society of Cardiology (ESC). 2013 ESH/ESC guidelines for the management of arterial hypertension. Blood Press. 2013;22:193–278.
50. Healey JS, Baranchuk A, Crystal E, Morillo CA, Garfinkle M, Yusuf S, Connolly SJ. Prevention of atrial fibrillation with angiotensin-converting enzyme inhibitors and angiotensin receptor blockers: a meta-analysis. J Am Coll Cardiol. 2005;45:1832–9.
51. Aksnes TA, Flaa A, Strand A, Kjeldsen SE. Prevention of new-onset atrial fibrillation and it's predictors with ARBs in the treatment of hypertension and heart failure. J Hypertens. 2007;25:15–23.
52. Kalus JS, Coleman CI, White CM. The impact of suppressing the renin-angiotensin system on atrial fibrillation. J Clin Pharmacol. 2006;46:21–8.
53. Schneider MP, Hua TA, Bohm M, Wachtell K, Kjeldsen SE, Schmieder RE. Prevention of atrial fibrillation by Renin-Angiotensin system-inhibition a meta-analysis. J Am Coll Cardiol. 2010;55:2299–307.
54. Mancia G, De Backer G, Dominiczak A, Cifkova R, Fagard R, Germano G, et al. 2007 guidelines for the management of arterial hypertension: the Task Force for the Management of Arterial Hypertension of the European Society of Hypertension (ESH) and of the European Society of Cardiology (ESC). J Hypertens. 2007;25:1105–87.
55. Gerdts E, Wachtell K, Omvik P, Otterstad JE, Oikarinen L, Boman K, et al. Left atrial size and risk of major cardiovascular events during antihypertensive treatment: losartan intervention for endpoint reduction in hypertension trial. Hypertension. 2007;49:311–6.
56. Okin PM, Wachtell K, Devereux RB, Harris KE, Jern S, Kjeldsen SE, et al. Regression of electrocardiographic left ventricular hypertrophy and decreased incidence of new-onset atrial fibrillation in patients with hypertension. JAMA. 2006;296:1242–8.
57. ONTARGET Investigators, Yusuf S, Teo KK, Pogue J, Dyal L, Copland I, Schumacher H, et al. Telmisartan, ramipril, or both in patients at high risk for vascular events. N Engl J Med. 2008;358:1547–59.
58. Telmisartan Randomised AssessmeNt Study in ACE iNtolerant subjects with cardiovascular Disease (TRANSCEND) Investigators, Yusuf S, Teo K, Anderson C, Pogue J, Dyal L, Copland I, et al. Effects of the angiotensin-receptor blocker telmisartan on cardiovascular events in high-risk patients intolerant to angiotensin-converting enzyme inhibitors: a randomised controlled trial. Lancet. 2008;372:1174–83.
59. Yusuf S, Diener HC, Sacco RL, Cotton D, Ounpuu S, Lawton WA, PRoFESS Study Group, et al. Telmisartan to prevent recurrent stroke and cardiovascular events. N Engl J Med. 2008;359:1225–37.
60. Salehian O, Healey J, Stambler B, Alnemer K, Almerri K, Grover J, et al. Impact of ramipril on the incidence of atrial fibrillation: results of the Heart Outcomes Prevention Evaluation study. Am Heart J. 2007;154:448–53.
61. Madrid AH, Bueno MG, Rebollo JM, Marin I, Pena G, Bernal E, et al. Use of irbesartan to maintain sinus rhythm in patients with long-lasting persistent atrial fibrillation: a prospective and randomized study. Circulation. 2002;106:331–6.

62. Ueng KC, Tsai TP, Yu WC, Tsai CF, Lin MC, Chan KC, et al. Use of enalapril to facilitate sinus rhythm maintenance after external cardioversion of long-standing persistent atrial fibrillation. Results of a prospective and controlled study. Eur Heart J. 2003;24:2090–8.
63. Jibrini MB, Molnar J, Arora RR. Prevention of atrial fibrillation by way of abrogation of the rennin-angiotensin system: a systematic review and meta-analysis. Am J Ther. 2008;15:36–43.
64. Anand K, Mooss AN, Hee TT, Mohiuddin SM. Meta-analysis: inhibition of rennin-angiotensin system prevents new-onset atrial fibrillation. Am Heart J. 2006;152:217–22.
65. Tveit A, Seljeflot I, Grundvold I, Abdelnoor M, Smith P, Arnesen H. Effect of candesartan and various inflammatory markers on maintenance of sinus rhythm after electrical cardioversion for atrial fibrillation. Am J Cardiol. 2007;99:1544–8.
66. GISSI-AF Investigators, Disertori M, Latini R, Barlera S, Franzosi MG, Staszewsky L, et al. Valsartan for prevention of recurrent atrial fibrillation. N Engl J Med. 2009;360:1606–17.
67. Kühlkamp V, Schirdewan A, Stangl K, Homberg M, Ploch M, Beck OA. Use of metoprolol CR/XL to maintain sinus rhythm after conversion from persistent atrial fibrillation: a randomized, double-blind, placebo-controlled study. J Am Coll Cardiol. 2000;36:139–46.
68. Nasr IA, Bouzamondo A, Hulot JS, Dubourg O, Le Heuzey JY, Lechat P. Prevention of atrial fibrillation onset by beta-blocker treatment in heart failure: a meta-analysis. Eur Heart J. 2007;28:457–62.
69. Schaer BA, Schneider C, Jick SS, Conen D, Osswald S, Meier CR. Risk for incident atrial fibrillation in patients who receive antihypertensive drugs: a nested case–control study. Ann Intern Med. 2010;152:78–84.
70. Van Noord T, Van Gelder IC, Tieleman RG, Bosker HA, Tuinenburg AE, Volkers C, et al. VERDICT: the Verapamil versus Digoxin Cardioversion Trial: A randomized study on the role of calcium lowering for maintenance of sinus rhythm after cardioversion of persistent atrial fibrillation. J Cardiovasc Electrophysiol. 2001;12:766–9.
71. De Simone A, Stabile G, Vitale DF, Turco P, Di Stasio M, Petrazzuoli F, et al. Pretreatment with verapamil in patients with persistent or chronic atrial fibrillation who underwent electrical cardioversion. J Am Coll Cardiol. 1999;34:810–4.
72. Lee SH, Yu WC, Cheng JJ, Hung CR, Ding YA, Chang MS, Chen SA. Effect of verapamil on long-term tachycardia-induced atrial electrical remodelling. Circulation. 2000;101:200–6.
73. L'Allier PL, Ducharme A, Keller PF, Yu H, Guertin MC, Tardif JC. Angiotensin-converting enzyme inhibition in hypertensive patients is associated with a reduction in the occurrence of atrial fibrillation. J Am Coll Cardiol. 2004;44:159–64.
74. Swedberg K, Zannad F, McMurray JJ, Krum H, van Veldhuisen DJ, Shi H, for the EMPHASIS-HF Study Investigators, et al. Eplerenone and atrial fibrillation in mild systolic heart failure: results from the EMPHASIS-HF (Eplerenone in Mild Patients Hospitalization And SurvIval Study in Heart Failure) study. J Am Coll Cardiol. 2012;59:1598–603.

Chapter 10
Echocardiographic Assessment of Hypertensive Patients

Ioannis Felekos, Costas Tsioufis, and Petros Nihoyannopoulos

Introduction

Echocardiography is the reference method for evaluating the structural and functional adaptations in the remodelling of the heart due to systemic hypertension. It provides valuable information regarding left ventricular geometry, systolic, and diastolic function, as well as left atrial and ascending aorta dimensions and function.

Two Dimensional Echo Anatomic Assessment

The standard echocardiographic evaluation involves measurements of cardiac chambers, including the interventricular septum, posterior wall thickness, left atrial size, end-systolic and end-diastolic diameters. From these measurements, left ventricular mass can be derived according to available formulas indexing for body surface area but for the most cases calculation of LVM is currently performed using the American

I. Felekos, M.D.
Department of Cardiology, Hippokrateion Hospital, Athens, Greece
e-mail: yannisfd@hotmail.com

C. Tsioufis, M.D., Ph.D., FESC, FACC
First Cardiology Clinic, Department of Cardiology, University of Athens, Hippokration Hospital, Athens, Greece

Department of Medicine, Georgetown University, Washington, DC, USA

P. Nihoyannopoulos, M.D., FRCP, FESC, FACC, FAHA (✉)
Department of Cardiology, Imperial College London, London, UK

National Kapodistrian University of Athens, Athens, Greece
e-mail: p.nihoyannopoulos@imperial.ac.uk

E.A. Andreadis (ed.), *Hypertension and Cardiovascular Disease*,
DOI 10.1007/978-3-319-39599-9_10

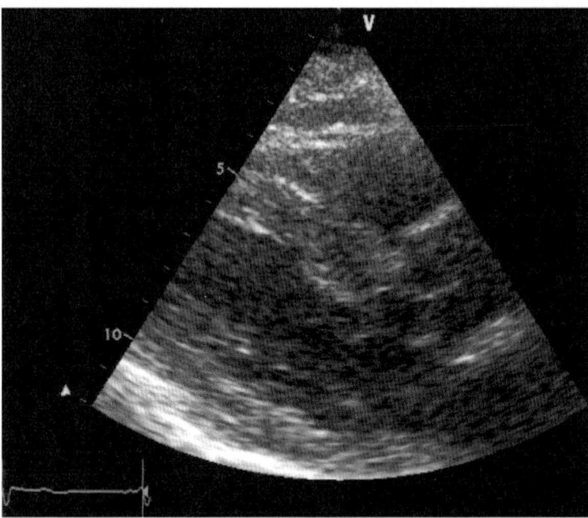

Fig. 10.1 Parasternal long-axis view in a hypertensive patient (end-diastolic frame), illustrating increased wall thickness

Society of Echocardiography formula: LV mass = [1.04(STd + PWTd + LVIDd)^3 − LVIDd^3] + 0.6 g. It is well established that one of the major characteristics and prognostic determinants of long-standing systemic hypertension is left ventricular hypertrophy (LVH), which can be accurately assessed by two-dimensional echocardiography (Fig. 10.1). Indexation of LVM for height, in which height to the allometric power of 1.7 or 2.7 has been used, can be considered in overweight and obese patients in order to scale LVM to body size and avoid under-diagnosis of LVH. It has recently been shown that the optimal method is to scale allometrically by body height to the exponent 1.7 (g/m1.7) and that different cut-offs for men and women should be used. Scaling LVM by height exponent 2.7 could overestimate LVH in small subjects and underestimate in tall subjects. The most used scaling for evaluating LVH in hypertension is to divide LVM by BSA, so that the effects on LVM of body size and obesity are largely eliminated. Despite largely derived from control study populations with the obvious possibility for bias, these parameters recommended by the American Society of Echocardiography and the European Association of Echocardiography are used in the majority of laboratories for echocardiography [1].

Apart from the linear dimensions of the septum and posterior wall, relative wall thickness can be easily calculated, which will aid in the echocardiographic distinction between eccentric and concentric hypertrophy. The determination of LV geometry according to LV mass index and relative wall thickness ($\geq$0.43 or <0.43) provides further prognostic data. More specifically, there is a graded continuous incremental effect of left ventricle geometrical adaptations on cardiovascular risk, ranging from normal LV pattern, to LV concentric remodelling, LV eccentric hypertrophy, and finally, LV concentric hypertrophy [2]. Concentric LVH is the strongest predictor of increased risk. Echocardiography is more sensitive than electrocardiography in diagnosing LVH and is useful to refine cardiovascular and renal risk. The prevalence of LVH increases with the duration and the severity of systemic hypertension and ranges from <10% in subjects with stage 1 hypertension to 90% among those with stage 3. Risk increases proportionally, even in the conventionally normal range of LV mass index, according to gender-specific criteria Although the relation between LVM and CV risk is continuous, thresholds of 95 g/m^2 for women and 115 g/m^2 for men are widely used for estimates of clear-cut LVH.

More interestingly the dipping status of the hypertensive patients has a direct effect on LV structural remodelling. According to a recent large metanalysis, left ventricular (LV) mass index, as well as relative wall thickness was significantly higher in non-dipping than in dipping hypertensives [3]. While among different antihypertensive drugs the efficacy on LVH regression varies, renal sympathetic denervation, a new approach for patients with resistant hypertension, reduces LVH, exhibits a favourable impact on LA volume and improves cardiac function in patients with resistant hypertension [4].

Left atrium (LA) dilatation is an early and common finding in hypertensive heart disease: in the LIFE study [5], 56% of female and 38% of males had increased LA size. The left atrium enlarges asymmetrically and not only in the anteroposterior diameter. Therefore, a plain measurement of 2D atrial linear dimension underestimates its true size. Current chamber quantification guidelines recommend the calculation of LA volumes, as this represent more accurately the actual dimensions (Fig. 10.2). LA volume measurements are simple and reproducible. LA volume index (an echocardiographic measurement of LA volume indexed or the body surface area—normal values: 34 ml/m^2 the upper limit) was found closely associated with advanced age, high systolic BP, increased LV mass index, and BNP levels [6]. Determination of left atrial dilatation can provide additional information and is a prerequisite for the diagnosis of diastolic dysfunction. Left atrial size has been shown to be an independent predictor of death, heart failure, atrial fibrillation and ischaemic stroke. LA volume is a more robust marker of CV events than LA area or diameter, while, in subjects with AF, the predictive value of LA size for CV events was poor, irrespective of the method of LA size quantization. Left atrial mechanics seem to be in close relation to alteration in LV geometry. It was recently demonstrated that LV geometric patterns significantly influence LA phasic function. Concentric and dilated LVH patterns have the most prominent negative effect on LA enlargement assessed by both 2D and 3D echocardiography [7].

Systolic and Diastolic Function Evaluation

Long standing and poorly-controlled hypertension eventually leads to left ventricular remodelling and dilatation with concomitant systolic function impairment, even in the absence of coronary artery disease. End-stage hypertensive heart-disease has an echocardiographic appearance similar to end-stage dilated cardiomyopathy, due to chronic afterload elevation.

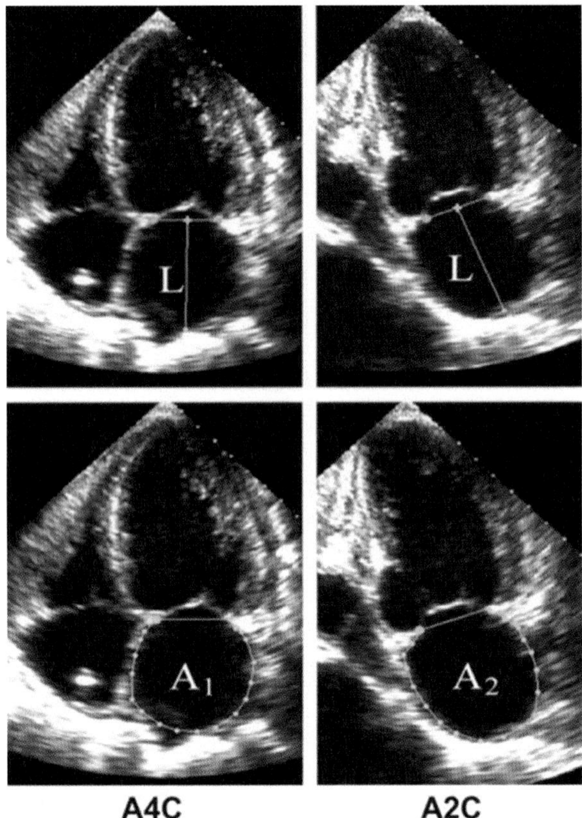

Fig. 10.2 Assessment of LA volumes by 2D echocardiography

Even prior to the establishment of LVH and depressed systolic function, hypertension mediates diastolic dysfunction (Table 10.1) which is associated with concentric remodelling, leading to impaired relaxation and increased stiffening of the left ventricle. This in turn results in a clinical situation of diastolic heart failure with preserved ejection fraction. Diastolic function can be assessed by Doppler measurement of the E/A ratio of transmitral blood flow. Additional measurements include deceleration time of E wave and isovolumic relaxation time [8]. The first abnormality encountered on the hypertensive patient is abnormal relaxation, manifesting as low E/A ratio, prolonged isovolumic relaxation time and E deceleration slope. Disease progression results in further diastolic function deterioration and filling pressure elevation. The second type of diastolic function also referred as pseudonormalization illustrates normal E/A ratio. However, Valsalva manoeuvres and pulmonary vein flow patterns may uncover diastolic dysfunction in the setting of pseudo-normalized transmitral patterns. One major disadvantage of this approach is that all these measurements are load-dependent and they should be interpreted in the context of loading conditions.

Table 10.1 Cut-off values for parameters used in the assessment of LV remodeling and diastolic function in patients with hypertension

Parameter	Abnormal if
LV mass index (g/m²)	>95 (women) >115 (men)
Relative wall thickness (RWT)	≥0.42
Diastolic function:	
Mitral valve inflow	E<A or E>>A E_{DT}>200 ms or <140 ms
Septal e' velocity (cm/s)	<8
Lateral e' (cm/s)	<10
LA volume index (mL/m²)	≥34
Pulmonic veins	S<<D
	A velocity >0.35 m/s
	adur- Adur>0.20 s
LV Filling pressures:	
E/e' (averaged) ratio	≥13

Based on Lang et al. and Nagueh et al.

The Doppler transmitral inflow pattern can quantify filling abnormalities and predict subsequent heart failure and all-cause mortality, but is not sufficient to stratify completely the hypertensive clinical status and prognosis. According to recent echocardiographic recommendations it should therefore be combined with pulsed tissue Doppler of the mitral annulus.

Additionally, TDI derived parameters seem to be less dependent on loading conditions as they reflect only the amount of blood passing through the LV inflow tract. This method accurately describes left ventricle systolic and diastolic function, with reproducible measurements of the systolic (S wave) and diastolic waves (e' and a') from the diaphragmatic, lateral, anterior, and inferior wall proximally to mitral annulus. Reduction of the Tissue Doppler derived early diastolic velocity (e') is typical of hypertensive heart disease and often the septal e' is reduced more than the lateral e'. Diagnosis and grading of diastolic dysfunction is based on e' (average of septal and lateral mitral annulus) and additional measurements including the ratio between transmitral E and e' (E/e' ratio) and left atrial size. This grading is an important predictor of all-cause mortality in a large epidemiologic study. The values of e' velocity and of E/e' ratio are highly dependent on age and somewhat less on gender. The E/e' ratio is able to detect an increase of LV filling pressures. The prognostic value of e' velocity is recognized in the hypertensive setting and E/e' ratio (upper cut-off value ≥ 13) is associated with increased cardiac risk independent of LVM and relative wall thickness in hypertensive patients [9]. In a recent study involving 80 multiethnic hypertensive children, TDI imaging was able to detect premature diastolic dysfunction. According to the investigators, hypertensive children had lower e' and a' velocities of anterior and posterior walls and higher lateral wall E/e' ratio, in comparison to controls. The authors concluded that decreased regional TDI velocities were seen with preserved left ventricular systolic function even when other measures of diastolic dysfunction remained unchanged in untreated hypertensive children. Hypertension and serum insulin levels had strong associations with preclinical diastolic alterations in children [10]. Normal ranges and cut-off values for hypertensive heart disease for key echocardiographic parameters are summarized in Table 10.1.

Differential Diagnosis from Other Causes of LVH

Apart from hypertensive heart disease, there are other causes of left ventricular hypertrophy. Prompt and accurate diagnosis is crucial in order to offer the patient optimal therapeutic management.

Hypertrophic cardiomyopathy is a major cause of LVH. Still, the pattern and the magnitude of LVH aid in differentiation from hypertensive LVH. HCM illustrates an asymmetric pattern, affecting mainly the IVS, the lateral wall and less commonly LV apex. Moreover, the RV wall can be also involved. However, the posterior wall is usually unaffected by the disease. In addition the size of the hypertrophied segments most commonly exceeds 15 mm.

Another differential diagnosis that can be made by studying the patterns of hypertrophy along with diastolic function is that of athletic heart. The athlete's heart exhibits mild LV dilatation, with normal diastolic function indices, as opposed to the diastolic dysfunction caused by hypertension. These changes reflect adaptive mechanisms of the athletic heart to augment LV filling in order to enhance cardiac output. Table 10.2 illustrates the major differences among entities that cause increased wall thickness.

Echocardiographic Evaluation of the Aorta

Evaluation of the aorta is a routine part of the standard echocardiographic examination, especially in patients with hypertension. Elevated blood pressure poses an increased shear stress in the aortic wall, causing vessel dilatation. Therefore a

Table 10.2 Echocardiographic differentiation of increased wall thickness

Parameter	Hypertension	HCM	Athlete's heart
Hypertrophy	Concentric	Asymmetric	Normal wall thickness
LV systolic function	Normal	Normal	Normal
Chamber dilatation	Biatrial dilatation, especially if AF is present	None	LV dilatation
LV diastolic function	Abnormal	Abnormal	Normal
RV hypertrophy	Absent	May be present	Absent
Pulmonary hypertension	Mild	Mild	None
LV end-diastolic pressure	Elevated	Elevated	Normal

comprehensive assessment of the aorta is crucial. The commonly and erroneously used term “aortic root” consists of various anatomic components including the annulus, Valsalva sinuses, sinotubular junction and ascending aorta (Fig. 10.3), which should be meticulously measured and reported in the echocardiographic assessment of the hypertensive patient. Using different acoustic windows the proximal ascending aorta is visualized [11]. The suprasternal view is of paramount importance for evaluation of the thoracic aorta. This view primarily depicts the aortic arch and its spatial relationship with the three major supra-aortic vessels (innominate, left carotid and left subclavian arteries), as well as variable lengths of the descending and, to a lesser degree, the ascending aorta. Although this view may be obstructed, particularly in patients with emphysema or short wide necks, it should be systematically sought when aortic disease is evaluated. Still, the clinician should bear in mind that transthoracic echo cannot depict the entire thoracic descending aorta in not well visualized by TTE. Moreover, suboptimal image quality can cause diagnostic dilemmas to the inexperienced operator. TOE on the other hand uses high frequency transducers, improving image resolution and providing more accurate anatomic data. This is extremely important in cases where acute aortic syndromes

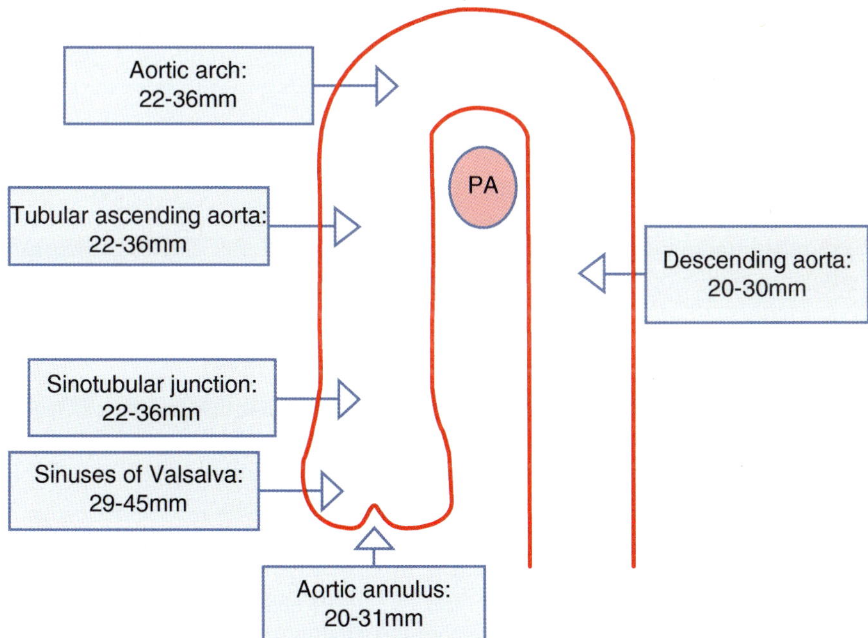

Fig. 10.3 The thoracic aorta can be divided into three segments: the ascending aorta that extends from the aortic annulus to the innominate artery and is typically measured at the level of the aortic annulus, the sinuses of Valsalva, the sinotubular junction and the proximal ascending aorta; the aortic arch that extends from the innominate artery to the ligamentum arteriosum; and the descending aorta that extends from the ligamentum arteriosum to the level of the diaphragm. *PA* right pulmonary artery

are suspected. In this instance, transoesophageal echo can provide a fast and secure the diagnosis [12].

Apart from the assessment of chronic loading effects of hypertension on the aortic wall, congenital abnormalities of the aorta that are related to hypertension can be excluded. Coarctation of the aorta can be diagnosed from the suprasternal view, although imaging of the coarctation site is difficult from transthoracic or suprasternal notch windows in adults. From the suprasternal notch approach, the descending thoracic aorta has a tapering appearance, even in normal individuals, because of the oblique tomographic view of the descending aorta obtained as the descending aorta leaves the image plane. This could erroneously lea to the diagnosis of coarctation even in a normal individual. Doppler interrogation can reveal an increased velocity across the coarctation and, if the obstruction is severe, persistent ante grade flow into diastole ("diastolic run-off"). If the velocity proximal to the coarctation is elevated, proximal velocity should be included in the Bernoulli equation for pressure gradient estimation.

Functional Assessment of Coronary Circulation and Micro-circulation in Hypertensive Patients

As a major risk factor for the development of coronary artery disease (CAD), the screening of the hypertensive for inducible ischemia is of paramount importance (Fig. 10.4). Traditionally this has been performed by means of treadmill stress test. However, this method suffers from inherent limitations involving its low sensitivity rates in women and in patients with single-vessel CAD. In addition electrocardiographic abnormalities such as LVH, strain and LBBB, which can frequently be recorded in hypertensives, make result interpretation challenging at times. In this context, imaging techniques offer an alternative option, with higher sensitivity and specificity Stress echocardiography is a well-established technique for the diagnosis and prognosis of patients suspected for CAD. It is based on the interpretation of inducible wall motion abnormalities/and or perfusion defects. Various stressors can be used; both exercise and pharmacological agents (dobutamine, dipyridamole and adenosine). All stress echo modalities exhibit similar sensitivity and specificity rates. In terms of diagnostic performance, it has been found that stress echocardiography has similar accuracy in hypertensive patients with and without left ventricular hypertrophy. Furthermore, stress echo has been used as a risk stratification tool in various study population, including patients with hypertension. The efficacy of dipyridamole stress echocardiography in risk stratification of hypertensive patients with chest pain, on the basis of presence/absence of the induced new wall motion abnormalities was previously illustrated. In particular, a negative echocardiographic result was found to be associated with only 3 % and 4 % event rates over 3 years of follow-up in a large multicentre study [13].

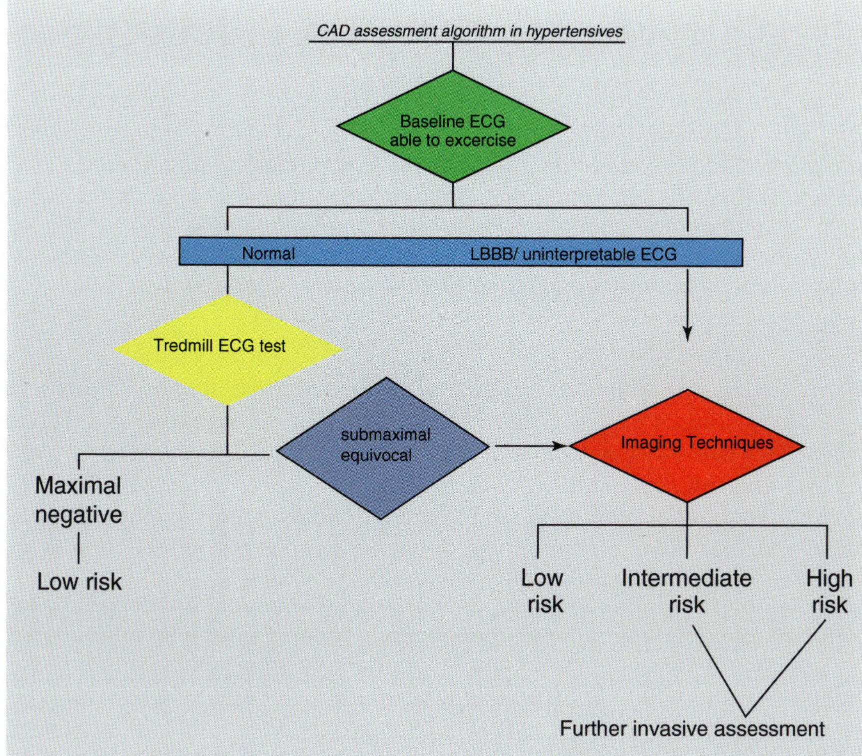

Fig. 10.4 Proposed algorithm for CAD diagnostic approach in hypertensives

Apart from CAD and macrovascular complications, hypertension can also affect the microcirculation. Evidence of endothelial dysfunction in human hypertension is well established. Experimental studies have shown that the endothelial cells exposed to a chronic elevation in arterial blood pressure age prematurely, their turnover is accelerated, and they are replaced by regenerated endothelial cells. However, the regenerated endothelium seems to be functionally impaired [14]. In clinical practice coronary flow reserve assessment by means of Doppler and the implementation of contrast agents serve as valuable adjuncts in the study of microcirculation.

The introduction of Doppler velocity measurements has allowed the functional assessment of coronary arteries and TTE has been introduced in the detection of coronary flow velocity and coronary flow velocity reserve (CFR) [15]. CFR can be quantified using flow velocity-derived methods. This in turn can be achieved by inducing maximal hyperaemia with the use of pharmacological agents such as adenosine and dipyridamole. The rationale for CFR application is that it can be affected by epicardial stenosis and microcirculation. In the absence of epicardial artery stenosis, CFR depicts the reactivity of the microcirculation. To level out the effect of microcirculation on CFR measurements in stenosed vessels the relative flow reserve has been developed. It is calculated by comparing the flow velocity reserve distal to the stenosis in the target vessel with the velocity reserve to a non-stenosed reference vessel [15].

Notably, abnormal CFR often accompanies hypertension even in the absence of left ventricular hypertrophy [16]. The observed reduction in CFR in hypertension is attributed to remodelling of the coronary small arteries and arterioles as well as to interstitial fibrosis [16]. This pathological alteration has been suggested to cause angina-like chest pain in non-coronary artery disease patients with or without hypertension [17, 18] and is regarded as a microvascular disturbance. End organ damage in the form of left ventricular hypertrophy has a strong contribution to the attenuation of CFR [19]. Carotid intima-media thickness (IMT) has been shown to correlate with traditional risk factors for atherosclerosis and the presence and severity of coronary artery disease, as well as with left ventricular mass in patients with hypertension [20, 21]. Interestingly, carotid atherosclerosis, measured by IMT, not only reflects coronary morphological changes (coronary IMT measured by intravascular ultrasound) [22] but also coronary functional changes (reduced CFR) [23]. Using the more sensitive method of Optical Coherence Tomography (OCT) in untreated hypertensive patients, it was again confirmed that reduced CFR was not related to increased coronary IMT in the absence of echocardiographically evident left ventricular hypertrophy. Moreover, no significant difference was found between patients with low and normal CFR with respect to OCT-measured IMT and IT with the values of the latter being in agreement with past reports [24, 25]. Therefore, adverse functional microcirculatory changes occur independently from and possibly precede vascular remodelling in hypertension.

In addition, both coronary circulation and microcirculation can be assessed by contrast agents. Contrast agents are microbubbles which primarily act as intravascular markers. The ischemic cascade illustrates that perfusion defects occur prior to systolic thickening abnormalities and ECG alterations. Moreover, perfusion defects appear in lower doses than those needed to provoke pathologic wall-motion response. As a result, perfusion assessment is a precise approach for CAD diagnosis. It was previously demonstrated that patients with malignant hypertension had abnormal perfusion during MCE as compared to healthy subjects, suggesting microvascular injury [14]. Myocardial blood flow impairment has been shown as prognostic indicator in hypertensive patients, without overt CAD. Last but not least, clinical studies based on real life echo protocols, demonstrated excellent safety profiles, thus rendering contrast agents an indispensable tool in clinical practice.

Novel Imaging Techniques

Echocardiography over the last decade has been marked by revolutionary changes, involving novel imaging techniques such as three-dimensional echo and speckle tracking echocardiography.

An early use and probably the most common clinical application of 3DE is the measurement of cardiac chamber dimensions and volumes. A firmly established advantage of 3D imaging over cross-sectional slices of the heart is the improvement in the accuracy of the evaluation of left ventricular volumes and ejection fraction by eliminating the need for geometric modeling, which is inaccurate in the presence of aneurysms, asymmetrical ventricles, or wall motion abnormalities. Three-dimensional echocardiography can depict the whole extent of the left ventricle, allowing accurate offline assessment of left ventricular mass and volumes with the implementation of dedicated software that all vendors have developed. The results have been validated against cardiac magnetic resonance imaging (MRI) which is regarded as the standard of reference for the assessment of left ventricle volumes and ejection fraction (EF) [26]. Conversely, 3DE offers more accurate measurements of the left atrium as compared to MRI (Fig. 10.5) [18]. Recent advances on 3DE have focused on specific software for each particular chamber resulting in more accurate evaluation of shape and function.

Speckle tracking implementing rotational and longitudinal deformation parameters, has offered valuable insights into the pathophysiologic processes of various disease stares, including hypertension. Moreover, deformation imaging can diagnose early cardiac dysfunction, even before the conventional assessment of diastolic indices and ejection fraction show sign of impairment. One should bear in mind that systolic function assessment by means of EF, is a rather simplistic approach as only refers to the radial component of deformation, and does not account for the complex three-dimensional heart deformation throughout systole. It was previously shown that in hypertensive patients longitudinal systolic dysfunction may be present in hypertensive patients with diastolic dysfunction, especially when septal Ea, 5.9 cm/s [27]. In general, longitudinal LV mechanics, which are predominantly governed by

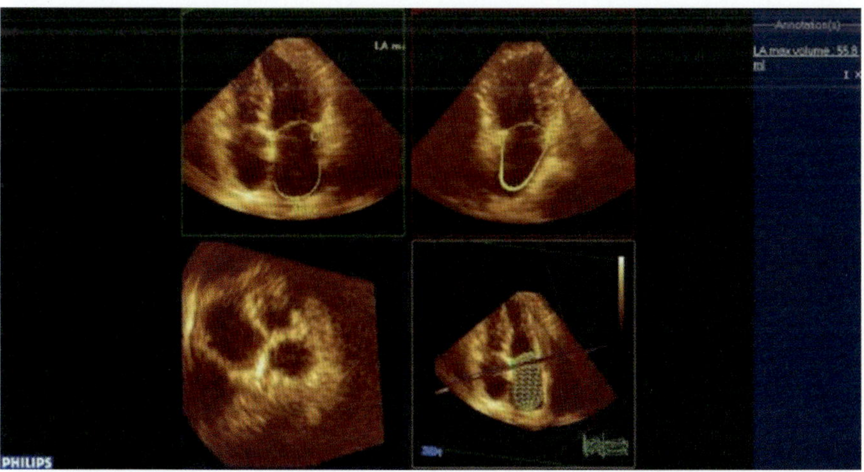

Fig. 10.5 Assessment of LA volumes using RT3DE. The figure captures an end-systolic frame, from which left atrial maximum volume is derived

the sub endocardial layer, are the most vulnerable and most sensitive to the presence of myocardial disease. If unaffected, midmyocardial and epicardial function may result in normal or nearly normal circumferential and twist mechanics with relatively preserved LV pump function and EF. However, compromised early diastolic longitudinal mechanics and reduced and/or delayed LV untwisting may elevate LV filling pressures and result in diastolic dysfunction. In hypertensives abnormal relaxation appears to have a particular distribution over the myocardial walls. Basal parts are generally more heavily affected, particularly the septal and inferior walls. The lateral wall and apical regions are more resistant to diastolic abnormalities. This pattern assists in differentiation of diastolic changes attributed to age. Furthermore, speckle tracking can assess the efficacy of various treatments in myocardial mechanics. Additionally, strain assessment can distinguish between hypertrophic cardiomyopathy, hypertensive heart disease and athlete's heart. This differentiation is possible because regional deformation may be reduced in hypertrophic cardiomyopathy, whereas it may be unchanged or hyper contractile in athletes' hearts. A recent study has demonstrated that in hypertensives, peak systolic strain is reduced even when conventional indices of systolic function such as EF and FS remain unaffected. These changes seem to be more prominent during physical stress. Longitudinal strain has been correlated to pulse-wave velocity measurements. The results of a recent study suggest that PWV may be independently associated with LV GLS, supporting the evidence of a close interaction between arterial stiffness and LV function. Increased arterial stiffness may result in impaired LV longitudinal function [28].

Current Practice Guidelines

In clinical practice, echocardiography should be considered in hypertensive patients in different clinical contexts and with different purposes: in hypertensive patients at moderate total CV risk, it may refine the risk evaluation by detecting LVH undetected by ECG; in hypertensive patients with ECG evidence of LVH it may more precisely assess the hypertrophy quantitatively and define its geometry and risk; in hypertensive patients with cardiac symptoms, it may help to diagnose underlying disease. It is obvious that echocardiography, including assessment of ascending aorta and vascular screening, may be of significant diagnostic value in most patients with hypertension and should ideally be recommended in all hypertensive patients at the initial evaluation. However, a wider or more restricted use will depend on availability and cost [29].

References

1. Lang RM, Bierig M, Devereux RB, et al. Recommendations for chamber quantification: a report from the American Society of Echocardiography's Guidelines and Standards Committee and the Chamber Quantification Writing Group, developed in conjunction with the European

Association of Echocardiography, a branch of the European Society of Cardiology. J Am Soc Echocardiogr. 2005;18:1440–63.

2. Schillacci G, Verdecchia P, Porcellati C, Cuccurullo O, Cosco C, Petricone F. Continuous relation between left ventricular mass and cardiovascular risk in essential hypertension. Hypertension. 2000;35:580–6. 20.
3. Cuspidi C, Sala C, Tadic M, Rescaldani M, Grassi G, Mancia G. Non-dipping pattern and subclinical cardiac damage in untreated hypertension: a systematic review and meta-analysis of echocardiographic studies. Am J Hypertens. 2015;28(12):1392–402. pii: hpv094.
4. Schirmer SH, Sayed MM, Reil JC, Lavall D, Ukena C, Linz D, Mahfoud F, Böhm M. Atrial remodeling following catheter-based renal denervation occurs in a blood pressure- and heart rate-independent manner. JACC Cardiovasc Interv. 2015;8(7):972–80. doi:10.1016/j.jcin.2015.02.014.
5. Wachtell K, Gerdts E, Aurigemma GP, Boman K, Dahlöf B, Nieminen MS, Olsen MH, Okin PM, Palmieri V, Rokkedal JE, Devereux RB. In-treatment reduced left atrial diameter during antihypertensive treatment is associated with reduced new-onset atrial fibrillation in hypertensive patients with left ventricular hypertrophy: The LIFE Study. Blood Press. 2010;19(3):169–75.
6. Tsioufis C, Stougiannos P, Taxiarxou E, et al. The interplay between haemodynamic load, brain natriuretic peptide and left atrial size in the early stages of essential hypertension. J Hypertens. 2006;24(5):965–72.
7. Tadic M, Cuspidi C, Pencic B, Kocijancic V, Celic V. The influence of left ventricular geometry on left atrial phasic function in hypertensive patients. Blood Press. 2015;27:1–8.
8. Nagueh SF, Appleton CP, Gillebert TC, et al. Recommendations for the evaluation of left ventricular diastolic function by echocardiography. J Am Soc Echocardiogr. 2009;10:165–93.
9. Wang M, Yip GW, Wang AY, et al. Tissue Doppler imaging provides incremental prognostic value in patients with systemic hypertension and left ventricular hypertrophy. J Hypertens. 2005;23(1):183–91.
10. Agu NC, McNiece Redwine K, Bell C, Garcia KM, Martin DS, Poffenbarger TS, Bricker JT, Portman RJ, Gupta-Malhotra M. Detection of early diastolic alterations by tissue Doppler imaging in untreated childhood-onset essential hypertension. J Am Soc Hypertens. 2014;8(5):303–11.
11. Evangelista A, Flachskampf FA, Erbel R, Antonini-Canterin F, Nihoyannopoulos P, et al. Echocardiography in aortic diseases: EAE recommendations for clinical practice. Eur J Echocardiogr. 2010;11:645–58.
12. Pearson AC, Guo R, Orsinelli DA, Binkley PF, Pasierski TJ. Transoesophageal echocardiographic assessment of the effects of age, gender, and hypertension on thoracic aortic wall size, thickness and stiffness. Am Heart J. 1994;128(2):344–5.
13. Cortigiani L, Paolini EA, Nannini E. Dipyridamole stress echocardiography for risk stratification in hypertensive patients with chest pain. Circulation. 1998;98(25):2855–9.
14. Shantsila A, Dwivedi G, Shantsila E, Butt M, Beevers DG, Lip GY. Persistent macrovascular and microvascular dysfunction in patients with malignant hypertension. Hypertension. 2011;57(3):490–6.
15. Brush Jr JE, Cannon 3rd RO, Schenke WH, Bonow RO, Leon MB, Maron BJ, Epstein SE. Angina due to coronary microvascular disease in hypertensive patients without left ventricular hypertrophy. N Engl J Med. 1988;319(20):1302–7.
16. Schwartzkopff B, Motz W, Frenzel H, Vogt M, Knauer S, Strauer BE. Structural and functional alterations of the intramyocardial coronary arterioles in patients with arterial hypertension. Circulation. 1993;88(3):993–1003.
17. Reis SE, Holubkov R, Lee JS, Sharaf B, Reichek N, Rogers WJ, Walsh EG, Fuisz AR, Kerensky R, Detre KM, Sopko G, Pepine CJ. Coronary flow velocity response to adenosine characterizes coronary microvascular function in women with chest pain and no obstructive coronary disease. Results from the pilot phase of the Women's Ischemia Syndrome Evaluation (WISE) study. J Am Coll Cardiol. 1999;33(6):1469–75.
18. Camici PG. Is the chest pain in cardiac syndrome X due to subendocardial ischaemia? Eur Heart J. 2007;28(13):1539–40.

19. Hamasaki S, Al Suwaidi J, Higano ST, Miyauchi K, Holmes Jr DR, Lerman A. Attenuated coronary flow reserve and vascular remodeling in patients with hypertension and left ventricular hypertrophy. J Am Coll Cardiol. 2000;35(6):1654–60.
20. Kallikazaros I, Tsioufis C, Sideris S, Stefanadis C, Toutouzas P. Carotid artery disease as a marker for the presence of severe coronary artery disease in patients evaluated for chest pain. Stroke. 1999;30(5):1002–7.
21. Chambless LE, Heiss G, Folsom AR, Rosamond W, Szklo M, Sharrett AR, Clegg LX. Association of coronary heart disease incidence with carotid arterial wall thickness and major risk factors: the Atherosclerosis Risk in Communities (ARIC) Study, 1987-1993. Am J Epidemiol. 1997;146(6):483–94.
22. Amato M, Montorsi P, Ravani A, Oldani E, Galli S, Ravagnani PM, Tremoli E, Baldassarre D. Carotid intima-media thickness by B-mode ultrasound as surrogate of coronary atherosclerosis: correlation with quantitative coronary angiography and coronary intravascular ultrasound findings. Eur Heart J. 2007;28(17):2094–101. Epub 2007 Jun 27.
23. Campuzano R, Moya JL, Garcia-Lledo A, Tomas JP, Ruiz S, Megias A, Balaguer J, Asín E. Endothelial dysfunction, intima-media thickness and coronary reserve in relation to risk factors and Framingham score in patients without clinical atherosclerosis. J Hypertens. 2006;24(8):1581–8.
24. Prati F, Regar E, Mintz GS, Arbustini E, Di Mario C, Jang IK, Akasaka T, Costa M, Guagliumi G, Grube E, Ozaki Y, Pinto F, Serruys PW, Expert's OCT Review Document. Expert review document on methodology, terminology, and clinical applications of optical coherence tomography: physical principles, methodology of image acquisition, and clinical application for assessment of coronary arteries and atherosclerosis. Eur Heart J. 2010;31(4):401–15.
25. Kume T, Akasaka T, Kawamoto T, Watanabe N, Toyota E, Neishi Y, Sukmawan R, Sadahira Y, Yoshida K. Assessment of coronary intima–media thickness by optical coherence tomography: comparison with intravascular ultrasound. Circ J. 2005;69(8):903–7.
26. Aggeli C, Felekos I, Kastellanos S, Panagopoulou V, Oikonomou E, Tsiamis E, Tousoulis D. Real-time three-dimensional echocardiography: never before clinical efficacy looked so picturesque. Int J Cardiol. 2015;198:15–21.
27. Pavlopoulos H, Grapsa J, Stefanadi E, Philippou E, Dawson D, Nihoyannopoulos P. Is it only diastolic dysfunction? Segmental relaxation patterns and longitudinal systolic deformation in systemic hypertension. Eur J Echocardiogr. 2008;9(6):741–7.
28. Kim HL, Seo JB, Chung WY, Kim SH, Kim MA, Zo JH. Independent association between brachial-ankle pulse wave velocity and global longitudinal strain of left ventricle. Int J Cardiovasc Imaging. 2015;31(8):1563–70.
29. Mancia G, Fagard R, Narkiewicz K, et al. 2013 ESH/ESC Guidelines for the management of arterial hypertension. Eur Heart J. 2013;34(28):2159–219.

Chapter 11
Biomarkers of Oxidative Stress in Human Hypertension

Sofia Tsiropoulou, Maria Dulak-Lis, Augusto C. Montezano, and Rhian M. Touyz

Introduction

Hypertension is a common chronic condition and a leading cause of morbidity and mortality worldwide [1]. Pathophysiological mechanisms contributing to high blood pressure are complex involving many systems including genetics, the sympathetic nervous system, activation of the renin-angiotensin-aldosterone system, adaptive and innate immunity and inflammation [2, 3]. Common to these processes is oxidative stress, defined as an increase in the bioavailability of reactive oxygen species (ROS), which causes activation and dysregulation of redox-sensitive signaling pathways leading to cellular damage and impaired function [4, 5].

Increased ROS levels have been described in many organs in experimental and human hypertension including the heart, kidneys, vasculature and brain [6–8]. In addition, ROS are detected in the circulation, and levels of plasma, erythrocyte and lymphocyte ROS are elevated in hypertension [9, 10]. Similarly too, urine ROS levels are increased in hypertension [11]. Mechanisms underlying oxidative stress in hypertension include increased ROS generation through pro-oxidant enzymes, such as NADPH oxidase, mitochondrial oxidases, xanthine oxidase and uncoupled nitric oxide synthase (NOS), as well as reduced degradation due to decreased activity of antioxidant systems, such as superoxide dismutase (SOD), catalase, peroxidases and Nrf-2-regulated antioxidants [12–14].

Oxidative stress plays an important role in the pathophysiology of hypertension through its damaging actions at the cellular and DNA levels. Cardiac, vascular and renal injury and inflammation in experimental hypertension are redox-sensitive processes, because treatment with NADPH oxidase inhibitors, ROS scavengers and

S. Tsiropoulou, Ph.D. • M. Dulak-Lis, Ph.D. • A.C. Montezano, Ph.D.
• R.M. Touyz, M.D., Ph.D. (✉)
Institute of Cardiovascular and Medical Sciences, BHF Glasgow Cardiovascular Research Centre, University of Glasgow, 126 University Place, Glasgow G12 8TA, UK
e-mail: Rhian.Touyz@glasgow.ac.uk

E.A. Andreadis (ed.), *Hypertension and Cardiovascular Disease*,
DOI 10.1007/978-3-319-39599-9_11

anti-oxidant vitamins normalize blood pressure and are cardiovascular- and renal-protective [15, 16]. At the molecular level increased ROS stimulate signaling pathways such as mitogen-activated protein kinases (MAPK), protein tyrosine phosphatases (PTP), Rho kinases, ion channels and transcription factors that induce cell growth, fibrosis, inflammation, de-differentiation and apoptosis [17–19]. In addition protein tyrosine phosphatases (PTP) are highly sensitive to oxidation [17, 18]. Oxidised PTP leads to inactivation of PTP with consequent increased phosphorylation of downstream kinases, including MAPK [17, 18], These phenomena are reversible when intracellular ROS levels are tightly regulated. However, sustained oxidative stress leads to irreversible DNA injury and cell death, important processes underlying target organ damage in hypertension.

While there is convincing data implicating oxidative stress in the pathophysiology of experimental hypertension, the evidence in human hypertension is less robust. Epidemiological studies suggest a relationship between plasma ROS levels and blood pressure [20]. Small clinical studies have demonstrated increased activation of ROS-producing enzymes, elevated ROS levels and decreased antioxidant capacity in vascular tissue, plasma and urine in hypertensive patients [21–24]. Despite these studies supporting a role for oxidative stress in clinical hypertension, large antioxidant trials failed to demonstrate cardiovascular protection and reduction in risk of cardiovascular disease [25, 26]. Reasons for these negative results include: (1) complex regulation of ROS and redox signaling in the cardiovascular system, (2) possibility of inappropriate antioxidants used because some antioxidant vitamins may be pro-oxidant, e.g., vitamin E, (3) sub-optimal doses of antioxidants tested, (4) timing of anti-oxidant therapy administration may be too late and introduced at a time when cardiovascular injury is irreversible and (5) challenges related to direct measurement of ROS in the clinical setting.

With an increased understanding of the redox biology underlying hypertension and advancements in the field of free radicals, new approaches to assess oxidative status in (patho) physiological conditions have been developed [27, 28]. While many of these approaches are still used in the experimental setting, there is a growing trend to exploit these in the clinic. In particular oxidative stress biomarkers are increasingly been measured as an indirect assessment of redox status in patients. To appreciate exactly what circulating biomarkers reflect, it is necessary to introduce the concept of oxidative stress and to briefly discuss redox signaling. Here we provide an overview of the biology of reactive oxygen species in the cardiovascular system, focusing particularly on human hypertension. We also highlight methods to assess redox status and discuss some biomarkers of oxidative stress in the clinical setting.

Oxidative Stress, ROS Generation and Redox Signaling in the Cardiovascular System: A Brief Overview

The notion of 'oxidative stress' was originally defined as an imbalance between pro-oxidants and anti-oxidants, with consequent increased ROS bioavailability leading to tissue damage [29]. More recently it has become clear that ROS also play an important physiological role in cellular signaling and cell function. In the vascular system, ROS influence vascular contraction/dilation and are critically involved in regulating endothelial function [30]. Accordingly, ROS are now considered as molecules or second messengers that influence redox signaling, defined as the specific oxidation-reduction modification of signaling molecules by a reactive species [31, 32]. Major ROS important in the cardiovascular and renal systems are superoxide anion (O_2^-), hydrogen peroxide (H_2O_2) and nitric oxide (NO) [31, 32].

In the kidney and vasculature ROS are produced mainly by non-phagocytic nicotinamide adenine dinucleotide phosphate (NADPH) oxidases (Nox) [33, 34]. In human hypertension the Noxs appear to be particularly important in vascular and renal dysfunction (Fig. 11.1).

Nox Family of Oxidases

Seven Nox isoforms have been identified (Nox1-5, Duox1, Duox2) of which Nox 1,2,4 and 5 are present in the human kidney and vessels [35]. The prototype Nox, is Nox2, also called gp91phox, and was originally identified in phagocytic cells as an important generator of ROS in host defense responses [36]. The main function of Nox enzymes is the production of ROS. Nox catalyze the reduction of O_2 by NADPH as electron donor thereby generating O_2-. Nox themselves are regulated by binding to various NADPH oxidase subunits, including p22phox, p47phox (isoform, NOXO1), p67phox (isoform, NOXA1) and p40phox. Whereas Nox1, Nox2 and Nox4 require p22phox as a membrane stabilizing subunit, Nox5, which is Ca^{2+}-sensitive, is unique in that it does not require any NADPH oxidase subunits for its activation [37, 38]. Vascular Nox activity is increased in hypertension and is highly sensitive to pro-hypertensive factors such as Ang II, ET-1 and aldosterone. In vascular cells from small arteries of hypertensive patients, expression of Nox 1,2,4 and 5 is upregulated with increased generation of ROS [6, 39–41]. These processes are associated with oxidative stress and altered redox signaling through MAP kinases and phosphatases leading to endothelial dysfunction and vascular remodeling [17–19, 42]. In vascular injury associated with diabetes, Nox1 is upregulated and in renal pathologies, activity and expression of Nox4, also known as renox, are increased [43, 44].

Antioxidant Enzymes

Antioxidant enzymes, which reduce ROS bioavailability include superoxide dismutase (SOD), catalase, peroxidases, and glutathione and thioredoxin antioxidant systems [45]. SOD, of which there are three isoforms, are particularly important because they catalyze dismutation of O_2^- to H_2O_2 and localize in discrete vascular compartments: cytosol for SOD1, mitochondria for SOD2 and extracellular matrix for SOD3 [46]. Accordingly SOD influences vascular redox signaling in a highly regulated and compartmentalized manner.

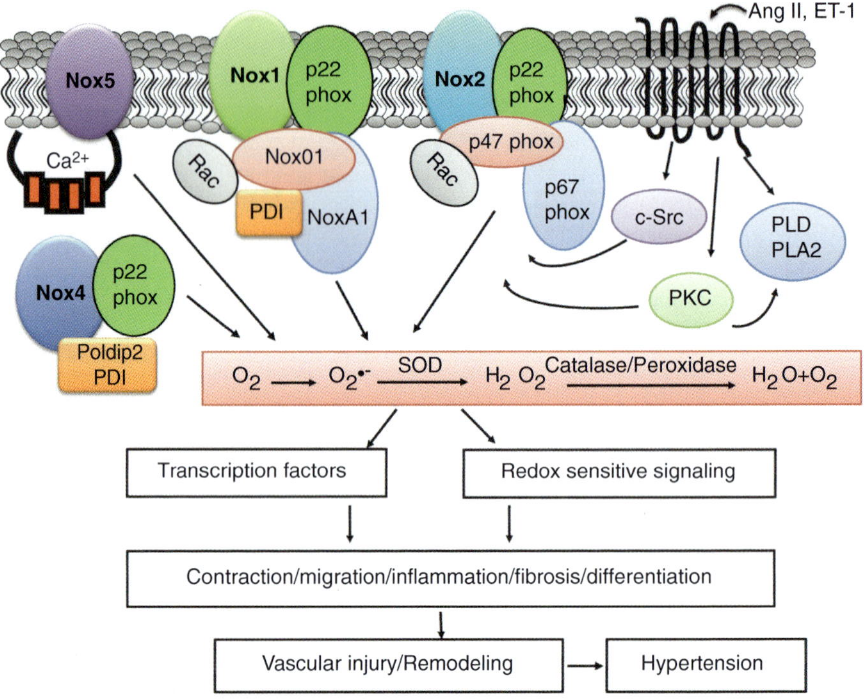

Fig. 11.1 Schematic demonstrating major Nox mechanisms responsible for ROS production in vascular cells in hypertension. Human vascular smooth muscle cells possess multiple Nox isoforms, including Nox1, 2,4 and 5. The expression and activity of these isoforms may be variable in physiological and pathological conditions. Activation of Noxs by pro-hypertensive factors, such as Ang II and ET-1, induces increased generation of ROS, which stimulate transcription factors and redox-sensitive signaling pathways that influence vascular function and structure in hypertension

Nrf-2 Transcription Factor

The pleiotropic transcription factor nuclear factor-erythroid 2 p45-related factor (Nrf)2 is also important in redox balance, as it is a key player in anti-oxidant protein production, through its regulation of genes that contain antioxidant response element (ARE) [47]. Nrf-2 induces transcriptional activation of antioxidant genes containing ARE, including NADPH dehydrogenase (quinone 1), glutathione peroxidases, heme oxygenase-1, thioredoxin reductase, glutathione-S-transferase, and SOD [48]. Nrf2 is constitutively controlled by ROS and by repressor protein Keap1 (Kelch-like ECH-associated protein 1) and induces upregulation of antioxidant defense mechanisms in states of cellular stress as a protective response [47, 48]. Nrf-2 activity appears to be downregulated in patients with cardiovascular disease and we demonstrated that pro-hypertensive factors, like Ang II, reduce Nrf-2 activity [49, 50]. Moreover in experimental hypertension, expression and activity of vascular Nrf-2 are attenuated, thereby contributing to reduced antioxidant capacity and increased oxidative stress. Treatment of hypertensive rats with a Nrf-2 inducer decreased blood pressure [51]. Cardiovascular and renal protective effects of Nrf-2 activators have also been demonstrated in human studies. For example, early studies in patients with diabetic nephropathy who were treated with the Nrf-2 activator bardoxolone methyl, showed significant improvement in renal function [52]. However later studies failed to demonstrate such protective actions [53].

Importance of Redox Signaling in Hypertension

To appreciate how ROS regulate signaling and cardiovascular function, it is important to know how ROS influence protein activity and cell function. It is also important to understand how ROS modify proteins, because the products of many of these processes are now being used as biomarkers of redox status. Briefly, proteins that contain cysteine or methionine residues are highly sensitive to oxidative modifications, which lead to changes in structure, activity and function of target proteins [54]. Reversible modifications of cysteine residues include S-nitrosylation/S-nitrosation, S-sulfenylation, disulfide bonds and S-glutathionylation [55]. These redox-induced changes target ion transporters, receptors, kinases, phosphatases, transcription factors, structural proteins and matrix metalloproteases (MMP), important in regulating cardiac, endothelial and vascular smooth muscle cell function [56]. Redox signaling is also important in the kidney. Oxidative stress may lead to irreversible oxidation of proteins leading to cell death. ROS-induced modification of proteins is increasingly been used as biomarker of oxidative stress.

Clinical Significance of Biomarkers of Oxidative Stress

By definition, a biomarker has the following characteristics: it is objectively measured and evaluated as an indicator of normal biological processes, pathogenic processes or pharmacologic responses to a therapeutic intervention [57]. In cardiovascular medicine, biomarkers are currently used to identify high-risk individuals and to predict cardiovascular risk. While there is extensive research in the field of biomarkers of cardiovascular risk, including markers of angiogenesis, fibrosis, inflammation, necrosis and oxidative stress, there is still some debate as to whether these novel circulating biomarkers are superior in predicting risk compared with traditional risk factors of age, sex, body mass index etc. However growing evidence indicates that risk evaluation may be improved if traditional factors are combined with circulating biomarkers. With respect to oxidative stress biomarkers, it is currently too premature to consider these as useful markers of cardiovascular risk in the clinical setting. New robust assays to measure oxidative status in the clinic together with large clinical studies to prove that biomarkers of oxidative stress truly and accurately reflect redox status are urgently needed. Nevertheless, the many biomarkers of oxidative stress discussed in this chapter are very useful in providing insights into mechanisms and pathophysiology of disease processes associated with redox imbalance in experimental and human hypertension.

Biomarkers of Oxidative Stress in Human Hypertension

ROS are unstable and have a very short half-life and as such accurately measuring $O_2^{\bullet-}$ and H_2O_2 is very challenging, particularly in the clinic. To address this, methods have been developed to measure stable markers of ROS that reflect oxidative status [27, 58]. The most common biomarkers of oxidative stress that are currently used to evaluate the redox state in human samples are (1) oxidation products of lipids, (2) oxidative modification of proteins, and (3) oxidative modification of DNA/RNA [59, 60] (Table 11.1).

Oxidation Products of Lipids

Polyunsaturated fatty acids (PUFAs), including phospholipids, glycolipids and cholesterol are important targets of lipid peroxidation. Increased ROS levels trigger the process of lipid peroxidation during which lipid peroxyl radicals act as chain-carrying radicals and lipid hydroperoxides are generated as the main end products [61, 62]. Lipid hydroperoxides are further processed into different reactive aldehydes that influence signaling and cell function. Major reactive aldehydes include trans-4-hydroxy-2-nonenal (4-HNE) and malondialdehyde (MDA). ROS-induced oxidation of arachidonic acid gives rise to isoprostanes [63–65].

Malondialdehyde (MDA)

MDA can be detected by thiobarbituric acid (TBA) using a colorimetric method based on the reaction between MDA and TBA that gives a pink colour [66]. The products that are measured are called TBA reactive species (TBARS). The TBARS assay is amongst the most widely employed to evaluate lipid peroxidation in human plasma and urine samples. Plasma TBARS levels are increased in patients with hypertension, atherosclerosis, diabetes, heart failure, stroke and aging [67, 68]. Cigarette smokers also have elevated levels of TBARS [69].

Table 11.1 Biomarkers of oxidative stress

Lipid peroxidation
Malondialdehyde (TBARS)
F2-isoprostanes
4-hydroxynonenal (4-HNE)
OxLDL
Protein oxidation
Carbonyls
Sulfur oxidation
DNA oxidation
7,8-dihydro-8-oxo-2'-deoxyguanosine (8oxodG)
RNA oxidation
7,8-dihydro-8-oxo-guanosine (8oxoGuo)
Pro-oxidant enzymes
Xanthine oxidase
Mitochondrial oxidases
Myeloperoxidases
NADPH oxidases (Nox)
Antioxidant enzymes
Superoxide dismutase
Catalase
Glutathione peroxidase
GSH/GSSG ratio
Non-enzymatic antioxidants
Total antioxidant capacity
Vitamin C
Vitamin A
Urate
Bilirubin
Thiols
Flavonoids
Carotenoids

4-hydroxynonenal (4-HNE)

4-HNE is produced by lipid peroxidation in cells and is considered as one of the most specific and sensitive measures of lipid auto-oxidation. Various methods have been developed to measure 4-HNE including HPLC and immune-based methods. Higher circulating 4-HNE levels correlate with more severe diastolic dysfunction in experimental models of hypertension [70]. 4-HNE has also been associated with stroke, ischaemia-reperfusion injury and cardiac hypertrophy. Increasing experimental evidence indicates that 4-HNE may have a dual role in that it may be a marker of systemic oxidative stress and also contribute directly to the pathogenesis of cardiovascular disease [71, 72]. Despite experimental evidence linking 4-HNE and cardiovascular disease, there is a paucity of information in humans. A few studies in dialyzed patients demonstrated that MDA and 4-HNE thiols correlated with severity of cardiovascular disease [73, 74].

Isoprostanes

Oxidation of arichidonic acid forms a family of stereoisomers termed H-isoprostanes. Rearrangement of these H2-isoprostanes form stable F2-isoprostanes and highly reactive isoketals [75]. F2-isoprostanes are stable end products of lipid peroxidation and can be measured in all human tissues and biological fluids, including urine, plasma and cerebrospinal fluid [76]. Because of their stability and sensitivity to changes in redox state, F2-isoprostanes are considered the most reliable markers for tracking oxidative stress in vivo.

Formation of isoprostanes is independent of the COX enzymes that catalyse production of prostaglandins. A metabolite of F2-isoprostanes, 8-iso-prostaglandin F2α (8-iso-PGF2α) has vasoconstrictor, mitogenic and pro-thrombotic actions and as such is biologically active independently of its biomarker status [77, 78]. Levels of F2-isoprostanes in plasma and urine correlate with circulating ROS levels in experimental and human hypertension [79]. In healthy individuals with risk factors, such as obesity, hyperlipidaemia and hyperhomocysteinaemia, plasma concentrations of F2-isoprostanes are elevated, suggesting that indices of lipid peroxidation may be clinically relevant biomarkers of cardiovascular risk [80]. In support of this, a prospective study including 1,002 anticoagulated patients with atrial fibrillation studied over 2 years demonstrated that 8-iso-PGF2α and sNOX2-dp (a marker of Nox2 levels) correlated with cardiovascular events [81]. Using various modelling paradigms it was shown that 8-iso-PGF2α predicted cardiovascular events and death. Accordingly it was suggested that F2-IsoP may complement traditional risk factors in prediction of cardiovascular events.

Oxidative Modification of Proteins

DNA and proteins are highly susceptible to modifications by changes in the redox state. Protein oxidation, which can be reversible or irreversible, leads to changes in the biological function of the target protein [82] (Table 11.2). Assessment of the extent of such a general type of oxidation serves as a marker of increased oxidative stress.

Irreversible Oxidative Modification of Proteins- Carbonylation

The most common type of irreversible modification is the formation of carbonyl groups, which are generated when there is oxidative cleavage of protein backbones. Amino acids prone to carbonylation include proline, arginine, threonine, lysine, histidine and cysteine [83]. Protein carbonyls (having aldehyde and ketone

Table 11.2 Some common protein oxidative modifications detected in cells of the cardiovascular and renal systems

Type of oxidation	Reversible/Irreversible	Target amino acid
Carbonylation	Irreversible	Arg, Cys, His, Lys, Pro.
Sulfur Oxidation	Reversible/irreversible	Cys/Met
S-glutathionylation S-nitrosylation Disulfide linkage Sulfenic/sulfinic acid	Reversible	Cys
Sulfonic acid	Irreversible	Cys
Methionine sulfoxide	Reversible	Met
Tyrosine oxidation	Reversible	Tyr
Lipid peroxidation adducts	Reversible	Lys, His, Cys

moieties) are detected after derivatization and the products are measured spectrophotometrically, by HPLC or by immune-based approaches. Elevated protein carbonyl levels have been reported in a number of conditions, including aging, obesity, diabetes, cancer and cardiovascular diseases [84, 85]. Protein carbonylation is an irreversible process and as such increased levels of protein carbonyls reflect increased irreversible oxidation.

Reversible Oxidation of Proteins

Cysteine Thiol Oxidation

The main thiol compound in the body is cysteine, which is highly susceptible to oxidation. Biologically occurring thiols include low molecular weight thiols, such as cysteine and glutathione (GSH), and protein thiols [86]. Cysteine thiol oxidation, which is reversible or irreversible, results in structural and functional changes of proteins and as such may have significant impact on cell signaling and function [87]. The most commonly used approach to measure thiol cysteine oxidation involves alkylation of free thiols with subsequent reduction of the reversibly oxidized thiols and labeling with a probe [82, 88]. Increase in the signal is indicative of elevated reversible oxidation. This approach can assess either global or specific types of reversible thiol modifications, depending on the selectivity of the reductant being used. A more direct approach in assessing cysteine thiol oxidation under non-reducing conditions is an antibody-based strategy [89].

Protein cysteine residues can exist in various oxidation states, including S-glutathionylation, S-sulfenylation and S-nitrosylation. These modifications are increasingly recognized as important specific signaling events in cardiovascular physiology and disease [90]. The significance of protein S-glutathiolation and S-sulfenylation in cardiovascular disease has been suggested in various experimental models [91–93]. In addition, mitochondrial-selective S-nitrosylation has been shown to protect against heart failure and cardiac injury in a mouse model of infarction [91, 93].

Methionine Oxidation

Similar to cysteine, methionine is a sulfur-containing amino acid, which is also highly sensitive to oxidative modification [94]. Sulfur in methionine can be reversibly oxidized to a sulfoxide. Emerging evidence suggests that methionine oxidation can directly influence protein function and may be associated with cardiovascular disease [95]. Increased plasma levels of methionine sulfoxide have been reported in inflammatory processes and diabetes. A recent study demonstrated that methionine sulfoxide reductase A acts as a negative modulator of vascular smooth muscle cell proliferation and neointimal hyperplasia after vascular injury through regulation of MAP kinases [95]. Whether methionine oxidation is altered in hypertension is unclear.

Oxidative Modification of DNA and RNA

Oxidation of DNA and RNA by ROS, are also biomarkers of redox status. Oxidative changes of DNA can lead to mutations due to mispair of bases and levels are increased in cancer [96]. RNA oxidation is a relatively new biomarker of oxidative stress and has been associated with increased risk of diabetes. Oxidised nucleotides are excreted into urine and reflect cumulative total body oxidative stress [97]. Hence, as urinary biomarkers, oxidized nucleotides are reflective of systemic oxidative stress rather than localized tissue-specific increased levels of ROS. Urinary assays to measure 7,8-dihydro-8-oxo-2'-deoxyguanosine (8oxodG) (DNA oxidation) and 7,8-dihydro-8-oxo-guanosine (8oxoGuo) (RNA oxidation) are now commercially available as ELISA kits.

Biomarkers of ROS-Generating Enzymes

Myeloperoxidase and Xanthine Oxidase

Some ROS-generating enzymes, such as myeloperoxidase and xanthine oxidase, have been detected in the circulation [98]. Elevated circulating levels of xanthine oxidase and myeloperoxidase, possibly due to increased release from damaged cells have been described in hypertension [99, 100]. Myeloperoxidase catalyzes the reaction between H_2O_2 and chloride ions producing HOCl, important oxidants in innate immunity and vascular inflammation associated with atherosclerosis, hypertension and ischemia-reperfusion injury [100].

Xanthine oxidase, which itself is redox-sensitive, is responsible for purine catabolism. It catalyses the oxidation of hypoxanthine to xanthine, and xanthine to uric acid. Plasma levels of xanthine oxidase are normally very low in humans, but are elevated in pathological condition when injured cells release xanthine oxidase into the circulation. Uric acid gives rise to free radicals by interacting with $O_2^{\cdot-}$, NO and

$ONOO^-$ [101]. Increased plasma levels of uric acid may thus reflect underlying oxidation and as such may be a useful biomarker of oxidative stress. This may be particularly relevant in hypertension, where hyperuricemia is an independent risk factor for cardiovascular disease and is predictive of mortality if associated with diabetes and hypertension [102]. To further support a relationship between hyperuricemia and hypertension, increasing evidence indicates that allopurinol, a xanthine oxidase inhibitor reduces blood pressure in hypertensive adolescents and adults and protects against hypertension-associated target organ damage and stroke [103, 104].

NADPH Oxidase (Nox) in Circulating Cells

Of the many ROS-generating enzymes in biological systems, the Nox isoforms appear to be amongst the most important in the cardiovascular and renal systems. Nox2 (gp91phox-NADPH oxidase) is characteristically expressed in circulating phagocytic cells and its expression and activity are increased in experimental and human hypertension, and as such may be a marker of global oxidative stress [81, 105, 106]. Increased expression of NADPH oxidase subunits p47phox and p67phox as well as other Nox isoforms (Nox4, 5) has also been demonstrated in hypertensive patients [107, 108].

Plasma/Urine Anti-oxidants and Total Antioxidant Capacity

Because of the highly reactive nature of ROS, the human body must have systems that tightly regulate ROS to maintain redox homeostasis. This is achieved through complex enzymatic and non-enzymatic anti-oxidant systems. The major enzymatic systems include SOD, catalase, peroxidases and oxireductases, such as thioredoxin, peroxiredoxins and glutathione, which function to keep thiols in the reduced state [109]. Non-enzymatic systems include small molecules and anti-oxidant vitamins. Most of these antioxidants can be measured in plasma, urine and circulating cells. Reduced plasma and urine levels of various antioxidants have been demonstrated in experimental and human hypertension, which may reflect underlying systemic oxidative stress [110].

In addition to measuring plasma concentrations of individual enzymatic antioxidants as biomarkers of the oxidative state, it is now possible to assess total antioxidant capacity, which is a measure of the combined antioxidant effect of the non-enzymatic defenses in biological fluids and does not take into account the enzymatic anti-oxidant systems [111]. The assay measures low molecular weight water-soluble and lipid soluble antioxidants and includes urate, bilirubin, vitamin C, thiols, flavonoids, carotenoids and vitamin E [111]. Experimental and clinical studies have shown, for the most part, low levels of total antioxidant capacity in various cardiovascular diseases including hypertension [112–114]. Total antioxidant capacity assays have also been used extensively in human studies evaluating effects of dietary antioxidants [115].

Oxidative Stress Biomarkers and Human Hypertension

Clinical studies in patients with essential hypertension demonstrated that blood pressure correlates positively with markers of oxidative stress (e.g. TBARS and isoprostane levels) and negatively with anti-oxidant capacity, indicating an association between increased ROS bioavailability, vascular dysfunction and hypertension [116, 117] (Fig. 11.2). Endothelial dysfunction, a hallmark of hypertension, is associated with increased vascular ROS production, oxidative stress and vascular inflammation [116–118]. This is supported by an inverse association between acetylcholine-dependent vasodilation and plasma levels of soluble adhesion molecules (e-selectin, p-selectin), cytokines (interleukins, monocyte chemotactic protein type 1), metalloproteinases type 1 (TIMP-1) and TBARS and positive associations with serum levels of antioxidants [119]. We showed that ROS production in vascular smooth muscle cells from resistance arteries of patients with essential hypertension have higher levels of ROS, increased activation and expression of Noxs and enhanced redox-dependent signaling, versus cells from normotensive healthy subjects [39, 40].

Increased plasma levels of reactive carbonyl species (RCS) has been demonstrated in hypertensive patients, and blood pressure was found to be significantly correlated with plasma RCS levels [120]. In untreated mild hypertensive patients the lipid peroxidation (TBARS levels) and stable end products of nitric oxide are increased [121]. To further support an association between oxidative stress and cardiovascular risk, anti-oxLDL antibody levels were increased after antihypertensive therapy in primary prevention of hypertension, suggesting that the results are in agreement with the concept that the susceptibility to oxidation is increased by hypertension and that anti-oxLDL antibodies may be protective and also have potential as a biomarker of oxidative stress [122].

Population-based observational studies showed an inverse relationship between plasma antioxidant levels and blood pressure. Decreased antioxidant activity (SOD, catalase) and reduced concentrations of ROS scavengers (vitamin E, glutathione) may contribute to oxidative stress in human hypertension [123, 124]. Plasma vitamin C levels are inversely related to blood pressure in normotensive and hypertensive cohorts. Causes of reduced cellular antioxidants in hypertension are unclear but may relate, in part, to genetic factors. Polymorphisms of Noxs and the NADPH oxidase subunits have been identified in hypertensive patients [125, 126].

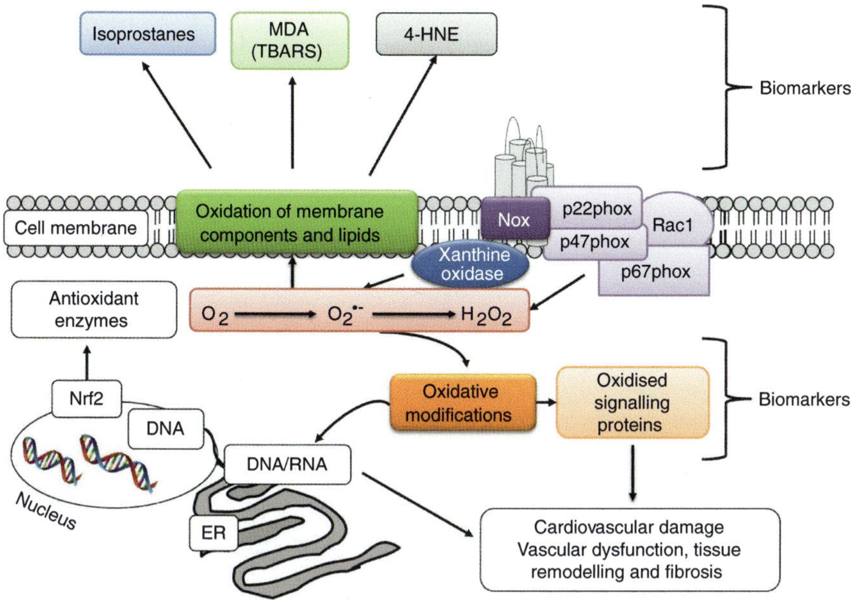

Fig. 11.2 Diagram demonstrating molecular and cellular redox-sensitive processes that can be tracked as biomarkers of oxidative stress. Major biomarkers that can be measured in human samples include markers of lipid peroxidation, markers of protein, DNA and RNA oxidation, as well as indices of pro-oxidant and anti-oxidant enzymes. *4-HNE* 4-hydroxynonenal, *MDA* malondialdehyde, *ER* endoplasmic reticulum

Conclusions

Physiologically, ROS play an important role in regulating cardiovascular function through tightly controlled redox-sensitive signaling pathways. Uncontrolled production/degradation of ROS results in oxidative stress, which induces cardiovascular injury with associated increase in blood pressure. Convincing evidence from experimental and animal studies indicate a causative role for ROS and ROS-generating Noxs in the pathogenesis of hypertension. However in humans it is still unclear whether oxidative stress is a prime cause of hypertension, although biomarkers of oxidative stress correlate positively with blood pressure in essential hypertension. Although numerous redox biomarkers including markers of lipid peroxidation, oxidation of proteins and DNA, thiol modifications and antioxidant status, have been identified in hypertension and cardiovascular disease, these still need to be validated clinically in large cohorts. Moreover, these biomarkers, which are an indirect index of oxidative status need to be correlated directly with oxidative changes and disease pathogenesis. Considering the complexity of hypertension and cardiovascular disease, it is likely that there will not be one oxidative biomarker, but rather an array or platform of various markers that will define the redox-oxidative phenotype in health and disease. Finally, although many of the described biomarkers of oxidative stress have provided important mechanistic insights into disease processes, well controlled studies with currently available biomarkers still need to be validated in large clinical cohorts and compared with current clinical standards to establish their utility in clinical diagnostics.

Acknowledgements Work from the author's laboratory was supported by grants 44018 and 57886, from the Canadian Institutes of Health Research (CIHR) and grants from the British Heart Foundation (BHF). RMT is supported through a BHF Chair. ACM is supported through a Leadership Fellowship from the University of Glasgow. MDL is supported through a Marie Curie ITN (RADOX).

Disclosures None

References

1. Bromfield S, Muntner P. High blood pressure: the leading global burden of disease risk factor and the need for worldwide prevention programs. Curr Hypertens Rep. 2013;15(3):134–6.
2. Caillon A, Schiffrin EL. Role of inflammation and immunity in hypertension: recent epidemiological, laboratory, and clinical evidence. Curr Hypertens Rep. 2016;18(3):21.
3. Montezano AC, Nguyen Dinh Cat A, Rios FJ, Touyz RM. Angiotensin II and vascular injury. Curr Hypertens Rep. 2014;16(6):431.
4. Ray PD, Huang BW, Tsuji Y. Reactive oxygen species (ROS) homeostasis and redox regulation in cellular signaling. Cell Signal. 2012;24(5):981–90.
5. Jones DP. Redefining oxidative stress. Antioxid Redox Signal. 2006;8(9–10):1865–7.
6. Nguyen Dinh Cat A, Montezano AC, Burger D, Touyz RM. Angiotensin II, NADPH oxidase, and redox signaling in the vasculature. Antioxid Redox Signal. 2013;19(10):1110–20.
7. Sahoo S, Meijles DN, Pagano PJ. NADPH oxidases: key modulators in aging and age-related cardiovascular diseases? Clin Sci (Lond). 2016;130(5):317–35.
8. Callera GE, Tostes RC, Yogi A, Montezano AC, Touyz RM. Endothelin-1-induced oxidative stress in DOCA-salt hypertension involves NADPH-oxidase-independent mechanisms. Clin Sci (Lond). 2006;110(2):243–53.
9. Montezano AC, Dulak-Lis M, Tsiropoulou S, Harvey A, Briones AM, Touyz RM. Oxidative stress and human hypertension: vascular mechanisms, biomarkers, and novel therapies. Can J Cardiol. 2015;31(5):631–41.
10. De Ciuceis C, Flati V, Rossini C, Rufo A, Porteri E, Di Gregorio J, Petroboni B, La Boria E, Donini C, Pasini E, Agabiti Rosei E, Rizzoni D. Effect of antihypertensive treatments on insulin signalling in lympho-monocytes of essential hypertensive patients: a pilot study. Blood Press. 2014;23(6):330–8.
11. Rodrigo R, Libuy M, Feliú F, Hasson D. Oxidative stress-related biomarkers in essential hypertension and ischemia-reperfusion myocardial damage. Dis Markers. 2013;35(6):773–90.
12. Gómez-Marcos MA, Blázquez-Medela AM, Gamella-Pozuelo L, Recio-Rodriguez JI, García-Ortiz L, Martínez-Salgado C. Serum superoxide dismutase is associated with vascular

structure and function in hypertensive and diabetic patients. Oxid Med Cell Longev. 2016;2016:9124676.

13. Lassègue B, San Martín A, Griendling KK. Biochemistry, physiology, and pathophysiology of NADPH oxidases in the cardiovascular system. Circ Res. 2012;110(10):1364–90.
14. Lopes RA, Neves KB, Tostes RC, Montezano AC, Touyz RM. Downregulation of nuclear factor erythroid 2-related factor and associated antioxidant genes contributes to redox-sensitive vascular dysfunction in hypertension. Hypertension. 2015;66(6):1240–50.
15. Chen X, Touyz RM, Park JB, Schiffrin EL. Antioxidant effects of vitamins C and E are associated with altered activation of vascular NADPH oxidase and superoxide dismutase in stroke-prone SHR. Hypertension. 2001;38(3 Pt 2):606–11.
16. Virdis A, Neves MF, Amiri F, Touyz RM, Schiffrin EL. Role of NAD(P)H oxidase on vascular alterations in angiotensin II-infused mice. J Hypertens. 2004;22(3):535–42.
17. Droge W. Free radicals in the physiological control of cell function. Physiol Rev. 2002;82(1):47–95.
18. Tabet F, Schiffrin EL, Callera GE, He Y, Yao G, Ostman A, Kappert K, Tonks NK, Touyz RM. Redox-sensitive signaling by angiotensin II involves oxidative inactivation and blunted phosphorylation of protein tyrosine phosphatase SHP-2 in vascular smooth muscle cells from SHR. Circ Res. 2008;103(2):149–58.
19. Bruder-Nascimento T, Callera GE, Montezano AC, He Y, Antunes TT, Cat AN, Tostes RC, Touyz RM. Vascular injury in diabetic db/db mice is ameliorated by atorvastatin: role of Rac1/2-sensitive Nox-dependent pathways. Clin Sci (Lond). 2015;128(7):411–23.
20. Schöttker B, Saum KU, Jansen EH, Holleczek B, Brenner H. Associations of metabolic, inflammatory and oxidative stress markers with total morbidity and multi-morbidity in a large cohort of older German adults. Age Ageing. 2016;45(1):127–35.
21. Annor FB, Goodman M, Okosun IS, Wilmot DW, Il'yasova D, Ndirangu M, Lakkur S. Oxidative stress, oxidative balance score, and hypertension among a racially diverse population. J Am Soc Hypertens. 2015;9(8):592–9.
22. Montezano AC, Touyz RM. Reactive oxygen species, vascular Noxs, and hypertension: focus on translational and clinical research. Antioxid Redox Signal. 2014;20(1):164–82.
23. Yu P, Han W, Villar VA, Yang Y, Lu Q, Lee H, Li F, Quinn MT, Gildea JJ, Felder RA, Jose PA. Unique role of NADPH oxidase 5 in oxidative stress in human renal proximal tubule cells. Redox Biol. 2014;2:570–9.
24. Kröller-Schön S, Steven S, Kossmann S, Scholz A, Daub S, Oelze M, Xia N, Hausding M, Mikhed Y, Zinssius E, Mader M, Stamm P, Treiber N, Scharffetter-Kochanek K, Li H, Schulz E, Wenzel P, Münzel T, Daiber A. Molecular mechanisms of the crosstalk between mitochondria and NADPH oxidase through reactive oxygen species-studies in white blood cells and in animal models. Antioxid Redox Signal. 2014;20(2):247–66.
25. Schiffrin EL. Antioxidants in hypertension and cardiovascular disease. Mol Interv. 2010;10(6):354–62.
26. Juraschek SP, Guallar E, Appel LJ, Miller 3rd ER. Effects of vitamin C supplementation on blood pressure: a meta-analysis of randomized controlled trials. Am J Clin Nutr. 2012;95(5):1079–88.
27. Apak R, Özyürek M, Güçlü K, Çapanoğlu E. Antioxidant activity/capacity measurement. 3. Reactive oxygen and nitrogen species (ROS/RNS) scavenging assays, oxidative stress biomarkers, and chromatographic/chemometric assays. J Agric Food Chem. 2016;64(5):1046–70.
28. Ho E, Karimi Galougahi K, Liu CC, Bhindi R, Figtree GA. Biological markers of oxidative stress: applications to cardiovascular research and practice. Redox Biol. 2013;1(1):483–91.
29. Lushchak VI. Free radicals, reactive oxygen species, oxidative stress and its classification. Chem Biol Interact. 2014;224C:164–75.
30. Touyz RM. Reactive oxygen species as mediators of calcium signalling by angiotensin II: implications in vascular physiology and pathophysiology. Antioxid Redox Signal. 2005;7(9–10):1302–14.

31. Tsimikas S. Oxidative biomarkers in the diagnosis and prognosis of cardiovascular disease. Am J Cardiol. 2006;98(11A):9P–17.
32. Valko M, Jomova K, Rhodes CJ, Kuča K, Musílek K. Redox- and non-redox-metal-induced formation of free radicals and their role in human disease. Arch Toxicol. 2016;90(1):1–37.
33. Holterman CE, Read NC, Kennedy CR. Nox and renal disease. Clin Sci (Lond). 2015;128(8):465–81.
34. Montezano AC, Touyz RM. Reactive oxygen species and endothelial function–role of nitric oxide synthase uncoupling and Nox family nicotinamide adenine dinucleotide phosphate oxidases. Basic Clin Pharmacol Toxicol. 2012;110(1):87–94.
35. Brandes RP, Weissmann N, Schröder K. Nox family NADPH oxidases: molecular mechanisms of activation. Free Radic Biol Med. 2014;76C:208–26.
36. Cachat J, Deffert C, Hugues S, Krause KH. Phagocyte NADPH oxidase and specific immunity. Clin Sci (Lond). 2015;128(10):635–48.
37. Chen F, Wang Y, Barman S, Fulton DJ. Enzymatic regulation and functional relevance of NOX5. Curr Pharm Des. 2015;21(41):5999–6008.
38. Holterman CE, Thibodeau JF, Towaij C, Gutsol A, Montezano AC, Parks RJ, Cooper ME, Touyz RM, Kennedy CR. Nephropathy and elevated BP in mice with podocyte-specific NADPH oxidase 5 expression. J Am Soc Nephrol. 2014;25(4):784–97.
39. Touyz RM, Schiffrin EL. Increased generation of superoxide by angiotensin II in smooth muscle cells from resistance arteries of hypertensive patients: role of phospholipase D-dependent NAD(P)H oxidase-sensitive pathways. J Hypertens. 2001;19(7):1245–54.
40. Touyz RM, Chen X, Tabet F, Yao G, He G, Quinn MT, Pagano PJ, Schiffrin EL. Expression of a functionally active gp91phox-containing neutrophil-type NAD(P)H oxidase in smooth muscle cells from human resistance arteries: regulation by angiotensin II. Circ Res. 2002;90(11):1205–13.
41. Touyz RM, Yao G, Schiffrin EL. c-Src induces phosphorylation and translocation of p47phox: role in superoxide generation by angiotensin II in human vascular smooth muscle cells. Arterioscler Thromb Vasc Biol. 2003;23(6):981–7.
42. Dikalov SI, Nazarewicz RR, Bikineyeva A, Hilenski L, Lassègue B, Griendling KK, Harrison DG, Dikalova AE. Nox2-induced production of mitochondrial superoxide in angiotensin II-mediated endothelial oxidative stress and hypertension. Antioxid Redox Signal. 2014;20(2):281–94.
43. Gray SP, Di Marco E, Okabe J, Szyndralewiez C, Heitz F, Montezano AC, de Haan JB, Koulis C, El-Osta A, Andrews KL, Chin-Dusting JP, Touyz RM, Wingler K, Cooper ME, Schmidt HH, Jandeleit-Dahm KA. NADPH oxidase 1 plays a key role in diabetes mellitus-accelerated atherosclerosis. Circulation. 2013;127(18):1888–902.
44. Araujo M, Wilcox CS. Oxidative stress in hypertension: role of the kidney. Antioxid Redox Signal. 2014;20(1):74–101.
45. Maksimenko AV. Experimental antioxidant biotherapy for protection of the vascular wall by modified forms of superoxide dismutase and catalase. Curr Pharm Des. 2005;11(16):2007–16.
46. Fukai T, Ushio-Fukai M. Superoxide dismutases: role in redox signaling, vascular function, and diseases. Antioxid Redox Signal. 2011;15(6):1583–606.
47. Hayes JD, Dinkova-Kostova AT. The Nrf2 regulatory network provides an interface between redox and intermediary metabolism. Trends Biochem Sci. 2014;39(4):199–218.
48. Hybertson BM, Gao B, Bose SK, McCord JM. Oxidative stress in health and disease: the therapeutic potential of Nrf2 activation. Mol Aspects Med. 2011;32(4–6):234–46.
49. Howden R. Nrf2 and cardiovascular defense. Oxid Med Cell Longev. 2013;2013:104308.
50. Wang YY, Yang YX, Zhe H, He ZX, Zhou SF. Bardoxolone methyl (CDDO-Me) as a therapeutic agent: an update on its pharmacokinetic and pharmacodynamic properties. Drug Des Devel Ther. 2014;8:2075–88.
51. Gomez-Guzman M, Jimenez R, Sanchez M. Epicatechin lowers blood pressure, restores endothelial function, and decreases oxidative stress and endothelin-1 and NADPH oxidase activity in DOCA-salt hypertension. Free Radic Biol Med. 2012;52:70–9.

52. de Zeeuw D, Akizawa T, Audhya P, Bakris GL, Chin M, Christ-Schmidt H, Goldsberry A, Houser M, Krauth M, Lambers Heerspink HJ, McMurray JJ, Meyer CJ, Parving HH, Remuzzi G, Toto RD, Vaziri ND, Wanner C, Wittes J, Wrolstad D, Chertow GM, BEACON Trial Investigators. Bardoxolone methyl in type 2 diabetes and stage 4 chronic kidney disease. N Engl J Med. 2013;369(26):2492–503.
53. Chen J, Zhang Z, Cai L. Diabetic cardiomyopathy and its prevention by nrf2: current status. Diabetes Metab J. 2014;38(5):337–45.
54. Go YM, Jones DP. Cysteine/cystine redox signaling in cardiovascular disease. Free Radic Biol Med. 2011;50(4):495–509.
55. Go YM, Jones DP. Thiol/disulfide redox states in signaling and sensing. Crit Rev Biochem Mol Biol. 2013;48(2):173–81.
56. Jones DP, Go YM. Redox compartmentalization and cellular stress. Diabetes Obes Metab. 2010;12:116–25.
57. Biomarkers Definition Working Group. Biomarkers and surrogate endpoints: preferred definitions and conceptual framework. Clin Pharmacol Ther. 2001;69:89–95.
58. Lee R, Margaritis M, Channon KM, Antoniades C. Evaluating oxidative stress in human cardiovascular disease: methodological aspects and considerations. Curr Med Chem. 2012;19(16):2504–20.
59. Yagi K. Simple assay for the level of total lipid peroxides in serum or plasma. Methods Mol Biol. 1998;108:101–6.
60. Arai H. Oxidative modification of lipoproteins. Subcell Biochem. 2014;77:103–14.
61. Niki E. Biomarkers of lipid peroxidation in clinical material. Biochim Biophys Acta. 2014;1840(2):809–17.
62. Bairova TA, Kolesnikov SI, Kolesnikova LI, Pervushina OA, Darenskaya MA, Grebenkina LA. Lipid peroxidation and mitochondrial superoxide dismutase-2 gene in adolescents with essential hypertension. Bull Exp Biol Med. 2014;158(2):181–4.
63. Spickett CM. The lipid peroxidation product 4-hydroxy-2-nonenal: advances in chemistry and analysis. Redox Biol. 2013;1(1):145–52.
64. Davies SS, Roberts 2nd LJ. F2-isoprostanes as an indicator and risk factor for coronary heart disease. Free Radic Biol Med. 2011;50(5):559–66.
65. Basu S. Bioactive eicosanoids: role of prostaglandin F(2α) and F_2-isoprostanes in inflammation and oxidative stress related pathology. Mol Cells. 2010;30(5):383–91.
66. Del Rio D, Stewart AJ, Pellegrini N. A review of recent studies on malondialdehyde as toxic molecule and biological marker of oxidative stress. Nutr Metab Cardiovasc Dis. 2005;15(4):316–28.
67. Konukoglu D, Serin O, Turhan MS. Plasma leptin and its relationship with lipid peroxidation and nitric oxide in obese female patients with or without hypertension. Arch Med Res. 2006;37(5):602–6.
68. da Cruz AC, Petronilho F, Heluany CC, Vuolo F, Miguel SP, Quevedo J, Romano-Silva MA, Dal-Pizzol F. Oxidative stress and aging: correlation with clinical parameters. Aging Clin Exp Res. 2014;26(1):7–12.
69. Campos C, Guzmán R, López-Fernández E, Casado Á. Urinary biomarkers of oxidative/nitrosative stress in healthy smokers. Inhal Toxicol. 2011;23(3):148–56.
70. Asselin C, Shi Y, Clément R, Tardif JC, Des Rosiers C. Higher circulating 4-hydroxynonenal-protein thioether adducts correlate with more severe diastolic dysfunction in spontaneously hypertensive rats. Redox Rep. 2007;12(1):68–72.
71. Mali VR, Ning R, Chen J, Yang XP, Xu J, Palaniyandi SS. Impairment of aldehyde dehydrogenase-2 by 4-hydroxy-2-nonenal adduct formation and cardiomyocyte hypertrophy in mice fed a high-fat diet and injected with low-dose streptozotocin. Exp Biol Med. 2014;239(5):610–8.
72. Zhang Y, Sano M, Shinmura K, Tamaki K, Katsumata Y, Matsuhashi T, Morizane S, Ito H, Hishiki T, Endo J, Zhou H, Yuasa S, Kaneda R, Suematsu M, Fukuda K. 4-hydroxy-2-nonenal protects against cardiac ischemia-reperfusion injury via the Nrf2-dependent pathway. J Mol Cell Cardiol. 2010;49(4):576–86.

73. Usberti M, Gerardi GM, Gazzotti RM, Benedini S, Archetti S, Sugherini L, Valentini M, Tira P, Bufano G, Albertini A, Di Lorenzo D. Oxidative stress and cardiovascular disease in dialyzed patients. Nephron. 2002;91(1):25–33.
74. Gerardi G, Usberti M, Martini G, Albertini A, Sugherini L, Pompella A, Di LD. Plasma total antioxidant capacity in hemodialyzed patients and its relationships to other biomarkers of oxidative stress and lipid peroxidation. Clin Chem Lab Med. 2002;40(2):104–10.
75. Galano JM, Mas E, Barden A, Mori TA, Signorini C, De Felice C, Barrett A, Opere C, Pinot E, Schwedhelm E, Benndorf R, Roy J, Le Guennec JY, Oger C, Durand T. Isoprostanes and neuroprostanes: total synthesis, biological activity and biomarkers of oxidative stress in humans. Prostaglandins Other Lipid Mediat. 2013;107:95–102.
76. Roberts LJ, Morrow JD. Measurement of F(2)-isoprostanes as an index of oxidative stress in vivo. Free Radic Biol Med. 2000;28(4):505–13.
77. Bauer J, Ripperger A, Frantz S, Ergün S, Schwedhelm E, Benndorf RA. Pathophysiology of isoprostanes in the cardiovascular system: implications of isoprostane-mediated thromboxane A2 receptor activation. Br J Pharmacol. 2014;171(13):3115–31.
78. Praticò D, Dogné JM. Vascular biology of eicosanoids and atherogenesis. Expert Rev Cardiovasc Ther. 2009;7(9):1079–89.
79. Zhang ZJ. Systematic review on the association between F2-isoprostanes and cardiovascular disease. Ann Clin Biochem. 2013;50(Pt 2):108–14.
80. Liu CK, Lyass A, Larson MG, Massaro JM, Wang N, D'Agostino Sr RB, Benjamin EJ, Murabito JM. Biomarkers of oxidative stress are associated with frailty: the Framingham Offspring Study. Age (Dordr). 2016;38(1):1.
81. Pignatelli P, Pastori D, Carnevale R, Farcomeni A, Cangemi R, Nocella C, Bartimoccia S, Vicario T, Saliola M, Lip GY, Violi F. Serum NOX2 and urinary isoprostanes predict vascular events in patients with atrial fibrillation. Thromb Haemost. 2015;113(3):617–24.
82. Shacter E. Quantification and significance of protein oxidation in biological samples. Drug Metab Rev. 2000;32(3–4):307–26.
83. Dalle-Donne I, Giustarini D, Colombo R, Rossi R, Milzani A. Protein carbonylation in human diseases. Trends Mol Med. 2003;9:169–76.
84. Jones DA, Prior SL, Barry JD, Caplin S, Baxter JN, Stephens JW. Changes in markers of oxidative stress and DNA damage in human visceral adipose tissue from subjects with obesity and type 2 diabetes. Diabetes Res Clin Pract. 2014;106(3):627–33.
85. Chen X, Mori T, Guo Q, Hu C, Ohsaki Y, Yoneki Y, Zhu W, Jiang Y, Endo S, Nakayama K, Ogawa S, Nakayama M, Miyata T, Ito S. Carbonyl stress induces hypertension and cardiorenal vascular injury in Dahl salt-sensitive rats. Hypertens Res. 2013;36(4):361–7.
86. Dean RT, Fu S, Stocker R, Davies MJ. Biochemistry and pathology of radical-mediated protein oxidation. Biochem J. 1997;324:1–18.
87. Cai Z, Yan LJ. Protein oxidative modifications: beneficial roles in disease and health. J Biochem Pharmacol Res. 2013;1(1):15–26.
88. Wang J, Sevier CS. Formation and reversibility of BiP cysteine oxidation facilitates cell survival during and post oxidative stress. J Biol Chem. 2016;291(14):7541–57. pii: jbc.M115.694810.
89. Haque A, Andersen JN, Salmeen A, Barford D, Tonks NK. Conformation - sensing antibodies stabilize the oxidized form of PTP1B and inhibit its phosphatase activity. Cell. 2011;147(1):185–98.
90. Paulsen CE, Truong TH, Garcia FJ, Homann A, Gupta V, Leonard SE, Carroll KS. Peroxide-dependent sulfenylation of the EGFR catalytic site enhances kinase activity. Nat Chem Biol. 2011;8(1):57–64.
91. Methner C, Chouchani ET, Buonincontri G, Pell VR, Sawiak SJ, Murphy MP, Krieg T. Mitochondria selective S-nitrosation by mitochondria-targeted S-nitrosothiol protects against post-infarct heart failure in mouse hearts. Eur J Heart Fail. 2014;16(7):712–7.
92. Pastore A, Piemonte F. Protein glutathionylation in cardiovascular diseases. Int J Mol Sci. 2013;14(10):20845–76.

93. Chouchani ET, Methner C, Nadtochiy SM, Logan A, Pell VR, Ding S, James AM, Cochemé HM, Reinhold J, Lilley KS, Partridge L, Fearnley IM, Robinson AJ, Hartley RC, Smith RA, Krieg T, Brookes PS, Murphy MP. Cardioprotection by S-nitrosation of a cysteine switch on mitochondrial complex I. Nat Med. 2013;19(6):753–9.
94. Tarrago L, Péterfi Z, Lee BC, Michel T, Gladyshev VN. Monitoring methionine sulfoxide with stereospecific mechanism-based fluorescent sensors. Nat Chem Biol. 2015;11(5):332–8.
95. Klutho PJ, Pennington SM, Scott JA, Wilson KM, Gu SX, Doddapattar P, Xie L, Venema AN, Zhu LJ, Chauhan AK, Lentz SR, Grumbach IM. Deletion of methionine sulfoxide reductase A does not affect atherothrombosis but promotes neointimal hyperplasia and extracellular signal-regulated kinase 1/2 signaling. Arterioscler Thromb Vasc Biol. 2015;35(12):2594–604.
96. Subash P, Premagurumurthy K, Sarasabharathi A, Cherian KM. Total antioxidant status and oxidative DNA damage in a South Indian population of essential hypertensives. J Hum Hypertens. 2010;24(7):475–82.
97. Kim JY, Prouty LA, Fang SC, Rodrigues EG, Magari SR, Modest GA, Christiani DC. Association between fine particulate matter and oxidative DNA damage may be modified in individuals with hypertension. J Occup Environ Med. 2009;51(10):1158–66.
98. Battelli MG, Bolognesi A, Polito L. Pathophysiology of circulating xanthine oxidoreductase: new emerging roles for a multi-tasking enzyme. Biochim Biophys Acta. 2014;1842(9):1502–17.
99. Bushueva O, Solodilova M, Ivanov V, Polonikov A. Gender-specific protective effect of the -463G>A polymorphism of myeloperoxidase gene against the risk of essential hypertension in Russians. J Am Soc Hypertens. 2015;9(11):902–6.
100. Berry CE, Hare JM. Xanthine oxidoreductase and cardiovascular disease: molecular mechanisms and pathophysiological implications. J Physiol. 2004;555(Pt 3):589–606.
101. Cantu-Medellin N, Kelley EE. Xanthine oxidoreductase-catalyzed reactive species generation: a process in critical need of reevaluation. Redox Biol. 2013;1(1):353–8.
102. Wang J, Qin T, Chen J, Li Y, Wang L, Huang H, Li J. Hyperuricemia and risk of incident hypertension: a systematic review and meta-analysis of observational studies. PLoS One. 2014;9(12):e114259.
103. MacIsaac RL, Salatzki J, Higgins P, Walters MR, Padmanabhan S, Dominiczak AF, Touyz RM, Dawson J. Allopurinol and cardiovascular outcomes in adults with hypertension. Hypertension. 2016;67(3):535–40.
104. Agarwal V, Hans N, Messerli FH. Effect of allopurinol on blood pressure: a systematic review and meta-analysis. J Clin Hypertens (Greenwich). 2013;15(6):435–42.
105. Maghzal GJ, Krause KH, Stocker R, Jaquet V. Detection of reactive oxygen species derived from the family of NOX NADPH oxidases. Free Radic Biol Med. 2012;53(10):1903–18.
106. Drummond GR, Sobey CG. Endothelial NADPH oxidases: which NOX to target in vascular disease? Trends Endocrinol Metab. 2014;25(9):452–63.
107. Kaludercic N, Deshwal S, Di Lisa F. Reactive oxygen species and redox compartmentalization. Front Physiol. 2014;5:285.
108. Montezano AC, Tsiropoulou S, Dulak-Lis M, Harvey A, Camargo Lde L, Touyz RM. Redox signaling, Nox5 and vascular remodeling in hypertension. Curr Opin Nephrol Hypertens. 2015;24(5):425–33.
109. Al Ghouleh I, Khoo NK, Knaus UG, Griendling KK, Touyz RM, Thannickal VJ, Barchowsky A, Nauseef WM, Kelley EE, Bauer PM, Darley-Usmar V, Shiva S, Cifuentes-Pagano E, Freeman BA, Gladwin MT, Pagano PJ. Oxidases and peroxidases in cardiovascular and lung disease: new concepts in reactive oxygen species signaling. Free Radic Biol Med. 2011;51(7):1271–88.
110. Maxwell S, Greig L. Anti-oxidants- a protective role in cardiovascular disease? Expert Opin Pharmacother. 2001;2(11):1737–50.
111. Fraga CG, Oteiza PI, Galleano M. In vitro measurements and interpretation of total antioxidant capacity. Biochim Biophys Acta. 2014;1840(2):931–4.

112. Pinchuk I, Shoval H, Dotan Y, Lichtenberg D. Evaluation of antioxidants: scope, limitations and relevance of assays. Chem Phys Lipids. 2012;165(6):638–47.
113. Popolo A, Autore G, Pinto A, Marzocco S. Oxidative stress in patients with cardiovascular disease and chronic renal failure. Free Radic Res. 2013;47(5):346–56.
114. Hendre AS, Shariff AK, Patil SR, Durgawale PP, Sontakke AV, Suryakar AN. Evaluation of oxidative stress and anti-oxidant status in essential hypertension. J Indian Med Assoc. 2013;111(6):377–8, 380–1.
115. Hollman PC, Cassidy A, Comte B, Heinonen M, Richelle M, Richling E, Serafini M, Scalbert A, Sies H, Vidry S. The biological relevance of direct antioxidant effects of polyphenols for cardiovascular health in humans is not established. J Nutr. 2011;141(5):989S–1009.
116. González J, Valls N, Brito R, Rodrigo R. Essential hypertension and oxidative stress: new insights. World J Cardiol. 2014;6(6):353–66.
117. Loukogeorgakis SP, van den Berg MJ, Sofat R, Nitsch D, Charakida M, Haiyee B, de Groot E, MacAllister RJ, Kuijpers TW, Deanfield JE. Role of NADPH oxidase in endothelial ischemia/reperfusion injury in humans. Circulation. 2010;121(21):2310–6.
118. Gutterman DD, Chabowski DS, Kadlec AO, Durand MJ, Freed JK, Ait-Aissa K, Beyer AM. The human microcirculation: regulation of flow and beyond. Circ Res. 2016;118(1):157–72.
119. Caimi G, Mulè G, Hopps E, Carollo C, Lo Presti R. Nitric oxide metabolites and oxidative stress in mild essential hypertension. Clin Hemorheol Microcirc. 2010;46(4):321–5.
120. Chen K, Xie F, Liu S, Li G, Chen Y, Shi W, Hu H, Liu L, Yin D. Plasma reactive carbonyl species: potential risk factor for hypertension. Free Radic Res. 2011;45(5):568–74.
121. Chen X, Wu Y, Liu L, Su Y, Peng Y, Jiang L, Liu X. Huang D relationship between high density lipoprotein antioxidant activity and carotid arterial intima-media thickness in patients with essential hypertension. Clin Exp Hypertens. 2010;32(1):13–20.
122. Brandão SA, Izar MC, Fischer SM, Santos AO, Monteiro CM, Póvoa RM, Helfenstein T, Carvalho AC, Monteiro AM, Ramos E, Gidlund M, Figueiredo Neto AM, Fonseca FA. Early increase in autoantibodies against human oxidized low-density lipoprotein in hypertensive patients after blood pressure control. Am J Hypertens. 2010;23(2):208–14.
123. Qin Z, Reszka KJ, Fukai T, Weintraub NL. Extracellular superoxide dismutase (ecSOD) in vascular biology: an update on exogenous gene transfer and endogenous regulators of ecSOD. Transl Res. 2008;151(2):68–78.
124. Ahmad A, Singhal U, Hossain MM, Islam N, Rizvi I. The role of the endogenous antioxidant enzymes and malondialdehyde in essential hypertension. J Clin Diagn Res. 2013;7(6):987–90.
125. Rafiq A, Aslam K, Malik R, Afroze D. C242T polymorphism of the NADPH oxidase p22PHOX gene and its association with endothelial dysfunction in asymptomatic individuals with essential systemic hypertension. Mol Med Rep. 2014;9(5):1857–62.
126. Qin YW, Peng J, Liang BY, Su L, Chen Q, Xie JJ, Gu L. The A930G polymorphism ofP-22phox (CYBA) gene but not C242T variation is associated with hypertension: a meta-analysis. PLoS One. 2013;8(12):e82465.

Chapter 12
The Role of Diet in the Prevention of Cardiovascular Disease

Mónica Domenech and Antonio Coca

Hypertension (HT) remains the main risk factor for developing coronary artery disease, congestive heart failure, stroke and kidney disease [1]. Its prevalence continues to increase exponentially due to better detection and an increase in associated factors such as obesity, physical inactivity and diabetes mellitus. Data from the National Health and Nutritional Examination Survey (NHANES) between 2007 and 2010 show that HT affects 33 % (77.9 million) of people aged ≥ 20 years in the United States [2] and the prevalence is estimated to increase to 37.3 % by 2030 [3]. This trend is spreading, even in countries that traditionally have a lower cardiovascular risk, such as Spain, where, in a cohort of 11,957 persons aged ≥ 18 years, 33 % (3983 persons) had a BP ≥ 140/90 mmHg, but > 40 % were unaware of this [4]. These data alert us to the magnitude of the problem and the need for increased efforts to improve the diagnosis, treatment and, especially, the prevention of hypertensive disease.

By 1970, Keys et al. were already highlighting the influence of lifestyles on the development and/or prevention of cardiovascular disease (CVD), with particular emphasis on the important role of diet. This was the basis for the Seven Countries Study [5], an ecological study of 12,770 participants aged 40–59 years from Finland, Greece, Italy, Japan, Netherlands, Norway, the United States and Yugoslavia, who were followed for 5 years. The study found significant differences between cohorts, with a higher incidence of CVD in Finland, the USA and the Netherlands compared with the Southern European countries and Japan. The differences were not accounted for by other traditional risk factors, such as smoking, obesity or physical activity. However, when dietary aspects were analysed, the authors found a significant association between the consumption of mono- and polyunsaturated fats and a lower

M. Domenech, M.D., Ph.D. • A. Coca, M.D., Ph.D. (✉)
Hypertension and Vascular Risk Unit, Hypertension, Nutrition and Aging Unit, Department of Internal Medicine, Hospital Clínic, IDIBAPS (Institut d'Investigacions Biomèdiques August Pi i Sunyer), University of Barcelona, Barcelona, Spain
e-mail: acoca@clinic.ub.es

E.A. Andreadis (ed.), *Hypertension and Cardiovascular Disease*,
DOI 10.1007/978-3-319-39599-9_12

incidence of CVD, suggesting that Southern European dietary patterns, with a low intake of saturated fat and a high intake of fruits and vegetables, was a key factor in lower cardiovascular mortality [6]. The results of this study are the pillar that supports today's growing evidence of the benefits associated with the so-called "Mediterranean Diet" (MD).

The north–south gradient with respect to CVD has been confirmed in several epidemiological studies, as evidenced by data from the MONICA Project (multinational monitoring of trends and determinants in cardiovascular disease) [7], which showed that Catalonia, the South of France and Italy had a lower incidence of mortality due to coronary heart disease (CHD) (in both men and women) than Northern European countries and the United States. Subsequently, numerous studies have shown the benefits of adherence to a "healthy diet" in reducing CVD. The results of the CARDIA study (Coronary Artery Risk Development in Young Adults) by Liu et al. [8] which was conducted in 3154 participants aged 18–30 years, underline the importance of maintaining a healthy lifestyle over a 20-year follow-up. In this study, adherence to a "healthy diet" increased the maintenance of a low cardiovascular risk profile (28.3 % for a healthy diet vs. 22.4 % for an unhealthy diet; $P<0.01$) on reaching adulthood, thus reducing, the likelihood of future CVD (Fig. 12.1).

Furthermore, the results of a systematic review by Mente et al. [9] on the effect of different dietary patterns on CHD, including prospective cohort studies and fewer randomized clinical trials (the latter only exploring effects of the Mediterranean diet) support the beneficial link between healthy dietary factors characterized by a high intake of vegetables, fruits, legumes, whole grains, fish and other seafood (healthy diet), a higher consumption of monounsaturated fatty acids (MUFA) and polyunsaturated fatty acids (PUFA) than saturated fatty acids, and reductions in CHD. More recently, a meta-analysis by Martinez-Gonzalez et al. [10] reinforced the beneficial effect of the MD, showing that a two-point increase in adherence to the MD (0–9 score) was associated with a significant reduction in cardiovascular events (pooled risk ratio: 0.87; 95 % CI: 0.85–0.90) with no evidence of heterogeneity between studies.

The strongest evidence for the benefits of the MD comes from the multicentre, randomized PREDIMED study in 4,774 patients at high cardiovascular risk. Patients

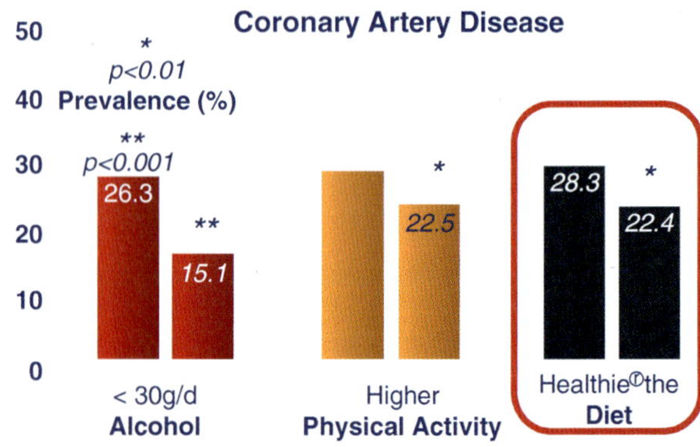

Fig. 12.1 Age-, sex-, and race-adjusted prevalence of low risk profile at year 20 by individual healthy lifestyle factors among Coronary Artery Risk Development in Young Adults (CARDIA) Study Participants. *P* value was computed with logistic regression

were assigned to one of three arms of a dietary intervention: MD supplemented with extra-virgin olive oil (VOO), MD supplemented with nuts, or a control low fat diet. The study was halted prematurely at 4.8 years of follow up in accordance with data obtained in an interim analysis. The PREDIMED [11] study is the first randomized trial in primary prevention of CVD to show that the MD supplemented with VOO or nuts significantly reduced the incidence of major cardiovascular events, with a HR of 0.70 (95 % CI, 0.54–0.92) and 0.72 (95 % CI, 0.54–0.96), respectively.

Better understanding of the contribution of risk factors to the disease burden has motivated several comparative studies in the past few decades. Although these risk factor-specific or cause-specific analyses are useful for policy, a more comprehensive global assessment of the disease burden attributable to risk factors could strengthen the rationale for actions to reduce the disease burden and promote health. The latest review by Lim et al. [12] estimated global attributable mortality and disability adjusted life-years in 1990 and 2010 for each of the 67 risk factors and clusters of risk factors. In 2010, the three leading risk factors for the global disease burden were high blood pressure (7.0 %; 95 % CI 6.2–7.7), smoking, including second-hand smoke (6.3 %; 95 % CI 5.5–7.0), and dietary risk factors and physical inactivity (10.0 %; 95 % CI 9.2–10.8), with the most prominent dietary risks being diets low in fruit or high in sodium (Fig. 12.2).

Despite worldwide clinical and therapeutic efforts to improve BP control, it remains low and persists as a leading risk factor associated with cardiovascular mortality. The strong evidence on the effect of diet on CV disease has motivated the inclusion of specific dietary recommendations in all cardiovascular prevention guidelines, making diet and lifestyle a cornerstone in the reduction and prevention

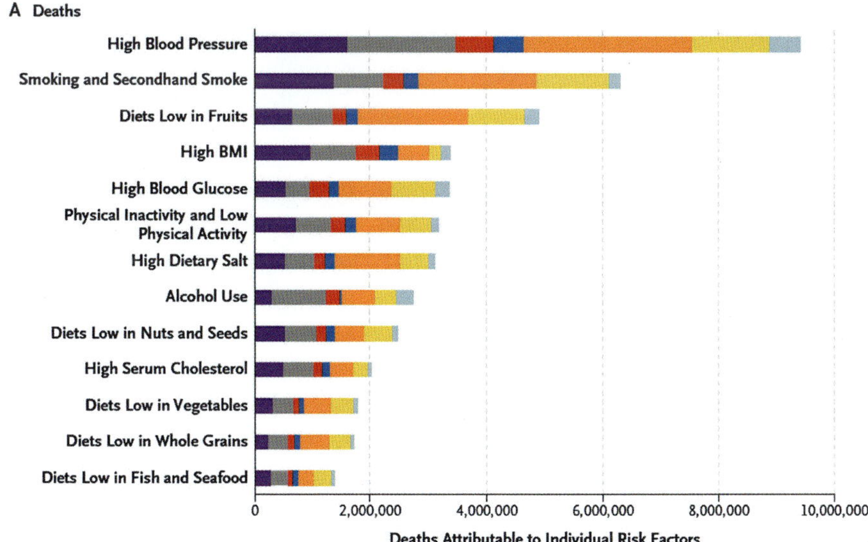

Fig. 12.2 Burden of disease attributable to 20 leading risk factors in 2010, expressed as a percentage of global disability-adjusted life-years

of CVD [13]. Lifestyle changes that have shown benefits in reducing BP values include reduction of body weight, low sodium intake, high potassium intake, reduction of excessive alcohol intake, and the DASH diet (Dietary Approaches to Stop Hypertension) [14, 15], which initially, potentiated increased consumption of fruits, vegetables and fatty dairy products, with a relatively low intake of total and saturated fat [16], although restrictions in sodium intake were later added in order to achieve greater reductions in BP values [17].

A total of 412 participants were randomly assigned to eat either a control diet (typical or usual diet in the United States) or the DASH diet. Within the assigned diet, participants ate foods with high, intermediate, and low levels of sodium for 30 consecutive days each, in random order. The three sodium levels were defined as high (a target of 150 mmol per day with an energy intake of 2,100 kcal, reflecting typical consumption in the USA), intermediate (a target of 100 mmol per day, reflecting the upper limit of current USA recommendations), and low (a target of 50 mmol per day, reflecting a level that might produce an additional lowering of blood pressure). Progressively-lower levels of sodium intake produced a greater BP response. In the control diet, a reduction in sodium intake of about 40 mmol per day from the intermediate sodium level lowered BP more than a similar reduction in sodium intake from the high level (P=0.03 for systolic BP, P=0.045 for diastolic BP). The DASH diet, as compared with the control diet, resulted in significantly-lower systolic BP (SBP) at every sodium level and in significantly-lower diastolic BP (DBP) at high and intermediate sodium levels (Fig. 12.3), with a larger effect on both SBP and DBP at high sodium levels than at low ones (P<0.001 for the interaction).

Subsequently, the Optimal Macronutrient Intake Trial to Prevent Heart Disease (OmniHeart) evaluated the effect of a dietary intervention based on modifications of the DASH diet aimed at maximizing the hypotensive effect on BP in individuals with prehypertension or established hypertension. The results showed that, compared with a diet rich in carbohydrates, increased consumption of vegetable protein significantly reduced SBP by 1.4 mmHg (p=0.002), with a reduction of 3.5 mmHg (p=0.006) in subjects with hypertension, while a diet rich in unsaturated fat, with

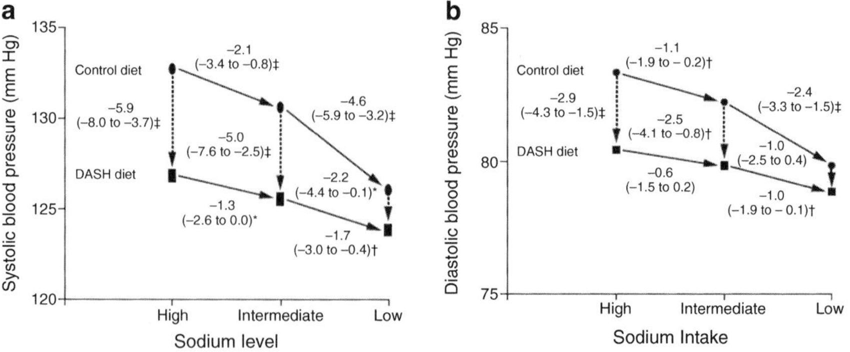

Fig. 12.3 Effect of reduced sodium intake and the *DASH diet* on systolic BP (**a**) and diastolic BP (**b**)

an increase in monounsaturated fatty acids (MUFA), was associated with a reduction in SBP of 1.3 mmHg ($p=0.005$) in the overall cohort and 2.9 mmHg ($p=0.02$) in hypertensives compared with the diet rich in carbohydrates [18].

In recent decades, the vasculoprotective potential of diet and nutrients has been increasingly recognized, with more solid evidence on the benefits of the MD emerging in recent years, although there is little data on its effect on BP reduction. Since the 1990s, evidence on the benefits of the MD in the prevention of CVD and the reduction of BP and cholesterol levels and/or diabetes has become stronger, although the level of evidence remains very heterogeneous. The MD is characterized by a diet rich in fruits, vegetables and cereals, with a high intake of mono- and polyunsaturated fats, and with olive oil being the main source of fat. Likewise, the MD encourages moderate fish and poultry consumption and a low consumption of dairy products, red meat, prepared meats and sweets and pastries. The MD also promotes moderate consumption of wine, preferably red, during meals [19].

Since the pioneering study by Keys et al. [5], data have been collected from more than 12 cross-sectional studies included in the ATTICA registry, which enrolled nearly 3,000 participants aged 18–89 years from the Greek region of Attica between 2001 and 2002. Overall, the studies showed that adherence to the MD is associated with a reduction in the incidence of diabetes, obesity, and CVD, and an improvement in the lipid profile and BP values. The data from two large cohort studies provide similar results: the Greek European Prospective Investigation into Cancer and Nutrition cohort (EPIC) and the Seguimiento Universidad de Navarra (SUN) study. The EPIC study now encompasses nearly half a million persons from 10 European countries and is the largest population-based cohort study focused on the beneficial effects of the MD on cardiovascular health. Substudies in Greece, Italy and Spain have found an inverse relationship between adherence to the MD and BP values, the BMI, the incidence of type-2 diabetes [20] and the tendency to obesity. More recent data from the Greek-EPIC cohort of 23,601 participants free of CVD showed that increasing adherence to the MD (determined by an increase of 2 points in the MD score) was inversely associated with the incidence of stroke (HR 0.85; 95 % CI 0.74–0.96), an association that was even stronger for women and for ischemic stroke vs. haemorrhagic stroke [21].

The SUN study of more than 15,000 Spanish university students without cardiovascular risk factors showed that adherence to the MD conditioned a lower incidence of metabolic syndrome (MetS) and type-2 diabetes, and a reduction in BP values [22]. Similar results were observed in the randomized, parallel Medi-RIVAGE study [23] which compared the effects of the MD in 180 patients with MetS compared with a control diet (carbohydrates 50–60 %, proteins 15–20 %, total fat <30 %). After 2 years follow up, patients assigned to the MD had a significant reduction in the prevalence of MetS and associated cardiovascular risk factors. Data from the first randomized study in secondary prevention, the Lyon Diet Heart Study [24], confirmed the benefits of the MD in reducing cardiovascular risk.

The cardioprotective role of the MD was confirmed in the meta-analysis by Sofi et al. [25]. Although evidence on the effects of the MD on BP has been scarce, probably because BP was usually a secondary outcome in nutritional studies, the preliminary results of the PREDIMED study [26] and the final results in the entire cohort [11] showed that adherence to the traditional MD significantly reduced the risk of cardiovascular disease. The risk reduction was highly significant for stroke, whose association with BP values is well established. Preliminary data from the PREDIMED study after the first 3 months of follow-up showed that, compared with the low-fat diet, the MD supplemented with VOO or nuts reduced office SBP by 5.9 mmHg (95 % CI: –8.7 to –3.1 mmHg) and 7.1 mmHg (95 % CI: –10.0 to –4.1 mmHg), respectively, and office DBP by 0.38 (95 % CI: –0.55 to–0.22) and 0.26 mmHg (95 % CI: –0.42 to –0.10), respectively [26]. However, in later results encompassing the whole PREDIMED cohort, the changes in office BP in 7,158 participants (mean age 67 years) were lower, although a trend to BP reduction was observed throughout the follow up [27]. The percentage of participants achieving good BP control increased significantly during the follow up in the three intervention groups, without between-group differences (31.9 % at baseline versus 41.3 % at study end; p <0.001). However, compared with patients assigned to the control diet, significantly-reduced DBP was observed in participants assigned to the MD supplemented with VOO (1.53 mmHg, 95 % CI: –2.01 to –1.04) and the MD supplemented with nuts (0.65 mmHg, 95 % CI: –1.15 to –0.15). No significant between-group differences in SBP were observed [27]. As the authors mention, a longer follow up, poor data with respect to changes in antihypertensive treatment during the study and a trend to greater adherence to the MD in the control group in the last years of follow-up may partly explain the differences in the results of long-term office BP. The other limitation was the technique for measuring office BP itself.

Prior studies of the effects of the MD on BP have relied on clinic (office) BP measurements, which are limited by poor reproducibility, the white-coat effect and observer and patient variability. Twenty-four hour ambulatory BP monitoring (ABPM) is considered the gold standard for the assessment of the effects of interventions on BP, as repeated measurements more accurately reflect usual BP than isolated office measurements.

The latest evidence of the beneficial effect of the MD on BP comes from the recent substudy of the PREDIMED study by Domenech et al. [28], which included 235 subjects (56.5 % female; mean age, 66.5 years) at high cardiovascular risk (85.4 % with hypertension). The results showed that the MD supplemented with either VOO or nuts directly resulted in significant reductions in 24-h ABPM compared with a control diet in individuals at high risk of CVD (85 % under hypertensive treatment), without considering the confounding effects of weight loss or changes in physical activity, sodium intake or alcohol consumption. The net differences between the MD supplemented with VOO and nuts and the control diet were –4.0 for mean systolic BP, –4.3 mmHg for mean diastolic ABPM, and –1.9 mmHg for both MD after adjustment for between-diet imbalances in baseline BP and for trial changes in antihypertensive medication (Fig. 12.4).

The impact of such BP changes, even if their magnitude seems small, could be remarkable at the population level. It has been estimated that a reduction of 3 mmHg in office systolic BP would reduce stroke mortality by 8 % and coronary heart disease mortality by 5 % [29].

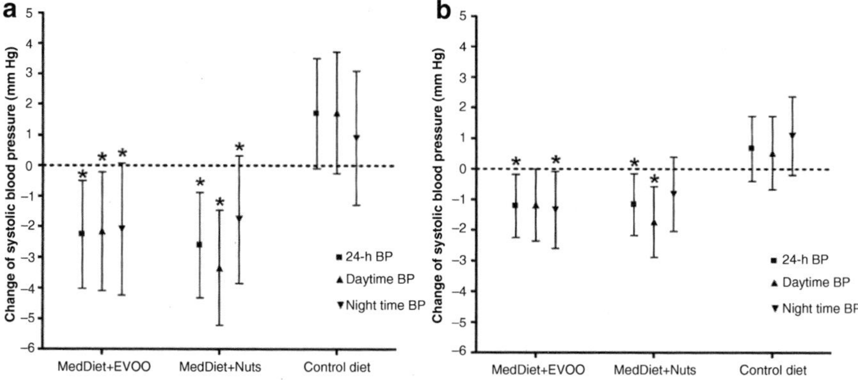

Fig. 12.4 Adjusted changes in ambulatory systolic (**a**) and diastolic (**b**) 24-h BP after 1 year of dietary intervention

Table 12.1 Degree of hypertension control by office and 24-h ambulatory blood pressure measurements

Variable	MedDiet + EVOO	P[a]	MedDiet + Nuts	P[a]	Control diet	P[a]	P[b]
Office BP control[c]							
Baseline	34.6		38.6		30.3		
1 year	42.3	0.238	41.0	0.815	38.2	0.238	<0.001
24 h-ABP control[d]							
Baseline	51.3		63.9		72.4		
1 year	62.8	0.049	69.9	0.302	61.8	0.115	0.008
Daytime ABP control[e]							
Baseline	61.5		63.9		69.7		
1 year	67.9	0.302	75.9	0.031	67.5	0.424	0.025
Nighttime ABP control[f]							
Baseline	54.2		57.1		69.7		
1 year	60.3	0.607	61.4	0.210	52.6	0.015	0.014

Values are percentages

[a]P value for comparisons between baseline and 1 year by McNemar test

[b]P value for comparisons between groups by Pearson's chi square test for categorical variables

[c]Office BP control defined by systolic BP ≤ 140 mm Hg and/or diastolic BP ≤ 90 mm Hg

[d]24h-ABP control defined by systolic BP ≤ 130 or diastolic BP ≤ 80 mmHg

[e]Daytime ABP control defined by systolic BP ≤ 135 or diastolic BP ≤ 85 mm Hg

[f]Nighttime ABP control defined by systolic BP ≤ 120 or diastolic BP ≤ 70 mm Hg

The known limitations of office BP measurement versus 24-h ABPM, with repeated measurements during usual living conditions, apply to the results of the total PREDIMED sample. The advantages of 24-h ABPM are well-known [13], especially for non-pharmacologic interventions with expected smaller individual BP effects. Table 12.1 shows the control rates of hypertension, defined by standard

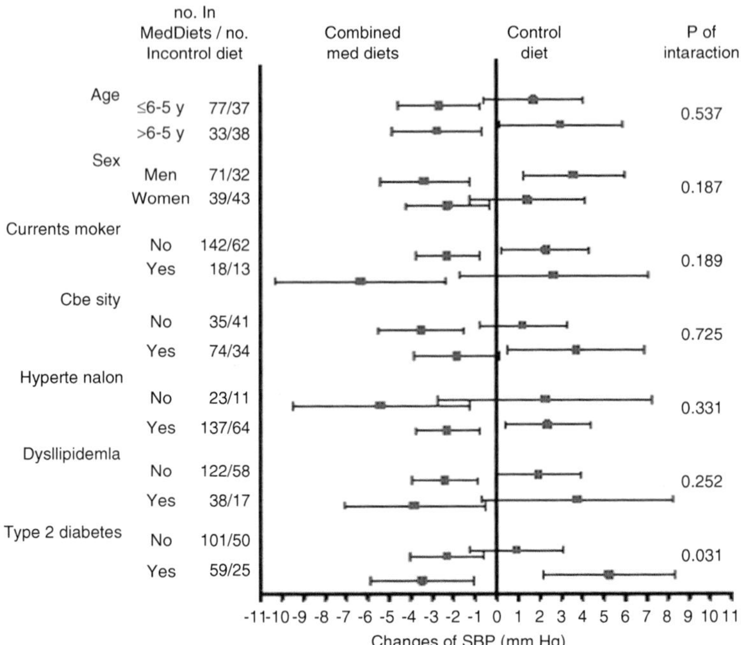

Fig. 12.5 Changes in systolic BP in the subgroup analysis

cutoffs, which were dissimilar between the three intervention groups in the PREDIMED substudy according to both office BP and 24-h ABPM measurements. In all groups, office BP control was similar at baseline and after the intervention. However, 24-h and daytime ABPM control improved variably from baseline in the MD groups, whereas nighttime ABPM control worsened in the control group. BP control was always better with ABPM monitoring compared with office BP, with the differences ranging between 16 % and 42, which can be equated with white-coat hypertension in the office setting.

The proportion of participants with good BP control at both baseline and after 1 year of the intervention was similar in PREDIMED substudy and in the full PREDIIMED cohort [26], further supporting the differential added value of the ABPM results. The reduction in ABPM associated with the MD in different subgroups defined by sex, age, and cardiovascular risk factors were comparable with those of the whole group for SBP except for diabetic participants, in whom greater reductions with the MD versus the control diet were observed compared with participants without diabetes mellitus (P for interaction, 0.031), reinforcing the global effect of adding dietary interventions in high risk populations (Fig. 12.5).

In conclusion, there is robust evidence that increasing adherence to the MD is associated with lower BP. Taking into account the lack of BP control rates despite pharmacological treatment, these results could have public health implications because the MD, a vegetable and high-unsaturated fat based dietary pattern, seems to be a useful adjunct to established dietary and pharmacological approaches to improving hypertension control while incurring little or no expense for the health system.

References

1. Ford ES. Trends in mortality from all causes and cardiovascular disease among hypertensive and nonhypertensive adults in the United States. Circulation. 2011;123:1737–44.
2. Go AS, Mozaffarian D, Roger VL, Benjamin EJ, Berry JD, Borden WB, et al. Heart disease and stroke statistics – 2013 update – a report from the American Heart Association. Circulation. 2013;127:143–52.
3. Heidenreich PA, Trogdon JG, Khavjou OA, Butler J, Dracup K, Ezekowitz MD, et al. Forecasting the future of cardiovascular disease in the United States: a policy statement from the American Heart Association. Circulation. 2011;123:933–44.
4. Banegas JR, Graciani A, de la Cruz-Troca JJ, León-Muñoz LM, Guallar-Castillón P, Coca A, et al. Achievement of cardiometabolic goals in aware hypertensive patients in Spain. A nationwide population-based study. Hypertension. 2012;60:898–905.
5. Keys A, et al. Coronary heart disease in seven countries. Circulation. 1970;41(Suppl I):1–211.
6. Menotti A, Keys A, Kromhout D, Nissinen A, Blackburn H, Fidanza F, et al. Twenty-five-year mortality from coronary heart disease and its prediction in five cohorts of middle-aged men in Finland, the Netherlands, and Italy. Prev Med. 1990;19:270–8.
7. Tunstall-Pedoe H, Kuulasmaa K, Amouyel P, Arveiler D, Rajakangas AM, Pajak A. Myocardial Infarction and coronary deaths in the World Health Organization MONICA Project. Registration procedures, event rates, and case-fatality rates in 38 populations from 21 countries in four continents. Circulation. 1994;90:583–612.
8. Liu K, Daviglus ML, Loria CM, Colangelo LA, Spring B, Moller AC, Donald M. Healthy lifestyle through young adulthood and the presence of low cardiovascular disease risk profile in middle age: the Coronary Artery Risk Development in (Young) Adults (CARDIA) Study. Circulation. 2012;125:996–1004.
9. Mente A, de Koning L, Shannon HS, Anand SS. A systematic review of the evidence supporting a causal link between dietary factors and coronary heart disease. Arch Intern Med. 2009;169(7):659–69.
10. Martinez-Gonzalez MA, Bes-Rastrollo M. Dietary patterns, Mediterranean diet, and cardiovascular disease. Curr Opin Lipidol. 2014;25:20–6.
11. Estruch R, Ros E, Salas-Salvado J, Covas MI, Corella D, Aros F, PREDIMED Study Investigators, et al. Primary prevention of cardiovascular disease with a Mediterranean diet. N Engl J Med. 2013;368:1279–90.
12. Lim SS, Voss T, Faxman AD, et al. A comparative risk assessment of burden of disease and injury attributable to 67 risk factors and risk factor clusters in 21 regions, 1990–2010: a systematic analysis for the Global Burden of Disease Study 2010. Lancet. 2012;380:2224–60.
13. Mancia G, Fagard R, Narkiewicz K, Redón J, Zanchetti A, Böhm M, et al. 2013 ESH/ESC Guidelines for the management of arterial hypertension: the Task Force for the management of arterial hypertension of the European Society of Hypertension (ESH) and of the European Society of Cardiology (ESC). 2013 ESH/ESC Guidelines for the management of arterial hypertension. J Hypertens. 2013;31:1281–357.
14. Appel LJ, Brands MW, Daniels SR, Karanja N, Elmer PJ, Sacks FM. Dietary approaches to prevent and treat hypertension: a scientific statement from the American Heart Association. Hypertension. 2006;47:296–308.
15. Sacks FM, Campos H. Dietary therapy in hypertension. N Engl J Med. 2010;362:2102–12.

16. Appel LJ, Moore TJ, Obarzanek E, Vollmer WM, Svetkey LP, Sacks FM, Bray GA, Vogt TM, Cutler JA, Windhauser MM, Lin PH, Karanja N. A clinical trial of the effects of dietary patterns on blood pressure: DASH Collaborative Research Group. N Engl J Med. 1997;336:1117–24.
17. Sacks FM, Svetkey LP, Vollmer WM, Appel LJ, Bray GA, Harsha D, Obarzanek E, Conlin PR, Miller 3rd ER, Simons-Morton DG, Karanja N, Lin PH, DASH-Sodium Collaborative Research Group. Effects on blood pressure of reduced dietary sodium and the Dietary Approaches to Stop Hypertension (DASH) diet. N Engl J Med. 2001;344:3–10.
18. Appel LJ, Sacks FM, Carey VJ, Obarzanek E, Swain JF, Miller 3rd ER, Conlin PR, Erlinger TP, Rosner BA, Laranjo NM, Charleston J, McCarron P, Bishop LM, OmniHeart Collaborative Research Group. Effects of protein, monounsatured fat, and carbohydrate intake on blood pressure and serum lipids. Results of the OmniHeart randomized trial. JAMA. 2005;294:2455–64.
19. Willett WC, Sacks F, Trichopoulou A, et al. Mediterranean diet pyramid: a cultural model for healthy eating. Am J Clin Nutr. 1995;61(Suppl):1402S–6.
20. Rossi M, Turati F, Lagiou P, Trichopoulos D, Augustin LS, La Vecchia C, Trichopoulou A. Mediterranean diet and glycaemic load in relation to incidence of type 2 diabetes: results from the Greek cohort of the population-based European Prospective Investigation into Cancer and Nutrition (EPIC). Diabetologia. 2013;56:2405–13.
21. Misirli G, Benetou V, Lagiou P, Bamia C, Trichopoulos D, Trichopoulou A. Relation of the traditional Mediterranean diet to cerebrovascular disease in a Mediterranean population. Am J Epidemiol. 2012;176(12):1185–92.
22. Núñez-Córdoba JM, Valencia-Serrano F, Toledo E, Alonso A, Martínez-González MA. The Mediterranean diet and incidence of hypertension: the Seguimiento Universidad de Navarra (SUN) study. Am J Epidemiol. 2009;169:339–46.
23. Esposito K, Marfella R, Ciotola M, Di Palo C, Giugliano F, Giugliano G, D'Armiento M, D'Andrea F, Giugliano D. Effect of a Mediterranean-style diet on endothelial dysfunction and markers of vascular inflammation in the metabolic syndrome: a randomized trial. JAMA. 2004;292(12):1440–6.
24. de Lorgeril M, Salen P, Martin JL, Monjaud I, Delaye J, Mamelle N. Mediterranean diet, traditional risk factors, and the rate of cardiovascular complications after myocardial infarction: final report of the Lyon Diet Heart Study. Circulation. 1999;99(6):779–85.
25. Sofi F, Abbate R, Gensini GF, et al. Accruing evidence on benefits of adherence to the Mediterranean diet on health: an updated systematic review and metaanalysis. Am J Clin Nutr. 2010;92:1189–96.
26. Estruch R, Martínez-González MA, Corella D, Salas-Salvadó J, Ruiz-Gutiérrez V, Covas MI, on behalf of the PREDIMED Study Investigators, et al. Effects of a Mediterranean-style diet on cardiovascular risk factors: a randomized trial. Ann Intern Med. 2006;145:1–11.
27. Toledo E, Hu FB, Estruch R, Buil-Cosiales P, Corella D, Salas-Salvadó J, on behalf of the PREDIMED Study Investigators, et al. Effect of the Mediterranean diet on blood pressure in the PREDIMED trial: results from a randomized controlled trial. BMC Med. 2013;11:207.
28. Doménech M, Roman P, Lapetra J, García de la Corte FJ, Sala-Vila A, de la Torre R, Corella D, Salas-Salvadó J, Ruiz-Gutiérrez V, Lamuela-Raventós RM, Toledo E, Estruch R, Coca A, Ros E. Mediterranean diet reduces 24-hour ambulatory blood pressure, blood glucose, and lipids: one-year randomized, clinical trial. Hypertension. 2014;64:69–76.
29. Stamler R. Implications of the INTERSALT study. Hypertension. 1991;17(1 Suppl):I16–20.

Chapter 13
The Role of Exercise and Physical Activity in the Prevention of Hypertensive Heart Disease

Peter Kokkinos, Puneet Narayan, Andreas Pittaras, and Charles Faselis

Introduction

Hypertensive heart disease is a constellation of structural and functional cardiac abnormalities caused by the direct and/or indirect effects of uncontrolled and prolonged elevations of arterial pressure [1, 2]. Such abnormalities include left ventricular hypertrophy (LVH), systolic and diastolic dysfunction, coronary artery disease (CAD), and their complications that manifest clinically as angina or myocardial infarction, cardiac arrhythmias (especially atrial fibrillation), and congestive heart failure (CHF).

P. Kokkinos, Ph.D., FACSM, FAHA (✉)
Cardiology Department, Veterans Affairs Medical Center,
50 Irving Street NW, Washington, DC 20422, USA

Georgetown University School of Medicine, 4000 Reservoir Road NW, Washington, DC, USA

Department of Exercise Science, Arnold School of Public Health,
University of South Carolina, Columbia, SC 29208, USA

George Washington University School of Medicine,
2121 I Street, Washington, DC 20052, USA
e-mail: peter.kokkinos@va.gov

P. Narayan, M.D.
Department of Medicine, Veterans Affairs Medical Center, 50 Irving Street NW,
Washington, DC 20422, USA

A. Pittaras, M.D.
Cardiology Department, Veterans Affairs Medical Center,
50 Irving Street NW, Washington, DC 20422, USA

Department of Medicine, George Washington University School of Medicine,
2121 I Street, Washington, DC 20052, USA

C. Faselis, M.D.
Cardiology Department, Veterans Affairs Medical Center, 50 Irving Street NW, Washington,
DC 20422, USA

George Washington University School of Medicine,
2121 I Street, Washington, DC 20052, USA

E.A. Andreadis (ed.), *Hypertension and Cardiovascular Disease*,
DOI 10.1007/978-3-319-39599-9_13

Concentric LVH, characterized by increased cardiac wall thickness, reduced left ventricular chamber size with normal left ventricular ejection fraction is the classic example of hypertensive heart disease [1] (Fig. 13.1). Chronically elevated blood pressure contributes significantly to the development of LVH [2, 3] and reductions in blood pressure with most antihypertensive agents are associated with LVH regression [4–8].

It is well-accepted that the presence of LVH caused by hypertension-induced increase in afterload is a strong and independent risk factor of future cardiac events and all-cause mortality. The risk of cardiovascular morbid events, including sudden cardiac death, increases three-fold in patients with LVH [9–11]. Conversely, regression of LVH is associated with a significant reduction in cardiovascular events and death [4–8, 12].

Increased physical activity or structured exercise programs have been shown to significantly lower blood pressure in individuals with mild to moderate hypertension.

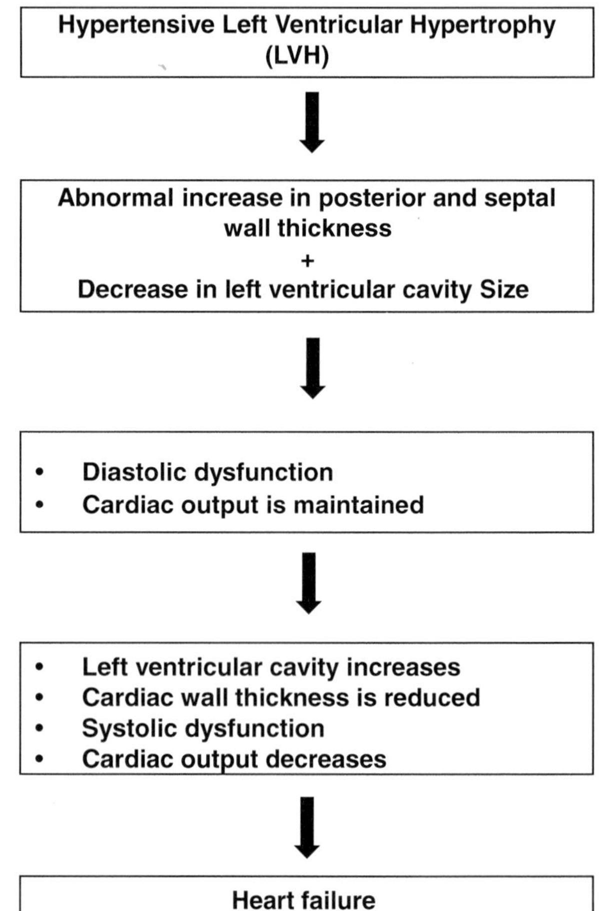

Fig. 13.1 Model of LVH development and exercise-induced regression

Some evidence also supports that the exercise-induced lowering of blood pressure leads to LVH regression. This chapter will address the effects of increased physical activity or structured exercise on blood pressure and hypertensive heart disease.

Physical Activity, Exercise and Hypertension

Hypertension, defined as systolic blood pressure ≥140 mmHg and/or diastolic blood pressure ≥90 mmHg, is a major and the most common risk factor for mortality and development of cardiovascular disease (CVD) [13, 14]. Approximately 1 billion people worldwide have hypertension [15] with an estimated 60 % increase in prevalence by the year 2025 [16].

The anti-hypertensive effects of increased cardiorespiratory fitness achieved either by structured exercise programs or a physically active lifestyle in general have been consistently documented by a number of well-controlled studies. Their findings are summarized by several reviews and meta-analyses [17–26]. In general, these studies support that structured aerobic exercise training programs of moderate intensity or increased physical activity of adequate volume and intensity result in an independent reduction of approximately 4–10 mmHg in systolic blood pressure and 3–8 mmHg in diastolic blood pressure in patients with Stage 1 hypertension. The magnitude of the reduction is likely related to the level of initial blood pressure [22–24] whereas the influences of age, gender or the independent contribution of each of the exercise components (intensity, duration and frequency) are not clear [20, 23, 24]. It is likely that an exercise volume threshold must be achieved before any favorable exercise-induced blood pressure changes are realized. This threshold is the result of the interaction between exercise duration, intensity, frequency and the length of exercise training. Moreover, this threshold is likely to be influenced by age, gender, genetic factors and the initial fitness status of the individual.

Limited information exists on the effects of exercise in individuals with stage 2 hypertension or in those with resistant hypertension, defined as blood pressure that remains above goal in spite of the concurrent use of 3 antihypertensive agents of different classes, one of which is a diuretic [27]. We reported that moderate-intensity aerobic exercise was well-tolerated by male veterans with stage 2 hypertension and leads to significant reductions in blood pressure just after 16 weeks of exercise training. At 32 weeks, blood pressure reduction was more pronounced even after a 33 % reduction in antihypertensive medication in the exercise group, while blood pressure in the no-exercise group increased substantially [28]. Similarly, in patients with resistant hypertension moderate-intensity exercise was effective in significantly lowering 24-h ambulatory blood pressure [29]. The reduction was similar to that reported by previous studies in individuals with mild to moderate hypertension [17, 19, 21, 24, 30, 31].

Information available on the effects of resistance or strength training on resting blood pressure is limited and conflicting and suggests that resistance training is less efficacious than aerobic exercise in lowering resting blood pressure [17, 21, 30–33].

The reasons for lack of blood pressure reductions resulting from resistance training are not clearly defined. Resistance exercise studies do not consistently support improvements in systemic vascular resistance, endothelium-dependent vasodilatation, and arterial compliance, mechanisms suspected to mediate the hypotensive effects of aerobic exercise [30]. The conclusions of a recent meta-analysis [32] and a review [33] suggest an average systolic blood pressure reduction as a result of resistance training of approximately 2–3 mmHg. Thus, it is recommended that resistance training may serve as an adjunct to an aerobic exercise program for blood pressure reduction and implemented as part of a complete exercise program [19, 24, 34, 35].

Exercise intervention studies that recorded blood pressure over a 24-h period (ambulatory blood pressure) are relatively few. In general, the exercise-induced 24-h blood pressure reductions appear less dramatic (mean 3.0 and 3.2 mmHg reduction for systolic and diastolic blood pressure, respectively) than for blood pressure assessed by auscultation [19, 36].

Antihypertensive Mechanisms of Exercise

The underlying mechanisms responsible for the reduction in blood pressure elicited by exercise training remain elusive and controversial. Current opinion is that the effects of exercise training must be multifactorial and the collective effects of these actions result in the reduction of total peripheral resistance, cardiac output or both (Fig. 13.2). It is generally agreed that the changes in blood pressure are independent of changes in body weight, body composition and dietary influences. In addition, diet and exercise-induced reductions in blood pressure do not appear to be additive [37]. However, it is likely that a combination of diet and exercise overall will lead to greater health benefits for the hypertensive individual than either one alone.

Reductions in cardiac output, sympathetic nerve activity and afterload (systemic vascular resistance) have been reported [38–40]. A meta-analysis involving 72 trials, comprising a total of 3,936 participants, reported reductions in systemic vascular resistance, plasma norepinephrine, and plasma renin activity as the main reasons for the decrease in blood pressure following exercise [18]. A reduction in systemic vascular resistance (SVR) is also suggested by arterial pressure changes observed in a group of hypertensive patients. Both systolic and diastolic blood pressures were reduced significantly at absolute submaximal workloads following 16 weeks of aerobic exercise [41]. Consequently, mean arterial pressure was reduced by 17–20 mmHg. More impressive were the significant reductions in peak exercise systolic (219 ± 24 mmHg vs 199 ± 34 mmHg), diastolic blood pressure (108 ± 10 mmHg vs 98 ± 13 mmHg) and mean arterial pressure (145 mmHg vs 131 mmHg) achieved after exercise training, despite a higher workload and similar maximal heart rate (153 ± 15 vs 153 ± 11 bpm) [41] (Fig. 13.3). Even if we assume that cardiac output at peak exercise did not increase despite the higher workload, the substantially lower mean arterial pressure is likely the outcome of a substantial

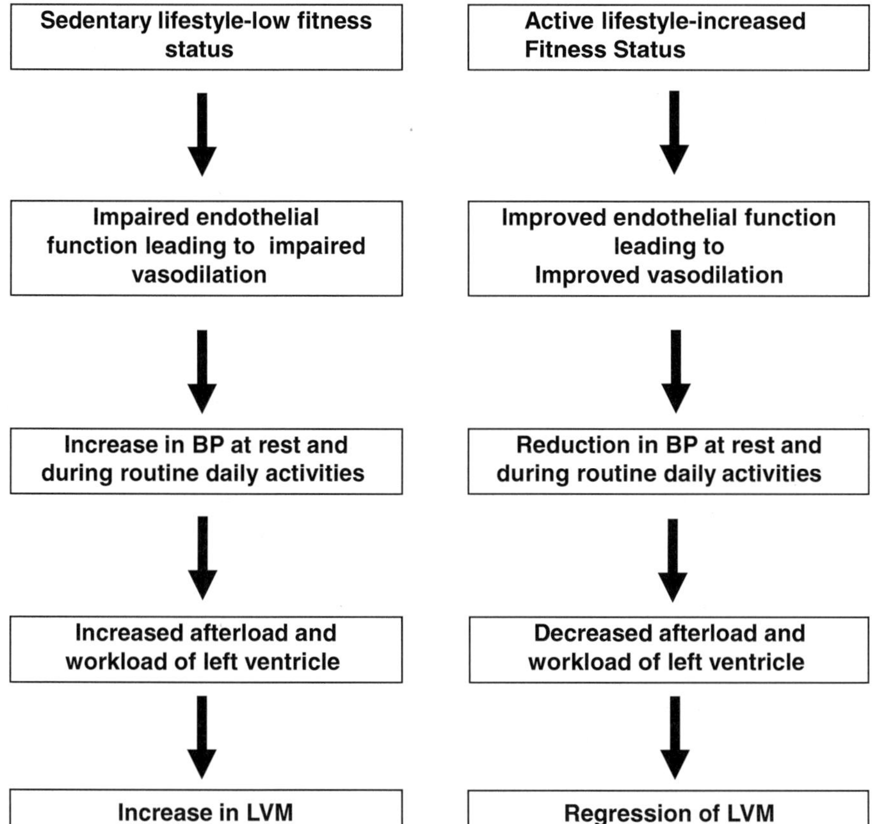

Fig. 13.2 Model of hypertensive LVH development and exercise-induced regression

reduction in SVR. The exercise-induced reduction in SVR is substantiated further by findings that the impaired endothelial function observed in hypertensive patients [42, 43] and older individuals with normal blood pressure is improved after just 12 weeks of moderate intensity exercise [44, 45].

Exercise and Cardiac Hypertrophy

Concentric LVH is considered an independent predictor of CV events and mortality [9–11]. Although various neurohormones, growth factors and cytokines have been identified as contributors in the development of concentric LVH [46, 47], the general consensus is that the mechanical stress from chronically elevated blood pressure in hypertensive states contributes significantly to the progressive increase in left ventricular mass (LVM) and consequent LVH [8]. Reductions in blood pressure with most antihypertensive agents are associated with LVH regression and

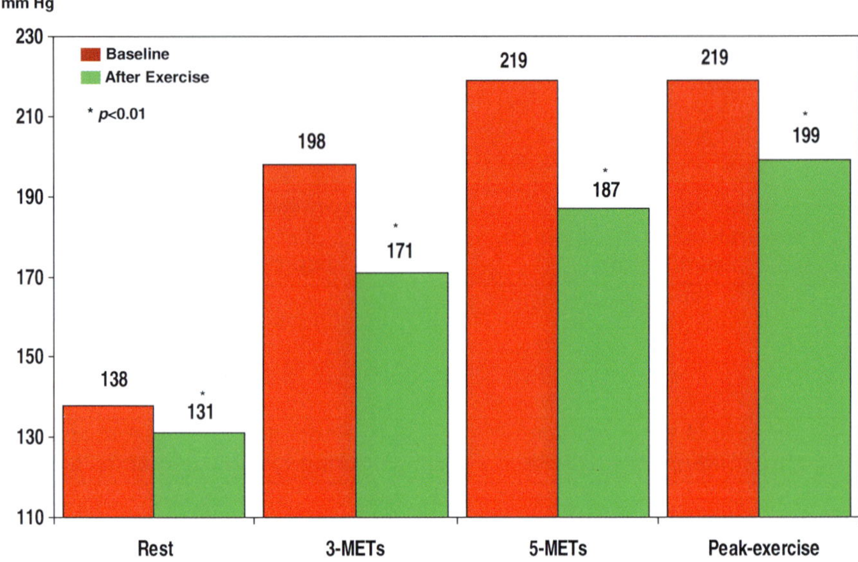

Fig. 13.3 Additional effects of aerobic exercise training on systolic BP at rest and during exercise in patients with treated hypertension (Adapted from Kokkinos et al. [41])

favorable CV prognosis [4–8, 12]. The degree of LVH regression is directly related to the degree of blood pressure reduction suggesting that at least in part, cardiac hypertrophy is mediated by pressure overload [4–8].

Thus, it is reasonable to assume that exercise-related reduction in blood pressure will lead to LV mass regression as a consequence of lower afterload. Support for this concept is provided by several interventional studies [28, 48–51]. Sixteen weeks of aerobic training in individuals with Stage 2 hypertension [28], resulted in a significant reduction in blood pressure, cardiac wall thickness, LVM and LVM index. The degree of LVH regression was similar in magnitude to that observed with most antihypertensive medications [52]. Similar findings were noted in a cohort of overweight hypertensive women (n=45) and men (n=37) undergoing 6 months of exercise training or behavioral modification for weight loss. Participants in both exercise and weight loss interventions exhibited significant reductions in blood pressure and cardiac wall thickness compared to the control group [48]. Significant reductions in cardiac wall thickness and LVM index with no significant changes in chamber size were also reported in 16 hypertensive individuals after 24 weeks of aerobic exercise training [50]. Similar findings were also observed in middle aged individuals with hypertension (n=11) who engaged in exercise and no changes in the control group [49]. Finally, in the Hypertension and Ambulatory Recording Venetia Study (HARVEST) [51], blood pressure decreased during a median follow up of 8.3 years in physically active individuals (n=173) and increased slightly in the sedentary group (n=281). In addition, physically active individuals were less likely to develop LVH compared to their sedentary counterparts.

It is noteworthy that LVH regression related to the exercise-induced reduction in blood pressure occurs relatively quickly, within weeks. This is not surprising since several studies have shown that blood pressure is lowered even after one bout of exercise and remains below baseline for approximately 12–24 h [26]. Thus, engaging in aerobic activity every other day (as is customary) favorably influences blood pressure, afterload and cardiac function. Consequently, the stimulus for cardiac hypertrophy is mitigated or removed and LV mass regression is initiated.

In contrast to the aforementioned studies, no structural or functional cardiac changes were noted after 24 weeks of aerobic exercise and resistance training in 51 overweight and obese individuals with an untreated baseline systolic blood pressure of 130–150 mmHg or diastolic blood pressure of 85–99 mmHg [52]. Similarly, no exercise-related changes in left ventricular mass were observed in 23 obese individuals with a mean baseline blood pressure of 131/84 mmHg, despite significant reductions in blood pressure [53]. However, the findings of these two studies should be interpreted with caution. In one study [52], it is not clear as to how many of the participants were truly hypertensive, since the baseline blood pressure range was 130–150 mmHg for systolic blood pressure or 85–99 mmHg for diastolic blood pressure. The exercise intervention was also a mixture of both aerobic and resistance training. Moreover, based on baseline LVM index normal values (63.6 g/m^2), cardiac remodeling was absent. Thus, exercise or any other intervention cannot "fix" what is not broken. In the other study [53], a closer scrutiny of the findings revealed that the LVM index decreased by approximately 8 % (baseline of 153–141 g/m^2 after exercise) in the exercise group, and increased by approximately 10 % (baseline of 141–155 g/m^2 after exercise) in the control group. Cardiac wall thickness also decreased after exercise, although statistical significance was not achieved, perhaps due to relatively small number of patients studied (n = 7). Collectively, evidence regarding the effects of aerobic exercises on cardiac remodeling supports that LVH regression is likely to occur, if the proper exercise modality is used, in populations with LVH.

Exercise Blood Pressure and LVH

A noteworthy observation is that the degree of LVH regression is disproportional to the degree of exercise-induced reduction in blood pressure. For example, in our study, resting blood pressure was lowered by 7/5 mmHg, reflecting a 12.3 % reduction in LV mass. Although the degree of LVH regression is comparable to what has been reported by most pharmacotherapies [54], the reduction in blood pressure was substantially greater (approximately 30/17 mmHg) with pharmacotherapies [55]. This suggests that exercise-induced LVH regression may be modulated not only by a lower resting blood pressure, but other factors. In this regard, we noted in our hypertensive patients that both systolic and diastolic exercise blood pressure at submaximal and peak workloads was significantly lower following 16 weeks of aerobic exercise training [28, 41]. Specifically, the exercise systolic blood pressures at submaximal workloads of approximately 3 and 5 METs and peak exercise were

27 mmHg, 32 mmHg and 20 mmHg, respectively (average 26 mmHg), lower after 16 weeks of exercise [41]. Consequently, the average rate-pressure product (RPP) at the same workloads was also 4,641 units lower. This is clinically significant because the metabolic demands of most daily chores fall within 3–5 METs [56]. Based on this, it is rational to assume that the daily hemodynamic load and metabolic demands of the myocardium of these subjects would be substantially lower after 16 weeks of exercise. Moreover, we can assume that the 24-h reduced hemodynamic load may have played a far greater role in the regression of LVH than the resting blood pressure. This assumption is further supported by the strong association noted between the blood pressure response at the submaximal workload of approximately 4–5 METs and LVH in 790 middle aged, individuals with prehypertension [57, 58] who underwent echocardiographic studies, 24 h ambulatory blood pressure monitoring, and a standard exercise stress test (Bruce protocol). Specifically, moderate and high-fit individuals had significantly lower LVM index, lower daytime blood pressure and lower exercise systolic blood pressure at the workload of approximately 4–5 METs compared to the low-fit individuals. Those who achieved systolic blood pressure ≥150 mmHg at the exercise intensity of 4–5 METs had a significantly higher LVM index and lower exercise capacity compared to those with a systolic blood pressure below this level. Furthermore, the risk of having LVH increased 4-fold for every 10 mmHg rise in systolic blood pressure beyond the threshold of 150 mmHg at approximately 5 METs. It is important to emphasize that the resting blood pressure in these two groups (i.e., exercise systolic blood pressure <150 mmHg and ≥150 mmHg) was similar.

The clinical significance of the blood pressure response to submaximal workloads of approximately 4–5 METs is that it reflects daytime blood pressure during most daily activities. This is supported by the similarity between systolic blood pressure of individuals with prehypertension (n=650) at the workload of 4–5 METs (148±12 mmHg) and daytime ambulatory systolic blood pressure (144±11 mmHg) [58]. Thus, the association between systolic blood pressure during physical exertion and LVM [57, 58] suggests that the daily exposure to relatively high systolic blood pressure (≥150 mmHg) provides the impetus for an increase in LVM even among those with prehypertension.

Others also reported similar findings among 49 individuals with hypertension at the exercise workload of approximately 7 METs. Systolic blood pressure at this workload was directly and independently associated with cardiac wall thickness and LVM index. This association was stronger than the association noted with office blood pressure and 24 h ambulatory systolic blood pressure [59].

Exercise Blood Pressure and Physical Fitness

A noteworthy finding of the above studies [57, 58] was that the peak exercise capacity of individuals with a systolic blood pressure response ≥ 150 mmHg at the workload of approximately 4–5 METs was significantly lower when compared to those with an exercise blood pressure <150 mmHg (i.e., 7.7 ± 1.6 METs vs 9.0 ± 1.1 METs, respectively). This finding suggests that the blood pressure response to exercise may be modulated by the physical fitness level of the individual. An inverse association was also observed between exercise capacity, the blood pressure response to exercise, and LVM [57, 58]. Furthermore, the systolic blood pressure of physically fit individuals at an exercise intensity of approximately 4–5 METs was significantly higher for the Low-Fit (155 ± 14 mmHg) compared to Moderate-Fit (146 ± 10 mmHg) and High-Fit (144 ± 10 mmHg) individuals. Similarly, Low-Fit individuals had significantly higher LVM index (48 ± 12 g/m$^{2.7}$) compared to Moderate-Fit (41 ± 10 g/m$^{2.7}$) and High-Fit (41 ± 9 g/m$^{2.7}$) (Fig. 13.4) In addition, for every 1-MET increase in the workload achieved, there was a 42 % reduction in the risk for LVH [57]. Finally, in a randomized controlled study, 16 weeks of aerobic training resulted in significantly lower blood pressure at the exercise intensity of approximately 3 and 5 METs [41] and a significant regression in LVM [28].

Collectively, the aforementioned findings suggest the following: (1) the systolic blood pressure response at the workloads of approximately 4–5 METs reflects the blood pressure during daily activities; (2) a systolic blood pressure ≥150 mmHg at this workload is associated with an increased risk for LVH; and (3) daily, intermittent exposure to a systolic blood pressure ≥150 mmHg provides the impetus for increases in LVM and progression to LVH; and (4) increased physical fitness status achieved by regularly performed exercises of moderate intensity modulates the blood pressure response, leading to a lower blood pressure at absolute submaximal and peak workloads. This is likely the outcome of favorable changes in SVR and afterload resulting from improved endothelial function. Consequently, relatively fit individuals are not likely to achieve systolic blood pressure ≥150 mmHg necessary

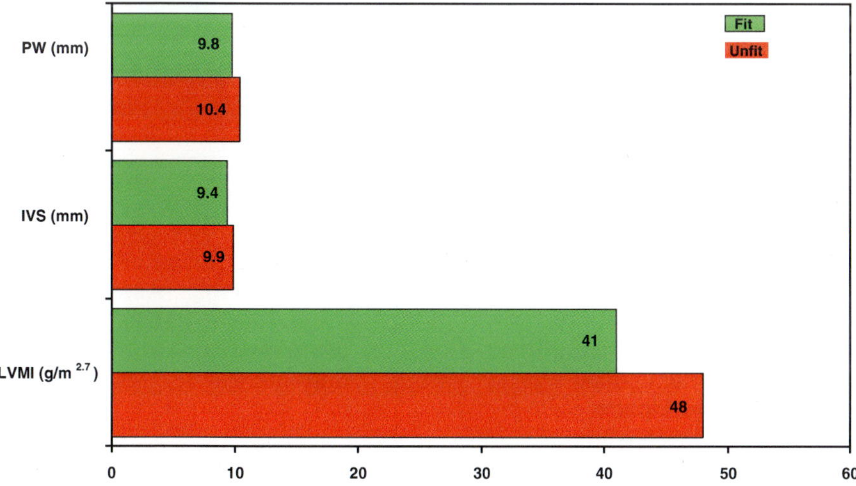

Fig. 13.4 Cardiac dimensions according to fitness status (Adapted from Kokkinos et al. [57])

to stimulate cardiac remodeling during normal daily activities and therefore, an increase in LVM is not likely to occur. For those with existing LVH, regularly performed aerobic exercise of moderate intensity improves fitness, lowers blood pressure at absolute workloads and the daily hemodynamic load, as is reflected by lower blood pressure. Consequently, the daily exposure to a substantially lower hemodynamic load removes the impetus for cardiac remodeling and eventually leads to LVM regression.

Exercise-Induced LVH

It is well-accepted that rigorous exercise as that endured by athletes promotes cardiac enlargement. The type of enlargement is specific to the type of activity or exercise performed (Fig. 13.5). The two traditional types of exercise training are: aerobic or endurance and anaerobic. Aerobic or endurance exercises include activities of relatively low-to-moderate intensity and long-duration that depend primarily on the aerobic energy-generating process. The classic examples of such activities include long distance running or swimming. Anaerobic exercises or activities are characterized by short-duration, high-intensity activities that derive most of the energy demands via the anaerobic pathways (glycolysis). The classic example of such activities is resistance or strength training.

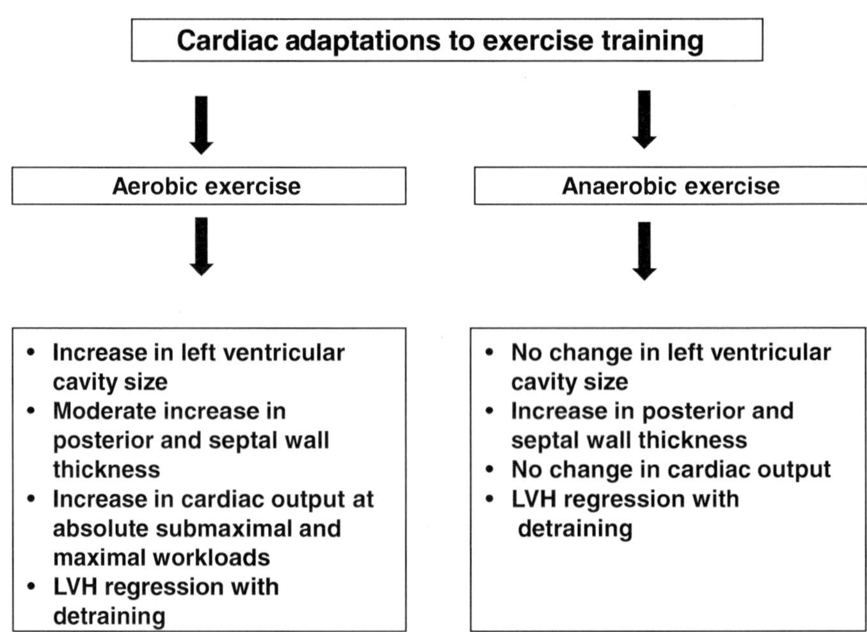

Fig. 13.5 Cardiac adaptations to aerobic and anaerobic exercises

The acute cardiovascular responses and chronic adaptations to these two types of activities differ considerably. Acute cardiovascular responses during aerobic exercises include a substantial increase in heart rate, stroke volume, cardiac output, systolic blood pressure, oxygen consumption and a marked decrease in peripheral vascular resistance with no significant changes in diastolic blood pressure. Cardiovascular responses to resistance training include a mild increase in cardiac output and oxygen consumption, but a substantial increase in heart rate, systolic and diastolic blood pressure and peripheral vascular resistance. Prolonged exposure to aerobic or resistance training results in cardiac adaptations specific to the type of training. Purely aerobic training leads to cardiac remodeling characterized by increases in left and right ventricular chamber dimensions and left atrial cavity size and normal systolic and diastolic function. Left ventricular wall thickness that exceeds normal upper limits of 13–15 mm is also evident in most athletes [60]. Anaerobic training alone results in a mild increase in wall thickness, often disproportionate compared to cavity size, but within the accepted normal range and no changes in left ventricular chamber size. Of note, some misunderstanding persists as to whether strength or resistance training alone results in concentric LVH [61]. Resistance exercises are associated with increased wall thicknesses, often disproportionate relative to cavity size. However, absolute values uncorrected for body surface area usually remain within the accepted normal range of ≤12 mm. It is also important to mention that most sports or daily activities are comprised of both aerobic and anaerobic types of activities. Consequently, structural and functional cardiac adaptations reflect the combined demands of the particular sport or activity. This is most evident in elite athletes participating in sports such as cycling, rowing and swimming that incorporate both aerobic and resistance components. These athletes have the most extreme increase in both LV wall thickness and cavity size [61]. It is important to emphasize that an increase in either alone (wall thickness or LV diastolic dimension) will not be physiologically desirable. LV dilatation without comparable increase in wall thickness will lead to an inappropriate increase in wall tension that is detrimental to the heart [62].

In general, chronic cardiac adaptations resulting from vigorous, chronic exercise as seen in athletes are considered normal physiologic responses to the hemodynamic demand of the particular sport or physical activity. They are not associated with diastolic dysfunction, arrhythmias or adverse prognosis, manifestation observed in hypertension-induced LVH [1, 2] and regress quickly when training is discontinued [62]. Less known are the long-term effects of rigorous exercise such as that demanded by competitive sports (basketball, soccer, etc.) and even non-competitive activities (long distance running, cycling, weight training, etc.) on cardiac structure and function in individuals with hypertension-induced LVH. However, from the available information, we can deduce that high-intensity activities are likely to impose an excessive demand on the cardiovascular system and perpetuate further maladaptations. Therefore, such activities should be avoided. Instead, the recommendations of the American College of Sports Medicine and the American Heart Association of low-to-moderate intensity aerobic exercise (brisk walk) of approximately 30 min per day, most if not all days of the week should be encouraged by health care providers [34, 63]. Such exercise is safe for almost all ages and populations with co-morbidities [28], has been shown to have a favorable effect on the traditional and novel cardiovascular risk factors [64], including LVH regression [28].

Collectively, the emerging concept is that a hemodynamic load threshold exists beyond which the cardiac muscle, as any muscle, will make the necessary adaptations to accommodate the increased demand. This hemodynamic load threshold is reflected by the systolic blood pressure of approximately ≥150 mmHg, as suggested by our findings [41, 57]. The level of physical activity that will elicit such response is relative to the individual's peak exercise capacity. For example, according to our finding, the systolic blood pressure ≥150 mmHg necessary to trigger cardiac remodeling was achieved by relatively low-fit individuals at the workload of 4–5 METs. This level of physical activity typically represents approximately 60 % of the peak exercise capacity of sedentary or relatively low-fit individuals (estimated peak exercise capacity 6–7 METs). If we assume that a 60 % of the peak workload is necessary to elicit a systolic blood pressure response ≥150 mmHg, this workload for a relatively fit individuals (estimated peak exercise capacity 12 METs) is 7.2 METs and for athletes (estimated peak exercise capacity 20 METs), 12 METs. Thus, for relatively fit individuals and athletes the workload of daily activities (4–5 METs) is not likely to elicit a systolic blood pressure response ≥150 mmHg necessary to elicit cardiac remodeling (Figs. 13.5 and 13.6). However, such blood pressure threshold is reached and well exceeded during the highly demanding exercise training endured by athletes and therefore, cardiac remodeling to accommodate the imposed demand is triggered.

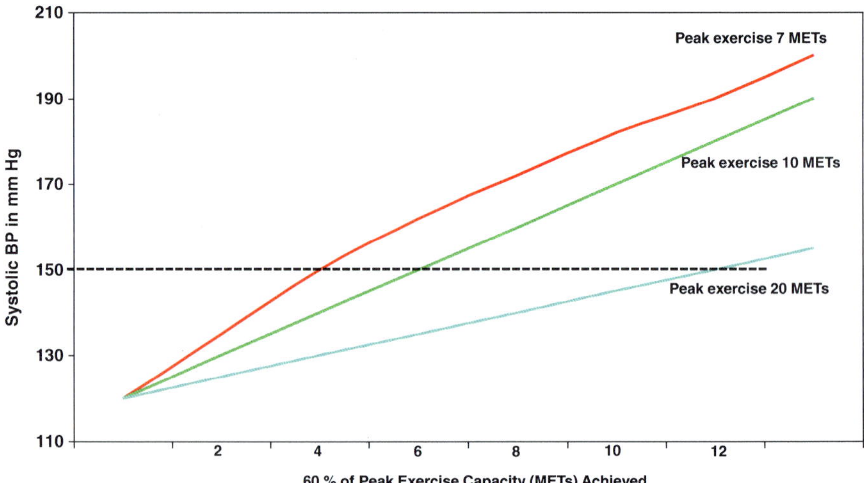

Fig. 13.6 Theoretical concept of exercise systolic BP threshold of 150 mmHg achieved according to fitness status. Note that low fit individuals achieve systolic BP of 150 mmHg (threshold) at 4 METs (within the metabolic demand for most daily activities). The same BP level is achieved at 6 METs for those with an exercise capacity of 10 METs and at 12 METs for highly individuals. Adapted from Kokkinos et al. [57]

Exercise, LVH and Related Cardiovascular Events

Exercise training studies addressing the efficacy of exercise in lowering the risk of mortality in individuals with hypertensive LVH have not been conducted. However, evidence from epidemiologic studies supports that physical activity and increased fitness status provide protection against cardiovascular events in patients with hypertensive LVH. In The Northern Manhattan Stroke Study [65] the risk of stroke in sedentary individuals with elevated LVM was 3.5 times greater when compared to sedentary individuals with normal LVM. Individuals with elevated LVM (presence of LVH), engaging in light intensity activities such as walking, had a similar risk of ischemic stroke to those with normal LVM. This is an important observation, since it suggests that the risk of stroke associated with increased LVM may be potentially attenuated by nonpharmacologic means such as moderate levels of physical activity.

It has been long known that LVH provokes tachyarrhythmias, including atrial fibrillation (AF). Individuals with evidence of LVH have a higher prevalence and greater complexity of ventricular premature beats and more serious arrhythmias compared with normotensive patients without LVH [66–68]. The frequency and complexity of premature ventricular complexes (PVCs), is related to the severity of LVH as well as chamber volume and indices of left ventricular contractility [69, 70]. LVM and age are the only independent predictors of developing AF. For every one standard deviation increase in LVM the risk of AF was increased 1.20 times [71]. Thus, left atrial remodeling resulting from prolonged elevation in blood pressure maybe the pathophysiological link between hypertension and AF [72, 73].

Several studies also suggest that atrial fibrillation is more common among currently or previously trained athletes than in their sedentary counterparts [74–80]. The association appears to be directly related to intensity, and hours or number of days per week engaged vigorous physical activity [77–81]. Potential mechanisms suggested for the higher risk of AF secondary to vigorous physical activity in athletes are speculative and include disruption in the balance between sympathetic and parasympathetic activity, an increase in left atrial size leading to atrial fibrosis, myocardial injury, and inflammation [76, 79, 82–85].

In contrast, moderate exercise had either no adverse effect on AF [86] or lowered the risk of AF [87]. The risk was inversely associated with fitness assessed by an exercise stress test in 6,390 middle-aged and older male veterans. For every 1-MET increase in exercise capacity, the AF risk was 21 % lower (hazard ratio, 0.79, 95 % CI, 0.76–0.82, $p<0.001$). When the cohort was stratified according to peak METs achieved, AF risk was 23 % lower for the Low-Fit; 46 % for Moderate-Fit and 64 % for High-Fit individuals compared to the Least-Fit [87].

Considerable evidence supports that concentric LVH is a common precursor of heart failure [88]. There is no direct evidence that increased fitness will attenuate the rate of progression form concentric LVH to heart failure. However, prospective epidemiologic evidence supports an association between low fitness with a higher prevalence of concentric remodeling and diastolic dysfunction. This suggests that the exercise-related favorable and long-term effects on cardiac remodeling and diastolic function may attenuate the rate of progression to heart failure [89]. At least 20 min of cycling or walking per day was associated with the largest reduction in HF risk [90]. However, an increase in heart failure was noted in those engaging in low and very high volume of exercise, a U-shape association.

Clinical Implications and Conclusions

The findings presented in this chapter support that regularly performed aerobic exercise of moderate intensity, adequate duration and volume that leads to improved fitness status can be implemented to lower blood pressure in hypertensive patients and modulate the associated hypertensive heart disease. Specifically, aerobic exercise training can prevent the development of concentric cardiac remodeling and lower LVM in those with LVH [28, 48–52]. In at least one study, exercise has been shown to lower the risk of stroke even in the presence of LVH and cardiac arrhythmias [65]. It is noteworthy that the aforementioned health benefits are achievable at a fitness level represented by an exercise capacity >5 METs. This has a significant clinical and public health impact because this level of fitness is achievable by a brisk walk of 20–40 min, most days of the week, an activity level attainable by most, including middle-aged and older individuals. Since walking requires virtually no instructions, has a relatively low cost, carries a low risk of injury, and can be easily implemented in large populations, it represents the ideal form of exercise for hypertensive individuals at any age. The effects of exercise have a favorable effect on a cardiovascular risk factors are additive to pharmacologic therapies and independent of body weight reduction and dietary factors [17, 25, 64, 91]. Thus, increased physical activity of moderate intensity should be an important component of any antihypertensive regimen and should be promoted by all health care providers.

References

1. Drazner MH. The progression of hypertensive heart disease. Circulation. 2011;123:327–34.
2. Frohlich ED, Apstein C, Chobanian AV, Devereux RB, Dustan HP, Dzau V, Fauad-Tarazi F, Horan MJ, Marcus M, Massie B, Pfeffer MA, Re RN, Roccella EJ, Savage D, Shub C. The heart in hypertension. N Engl J Med. 1992;327:998–1008.
3. Post WS, Larson MG, Levy D. Impact of left ventricular structure on the incidence of hypertension: the Framingham Heart Study. Circulation. 1994;90:179–85.
4. Mathew J, Sleight P, Lonn E, Johnstone D, Pogue J, Yi Q, et al. Reduction of cardiovascular risk by regression of electrocardiographic markers of left ventricular hypertrophy by the angiotensin-converting enzyme inhibitor ramipril. Circulation. 2001;104:1615–21.
5. Muiesan ML, Salvetti M, Monteduro C, Bonzi B, Paini A, Viola S, et al. Left ventricular concentric geometry during treatment adversely affects cardiovascular prognosis in hypertensive patients. Hypertension. 2004;43:731–8.

6. Muiesan ML, Salvetti M, Rizzoni D, Castellano M, Donato F, Agabiti-Rosei E. Association of change in left ventricular mass with prognosis during long-term antihypertensive treatment. J Hypertens. 1995;13:1091–5.
7. Verdecchia P, Angeli F, Borgioni C, Gattobigio R, de Simone G, Devereux RB, et al. Changes in cardiovascular risk by reduction of left ventricular mass in hypertension: a meta-analysis. Am J Hypertens. 2003;16:895–9.
8. Verdecchia P, Staessen JA, Angeli F, de Simone G, Achilli A, Ganau A, Mureddu G, Pede S, Maggioni AP, Lucci D, Reboldi G. Usual versus tight control of systolic blood pressure in non-diabetic patients with hypertension (Cardio-Sis): an open-label randomised trial. Lancet. 2009;374:525–33.
9. Levy D, Garrison RJ, Savage DD, Kannel WB, Castelli WP. Prognostic implications of echocardiographically determined left ventricular mass in the Framingham Heart Study. N Engl J Med. 1990;322:1561–6.
10. Vakili BA, Okin PM, Devereux RB. Prognostic implications of left ventricular hypertrophy. Am Heart J. 2001;141:334–41.
11. Bombelli M, Facchetti R, Carugo S, Madotto F, Arenare F, Quarti-Trevano F, Capra A, Giannattasio C, Dell'Oro R, Grassi G, Sega R, Mancia G. Left ventricular hypertrophy increases cardiovascular risk independently of in-office and out-of-office blood pressure values. J Hypertens. 2009;27(12):2458–64. doi:10.1097/HJH.0b013e328330b845.
12. Katholi RE, Couri DM. Left ventricular hypertrophy: major risk factor in patients with hypertension: update and practice clinical applications. Int J Hypertens. 2011;2011:1–10.
13. Chobanian AV, Bakris GL, Black HR, Cushman WC, Green LA, Izzo Jr JL, et al. The seventh report of the joint national committee on prevention, detection, evaluation, and treatment of high blood pressure: the JNC 7 report. JAMA. 2003;289:2560–72.
14. Go AS, Mozaffarian D, Roger VL, Benjamin EJ, Berry JD, Blaha MJ, et al. Heart disease and stroke statistics--2014 update: a report from the American Heart Association. Circulation. 2014;129:e28–292.
15. MacMahon S, Peto R, Cutler J, Collins R, Sorlie P, Neaton J, et al. Blood pressure, stroke, and coronary heart disease. Part 1. Prolonged differences in blood pressure: prospective observational studies corrected for the regression dilution bias. Lancet. 1990;335:765–74.
16. World Health Organization. The world health report 2002: reducing risks, promoting healthy life. World Health Organ. Geneva, Switzerland; 2002:57–8.
17. Kokkinos P. Cardiorespiratory fitness, exercise, and blood pressure. Hypertension. 2014;64:1160–4.
18. Cornelissen VA, Fagard RH. Effects of endurance training on blood pressure, blood pressure-regulating mechanisms, and cardiovascular risk factors. Hypertension. 2005;46:667–75.
19. Pescatello LS, Franklin BA, Fagard R, Farquhar WB, Kelley GA, Ray CA. American college of sports medicine position stand. Exercise and hypertension. Med Sci Sports Exerc. 2004;36:533–53.
20. Whelton SP, Chin A, Xin X, He J. Effect of aerobic exercise on blood pressure: a meta-analysis of randomized, controlled trials. Ann Intern Med. 2002;136:493–503.
21. Huai P, Xun H, Reilly KH, Wang Y, Ma W, Xi B. Physical activity and risk of hypertension: a meta-analysis of prospective cohort studies. Hypertension. 2013;62:1021–6.
22. Motoyama M, Sunami Y, Kinoshita F, et al. Blood pressure lowering effect of low intensity aerobic training in elderly hypertensive patients. Med Sci Sports Exerc. 1998;30(6):818–23.
23. Ishikawa K, Ohta T, Zhang J, Hashimoto S, Tanaka H. Influence of age and gender on exercise training induced blood pressure reduction in systemic hypertension. Am J Cardiol. 1999;84(2):192–6.
24. Cornelissen VA, Smart NA. Exercise training on blood pressure: a systematic review and meta-analysis. J Am Heart Assoc. 2013;2:e004473.
25. Kokkinos P. The impact of exercise and physical fitness on blood pressure, left ventricular hypertrophy, and mortality among individuals with prehypertension and hypertension. In: Pascatello LS, editors. Effects of exercise on hypertension: from cell to physiological systems. Cham: Humana Press; New York, 2015.

26. Pascatella LS. The effects of Aerobic exercise on hypertension: current consensus and emerging research. In: Pascatello LS, editor. Effects of exercise on hypertension: from cell to physiological systems. Cham: Humana Press; New York, 2015.
27. Calhoun DA, Jones D, Textor S, Goff DC, Murphy TP, Toto RD, White A, Cushman WC, White W, Sica D, Ferdinand K, Giles TD, Falkner B, Carey RM. Resistant hypertension: diagnosis, evaluation, and treatment. A scientific statement from the American Heart Association Professional Education Committee of the Council for High Blood Pressure Research. Hypertension. 2008;51:1403–19.
28. Kokkinos PF, Narayan P, Colleran J, Pittaras A, Notargiacomo A, Reda D, Papademetriou V. Effects of regular exercise on blood pressure and left ventricular hypertrophy in African-American men with severe hypertension. N Engl J Med. 1995;333:1462–7.
29. Dimeo F, Pagonas N, Seibert F, Arndt R, Zidek W, Westhoff TM. Aerobic exercise reduces blood pressure in resistant hypertension. Hypertension. 2012;60:653–8.
30. Brook RD, Appel LJ, Rubenfire M, Ogedegbe G, Bisognano JD, Elliott WJ, Fuchs FD, Hughes JW, Lackland DT, Staffileno BA, Townsend RR, Rajagopalan S. Beyond medications and diet: alternative approaches to lowering blood pressure. A scientific statement from the American Heart Association on behalf of the American Heart Association Professional Education Committee of the council for high blood pressure research, council on cardiovascular and stroke nursing, council on epidemiology and prevention, and council on nutrition, physical activity and metabolism. Hypertension. 2013;61:1360–83.
31. Cornelissen VA, Fagard RH, Coeckelberghs E, Vanhees L. Impact of resistance training on blood pressure and other cardiovascular risk factors: a meta-analysis of randomized, controlled trials. Hypertension. 2011;58:950–8.
32. Kelley GA, Kelley KS. Progressive resistance exercise and resting blood pressure: a meta-analysis of randomized controlled trials. Hypertension. 2000;35:838–43.
33. Hurley BF, Gillin AR. Can resistance training play a role in the prevention or treatment of hypertension?. In: Pascatello LS, editor. Effects of exercise on hypertension: from cell to physiological systems. Cham: Humana Press; New York, 2015.
34. Nelson ME, Rejeski WJ, Blair SN, Duncan PW, Judge JO, King AC, Macera CA, Castaneda-Sceppa C. Physical activity and public health in older adults: recommendation from the American College of Sports Medicine and the American Heart Association. Circulation. 2007;116:1094–105.
35. Williams MA, Haskell WL, Ades PA, Amsterdam EA, Bittner V, Franklin BA, Gulanick M, Laing ST, Stewart KJ. Resistance exercise in individuals with and without cardiovascular disease: 2007 update: a scientific statement from the American Heart Association Council on Clinical Cardiology and Council on Nutrition, Physical Activity, and Metabolism. Circulation. 2007;116:572–84.
36. Palatini P, et al. Relation between physical training and ambulatory blood pressure in stage I hypertensive subjects. Results of the HARVEST Trial. Hypertension and Ambulatory Recording Venetia Study. Circulation. 1994;90(6):2870–6.
37. Gordon NF, Scott CB, Levine BD. Comparison of single versus multiple lifestyle interventions: are the antihypertensive effects of exercise training and diet-induced weight loss additive? Am J Cardiol. 1997;79(6):763–7.
38. Seals DR, Reiling MJ. Effect of regular exercise on 24-hour arterial pressure in older hypertensive humans. Hypertension. 1991;18(5):583–92.
39. Cleroux J, et al. Aftereffects of exercise on regional and systemic hemodynamics in hypertension. Hypertension. 1992;19(2):183–91.
40. Floras JS, et al. Postexercise hypotension and sympathoinhibition in borderline hypertensive men. Hypertension. 1989;14(1):28–35.
41. Kokkinos PF, et al. Effects of aerobic training on exaggerated blood pressure response to exercise in African-Americans with severe systemic hypertension treated with indapamide +/– verapamil +/– enalapril. Am J Cardiol. 1997;79(10):1424–6.
42. Linder L, et al. Indirect evidence for release of endothelium-derived relaxing factor in human forearm circulation in vivo. Blunted response in essential hypertension. Circulation. 1990;81(6):1762–7.

43. Panza JA, et al. Abnormal endothelium-dependent vascular relaxation in patients with essential hypertension. N Engl J Med. 1990;323(1):22–7.
44. DeSouza CA, et al. Regular aerobic exercise prevents and restores age-related declines in endothelium-dependent vasodilation in healthy men. Circulation. 2000;102(12):1351–7.
45. Higashi Y, et al. Regular aerobic exercise augments endothelium-dependent vascular relaxation in normotensive as well as hypertensive subjects: role of endothelium-derived nitric oxide. Circulation. 1999;100(11):1194–202.
46. Hill JA, Olson EN. Cardiac plasticity. N Engl J Med. 2008;358:1370–80.
47. Diez J, Frohlich ED. A translational approach to hypertensive heart disease. Hypertension. 2010;55:1–8.
48. Hinderliter A, Sherwood A, Gullette EC, Babyak M, Waugh R, Georgiades A, et al. Reduction of left ventricular hypertrophy after exercise and weight loss in overweight patients with mild hypertension. Arch Intern Med. 2002;162:1333–9.
49. Turner MJ, Spina RJ, Kohrt WM, Ehsani AA. Effect of endurance exercise training on left ventricular size and remodeling in older adults with hypertension. J Gerontol A Biol Sci Med Sci. 2000;55:M245–51.
50. Rinder MR, Spina RJ, Peterson LR, Koenig CJ, Florence CR, Ehsani AA. Comparison of effects of exercise and diuretic on left ventricular geometry, mass, and insulin resistance in older hypertensive adults. Am J Physiol Regul Integr Comp Physiol. 2004;287: R360–8.
51. Palatini P, Visentin P, Dorigatti F, Guarnieri C, Santonastaso M, Cozzio S, et al. Regular physical activity prevents development of left ventricular hypertrophy in hypertension. Eur Heart J. 2009;30:225–32.
52. Reid CM, Dart AM, Dewar EM, Jennings GL. Interactions between the effects of exercise and weight loss on risk factors, cardiovascular haemodynamics and left ventricular structure in overweight subjects. J Hypertens. 1994;12:291–301.
53. Stewart KJ, Ouyang P, Bacher AC, Lima S, Shapiro EP. Exercise effects on cardiac size and left ventricular diastolic function: relationships to changes in fitness, fatness, blood pressure and insulin resistance. Heart. 2006;92:893–8.
54. Dahlöf B, Devereux RB, Kjeldsen SE, et al. Cardiovascular morbidity and mortality in the Losartan Intervention For Endpoint reduction in hypertension study (LIFE): a randomized trial against atenolol. Lancet. 2002;359(9311):995–1003.
55. Dahlöf B, Sever PS, Poulter NR, et al. Prevention of cardiovascular events with an antihypertensive regimen of amlodipine adding perindopril as required versus atenolol adding bendroflumethiazide as required, in the Anglo-Scandinavian Cardiac Outcomes Trial-Blood Pressure Lowering Arm (ASCOT-BPLA): a multicentre randomised controlled trial. Lancet. 2005;366(9489):895–906.
56. American College of Sports Medicine. ACSM's guidelines for exercise testing and prescription. 7th ed. Philadelphia: Lippincott Williams and Wilkins; 2005.
57. Kokkinos P, Pittaras A, Narayan P, Faselis C, Singh S, Manolis A. Exercise capacity and blood pressure associations with left ventricular mass in prehypertensive individuals. Hypertension. 2007;49:55–61.
58. Kokkinos P, Pittaras A, Manolis A, Panagiotakos D, Narayan P, Manjoros D, et al. Exercise capacity and 24-h blood pressure in prehypertensive men and women. Am J Hypertens. 2006;19:251–8.
59. Lim PO, Donnan PT, MacDonald TM. Blood pressure determinants of left ventricular wall thickness and mass index in hypertension: comparing office, ambulatory and exercise blood pressures. J Hum Hypertens. 2001;15:627–33.
60. Pelliccia A, Maron BJ, Spataro A, Proschan MA, Spirito P. The upper limit of physiologic cardiac hypertrophy in highly trained elite athletes. N Engl J Med. 1991;324:295–301.
61. Barry J, Maron BJ, Pelliccia A. The heart of trained athletes: cardiac remodeling and the risks of sports, including sudden death. Circulation. 2006;114:1633–44.
62. Martin III WH, Coyle EF, Bloomfield SA, Ehsani AA. Effects of physical deconditioning after intense endurance training on left ventricular dimensions and stroke volume. J Am Coll Cardiol. 1986;7:982–9.

63. American College of Sports Medicine, Chodzko-Zajko WJ, Proctor DN, et al. American College of Sports Medicine position stand. Exercise and physical activity for older adults. Med Sci Sports Exerc. 2009;41:1510–30.
64. Kokkinos P, Myers J. Exercise and physical activity: clinical outcomes and applications. Circulation. 2010;122:1637–48.
65. Rodriguez CJ, Sacco RL, Sciacca RR, Boden-Albala B, Homma S, Di Tullio MR. Physical activity attenuates the effect of increased left ventricular mass on the risk of ischemic stroke: The Northern Manhattan Stroke Study. J Am Coll Cardiol. 2002;39(9):1482–8.
66. Siegel D, Cheitlin MD, Black DM, et al. Risk of ventricular arrhythmias in hypertensive men with left ventricular hypertrophy. Am J Cardiol. 1990;65:742.
67. Vester EG, Kuhls S, Ochiulet-Vester J, et al. Electrophysiological and therapeutic implications of cardiac arrhythmias in hypertension. Eur Heart J. 1992;13(Suppl D):70.
68. Rials SJ, Wu Y, Ford N, et al. Effect of left ventricular hypertrophy and its regression on ventricular electrophysiology and vulnerability to inducible arrhythmia in the feline heart. Circulation. 1995;91:426.
69. Ghali JK, Kadakia S, Cooper RS, Liao YL. Impact of left ventricular hypertrophy on ventricular arrhythmias in the absence of coronary artery disease. J Am Coll Cardiol. 1991;17:1277.
70. Schmieder RE, Messerli FH. Determinants of ventricular ectopy in hypertensive cardiac hypertrophy. Am Heart J. 1992;123:89.
71. Verdecchia P, Reboldi G, Gattobigio R, et al. Atrial fibrillation in hypertension: predictors and outcome. Hypertension. 2003;41:218.
72. Kistler PM, Sanders P, Dodic M, Spence SJ, Samuel CS, Zhao C, Charles JA, Edwards GA, Kalman JM. Atrial electrical and structural abnormalities in an ovine model of chronic blood pressure elevation after prenatal corticosteroid exposure: implications for development of atrial fibrillation. Eur Heart J. 2006;27:3045–56.
73. Kirchhof P, Schotten U. Hypertension begets hypertrophy begets atrial fibrillation? Insights from yet another sheep model. Eur Heart J. 2006;27:2919–20.
74. Baldesberger S, Bauersfeld U, Candinas R, Seifert B, Zuber M, Ritter M, Jenni R, Oechslin E, Luthi P, Scharf C, Marti B, Attenhofer Jost CH. Sinus node disease and arrhythmias in the long-term follow-up of former professional cyclists. Eur Heart J. 2008;29:71–8.
75. Karjalainen J, Kujala UM, Kaprio J, Sarna S, Viitasalo M. Lone atrial fibrillation in vigorously exercising middle aged men: case–control study. BMJ. 1998;316:1784–5.
76. Mont L, Tamborero D, Elosua R, Molina I, Coll-Vinent B, Sitges M, Vidal B, Scalise A, Tejeira A, Berruezo A, Brugada J, Investigators G. Physical activity, height, and left atrial size are independent risk factors for lone atrial fibrillation in middle-aged healthy individuals. Europace. 2008;10:15–20.
77. Abdulla J, Nielsen JR. Is the risk of atrial fibrillation higher in athletes than in the general population? A systematic review and meta-analysis. Europace. 2009;11:1156–9.
78. Heidbüchel H, Anné W, Willems R, Adriaenssens B, Van de Werf F, Ector H. Endurance sports is a risk factor for atrial fibrillation after ablation for atrial flutter. Int J Cardiol. 2006;107:67–72.
79. Molina L, Mont L, Marrugat J, Berruezo A, Brugada J, Bruguera J, Rebato C, Elosua R. Long-term endurance sport practice increases the incidence of lone atrial fibrillation in men: a follow-up study. Europace. 2008;10:618–23.
80. Aizer A, Gaziano JM, Cook NR, Manson JE, Buring JE, Albert CM. Relation of vigorous exercise to risk of atrial fibrillation. Am J Cardiol. 2009;103:1572–7.
81. Kasper A, Finn R, Claes H, Martin N, Per T, Johan S. Exercise capacity and muscle strength and risk of vascular disease and arrhythmia in 1.1 million young Swedish men: cohort study. BMJ. 2015;351:h4543. doi:10.1136/bmj.h4543.
82. Naiara C, Josep B, Marta S, Lluís M. A trial fibrillation and atrial flutter in athletes. Br J Sports Med. 2012;46:i37–43. doi:10.1136/bjsports-2012-091171.
83. Pelliccia A, Maron BJ, Di Paolo FM, Biffi A, Quattrini FM, Pisicchio C, Roselli A, Caselli S, Culasso F. Prevalence and clinical significance of left atrial remodeling in competitive athletes. J Am Coll Cardiol. 2005;46:690–6.

84. Sorokin AV, Araujo CG, Zweibel S, Thompson PD. Atrial fibrillation in endurance-trained athletes. Br J Sports Med. 2011;45:185–8.
85. Basavarajaiah S, Makan J, Naghavi SH, Whyte G, Gati S, Sharma S. Physiological upper limits of left atrial diameter in highly trained adolescent athletes. J Am Coll Cardiol. 2006;47:2341–2.
86. Mozaffarian D, Furberg CD, Psaty BM, Siscovick D. Physical activity and incidence of atrial fibrillation in older adults: the cardiovascular health study. Circulation. 2008;118:800–7.
87. Faselis C, Kokkinos P, Tsimploulis A, et al. Exercise capacity and atrial fibrillation risk in veterans: a cohort study. Mayo Clin Proc. 2016;91(5):558–66.
88. Rosen DB, Edvardsen T, Shenghan Lai S, et al. Left ventricular concentric remodeling is associated with decreased global and regional systolic function the multi-ethnic study of atherosclerosis. Circulation. 2005;112:984–91.
89. Stephanie K, Brinker S, Pandey A, Ayers CR, et al. Association of cardiorespiratory fitness with left ventricular remodeling and diastolic function: the cooper center longitudinal study. J Am Coll Cardiol HF. 2014;2:238–46.
90. Rahman I, Bellavia A, Wolk A, Orsini N. Physical activity and heart failure risk in a prospective study of men. J Am Coll Cardiol HF. 2015;3(9):681–7. doi:10.1016/j.jchf.2015.05.006.
91. Mora S, Cook N, Buring JE, Ridker PM, Lee IM. Physical activity and reduced risk of cardiovascular events: potential mediating mechanisms. Circulation. 2007;116:2110–8.

Chapter 14
Hypertension and Atherosclerosis: Pathophysiology, Mechanisms and Benefits of BP Control

Misbah Zaheer, Paola Chrysostomou, and Vasilios Papademetriou

Introduction

Hypertension is a leading identifiable and reversible risk factor for myocardial infarction, heart failure, atrial fibrillation, aortic dissection, peripheral arterial disease, stroke and kidney failure [1, 2].· Hypertension is ranked first worldwide in an analysis of all risk factors for global disease burden in 2010 [2]. By the year 2025, hypertension is expected to increase in prevalence worldwide by 60 % and will affect 1.56 billion people [3]. Developing nations will experience an increase in the prevalence of hypertension by 80 % (from 639 million to 1.15 billion afflicted persons). As emerging countries have improved sanitation and other basic public health measures, cardiovascular (CV) disease has or soon will become the most common cause of death, and hypertension will be its most common reversible risk factor, as it already is in the United States.

Hypertension contributes to atherosclerosis at different levels: To the development of endothelial dysfunction, fatty streaks, early atherosclerotic plaque, plaque progression and plaque rapture. In this chapter we'll explore the pathophysiology,

M. Zaheer, M.D.
Department of Medicine, Georgetown University, Washington, DC, USA

P. Chrysostomou
Department of Veterans Affairs Medical Center, and National Institutes of Health (NIH), Intramural Research Program (IRP), Institute of Clinical Research, Washington, DC, USA

V. Papademetriou, M.D. (✉)
Department of Medicine, Georgetown University, Washington, DC, USA

Division of Hypertension and Vascular Medicine, Veteran Affairs Medical Center, Washington, DC, USA
e-mail: vpapademetriou@va.gov

E.A. Andreadis (ed.), *Hypertension and Cardiovascular Disease*,
DOI 10.1007/978-3-319-39599-9_14

the pathways by which hypertension contributes and accelerates atherosclerosis and final evidence that treatment and control of hypertension leads to reduced cardiovascular events.

HTN and Cardiovascular Risk

Hypertension is the most important modifiable risk factor for stroke [1]. Current estimates are that 77 % of those who have a first stroke have had a blood pressure (BP) above 140/90 mmHg. High BP is the leading antecedent condition for either the systolic or diastolic type of heart failure and the most common reason for acute care hospitalization among Medicare beneficiaries (approximately 1.023 million in 2010); approximately 74 % of people experiencing an initial hospitalization for heart failure either had or have BP of 140/90 mmHg or higher [1].

The risks attributable to elevated BP levels are documented in numerous epidemiologic studies, beginning in 1948 with the Framingham Heart Study and extending to the present [4, 5]. Meta-analyses of pooled data confirm the robust, continuous relationship between BP level and cerebrovascular disease and coronary heart disease in both Western and Eastern populations [6]. In addition, BP is linked directly in epidemiologic studies to incident left ventricular hypertrophy (LVH), heart failure, peripheral vascular disease, carotid atherosclerosis, end-stage kidney disease, and "subclinical CV disease." Out –of-office blood pressure measurements have also been shown to correlate with chronic kidney disease [7, 8]. The highest risk is at levels above the auto regulatory range of the kidney (i.e., a systolic BP > 180 mmHg). CV risk factors tend to cluster; thus hypertensive individuals are much more likely than normotensive people to have type 2 diabetes mellitus or dyslipidemia, especially elevated triglyceride levels and low high-density lipoprotein cholesterol levels.

Pathophysiology of HTN Leading to Atherosclerosis

Arterial Stiffness

In primary hypertension, the column of blood in the arterial tree between aortic valve and capillaries moves at abnormally high pressure throughout cardiac cycle of contraction and relaxation. However, cardiac output is usually normal or close to normal. Thus, the main determinant of the sustained elevated blood pressure is an increase in peripheral arterial resistance. Under normal circumstances, peripheral resistance is determined predominantly by precapillary vessels with a luminal diameter of approximately 100–300 μm [7, 8]. In human hypertension and in experimental animal models of hypertension, structural changes in these resistance vessels are commonly observed. Small artery remodeling is initiated by vasoconstriction, which normalizes wall stress and averts a trophic response. Normal smooth muscle cells rearrange themselves around a smaller lumen diameter, a process termed inward eutropic remodeling. The media-to-lumen ratio increases but the media cross sectional area remains unchanged. By decreasing lumen diameter in the peripheral circulation, inward eutropic remodeling increases systemic vascular resistance, the hemodynamic hall mark of diastolic hypertension.

In contrast large artery remodeling is characterized by the expression of hypertrophic changes, triggering increases in medial thickness as well as the media-to-lumen ratio. Such hypertrophic remodeling involves not only an increase in the size of vascular smooth muscle cells but also an accumulation of extracellular matrix proteins such as collagen and fibronectin, because of activation of TGF-β. The resultant large artery stiffness is the hemodynamic hall mark of isolated systolic hypertension. Increased Carotid pulse wave velocity hall mark of arterial stiffness PWV is associated with increased mortality and CV events [9], as well as with a variety of subclinical CV injury markers, such as coronary calcification, cerebral white matter lesions, ankle-brachial index, and albuminuria. The relationship with cardiac complications is easily grasped: increased impedance to left ventricular ejection results in LVH, diastolic dysfunction, and sub-endocardial myocardial ischemia

Anti-hypertensive therapy may not provide optimal cardiovascular protection and less vascular remodeling is prevented or reversed by normalizing hemodynamic load, restoring normal endothelial dysfunction and eliminating underlying neurohumoral activation [10].

Endothelial Dysfunction

The endothelial lining of blood vessels is critical to vascular health and constitutes a major defense against hypertension. Cyclic laminar sheer stress that accompanies hypertension, particularly with widened pulse pressure in isolated systolic hypertension leads to endothelial dysfunction.

Several elements are responsible for endothelial dysfunction in hypertension. Normotensive offspring of patients with hypertension have impaired endothelium dependent vasodilation despite normal endothelium-independent responses, thus suggesting a genetic component to the development of endothelial dysfunction. Besides direct pressure-induced injury in the setting of chronically elevated BP, a mechanism of major importance is increased oxidative stress. Reactive oxygen species are generated from enhanced activity of several enzyme systems, reduced nicotinamide adenine dinucleotide phosphate-oxidase (NADPH-oxidase), xanthine oxidase, and cyclo-oxygenase in particular, and decreased activity of the detoxifying enzyme superoxide dismutase (Fig. 14.1) [11–13]. Excess availability of superoxide anions leads to their binding to NO, leading to decreased NO bioavailability, in addition to generating the oxidant, proinflammatory peroxynitrite. It is the decreased NO bioavailability that links oxidative stress to endothelial dysfunction

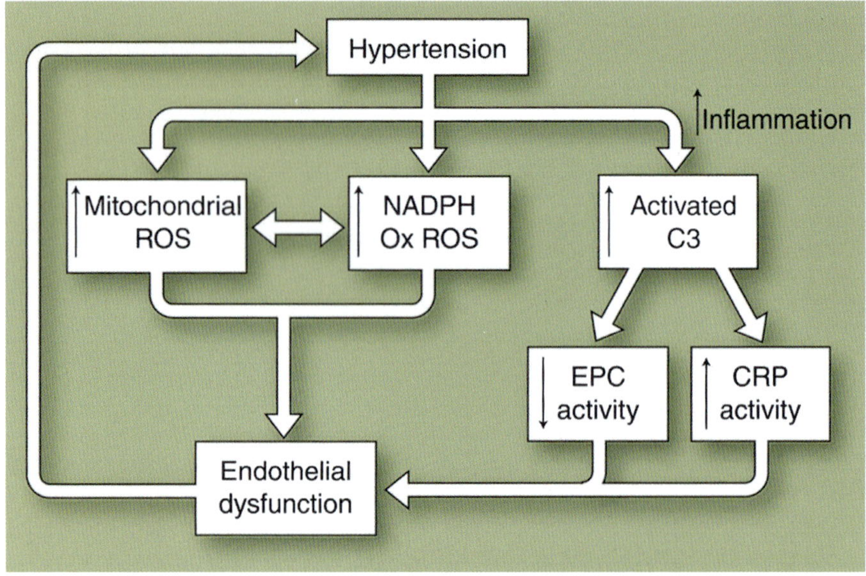

Fig. 14.1 Mechanism by which hypertension contributes to endothelial dysfunction [13]

and hypertension [13]. Angiotensin II is a major enhancer of NADPH-oxidase activity and plays a central role in the generation of oxidative stress in hypertension, although several other factors are also involved, including cyclic vascular stretch, ET-1, uric acid, systemic inflammation, norepinephrine, free fatty acids, and tobacco smoking [14]. ET-1 is the endothelial cell product that counteracts NO to maintain balance between vasodilation and vasoconstriction. ET-1 expression is increased by shear stress, catecholamines, angiotensin II, hypoxia, and several proinflammatory cytokines such as tumor necrosis factor-α, interleukins 1 and 2, and transforming growth factor-β [15]. ET-1 is a potent vasoconstrictor through stimulation of ET-A receptors in vascular smooth muscle. In hypertension, increased ET-1 levels are not consistently found. However, there is a trend of increased sensitivity to the vasoconstrictor effects of ET-1. ET-1 therefore is considered a relevant mediator of BP elevation, as ET-A and ET-B receptor antagonists attenuate or abolish hypertension in several experimental models of hypertension (angiotensin II–mediated models, deoxycorticosterone acetate–salt hypertension, and Dahl salt-sensitive rats) and are effective in lowering BP in humans [12]. Endothelial cells also secrete a variety of other vasoregulatory substances. These include the vasodilating prostaglandin prostacyclin and several vasodilating endothelium- derived hyperpolarizing factors, the identity of which remains uncertain. There are also endothelium-derived contracting factors besides ET-1, such as locally generated angiotensin II and vasoconstricting prostanoids such as thromboxane A2 and prostaglandin A2. The balance of these factors, along with NO and ET-1, determine the final impact of the endothelium on vascular tone.

In cross-sectional analyses, the lower the degree of forearm flow-mediated vasodilation, the greater the prevalence of hypertension [14, 16]. Prospective cohort studies have used flow-mediated vasodilation as a measure of endothelial dysfunction (regardless of specific mechanism) to evaluate its relationship with hypertension and test whether endothelial dysfunction is cause or consequence of hypertension, or both [17]. These studies have shown conflicting results, but the larger of them was unable to demonstrate an association between endothelial dysfunction and incident hypertension among 3500 patients followed for 4.8 years [17], so as it stands, the evidence is stronger for endothelial dysfunction as a consequence, not a cause, of hypertension [16].

Renin Angiotensin System

Activation of renin- angiotensin- aldosterone system (RAAS) is one of the most important mechanisms contributing to endothelial cell dysfunction, vascular remodeling, and hypertension. Activation of RAAS occurs by afferent arteriolar narrowing in kidneys [11]. This abnormality is characterized by a spectrum of histologic changes including focal spasm of otherwise normal afferent arterioles, endothelial edema, vascular smooth muscle hypertrophy and widening of internal elastic lamina with deposition of material that stains with periodic acid Schiff stain, and degenerative changes and hyalinization with focal luminal narrowing. In addition juxtaglomerular cells are hyperplastic, which signifies increased renin biosynthesis. However, it should be emphasized that these renal vascular changes are focal with relatively few obsolescent glomeruli being present, which supports the clinical observation that significant nephron loss and overt renal insufficiency are not major contributing factors in pathogenesis of uncomplicated primary hypertension.

The RAAS has wide-ranging effects on BP regulation. Figure 47.8 summarizes the most relevant elements of the RAAS and its role in the pathogenesis of hypertension and its complications. The different elements of the RAAS have key roles in mediating sodium retention, pressure natriuresis, salt sensitivity, vasoconstriction, endothelium dysfunction, and vascular injury. Taken together, the RAAS has an important role in the pathogenesis of hypertension. Renin and pro-renin are synthesized and stored in the juxtaglomerular cell apparatus and released in response to decreased renal afferent perfusion pressure, decreased sodium delivery to the macula densa, activation of renal nerves (via β1-adrenergic receptor stimulation), and a variety of metabolic products, including prostaglandin E2 and several others. Renin's main function is to cleave angiotensinogen into angiotensin I. Pro-renin, previously viewed as an inactive substrate for renin production, is now known to also stimulate the (pro)renin receptor (PRR). This receptor leads to more efficient cleavage of angiotensinogen and activates downstream intracellular signaling through the mitogen-activated protein (MAP) kinases extracellular signal–regulated kinases 1 and 2 (ERK1/2) pathways that have been associated with profibrotic effects in some, but not all, experimental models [18, 19] At this point, it is uncertain that the PRR is involved in the genesis or complications of hypertension in a manner that is independent of the effects of angiotensin II. Angiotensin II, formed by the cleavage of angiotensin I by the ACE, is at the center of the pathogenetic role of the RAAS in hypertension. Primarily through its actions mediated by the angiotensin II type 1 receptor (AT1R), angiotensin II is a potent vasoconstrictor of vascular smooth muscle, causing systemic vasoconstriction as well as increased renovascular resistance and decreased medullary flow, which is a mediator of salt sensitivity. It produces increased sodium reabsorption in the proximal tubule by increasing the activity of NHE3, the sodium-bicarbonate exchanger, and Na+–K+–ATPase and by inducing aldosterone synthesis and release from the adrenal zona glomerulosa. In addition, it is associated with endothelial cell dysfunction and produces extensive profibrotic and proinflammatory changes, largely mediated by increased oxidative stress, resulting in renal, cardiac, and vascular injury, thus giving angiotensin II a tight link to target-organ injury in hypertension [22]. Conversely, stimulation of the angiotensin II type 2 receptor (AT2R) is associated with opposite effects, resulting in vasodilation, natriuresis, and antiproliferative effects. The relative importance of the renal and vascular effects of angiotensin II was evaluated in classical crosstransplantation studies using both wild-type mice and mice lacking the AT1R [23, 24]. By cross transplanting the kidneys of wild-type mice into AT1R knockout mice and vice versa, investigators were able to generate animals that were selective renal AT1R knockouts or selective systemic (nonrenal) AT1R knockouts (Fig. 14.2). In physiologic conditions, renal, systemic, and total knockout animals had lower BP than wild-type animals, indicating a role of both renal and extrarenal AT1R in BP regulation [24]. The systemic AT1R absence was associated with approximately 50% lower aldosterone levels, but the lower BP observed in this group was independent of this lower aldosterone production, as BP remained low despite aldosterone infusions to supraphysiologic levels following adrenalectomy in the systemic knockout animals. In addition, the BP reduction in kidney knockout animals occurred despite normal aldosterone excretion, again confirming the independence of renal angiotensin II effects from aldosterone. In the hypertensive environment, it is the presence of renal AT1R that mediates both hypertension and organ injury [24] When animals were infused with angiotensin II for 4 weeks, animals lacking renal AT1R did not develop sustained hypertension, whereas wild-type and systemic knockout mice had a significant increase in BP. Additionally, only animals with elevated BP developed cardiac hypertrophy and fibrosis. This indicates that cardiac injury is largely dependent on hypertension and not on the presence of AT1R in the heart, as the (hypertensive) systemic knockout animals developed significant cardiac abnormalities despite the absence of AT1R in the heart. [22] In summary, these experiments indicate that both systemic and renal actions of angiotensin II are relevant to physiologic BP regulation, but in hypertension, the detrimental effects of angiotensin II are mediated via its renal effects. Aldosterone, the adrenocortical hormone synthesized in the zona glomerulosa, plays a critical role in hypertension through its well-known effects on sodium reabsorption that are largely mediated by genomic effects through the mineralocorticoid receptor leading to increased expression of ENaC. An extensive body of literature has identified other genomic and nongenomic effects of aldo-

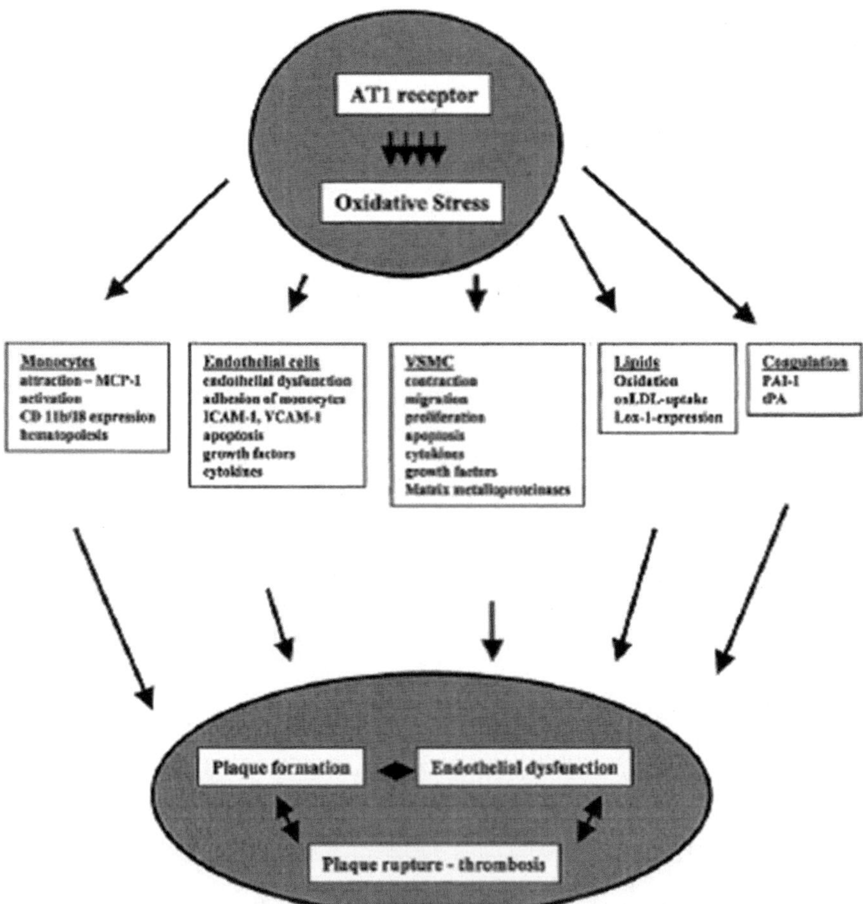

Fig. 14.2 AT_1 receptor-induced oxidative stress and atherosclerosis. AT_1 receptor activation leads to the release of reactive oxygen species in various vascular cells. Oxidative stress is in turn involved in monocyte attraction and activation. This involves increased production of monocyte chemoattractant protein-1 (*MCP-1*). In endothelial cells, adhesion molecules that are essential for the adhesion of monocytes, such as intercellular adhesion molecule-1 (*ICAM-1*) and the vascular adhesion molecule-1 (*VCAM-1*), are induced by angiotensin II via superoxide anions. In vascular smooth muscle cells (*VSMCs*), numerous biological processes are induced by reactive oxygen species. AT1 receptor activation increases expression of the oxLDL receptor LOX-1 resulting in an increased oxLDL uptake. Expression of plasminogen activator inhibitor-1 (*PAI-1*) is increased via AT1 receptor activation predisposing to a procoagulant state. The efects of angiotensin II on tissue plasminogen activator (*tPA*) are controversial

sterone with relevance to hypertension. Extensive nonepithelial effects include vascular smooth muscle cell proliferation, vascular extracellular matrix deposition, vascular remodeling and fibrosis, and increased oxidative stress leading to endothelial dysfunction and vasoconstriction [21, 23]. Several other elements of the RAAS have been identified as having potentially important roles in hypertension. The

Renovascular importance of ACE2 and angiotensin-(1–7) to BP regulation and angiotensin II–associated target-organ injury has become apparent. ACE2 is expressed largely in heart, kidney, and endothelium; it has partial homology to ACE and is unaffected directly by ACEIs [25]. It has a variety of substrates, but its most important action is the conversion of angiotensin II to angiotensin-(1–7). Angiotensin-(1–7) is formed primarily though the hydrolysis of angiotensin II by ACE2, and its actions are opposite to those of angiotensin II, including vasodilatory and anti- proliferative properties that are mediated by the Mas receptor, a G protein–coupled receptor that, upon activation, forms complexes with the AT1R, thus antagonizing the effects of angiotensin II. The vasodilatory effects are mediated by increased cyclic guanosine monophosphate, decreased norepinephrine release, and amplification of bradykinin effects. Studies have identified ACE2 and angiotensin-(1–7) as protective factors in the development of atherosclerosis and cardiac and renal injury [25, 26], and administration of recombinant ACE2 or its activator, xanthenone, has resulted in improved endothelial function, decreased BP, and improved renal, cardiac, and perivascular fibrosis in hypertensive animals [27–29].

Sympathetic Nervous System

The sympathetic nervous system (SNS) is activated consistently in patients with hypertension compared with normotensive individuals, particularly in the obese (Fig. 47.10). Many patients with hypertension are in a state of autonomic imbalance that encompasses increased sympathetic and decreased parasympathetic activity [30, 31]. SNS hyperactivity is relevant to both the generation and maintenance of hypertension and is observed in human hypertension from very early stages. Among patients with hypertension, increasing severity of hypertension is associated with increasing levels of sympathetic activity measured by microneurography [32, 33]. In human hypertension, plasma catecholamine levels, microneurographic recordings, and systemic catecholamine spillover studies have shown consistent elevation of these markers in obesity, the metabolic syndrome, and hypertension complicated by heart failure or kidney disease [31]. In addition, SNS hyperactivity is observed in most hypertensive subgroups, though it appears more pronounced in men than in women, and in younger than in older patients.

Several experimental models have outlined the importance of the SNS in generating hypertension. Different models of obesity-related hypertension indicate that the SNS is activated early in the development of increased adiposity [32], and the key factor in the maintenance of sustained hypertension is increased renal sympathetic nerve activity and its attendant sodium avidity [32]. Enhanced SNS activity results in α1-receptor–mediated endothelial dysfunction, vasoconstriction, vascular smooth muscle proliferation, and arterial stiffness, all of which contribute to the development of hypertension. Finally, evidence indicates that sympathetic overactivity results in salt sensitivity due to a reduction in the activity of WNK4. This results in increased sodium avidity through the thiazide-sensitive NCC [34].

Increased SNS activity is associated with vascular smooth muscle proliferation, LVH, large artery stiffness, myocardial ischemia, and arrhythmogenesis. There is also a mechanistic role for the SNS in the complications of hypertension. In support of this concept, there are several cohort studies reporting an association between physiologic or biochemical markers of SNS activation and adverse outcomes in heart failure, stroke, and end-stage kidney disease [31, 35]. However, there are no such studies among patients with hypertension, and the indirect evaluation of the impact of treatment-induced heart rate reduction in hypertension has yielded "paradoxical" results.

In a meta-analysis of hypertension trials, heart rate reduction during treatment with β-blockers was associated with increased risk for death and CV events in patients with hypertension [36]. In contrast, in a very large (n = 10,000) patient outcome trial, a post hoc analysis of heart rate at baseline demonstrated that those with a resting heart rate above 80 beats per minute even with a BP below 140/90 mmHg had a higher mortality rate [37]. Therefore, while apparent that SNS activation is deleterious to patients with CV disease, and presumably with hypertension, a cause for the over-activity should be sought and an attempt made to affect that mechanism.

Pathogenesis of Hypertensive Heart disease

Hypertension is a major risk factor not only for CAD but also for left ventricular hypertrophy (LVH) and heart failure. In hypertensive patients, LVH powerfully and independently predicts morbidity and mortality, predisposing them to heart failure, ventricular tachyarrhythmia, ischemic stroke, atrial fibrillation, and embolic stroke. Major advances have increased our understanding of the molecular signal transduction pathways underlying pressure overload cardiomyocyte hypertrophy [38]. Moreover, the structural abnormalities in the hypertensive heart extend beyond myocyte hypertrophy; they also include medial hypertrophy of the intra myocardial coronary arteries and collagen deposition, leading to cardiac fibrosis [39]. These changes result from pressure overload and the neurohormonal activation that contributes to hypertension. In animal models, A II, aldosterone, norepinephrine, and prorenin accelerate pressure overload cardiomyocyte hypertrophy and promote cardiac fibrosis, the hallmarks of pathologic LVH (in contrast with the physiologic hypertrophy of exercise training, which involves less fibrosis).

Impaired Coronary Vasodilator Reserve The hypertrophied hypertensive heart has normal resting coronary blood flow, but vasodilator reserve becomes impaired when myocyte mass outstrips the blood supply. Even in the absence of atherosclerosis, the hypertensive heart has blunted or absent coronary vasodilator reserve, leading to sub endocardial ischemia under conditions of increased myocardial oxygen demand. The combination of sub endocardial ischemia and cardiac fibrosis impairs diastolic relaxation, leading to exertional dyspnea and heart failure with preserved systolic function.

Before the advent of effective drug therapy for hypertension in the late 1950s, heart failure caused most deaths from hypertension. Better management has substantially reduced hypertension-related deaths from heart failure and significantly delayed its onset, but hypertension remains the most common cause of heart failure with preserved systolic function. In addition, hypertension indirectly leads to systolic heart failure as a major risk factor for MI. Whether mild or moderate hypertension without MI leads to systolic heart failure is unclear [39].

Treatment

Despite major progress in identifying the risks associated with elevated BP and demonstration that reducing BP to within a certain range reduces risk for death from CV disease and stroke as well as kidney disease progression, control rates are poor in the world. There are over 125 different medications encompassing eight different antihypertensive drug classes to help lower BP, as well as more than 20 single-pill combination agents for BP control. In spite of this, BP control remains suboptimal in many parts of the world [39–41]. BP control rates (to <140/90 mmHg) have improved substantially in the United States since 1974 (Fig. 47.6) and have stabilized at just over 50 % in the last three biennial NHANES reports [1]. Successful national efforts to increase hypertension treatment and control rates have been associated with significant reductions in CV hospitalizations or death in both Canada33 and the United Kingdom [42]. The prevalence of uncontrolled hypertension is greater for undiagnosed, untreated, or older individuals and for systolic (rather than diastolic) BP.

Meta-analyses of all commonly used antihypertensive drug classes demonstrate that, regardless of the agent used, reduction in BP corresponds to reduction in CV events if BP reduction is achieved [44, 45]. This reduction in CV risk, however, is predominantly seen in people with stage 2 hypertension with much less outcome data to support risk reduction in stage 1 hypertension. Events that drive the risk reduction are derived predominantly from reduced incidence of stroke, myocardial infarction, and heart failure. In all trials to date it is the group with the best overall BP control that has the best outcomes [46].

In large-scale randomized trials, it has been shown that reduction of BP by 5–6 mmHg diastolic or 10–12 mmHg systolic resulted in more than 50 % relative risk reduction in the incidence of heart failure, a 30–40 % relative risk reduction in stroke, and a 20–25 % relative risk reduction in myocardial infarction [46]

These relative risk reductions correspond to the following absolute benefits: antihypertensive therapy for 4–5 years prevents a coronary event in 0.7 % of patients and a cerebrovascular event in 1.3 % of patients for a total absolute benefit of approximately 2 % [47]. Thus, 100 patients must be treated for 4–5 years to prevent a complication in two patients. It is presumed that these statistics underestimate the true benefit of treating stage 1 hypertension since these data were derived from trials of relatively short duration (5–7 years); this may be insufficient to determine the efficacy of antihypertensive therapy on longer-term diseases such as atherosclerosis and heart failure. Equal if not greater relative risk reductions have been demonstrated with antihypertensive treatment of older hypertensive patients (over age 65 years), most of whom have isolated systolic hypertension. Because advanced age is associated with higher overall cardiovascular risk, even modest and relatively short-term reductions in blood pressure may provide absolute benefits that are greater than that observed in younger patients.

The benefits of antihypertensive therapy are less clear and more controversial in patients who have mild hypertension and no preexisting cardiovascular disease, and in elderly patients who are frail.

The benefit of blood pressure (BP) reduction in patients at increased risk of a cardiovascular event has been investigated in a number of major clinical trials of differing designs. Some of these trials compared one BP goal with a lower BP goal, while others compared an angiotensin converting enzyme (ACE) inhibitor or angiotensin receptor blocker (ARB) with placebo. Until recently evidence existed that reduction of systolic BP to around 140 mmHg systolic benefitted high risk patients bute the evidence was weak among elderly patients, diabetics and patients with CVD. Because of that, recent national guidelines accepted systolic BP up to 150 mmHg in patients >60 years of age.

However recent data from two large trials (SPRINT and ACCORD) may change guidelines [48, 49]. These two studies compared BP goals to test the hypothesis that lower attained systolic BPs (as low as less than 120 mmHg) improve patient outcomes in patients with cardiovascular disease or those at high risk. These trials provide support for the concept that the BP goal in patients with CVD or at high risk (this definition includes age >75 with no other cardiovascular risk factors) should be lower than that for the general population.

SPRINT randomly assigned 9361 patients aged 50 years or older with a systolic BP of 130–180 mmHg, and an increased risk of an adverse cardiovascular outcome (but without diabetes), to a systolic BP target of <120 mmHg (intensive treatment group) or <140 mmHg (standard treatment group). Increased cardiovascular risk was defined as: age greater than or equal to 75 years; clinically evident cardiovascular disease (i.e., previously documented coronary, peripheral arterial, or cerebrovascular disease [except for stroke]); subclinical cardiovascular disease (i.e., an elevated coronary artery calcification score by computerized tomography scan, left ventricular hypertrophy, or an ankle-brachial index <0.9); an estimated glomerular filtration rate of 20–59 mL/min/1.73 m^2; or a 10-year Framingham Risk Score greater than or equal to 15 %.

The primary composite outcome included myocardial infarction (MI), other acute coronary syndromes, stroke, heart failure, hospitalization, or death from cardiovascular causes. The mean BP at baseline was approximately 138/78 mmHg in patients treated with 2 antihypertensive agents.

The trial was stopped early for benefit after median follow-up of 3.26 years. The mean number of BP medications was 2.8 and 1.8 in the intensive and standard groups, respectively. At 1 year, the mean systolic BP was 121.4 and 136.2 mmHg in the intensive and standard treatment groups, respectively. There was a lower rate of the primary outcome in the intensive treatment group (1.65 versus 2.19 % per year; hazard ratio [HR] 0.75; 95 % CI 0.64–0.89). The primary outcome occurred in 562 patients. All-cause mortality was also significantly lower in the intensive treatment group (HR 0.73; 95 % CI 0.60–0.90). Rates of serious adverse events of hypotension, syncope, electrolyte abnormalities, and acute kidney injury were higher in the intensive treatment group presumably because of higher diuretic use. Patients with established cardiovascular disease accounted for approximately 20 % of enrollees and outcomes were similar in this subgroup relative to the entire population.

In The ACCORD BP trial 4733 patients were randomly assigned with type 2 diabetes who had cardiovascular disease or at least two additional risk factors for cardiovascular disease to systolic BP targets of either less than 120 mmHg or less than 140 mmHg. Patients were followed for mean of 4.7 years. The mean attained systolic pressures were 119 and 134 mmHg, respectively, compared to 139/76 mmHg at baseline. There was no significant difference in the annual rate of the primary composite outcome of nonfatal MI, nonfatal stroke, or death from cardiovascular causes between the intensive versus standard therapy groups (1.87 versus 2.09 %, hazard ratio [HR] 0.88, 95 % CI 0.73–1.06). There was no difference in the annual all-cause mortality rate between intensive and standard therapy groups (1.28 versus 1.19 %) or in the rate of death from cardiovascular causes between groups (0.52 versus 0.49 %). Intensive therapy was associated with significant reductions in the annual rates of total stroke and nonfatal stroke (0.32 versus 0.53 %, HR 0.59, 95 % CI 0.39–0.89 for total stroke and 0.3 versus 0.47 %, HR 0.63, 95 % CI 0.41–0.96 for nonfatal stroke). Serious adverse events attributable to antihypertensive drugs (eg, hypotension, syncope, bradycardia or arrhythmia, hyperkalemia, angioedema, and renal failure) occurred significantly more frequently in the intensive versus standard therapy group (3.3 versus 1.3 %). Intensive therapy was also associated with a significantly higher rate of an increase in serum creatinine of more than 1.5 mg/dL (133 micromol/L in men or more than 1.3 mg/dL [115 micromol/L] in women).

Placebo-controlled trials such as HOPE, EUROPA, PEACE, CAMELOT, TRANSCEND, and NAVIGATOR [50–55] evaluated the hypothesis that ACE inhibitors or ARBs might have a direct and clinically-significant cardiovascular benefit in patients with a mean baseline BP between (approximately) 130/75 and 140/90 mmHg. In addition, CAMELOT and ACTION compared long-acting dihydropyridine calcium channel blockers to placebo. However, these trials were not designed to determine the optimal BP. Any benefit seen might be due to another mechanism than BP lowering. In the aggregate, these trials suggest a benefit from the agents used in patients with a baseline BP between (approximately) 130/75 and 140/90 mmHg. As the decrease in BP was modest in these studies (average of 3–5 mmHg systolic), they do not provide evidence that BP lowering below 130 mmHg is of benefit. In addition, as the mean age in these trials was about 60 years, they do not provide evidence on how to manage older patients (>70 years) with diastolic BP levels below 65 or 70 mmHg.

A 2009 meta-analysis focused on seven trials that limited therapy to either an ACE inhibitor or an ARB to placebo in patients with ischemic heart disease and preserved left ventricular systolic function [56]. Six trials of ACE inhibitor therapy (including HOPE, EUROPA, CAMELOT, and PEACE) significantly reduced both total mortality (RR 0.87, 95 % CI 0.81–0.94) and nonfatal MI (RR 0.83, 95 % CI 0.73–0.94). A limitation to this meta-analysis is that it does not distinguish between angiotensin inhibition and lower attained BPs as the mechanism of benefit.

This limitation was overcome in a 2011 meta-analysis that included 25 placebo-controlled trials with more than 63,000 patients in which active treatment consisted of all major classes of antihypertensive drugs, including ACE inhibitors, ARBs, beta blockers, calcium channel blockers, diuretics, or combination therapy [57]. Drug therapy significantly lowered the risks of all-cause mortality and MI to the same degree as in the earlier meta-analysis (pooled relative risks 0.87, 95 % CI 0.80–0.95 and 0.80, 95 % CI 0.69–0.93, respectively), suggesting that there was no specific benefit from therapy with angiotensin inhibitors compared with other antihypertensive drugs. The absolute risk reductions in all-cause mortality and MI were 14 and 13 per 1000 persons treated.

Threshold for Low Blood Pressure

There is a blood pressure (BP) threshold for all patients below which tissue perfusion is reduced to vital organs. As long as the BP is lowered gradually, this threshold does not appear to occur at current BP goals [49].

For patients with coronary heart disease without heart failure, it is possible that a lower limit exists for desirable diastolic pressure because much of coronary filling occurs during diastole. Observations from the Framingham study and a post-hoc analysis from the INVEST trial suggested an increase in risk for patients with cardiovascular disease at a diastolic pressure below 70 to 75 mmHg [58, 59]. However in the ACCORD study diastolic BP was reduced to 62 mmHg in high risk diabetics with no evidence of J shape curve.

Other analyses from placebo-controlled trials of hypertension found a similar J-shaped curve for diastolic and systolic pressures in both treated and untreated groups and for both cardiovascular and non-cardiovascular mortality [60, 61]. These findings indicate that the worse outcomes at lower pressures are independent of antihypertensive therapy as long as the BP is lowered slowly. Although there must be a level of diastolic BP and perhaps systolic, that organ hypo perfusion occurs and CV mortality and cardiovascular events increase, but evidence suggest that it must be well below current targets.

In summary, presented evidence strongly suggest that hypertension is a major contributor to endothelial dysfunction, atherosclerosis and cardiovascular events. Treatment and gradual control of hypertension to levels below 120 mmHg systolic and below 65 mmHg diastolic continues to reduce cardiovascular events and improve survival. Implementation of wide scale programs to treat and control hypertension to these low levels it will improve longevity and reduce CV outcomes around the world

References

1. Mozaffarian D, Benjamin EJ, Go AS, et al. Executive summary: heart disease and stroke statistics—2015 update: a report from the American Heart Association. Circulation. 2015;131:434–41.
2. Lim SS, Vos T, Flaxman AD, et al. A comparative risk assessment of burden of disease and injury attributable to 67 risk factors and risk factor clusters in 21 regions, 1990–2010: a systematic analysis for the Global Burden of Disease Study 2010. Lancet. 2012;380:2224–60.
3. Kearney PM, Whelton M, Reynolds K, et al. Global burden of hypertension: analysis of worldwide data. Lancet. 2005;365:217–23.
4. Franklin SS, Jacobs MJ, Wong ND, et al. Predominance of isolated systolic hypertension among middle-aged and elderly US hypertensives: analysis based on National Health and Nutrition Examination Survey (NHANES) III. Hypertension. 2001;37:869–74.
5. Joffres M, Falaschetti E, Gillespie C, et al. Hypertension prevalence, awareness, treatment and control in national surveys from England, the USA and Canada, and correlation with stroke and ischaemic heart disease mortality: a cross-sectional study. BMJ Open. 2013;3:e003423.
6. Lewington S, Clarke R, Qizilbash N, et al. Age-specific relevance of usual blood pressure to vascular mortality: a meta-analysis of individual data for one million adults in 61 prospective studies. Lancet. 2002;360:1903–13.
7. Parati G, Ochoa JE, Bilo G, Agarwal R, Covic A, Dekker FW, Fliser D, Heine GH, Jager KJ, Gargani L, Kanbay M, Mallamaci F, Massy Z, Ortiz A, Picano E, Rossignol P, Sarafidis P, Sicari R, Vanholder R, Wiecek A, London G. Hypertension in chronic kidney disease part 1: out-of-office blood pressure monitoring: methods, thresholds, and patterns. Hypertension. 2016;67(6):1093–101. doi:10.1161/HYPERTENSIONAHA.115.06895.
8. Quinn U, Tomlinson LA, Cockcroft JR. Arterial stiffness. JRSM Cardiovasc Dis. 2012;1:cvd.2012.012024.
9. Zieman SJ, Melenovsky V, Kass DA. Mechanisms, pathophysiology, and therapy of arterial stiffness. Arterioscler Thromb Vasc Biol. 2005;25:932–43.
10. Ben-Shlomo Y, Spears M, Boustred C, et al. Aortic pulse wave velocity improves cardiovascular event prediction: an individual participant meta-analysis of prospective observational data from 17,635 subjects. J Am Coll Cardiol. 2014;63:636–46.
11. Duprez DA. Role of the renin-angiotensin-aldosterone system in vascular remodeling and inflammation: A clinical review. J Hypertens. 2006;24:983.
12. Spieker LE, Flammer AJ, Luscher TF. The vascular endothelium in hypertension. Handb Exp Pharmacol. 2006;249–283.
13. Dharmashankar K, Widlansky ME. Vascular endothelial function and hypertension: insights and directions. Curr Hypertens Rep. 2010;12:448–55.
14. Taddei S, Virdis A, Mattei P, et al. Endothelium-dependent forearm vasodilation is reduced in normotensive subjects with familial history of hypertension. J Cardiovasc Pharmacol. 1992;20 Suppl 12:S193–5.
15. Popolo A, Autore G, Pinto A, et al. Oxidative stress in patients with cardiovascular disease and chronic renal failure. Free Radic Res. 2013;47:346–56.
16. Quyyumi AA, Patel RS. Endothelial dysfunction and hypertension: cause or effect? Hypertension. 2010;55:1092–4.
17. Shimbo D, Muntner P, Mann D, et al. Endothelial dysfunction and the risk of hypertension: the multi-ethnic study of atherosclerosis. Hypertension. 2010;55:1210–6.
18. Rosendahl A, Niemann G, Lange S, et al. Increased expression of (pro)renin receptor does not cause hypertension or cardiac and renal fibrosis in mice. Lab Invest. 2014;94:863–72.
19. Peixoto AJ, Orias M. Is there a role for direct renin inhibitors in chronic kidney disease? Curr Opin Nephrol Hypertens. 2009;18:397–403.
20. Acelajado MC. Pathogenesis of hypertension. In: Black HR, Elliott W, editors. Hypertension: a companion to Braunwald's heart disease. Philadelphia: Elsevier; 2013.

21. Crowley SD, Gurley SB, Herrera MJ, et al. Angiotensin II causes hypertension and cardiac hypertrophy through its receptors in the kidney. Proc Natl Acad Sci U S A. 2006;103: 17985–90.
22. xxx
23. Crowley SD, Gurley SB, Oliverio MI, et al. Distinct roles for the kidney and systemic tissues in blood pressure regulation by the renin-angiotensin system. J Clin Invest. 2005;115:1092–9.
24. McCurley A, Jaffe IZ. Mineralocorticoid receptors in vascular function and disease. Mol Cell Endocrinol. 2012;350:256–65.
25. Tikellis C, Bernardi S, Burns WC. Angiotensin-converting enzyme 2 is a key modulator of the renin-angiotensin system in cardiovascular and renal disease. Curr Opin Nephrol Hypertens. 2011;20:62–8.
26. Ferrario CM. ACE2: more of Ang-(1–7) or less Ang II? Curr Opin Nephrol Hypertens. 2011;20:1–6.
27. Fraga-Silva RA, Costa-Fraga FP, Murca TM, et al. Angiotensinconverting enzyme 2 activation improves endothelial function. Hypertension. 2013;61:1233–8.
28. Hernandez Prada JA, Ferreira AJ, Katovich MJ, et al. Structurebased identification of small-molecule angiotensin-converting enzyme 2 activators as novel antihypertensive agents. Hypertension. 2008;51:1312–7.
29. Wysocki J, Ye M, Rodriguez E, et al. Targeting the degradation of angiotensin II with recombinant angiotensin-converting enzyme 2: prevention of angiotensin II-dependent hypertension. Hypertension. 2010;55:90–8.
30. Mancia G, Grassi G. The autonomic nervous system and hypertension. Circ Res. 2014;114:1804–14.
31. DiBona GF. Sympathetic nervous system and hypertension. Hypertension. 2013;61:556–60.
32. Grassi G, Cattaneo BM, Seravalle G, et al. Baroreflex control of sympathetic nerve activity in essential and secondary hypertension. Hypertension. 1998;31:68–72.
33. Smith PA, Graham LN, Mackintosh AF, et al. Relationship between central sympathetic activity and stages of human hypertension. Am J Hypertens. 2004;17:217–22.
34. Mu S, Shimosawa T, Ogura S, et al. Epigenetic modulation of the renal beta-adrenergic-WNK4 pathway in salt-sensitive hypertension. Nat Med. 2011;17:573–80.
35. Zoccali C, Mallamaci F, Parlongo S, et al. Plasma norepinephrine predicts survival and incident cardiovascular events in patients with end-stage renal disease. Circulation. 2002;105: 1354–9.
36. Bangalore S, Sawhney S, Messerli FH. Relation of beta-blockerinduced heart rate lowering and cardioprotection in hypertension. J Am Coll Cardiol. 2008;52:1482–9.
37. Julius S, Palatini P, Kjeldsen SE, et al. Usefulness of heart rate to predict cardiac events in treated patients with high-risk systemic hypertension. Am J Cardiol. 2012;109:685–92.
38. Hill JA, Olson EN. Cardiac plasticity. N Engl J Med. 2008;358:1370.
39. Gradman AH, Alfayoumi F. From left ventricular hypertrophy to congestive heart failure: management of hypertensive heart disease. Prog Cardiovasc Dis. 2006;48:326.
40. Chobanian AV, Bakris GL, Black HR, et al. Seventh report of the joint national committee on prevention, detection, evaluation, and treatment of high blood pressure. Hypertension. 2003;42:1206–52.
41. Nwankwo T, Yoon SS, Burt V, et al. Hypertension among adults in the United States: national health and nutrition examination survey, 2011–2012. NCHS Data Brief. 2013;133:1–8.
42. Chow CK, Teo KK, Rangarajan S, et al. Prevalence, awareness, treatment, and control of hypertension in rural and urban communities in high-, middle-, and low-income countries. JAMA. 2013;310:959–68.
43. Falaschetti E, Mindell J, Knott C, et al. Hypertension management in England: a serial cross-sectional study from 1994 to 2011. Lancet. 2014;383:1912–9.
44. Sundstrom J, Arima H, Woodward M, et al. Blood pressure– lowering treatment based on cardiovascular risk: a meta-analysis of individual patient data. Lancet. 2014;384:591–8.

45. Emdin CA, Rahimi K, Neal B, et al. Blood pressure lowering in type 2 diabetes: a systematic review and meta-analysis. JAMA. 2015;313:603–15.
46. Turnbull F, Neal B, Ninomiya T, et al. Effects of different regimens to lower blood pressure on major cardiovascular events in older and younger adults: meta-analysis of randomised trials. BMJ. 2008;336:1121–3.
47. Hebert PR, Moser M, Mayer J, et al. Recent evidence on drug therapy of mild to moderate hypertension and decreased risk of coronary heart disease. Arch Intern Med. 1993;153:578.
48. Wright Jr JT, Williamson JD, et al. A randomized trial of intensive versus standard blood-pressure control. N Engl J Med. 2015;373:2103.
49. Cushman WC, Evans GW, et al. Effects of intensive blood-pressure control in type 2 diabetes mellitus. N Engl J Med. 2010;362:1575.
50. Yusuf S, Sleight P, Pogue J, et al. Effects of an angiotensin-converting-enzyme inhibitor, ramipril, on cardiovascular events in high-risk patients. The Heart Outcomes Prevention Evaluation Study Investigators. N Engl J Med. 2000;342:145.
51. Fox KM, EURopean trial On reduction of cardiac events with Perindopril in stable coronary Artery disease Investigators. Efficacy of perindopril in reduction of cardiovascular events among patients with stable coronary artery disease: randomised, double-blind, placebo-controlled, multicentre trial (the EUROPA study). Lancet. 2003;362:782.
52. Nissen SE, Tuzcu EM, Libby P, et al. Effect of antihypertensive agents on cardiovascular events in patients with coronary disease and normal blood pressure: the CAMELOT study: a randomized controlled trial. JAMA. 2004;292:2217.
53. Braunwald E, Domanski MJ, Fowler SE, et al. Angiotensin-converting-enzyme inhibition in stable coronary artery disease. N Engl J Med. 2004;351:2058.
54. Telmisartan Randomised AssessmeNt Study in ACE iNtolerant subjects with cardiovascular Disease (TRANSCEND) Investigators, Yusuf S, Teo K, et al. Effects of the angiotensin-receptor blocker telmisartan on cardiovascular events in high-risk patients intolerant to angiotensin-converting enzyme inhibitors: a randomised controlled trial. Lancet. 2008; 372:1174.
55. NAVIGATOR Study Group, McMurray JJ, Holman RR, et al. Effect of valsartan on the incidence of diabetes and cardiovascular events. N Engl J Med. 2010;362:1477.
56. Baker WL, Coleman CI, Kluger J, et al. Systematic review: comparative effectiveness of angiotensin-converting enzyme inhibitors or angiotensin II-receptor blockers for ischemic heart disease. Ann Intern Med. 2009;151:861.
57. Thompson AM, Hu T, Eshelbrenner CL, et al. Antihypertensive treatment and secondary prevention of cardiovascular disease events among persons without hypertension: a meta-analysis. JAMA. 2011;305:913.
58. D'Agostino RB, Belanger AJ, Kannel WB, Cruickshank JM. Relation of low diastolic blood pressure to coronary heart disease death in presence of myocardial infarction: the Framingham Study. BMJ. 1991;303:385.
59. Messerli FH, Mancia G, Conti CR, et al. Dogma disputed: can aggressively lowering blood pressure in hypertensive patients with coronary artery disease be dangerous? Ann Intern Med. 2006;144:884.
60. Boutitie F, Gueyffier F, Pocock S, et al. J-shaped relationship between blood pressure and mortality in hypertensive patients: new insights from a meta-analysis of individual-patient data. Ann Intern Med. 2002;136:438.
61. Bangalore S, Messerli FH, Wun CC, et al. J-curve revisited: An analysis of blood pressure and cardiovascular events in the Treating to New Targets (TNT) Trial. Eur Heart J. 2010;31:2897.

Chapter 15
Selecting Optimum Antihypertensive Therapy

Vasilios Papademetriou and Michael Doumas

Introduction

The selection of optimum antihypertensive therapy for a particular patient represents a challenge, which the treating physician managing patients with arterial hypertension confronts every day. The choice involves not only the initial selection of antihypertensive drugs, but also the right dual, triple, or multiple combination therapy for the particular patient, since antihypertensive drugs as monotherapy are efficacious in the minority of cases (30–40 %) and blood pressure response is unpredictable. Therefore, the choice affects all hypertensive patients and is neither simple nor careless.

Undoubtedly, essential hypertension is not due to one cause and certainly there is no therapy that fits all. Arterial hypertension is a multi-factorial disease with several mechanisms implicated in blood pressure elevation. Each class of antihypertensive drugs targets one or more mechanisms but leaves unaffected or even has an adverse impact on the other mechanisms. Therefore, the selection of optimum therapy requires the identification of the specific mechanism(s) contributing to blood pressure elevation in each individual.

The aim of this chapter is to present the therapeutic strategies for the management of arterial hypertension (stepped-care, sequential monotherapy, individualized,

V. Papademetriou, M.D. (✉)
Department of Medicine (Cardiology), Veteran Affairs Medical Center and
Georgetown University, 50 Irving Street, NW, Washington, DC 20422, USA
e-mail: vpapademetriou@va.gov

M. Doumas, M.D., Ph.D.
Department of Medicine, Veteran Affairs Medical Center and George Washington University,
Washington, DC, USA

2nd Propedeutic Department of Internal Medicine, Aristotle University,
126, Vas. Olgas Street, Thessaloniki 54645, Greece

E.A. Andreadis (ed.), *Hypertension and Cardiovascular Disease*,
DOI 10.1007/978-3-319-39599-9_15

renin-based, hemodynamic), and critically discuss each approach highlighting its advantages and disadvantages. Moreover, several practical recommendations are provided on the build-up of optimum antihypertensive therapy in individual patients.

Therapeutic Strategies for the Management of Arterial Hypertension

The main therapeutic strategies for the management of arterial hypertension are depicted in Table 15.1. There are three main therapeutic approaches: (a) the stepped-care approach, (b) the sequential monotherapy approach, and (c) the individualized, patient-centered approach.

Last but not least, special emphasis needs to be placed in two particular approaches: (a) the renin approach, and (b) the hemodynamic approach. Although both approaches could be considered as part of the individualized approach, they merit discussion separately, since each one represents a complete particular concept with its own advantages and disadvantages, strengths and weaknesses.

The Stepped-Care Approach

The traditional stepped-care approach dominated the hypertension field at the beginning of antihypertensive drug therapy. According to this approach, when the first antihypertensive drug (titrated to maximum dose) fails to achieve blood pressure control, then a second drug is added and titrated to maximum dose, and so on, until successful blood pressure control occurs.

The efficacy of the stepped care approach in blood pressure reduction and the subsequent benefits in cardiovascular morbidity and mortality have been demonstrated very early in the antihypertensive era, with the first large clinical studies, such as the VA trials, the USPHS trial, the Australian trial, and the Oslo trial [1–5]. Moreover, the superiority of the stepped care approach over usual care has been confirmed in the HDFP trial [6].

The stepped care approach was designed as a simple algorithm that was found very effective, resulting in significant blood pressure reduction (mean 10/5 mmHg; maximum 20/10 mmHg, in patients with mild to moderate hypertension) [7]. The

Table 15.1 Therapeutic strategies for the management of arterial hypertension

Therapeutic strategies
Stepped-care approach
Sequential monotherapy
Individualized approach
Renin-based approach
Hemodynamic approach

stepped care approach was embraced by the Joint National Committee which issued the US guidelines for the management of arterial hypertension in 1977, 1980, 1984, and 1988 [8–10].

As every approach, the stepped care approach has its own advantages and disadvantages. It is easy to understand and thus can be widely implemented, it highlights the selection of drugs from different classes to attain synergistic actions, and it includes a gradual dose titration to identify the maximum tolerated dose of a drug. On the other hand, the stepped care approach ignores the different pathogenetic mechanisms contributing in blood pressure elevation in different patients, the hemodynamic and hormonal variability in hypertension, i.e., the heterogeneity in hypertension pathogenesis. Moreover, the stepped care approach does not take into account several factors, such as target organ damage, cardiovascular disease, cardiovascular risk factors, other comorbidities, concomitant medication, drug adverse effects, and adverse metabolic actions of antihypertensive drugs.

The stepped care approach was not the result of rigorous and extensive scientific clinical testing, but rather an expert opinion aiming to provide a standard management plan, appropriate for implementation in large populations in everyday clinical practice. Nevertheless it was simple enough, easy to follow and help in the wide spread of blood pressure treatment and control in the US and around the world.

Sequential Monotherapy

As the years passed by, however, it was realized that: (a) the various antihypertensive drug classes result in blood pressure control (<140/90 mmHg) in a limited percentage of hypertensive patients (30–40 %), and (b) not all patients respond the same way to each antihypertensive drug category, i.e., an individual patient may respond to one class of drugs, be totally unresponsive to another class, and experience a partial response to a third class. Therefore, the concept of sequential monotherapy has emerged, a classic interpretation of the 'trial and error' method. According to this approach, antihypertensive drug classes are consecutively tested in all hypertensive patients in order to discover effective drugs and uncover ineffective drugs for the individual patient. The rationale beneath this concept is solid and attractive, since antihypertensive therapy is life-long and it is therefore of utmost importance and clinically meaningful to detect the efficacy of each drug class for the individual patient. Like every concept however, sequential monotherapy has its own disadvantages. The main disadvantage is that the time required to test the efficacy of each class is long and at times unacceptable. In particular, drugs have to be administered for several weeks, at least 4–6 weeks and even longer for diuretics, to evaluate appropriately the full effect of each drug category. In addition a wash-out period of 3–4 weeks has to follow each drug-testing period to avoid the carry-over effect. Thus, it was soon realized that a very long period of 1–1.5 years is required to test the efficacy of the four main antihypertensive drug classes (diuretics, beta blockers, calcium antagonists, ACE-inhibitors), and an even longer period required if dose escalation or second line drugs (alpha blockers, centrally acting, direct vasodilators, mineralocorticoid receptor antagonists) are being tested as well.

The time consuming sequential monotherapy approach carries significant consequences. First, the patients get tired, may consider themselves 'testing objects', and thus exhibit poor adherence rates and high discontinuation rates. Then, the cost of medical visits (direct and indirect) both for the patient and the insurance system is high, and there is no guarantee (reassurance) that the response pattern to each drug will be maintained the same over the time. Moreover, this approach raises safety flags for several patient populations, especially high-risk patients with either established cardiovascular disease or a cluster of cardiovascular risk factors. In addition, available data suggests that the earlier the blood pressure control the better. For example, in the VALUE trial, it was found that cardiovascular event rates were lower in patients achieving early blood pressure control (during the first 6 months of the study) compared to patients with initially uncontrolled blood pressure, irrespective of the administered antihypertensive drug [11]. It is obvious that sequential monotherapy does not offer rapid, prompt and early blood pressure control. Finally, the efficacy of sequential monotherapy is questionable in more advanced stages of hypertension, since it is highly unlikely that blood pressure will be controlled with monotherapy in patients with severe hypertension, and rather unlikely in patients with moderate hypertension.

The Personalized Approach

It is therefore of no surprise that recent therapeutic strategies have moved towards individualized therapy for the reduction of elevated blood pressure in hypertensive patients. Indeed, individualized therapy represents the key element of the last European guidelines for the management of arterial hypertension [12–15]. According to this approach, the selection of an antihypertensive drug for each individual is based on: (a) several individual's baseline demographic characteristics (age, gender, race, and body mass index) and the heart rate, (b) the presence and the type of target organ damage, (c) the presence and the type of established cardiovascular disease, and (d) the presence and the type of other comorbidities.

In addition, the selection of optimum antihypertensive therapy is influenced by the specific characteristics of each antihypertensive drug and concomitant medications (pharmacokinetics, pharmacodynamics, adverse events, metabolic effects). Finally, the selection of optimum therapy has to take into account several other very significant factors, such as individual's prior experience with antihypertensive drugs (efficacy and safety), the quality of life with special emphasis on sexual function, adherence to antihypertensive therapy and discontinuation rates, the blood pressure pattern (isolated systolic hypertension, non-dippers), lifestyle factors (salt intake, exercise), and the cost (direct and indirect), especially in these times of financial constraints worldwide and recession in many parts of the world.

Another very important aspect is to evaluate whether the profile of the selected drug match the needs and the preferences of the specific individual. For example, a diuretic might not be the best choice for a young and highly active executive in a multi-national company; a beta blocker might not be the best choice for someone who is involved in intense physical activities [16].

Of major importance, the individualization of antihypertensive therapy has to fulfill several requirements: (a) to be effective, (b) to be safe and well tolerated, (c) to reduce the risk for cardiovascular morbidity and mortality, (d) to improve or at least attenuate target organ damage, and (e) to exert beneficial or at least neutral effects on traditional cardiovascular risk factors and/or other comorbidities.

A detailed analysis of the factors influencing the choice of antihypertensive therapy according to the individualized approach will be presented later in this chapter, after the presentation of the renin-based and the hemodynamic approach.

The Renin-Based Approach

Renin was identified at the very end of the nineteenth century by Tigerstedt, a Scandinavian physiologist, who extracted from rabbit kidneys a substance with pressor properties [17]. Its role however in blood pressure control was not established until more than three decades later, when Goldblatt performed his landmark experiments in one-clip and two-clip hypertension, and proposed the theory that renal ischemia (through clamping of renal artery) results in the production of a strong pressor molecule from the kidneys (renin), which is capable of producing blood pressure elevation [18]. It took almost two more decades to describe the renin-angiotensin system (RAS) [19] and realize the role of this system as a servo-control with crucial role in blood pressure, water, sodium, and potassium regulation [20–24]. In parallel, Jerome Conn has identified primary hyperaldosteronism and described its main characteristics [25, 26], long before aldosterone and renin could be actually measured, since the first clinical assays appeared in 1964 (10 years after Conn's first description).

The role the RAS was thus established in secondary hypertension (renovascular hypertension, primary hyperaldosteronism); however, its role in essential hypertension remained controversial. It is the life-time, persistent work of the late John Laragh, which highlighted the importance of renin in essential hypertension, and even proposed the renin-based management of hypertensive patients (Table 15.2). The renin approach is based in two simple assumptions: (a) hypertensive patients can be divided according to renin status in high and low renin groups, and (b) antihypertensive drugs are mainly effective in ore or the other category.

Plasma renin activity (PRA) is broadly distributed in hypertensive patients. About one third of hypertensive patients have low PRA levels, suggesting a functional renal response to elevated blood pressure and sodium overload. The remaining two thirds of hypertensive patients have inappropriately elevated renin for the blood pressure and sodium status, indicating a relative over-activation of the RAS

Table 15.2 The renin-based approach

Low renin levels	High & normal renin levels
PRA < 0.65 ngAI/ml/h	PRA > 0.65 ngAI/ml/h
Volume overload	RAS overactivation
More effective drugs	More effective drugs
Thiazides	ACE-inhibitors
Calcium antagonists	Angiotensin receptor blockers
Spironolactone	Beta blockers

both in patients with high PRA values (about 15 % of patients) or normal PRA values (about 50 % of patients) [27–29]. To sum up, one out of three hypertensive patients have low renin hypertension which is salt-mediated, while the other two out of three patients have inappropriately high renin levels (either normal or high in absolute values), and blood pressure elevation is due to RAS over-activation.

The second assumption regards the efficacy of antihypertensive drugs in these two patient subgroups. Hypertensive patients with high and normal PRA values tend to respond to drugs affecting the RAS, such as beta blockers and centrally acting drugs (directly affecting renin secretion), ACE-inhibitors, angiotensin receptor blockers, and direct renin inhibitors. In contrast, hypertensive patients with low PRA levels tend to respond to natriuretic drugs and subsequent volume depletion (diuretics, alpha blockers, calcium antagonists).

The efficacy of the renin approach has been tested and verified mainly by the Laragh group in New York. The selective efficacy of antihypertensive drugs according to baseline renin levels, with beta blockers being preferentially effective in normal and high renin patients, and diuretics being preferentially effective in low renin patients, have been shown in numerous studies during the 1970s [30–42]. An even more important set of data comes from two studies suggesting that diuretics in fact raise blood pressure in patients with elevated renin levels, and vice versa, beta blockers may raise blood pressure in patients with low renin levels [43, 44].

Another significant characteristic of the renin approach is that it can be applied not only to naïve (previously untreated) patients, but also to patients with uncontrolled blood pressure while on therapy with antihypertensive drugs. In the original small clinical study of 73 patients with uncontrolled blood pressure despite administration of at least one antihypertensive drug, it was found that a renin-based therapeutic strategy resulted in a significant blood pressure reduction, an additional reduction in the number of antihypertensive medications used by study participants, and even cost benefits [45].

More recently, the renin-based approach was compared with clinical hypertension specialist care in another small clinical study of 84 patients with treatment resistant hypertension [46]. It was found that blood pressure reduction was similar with both approaches, while the renin-based approach was superior to specialist care regarding the removal of antihypertensive drugs and dose reductions of some antihypertensive agents, in addition to a non-significant trend towards better blood pressure control. Therefore, the renin-based therapeutic strategy seems to be as effective as specialist care, and therefore represents an attractive alternative for primary care practice.

This year, the PATHWAY-2 trial provided also some evidence supporting the renin-based strategy. In this placebo-controlled, randomized, cross-over study, spironolactone was compared to alpha- and beta-blockers in a large number of patients with resistant hypertension [47]. It was found that the blood pressure response was strongly affected by baseline renin levels, with spironolactone being very effective and superior to comparator drugs in patients with low and normal renin levels, while beta blockers were more effective in patients with high renin levels, achieving the efficacy of spironolactone.

The renin approach has not been widely applied in the management of arterial hypertension for several reasons [48, 49]. PRA determination requires a well-equipped and specialized laboratory, is time consuming and not practical in everyday clinical practice. Moreover, the results may be inaccurate, present interpretation difficulties, and most importantly have reproducibility problems. [50–52] Indeed, one out of four patients classified in one renin group (high, normal, or low) is actually re-classified in another group on repeat testing [48]. In addition, PRA values have to be adjusted for age, gender, race, and several other parameters, in order to ensure the accuracy of each laboratory [48, 50, 51]. Moreover, PRA presents great variations according to sodium intake, potassium levels, posture and its duration, and timing of the sampling during the day. Of equal importance, renin concentrations are highly affected by antihypertensive drugs, which either reduce significantly renin levels (beta blockers, centrally acting drugs) or result in significant elevation of renin levels (diuretics). Of note, other drugs might also affect renin determination, such as non-steroidal anti-inflammatory drugs and fludrocortisone, while the effects of commonly used psychotropic drugs (such as anxiolytics and antidepressants) on renin levels have not been adequately clarified, despite the fact that such drugs may inhibit sympathetic activity and subsequently renin levels. Another very significant and clinically meaningful limitation of the renin approach regards the poor correlation (about 50 %) between renin categorization and subsequent blood pressure response to indicated drugs [51, 53].

The Hemodynamic Approach

Blood pressure equals the product of cardiac output (CO) and systemic vascular resistance (SVR). Aging is accompanied by significant hemodynamic changes in hypertensive patients. At the early stages of hypertension in young patients, the CO is increased due to sympathetic overactivity and the subsequent tachycardia (CO is the product of heart rate and stroke volume), while SVR is inappropriately high (relatively increased) [54–57]. Later on, when hypertension is established, the CO is usually slightly reduced by 10–15 %, whereas SVR is slightly increased by 15–20 % [54, 58, 59]. At the late stages of hypertension in the elderly, the CO is further decreased up to 25 %, while SVR is further increased up to 25–30 % [54, 58, 59]. Therefore, SVR is elevated in hypertensive patients and this represents the primary hemodynamic abnormality.

From the hemodynamic point of view, it seems rational to reduce blood pressure through the reduction of SVR, while maintaining the CO unaffected, in order to ensure adequate renal blood flow and the perfusion of vital organs. Ideally, these alterations should not be accompanied by compensatory changes, such as water and salt retention, reflex tachycardia, and vasoconstriction.

The hemodynamic effects of antihypertensive drugs (Table 15.3) can be divided in five groups according to their effects in SVR, CO, organ perfusion and arterial compliance [60–72]. RAS inhibitors (ACE-inhibitors, ARBs, and direct renin inhibitors), calcium antagonists, and vasodilatory beta blockers reduce SVR, while preserving CO and improving organ perfusion and arterial compliance. Alpha blockers and centrally acting agents reduce SVR and preserve CO and perfusion, while their effects on arterial compliance are not yet adequately clarified. Direct vasodilators and beta blockers with intrinsic sympathomimetic activity reduce SVR, preserve CO and organ perfusion, while worsening arterial compliance. Diuretics and ganglionic blocking agents reduce SVR, CO, and organ perfusion, whereas arterial compliance is worsened. Finally, traditional beta blockers (without intrinsic sympathomimetic activity or vasodilatory properties) increase SVR and reduce CO, organ perfusion, and worsen arterial compliance.

Table 15.3 Hemodynamic effects of antihypertensive drugs

Group A
SVR reduction, CO unaffected, organ perfusion & arterial compliance improved
RAS inhibitors (ACE-inhibitors, angiotensin receptor blockers)
Calcium antagonists
Vasodilatory beta blockers
Group B
SVR reduction, CO & organ perfusion unaffected, arterial compliance unclarified
Alpha blockers
Centrally acting agents
Group C
SVR reduction, CO & organ perfusion unaffected, arterial compliance worsened
Vasodilators (Hydralazine, minoxidil)
Beta blockers with intrinsic sympathomimetic activity
Group D
SVR & CO & organ perfusion reduction, arterial compliance worsened
Diuretics
Ganglionic blocking agents
Group E
SVR increased, CO & organ perfusion reduction, arterial compliance worsened
Traditional beta blockers

Some points regarding the hemodynamic effects of antihypertensive drugs need to be highlighted. First, the most favorable hemodynamic profile is expressed by RAS inhibitors and calcium antagonists. In contrast, diuretics and especially beta blockers seem to exhibit the most detrimental hemodynamic profile. Second, the hemodynamic effects of diuretics are time-dependent. During the first weeks, diuretic use is accompanied by sodium and water excretion and subsequent shrinkage of intravascular volume, a slight reduction of CO (by approximately 5 %) and renal perfusion with subsequent decrease of renal blood flow and glomerular filtration rate, and a slight increase of heart rate [62–65, 67, 73]. However, after some weeks of treatment (usually 8 up to 12 weeks), SVR is reduced, the CO tends to return in pre-treatment values, and the intravascular volume is slightly expanded (reduced by 5 % compared to pre-treatment values) [62–64, 66].

The determination of the hemodynamic status of a hypertensive patient provides valuable information, which in turn might guide the selection of antihypertensive therapy, based on the above-mentioned hemodynamic effects of antihypertensive drugs. However, the hemodynamic evaluation is invasive, carries some risks, and it is not applicable in everyday clinical practice, limiting its use only in experimental studies. Recent technologic advances however permitted for the development of devices that provide significant information about the hemodynamic status of patients, by using the thoracic bio-impedance [74]. Therefore, the hemodynamic profile of an individual patient can be evaluated using a non-invasive, accurate, cheap, and reproducible method, which can be widely applied in everyday clinical practice [75–79].

The non-invasive hemodynamic approach was introduced by the Mayo Clinic group (Sandra Taler and Stephen Textor) and adopted by Carlos Ferrario and others. Up to now, three small, single-center clinical studies have been performed using this approach. In the first study, 104 patients with resistant hypertension were randomized to hemodynamic-guided therapy or specialist care [80]. It was found that the hemodynamic approach was associated with lower blood pressure values and higher control rates compared to specialist care. Intensification of diuretic therapy and greater reductions in SVR seem to mediate the superiority of the hemodynamic approach over specialist care in this pilot study [80]. The second study included 164 patients with uncontrolled blood pressure while on three antihypertensive drugs [81]. Once again, the hemodynamic approach was associated with lower blood pressure values, better control rates (77 % vs 57 %; $p<0.01$), and lower SVR. The third study randomly assigned 128 patients with uncontrolled blood pressure (either untreated or taking up to two antihypertensive drugs) to hemodynamic-guided therapy or standard empiric care [82]. Similarly to the other studies, blood pressure values were lower with the hemodynamic approach both by office and ambulatory blood pressure measurements. A recent meta-analysis revealed a benefit for the hemodynamic approach with combined odds ratio of 2.4, and 67 % control rates in randomized studies, while a similar blood pressure control rate (68 %) was observed in single-arm studies [83].

The Individualized Approach

Attempts have been made to identify genes or SNPs that predict blood pressure response and/or outcomes, but the yield was rather poor. In the GenHat for example, more than 42,000 patients were genotyped and SNPs were identified that predicted better BP response to ACE inhibitors, diuretics and beta blockers. Certain genotypes also predicted better outcomes with certain drug therapies [84]. When the results however were corrected for cofounders the association was minimized. Thus gene guided treatment of hypertension still remains problematic.

Demographic factors, such as age, gender, race, and adiposity may provide useful information, which will help the orientation about the mechanisms involved in the pathogenesis of elevated blood pressure and subsequently help in the prediction of blood pressure response to a given therapy. It needs to be emphasized however that their contribution is soft and not very helpful in individual patients. Before treatment initiation (monotherapy or combination therapy) the cardiovascular status should be carefully assessed. In conjunction with blood pressure control, cardiovascular risk reduction necessitates the management of other cardiovascular risk factors as well.

The European guidelines for the management of arterial hypertension place significant emphasis on individualized (Table 15.4) antihypertensive therapy [12–15]. A lot of patients fail to achieve blood pressure goals due to inadequate blood pressure response to certain drugs, due to known variability in response with all currently available antihypertensive drugs. Therefore, a personalized approach to antihypertensive therapy seems particularly prudent for the astute physician.

Age

The pathophysiology of hypertension is highly age-dependent. In brief, younger patients tend to present hyperdynamic circulation, characterized by increased CO (increased heart rate and stroke volume), sympathetic and RAS over-activation, while SVR is usually normal. With increasing age, SVR tends to increase, whereas CO tends to return towards normal [85–87]. On the other hand, older hypertensive patients have elevated arterial stiffness, increased SVR, lower CO [88], and plasma renin levels tend to decrease with advancing age [53, 87, 89–91]. Whether these pathophysiological changes can predict blood pressure response to antihypertensive drugs remains a matter of debate.

Data support a favorable effect of diuretics and calcium antagonists in older hypertensive patients and a favorable effect of beta blockers and ACE-inhibitors in younger patients with hypertension. Indeed, diuretics seem to be particularly effective in older patients [37, 92, 93]. Similar effects have been reported for calcium antagonists as well [90, 91]. On the other hand, several studies indicate that beta blockers are very effective in younger patients [90, 91, 93–95], while older hypertensive patients show a poor blood pressure response to beta blockers, and

Table 15.4 Factors influencing the choice of antihypertensive therapy according to the individualized approach

1. Demographic
Age, race, gender, adiposity
2. Heart rate
3. Blood pressure pattern
Isolated systolic hypertension, non-dipping
4. Target organ damage
Left ventricular hypertrophy, arterial stiffness, albuminuria, carotid IMT
5. Comorbidities
Diabetes mellitus, metabolic syndrome, stroke, coronary artery disease, heart failure, atrial fibrillation, peripheral artery disease, chronic kidney disease
6. Concomitant medications
Drug interactions
7. Antihypertensive drug characteristics
Indications, contra-indications, adverse events, metabolic effects
8. Adherence to therapy
9. Lifestyle
Exercise, sodium intake
10. Quality of life
Especially sexual function
11. Cost
Direct and indirect
12. Patient's preference
13. Genetics, genomics

only 20 % of them achieve blood pressure goals [96]. In fact, the age-dependent efficacy of beta blockers seems gradual and remarkable: in one study diastolic blood pressure control was achieved in 80 % of younger patients (<40 years), 50 % in middle-aged patients (40–60 years), and only 20 % in older patients (>60 years) [94]. Finally, ACE-inhibitors seem also to be more effective in younger patients [90, 95, 97]. Further credence to the above-mentioned findings of small clinical studies comes from a post-hoc analysis of the MRC trial reporting that diuretics were more effective than beta blockers in older patients (>45 years) [93].

The findings of these older studies, performed in the 1970s and 1980s were verified in more recent studies performed by the Cambridge study group in UK. A double-blind, randomized, cross-over study of 56 young hypertensive patients evaluated the response rates to monotherapy with the four main categories of antihypertensive drugs (ACE-inhibitors, beta blockers, calcium antagonists, and diuretics) [98]. A marked variability in blood pressure response to the tested drugs was observed. However, significant correlations were reported in the blood pressure response between the ACE-inhibitors and beta blockers in one hand, and between the calcium antagonists and diuretics in the other hand. Another study of 34 young hypertensive patients of identical design with the previous study evaluated the effects of the five main categories (ACE-inhibitors, beta blockers, calcium antagonists, diuretics, and alpha blockers) compared to placebo [99]. This study replicated the results of the previous study. In addition, it was found that the majority of participating patients (two thirds of participants) responded best to a drug inhibiting the RAS (ACE-inhibitor or beta blocker).

More recently, the Identification of the Determinants of the Efficacy of Arterial blood pressure Lowering drugs (IDEAL) trial evaluated the effect of age and gender on blood pressure response to a diuretic (indapamide) and an ACE-inhibitor (perindopril). This randomized, double-blind, placebo-controlled, cross-over study included 112 untreated, middle aged hypertensive patients [100]. It was found that age and gender were important determinants of blood pressure response to these two drugs since: (a) the systolic blood pressure response to indapamide increased by 3 mmHg every 10 years of age gradient in women, and (b) the systolic blood pressure response to perindopril decreased by 2 mmHg every 10 years of age gradient in both sexes [100].

The group of Morris Brown in Cambridge has proposed a modified version of the renin concept [101], which was adopted by the British guidelines for the management of arterial hypertension [102]. Based on the differences in PRA levels according to age and race, the British version uses age and race as surrogates for renin, in order to overcome existing difficulties with renin determination. The basic assumption is that renin levels are more likely to be elevated in patients younger than 55 years of age, while renin levels are more likely to be low in older patients and patients of black race. Therefore, similar to the renin approach, antihypertensive drugs inhibiting the RAS are preferred in younger patients, while diuretics and calcium antagonists are preferred in older patients and blacks. The AB/CD algorithm (from the initials of ACE-inhibitors or ARBs, beta blockers, calcium antagonists, and diuretics) was recently modified to the A/CD algorithm, and the beta blockers are no longer considered as first line agents [102]. This modification was based on the results of the LIFE and the ASCOT studies that used atenolol as the comparator. Several meta-analyses suggest that beta blockers (primarily atenolol) are less effective than the other first line agents in cardiovascular protection [103–106].

This approach has strength in its simplicity. It's very easy to remember this algorithm and thus more likely to implement it in everyday clinical practice. This is very important if one takes into account that the vast majority of hypertensive patients are treated by primary care physicians and not by hypertension specialists. Therefore, a simple algorithm is of utmost importance. On the other hand, the British approach has disadvantages; it does not take into account any patient characteristic apart from age and race. Therefore, target organ damage and other comorbidities are left unaccounted by the British algorithm, a simple but mechanistic approach, in contrast to the European guidelines that promote a more sophisticated individualized approach.

Another significant concern is raised about the age categorization. Although renin levels are usually low in the elderly, it is not unusual to find high renin levels in older hypertensive patients. Diuretics have been found to be preferentially effective in elderly patients with low PRA levels, while beta blockers were more efficacious in elderly hypertensives with high PRA levels [107, 108]. Caution should be used however when diuretic therapy is administered as they can easily get dehydrated. Low doses are preferred [87].

Large randomized clinical trials suggest that most antihypertensive drugs work in the elderly. Evidence proving the beneficial effects of antihypertensive therapy in older hypertensive patients exists not only for diuretics [109–113] and calcium antagonists [114–116], but also for beta blockers [111, 117], ACE-inhibitors [116] and ARBs [118]. Of even greater importance, a large meta-analysis evaluating the effects of antihypertensive drug categories according to age revealed that there is no evidence supporting the concept that the various drug categories are differently effective in patients younger or older than 65 years of age [119]. The recently published SPRINT study showed greater benefit in patients >75 years with intensive BP control [120].

Race

The pathophysiology of hypertension presents some differences between African American and Caucasian patients. PRA is lower in African Americans, even after adjustments for sodium excretion and plasma volume, or after stimulation with orthostasis or diuresis [121–124]. In addition, plasma volume is relatively expanded in African American compared to Caucasian hypertensives [121, 125], suggesting an enhanced salt sensitivity in African Americans [121]. In summary, almost 50 % of African Americans with arterial hypertension have low PRA levels and volume-dependent hypertension, while low PRA levels are found in only 10–15 % hypertensive patients of Caucasian origin [121, 126–128].

The pathophysiology of hypertension in African Americans seems to affect blood pressure response to antihypertensive therapy. Beta blockers seem to be rather ineffective in African Americans and are consistently less effective compared to Caucasian patients [129–134]. Several studies revealed a poor blood pressure response to beta blockers compared with diuretics or other drugs in African Americans [41, 130, 133, 135–138]. Blood pressure response to beta blockers was found extremely poor in African Americans, even similar to placebo in one study [137] or of marginal benefit in another study (4 % response rates in low renin hypertensives) [135]. In another study using renin profiling, blood pressure control with beta blockers was achieved only in 2 % of African Americans who had either low or normal PRA values [139]. In the VA trial the mean blood pressure reduction was significantly less with propranolol (8/9 mmHg) compared to hydrochlorothiazide (20/13 mmHg) in the 643 African American study participants [130]. Thus, diastolic blood pressure control in African Americans was achieved more often with diuretics (71 %) than with beta blockers (53 %), while the beta blockers failed to reduce blood pressure to less than 160/100 mmHg in 18 % of African Americans [130].

An analogous lack of efficacy in African Americans was observed with ACE-inhibitors, while diuretics were more effective than ACE-inhibitors in African

Americans, and ACE-inhibitors were more effective in Caucasians [140–142]. On the other hand, calcium antagonists seemed to be more effective than beta blockers with similar efficacy to diuretics in African Americans [125, 143–145]. In summary, African Americans have a better blood pressure response to diuretics and calcium antagonists compared with RAS inhibitors and beta blockers [146].

Gender

Life expectancy is longer in females than in males; moreover, cardiovascular events are less frequent and occur later in life in females [147]. Several differences exist between genders regarding prevalence, awareness, treatment, and control of hypertension, and the observed differences are age-dependent [148]. The pathophysiology of hypertension seems to be different in females and males [149]. Estrogens seem to exert beneficial effects on blood pressure and the cardiovascular system, including vasorelaxation, sympathetic inhibition and subsequent attenuation of the RAS [150]. Along with the hormonal differences, the mechanical properties of the arteries differ as well, since more pronounced increments at older age are observed in females than in males [151]. Moreover, several differences between the two genders have been reported in target organ damage, comorbidities, and cardiovascular risk [149].

Data from small clinical studies suggested that the blood pressure response to antihypertensive therapy might be different in females than in males [152–154]. Furthermore, post-hoc analyses from some large trials (ALLHAT and VALUE, but not in others) suggested that either the blood pressure reduction with some drugs differed according to gender [155, 156] or the cardiovascular outcomes might be different between the two genders (Heart Attack trial, Hypertension Care Computing Project, Second ANBP) [157–159].

However, there is yet no firm evidence that a particular drug class is better suited than another for treating arterial hypertension according to gender. In fact, a recent meta-analysis of large clinical trials with antihypertensive drugs according to gender did not find any significant differences in blood pressure reduction and cardiovascular outcomes between males and females [160]. Moreover, no evidence was found that the different antihypertensive drug classes are more effective in one gender than the other [160].

Adiposity

The pathophysiological mechanisms underlying blood pressure elevation in lean and obese patients have significant differences [161, 162]. Therefore, the probability for different optimum antihypertensive therapy according to adiposity might be a credible assumption.

Very recently, the Blood Pressure Lowering Treatment Trialists Collaboration performed a meta-regression analysis to evaluate the cardiovascular effects of antihypertensive drugs according to baseline adiposity categories [163]. The authors analyzed the data of more than 135,000 patients participating in 22 trials and divided participants in obese, overweight, and lean according to baseline body mass index values. The categorical analysis of the outcome did not show any special protection from cardiovascular events across the three adiposity categories. In contrast, the analysis of the comparisons as continuous variables revealed that ACE-inhibitors provided greater protection from cardiovascular events over other drugs (calcium antagonists and diuretics) for each 5 kg/m^2 increase in baseline body mass index levels. The combined findings of continuous and categorical analyses led the Collaboration to conclude that the superiority of ACE inhibitors over other drugs in obese versus lean patients is probably a false-positive finding, and therefore the findings of previous clinical trials might be a play of chance [163].

On the other hand, a sub-analysis of the ACCOMPLISH trial revealed that the combination of a calcium antagonist with an ACE-inhibitor had similar outcome benefits across the baseline adiposity status (lean, overweight, and obese). In contrast, the combination of a diuretic with an ACE-inhibitor was associated with significantly greater benefits in obese patients than in overweight and especially in lean patients, suggesting that the diuretic combination might be less effective in lean hypertensive patients when compared with a calcium antagonist combination [164].

The findings of the ACCOMPLISH study are in line with the results of the Systolic Hypertension in the Elderly Programme (SHEP). In a post-hoc analysis of the SHEP study, chlorthalidone (a thiazide-like diuretic) was less effective in cardiovascular protection (stroke) and mortality reduction in lean elderly hypertensive patients, especially in women [165]. In contrast, no difference in cardiovascular events and mortality was observed between lean and obese patients randomized to placebo.

Left Ventricular Hypertrophy

Left ventricular hypertrophy is a strong and independent cardiovascular risk factor. Several observational studies have shown that the reversal of left ventricular hypertrophy is associated with significant reductions in cardiovascular morbidity and mortality, as well as all-cause mortality [166–168]. Recent findings from large clinical trials confirmed that: (a) regression of left ventricular hypertrophy with antihypertensive therapy can occur, but it takes up to 2–3 years to reach maximum left ventricular mass reduction and then remains stable [169, 170], and (b) reversal or regression of left ventricular hypertrophy is associated with significant cardiovascular benefits [171].

Antihypertensive drugs seem to exert different effects on left ventricular mass, with RAS inhibitors and calcium antagonist having the greatest efficacy and beta blockers the lowest. [172–180] The findings of these studies should be taken with a grain of salt, since some studies were not adequately blinded (operator reading bias), the sample size was usually small, the study duration short, and blood pressure differences between comparator drugs were not always reported. However, the large echocardiography sub-study of the LIFE trial with 960 hypertensive patients with left ventricular hypertrophy was devoid of the abovementioned problems, and revealed a significant superiority of angiotensin receptor blocker over the beta blocker on left ventricular hypertrophy reduction [170].

Arterial Stiffening

Large arteries stiffen with age, and arterial hypertension is a major contributor of enhanced stiffening along with other factors. Therefore, antihypertensive therapy results in improvement of arterial compliance through the reduction of blood pressure *per se* [181–183]. Whether differences between antihypertensive drug classes on their effect on arterial stiffness exist remains unknown. Although some studies suggested superiority of RAS inhibitors over the other antihypertensive drugs in reducing arterial stiffness [184–186], other high quality studies –such as the EXPLOR- failed to confirm it [187]. Of note, significant within-class differences seem to exist for beta blockers regarding their effects on arterial stiffness; however the clinical significance remains unclarified [188].

Diabetes Mellitus

Diabetes mellitus usually coexists with hypertension. Blood pressure control is more difficult to be attained in patients with diabetes mellitus, and the vast majority of diabetic patients require combination therapy to achieve target blood pressure [189]. Therefore, it seems meaningless to spend time in finding appropriate monotherapy since most patients will require two or more medications. From existing data it seems reasonable to start with a RAAS blocker with or without a diuretic depending on the level of baseline BP. ACE inhibitors or ARBs are particularly indicated in the presence of macro or micro-albuminuria [190]. Despite concerns about using beta blockers in diabetic patients, mainly due to the impairment of insulin sensitivity, beta blockers have been shown to be equally effective with ACE inhibitors in the UKPDS trial [191]. Overall, all antihypertensive drugs have a place in the treatment of patients with diabetes mellitus and can be used for effective BP control [192] but a RAAS blocker should be the first or second agent.

. Three studies that addressed combination therapy among diabetics produced variable results. The ONTARGET and ALTITUDE trials, found no benefit with the combinations of two RAAS inhibitors, while an increased risk of adverse events was reported [193, 194]. In the ACCOMPLISH study, the combination of an ACE inhibitor with a calcium antagonist was significantly superior to the combination with a diuretic in the whole study population, as well as in diabetics and in high-risk diabetic patients [195]. Therefore, the combination of two RAS inhibitors is contraindicated, while the combination of a RAS inhibitor with calcium antagonists seems to be more beneficial than the combination with diuretics but this is still debated. In the ACCORD trial combinations of RAAS blockers with diuretics did not seem to be inferior to other combinations.

Metabolic Syndrome

The metabolic syndrome is a disputable clinical entity, which represents a clustering of cardiovascular risk factors (obesity, hypertension, dyslipidemia, and glucose abnormalities) [196–198]. Patients with metabolic syndrome are at increased risk to develop diabetes mellitus. It appears therefore reasonable to try to avoid antihypertensive agents that increase insulin resistance in such patients. Consequently, RAS inhibitors and calcium antagonists are preferred instead of diuretics and beta blockers, and especially their combination. When the latter categories are used, it seems prudent: (a) to prefer vasodilatory beta blockers that do not share the adverse metabolic actions of traditional beta blockers, (b) to combine the diuretic with a potassium-sparing drug, since hypokalemia enhances glucose intolerance, and (c) to select low doses of these drugs, since their metabolic actions are dose-dependent [199–202].

Stroke

All antihypertensive agents are effective for primary stroke prevention, since arterial hypertension is a major risk factor for cerebrovascular disease and blood pressure reduction results in significant benefits [203]. Calcium antagonists seem to be more protective from stroke than the other antihypertensive drug classes, as shown in several meta-analyses and meta-regression analyses [204–206]. However, this does not hold true for the totality of CV complication protection and treatment should be individualized. Until accurate predictors of future cardiovascular events are identified, the relative superiority of one class over the other for a specific outcome remains meaningless.

Secondary stroke prevention has not been adequately studied [207]. Significant benefits with antihypertensive medication have been observed in two studies, one using a diuretic and the other an ACE inhibitor combined with a diuretic [208, 209]. In addition, better cerebrovascular protection with ARBs than with other antihypertensive agents has been also observed [210, 211].

Myocardial Infarction

Antihypertensive therapy has resulted in significant reduction of cardiovascular morbidity and mortality. However, the benefits on myocardial infarction risk reduction are less impressive as compared to the benefits on stroke reduction, a finding observed first in the VA trials and confirmed later in several large randomized trials [1, 5, 12]. This disparity in risk reduction may be due to the fact that hypertension plays a less important role in the pathogenesis of coronary artery disease. The INTERHEART study for example showed that only 25 % of the risk for myocardial infarction could be attributed to hypertension [212].

Beta blockers and RAS inhibitors have demonstrated significant benefits in many studies, in patients who suffered a recent myocardial infarction [204, 213, 214]. Later on, agents from every antihypertensive drug class can be used and exert similar benefits [204]. In hypertensive patients with symptomatic coronary artery disease, beta blockers and calcium antagonists should be preferred agents at least for symptom relief.

Heart Failure

Arterial hypertension is the major risk factor for heart failure and antihypertensive therapy has resulted in pronounced reduction of heart failure development [12]. Calcium antagonists seem to be inferior to other antihypertensive drugs in heart failure prevention [205], diuretics were more effective than ACE-inhibitors in ALLHAT [155], and ARBs were even less effective in some studies (ONTARGET, TRANSCEND, PROFESS) [194, 215, 216]. As mentioned above however, the relative benefits of one class over the other regarding a specific benefit remain without clinical significance, since prediction of a specific outcome in an individual is currently impossible.

Beta blockers, RAS inhibitors (ACE inhibitors and ARBs), and mineralocorticoid receptor antagonists (spironolactone and eplerenone) have all shown significant survival benefits in patients with heart failure and reduced ejection fraction. Therefore, these agents are recommended for the management of heart failure patients, independent of blood pressure level even in patients with low BP as long as they can be tolerated. Loop diuretics are used primarily for decongestion and symptom relief [12]. Calcium antagonists do not seem to have a place in the management of systolic heart failure unless needed for blood pressure control. In patients with heart failure and preserved ejection fraction, an entity with high prevalence of hypertension and left ventricular hypertrophy, optimal control of hypertension is the ultimate goal. Specific use antihypertensive drugs failed to show added benefit [12, 217].

Atrial Fibrillation

Hypertension is frequently encountered in patients with atrial fibrillation, and in fact hypertension may contribute to the development and maintenance of atrial fibrillation. In these patients ventricular rate is usually high [218, 219]. Therefore, antihypertensive agents reducing heart rate, such as beta blockers and non-dihydropyridine calcium antagonists (verapamil and diltiazem), are frequently used for rate control in this patient population.

From the clinical point of view, the prevention of incident atrial fibrillation or the attenuation of recurrences is of paramount importance. Several lines of evidence coming from post-hoc analyses of large clinical trials suggested that ARBs were superior to calcium antagonists and beta blockers for the prevention of incident atrial fibrillation [220–224], which however was not observed in other trials [215, 216]. Studies specifically addressing the effect of ARBs on atrial fibrillation failed to show either prevention of recurrences in paroxysmal and persistent atrial fibrillation or prevention of cardiovascular events in patients with established atrial fibrillation [225–229]. Finally, incident atrial fibrillation was prevented by beta blockers and mineralocorticoid receptor antagonists in patients with heart failure and reduced ejection fraction [230, 231].

In Summary

Selection of optimal antihypertensive therapy should have the following three generic goals in mind:

1. Control blood pressure with least intrusive means
2. Take into consideration co-morbidities and how to optimize symptom control
3. Contribute to improvement of health outcomes and life expectancy.

It is well known that most patients with hypertension will need more than one medication to achieve blood pressure control. Monotherapy is only adequate in 20–25 % of patients with hypertension. Achieving blood pressure control is probably much more important than what drug combination has been used. Although current guidelines allow for acceptable BP control a systolic up to 150 mmHg, the recently published SPRINT study demonstrated to all of us in an undisputed way that lower is better and goals of systolic BP <120 mmHg provide improvement in morbidity and mortality. The SPRINT study was not a drug focuses study; it was rather a blood pressure level focused study and yet surprised us all with impressive improvement in health outcomes with the intensive lowering of blood pressure.

Focusing on co-morbidities is important and will make patients feel better and live longer. For example, patients with high heart rate, angina and/or atrial fibrillation will benefit from beta blockers or heart rate lowering calcium antagonists. Rate control will make patients feel better and probably live longer. Similarly patients with heart failure will benefit from beta blockers, ACE-i/ARBs and MRAs and certainly most of them need diuretics for symptom control.

Since the early studies from the Veterans Administration that demonstrated marked improvement in health outcomes with blood pressure control, we came a long way in our understanding of optimal choice of antihypertensive therapy. Taking into consideration co-morbidities we can not only prolong life, but can pretty much eliminate symptoms and minimize complications of hypertension.

References

1. Smith WM. Treatment of mild hypertension: results of a ten-year interaction trial. US-PHS Hospital Cooperative Study Group. Circ Res. 1977;40 Suppl 1:98–105.
2. Veterans Administration Cooperative Study Group on Anti hypertensive Agents. Effects of treatment on morbidity in hypertension: results in patients with diastolic blood pressure averaged 115–129 mmHg. JAMA. 1976;202:1028–34.
3. The Australian therapeutic trial in mild hypertension. Report by the Management Committee. Lancet. 1980;1:1261.
4. Helgeland A. Treatment of mild hypertension; a 5-year controlled drug trial. The Oslo Study. Am J Med. 1980;69:725–32.
5. Veterans Administration Cooperative Study Group on Anti hypertensive Agents. Effects of treatment on morbidity in hypertension: results in patients with diastolic blood pressure averaging 90 through 114 mmHg. JAMA. 1970;213:1143–51.
6. Hypertension Detection and Follow-up Program Cooperative Group. Five-year findings of the hypertension detection and follow-up program: I. Reduction in mortality of persons with high blood pressure, including mild hypertension. JAMA. 1979;242:2562–71.
7. Whitworth JA, Kincaid-Smith P. Diuretics or beta blockers first for hypertension? Pract Ther Section Drugs. 1982;23:394–402.
8. Moser M, Guyther JR, Finnerty F. Joint National Committee report on detection, evaluation, and treatment of high blood pressure. JAMA. 1977;237:255–61.
9. The 1980 Report of the Joint National Committee on detection, evaluation, and treatment of high blood pressure. Arch Intern Med. 1980;140:1280–5.
10. The 1988 Report of the Joint National Committee on detection, evaluation, and treatment of high blood pressure. Arch Intern Med. 1988;148:1023–38.
11. Julius S, Kjeldsen SE, Weber M, Brunner HR, Ekman S, Hansson L, et al; VALUE trial group. Outcomes inhypertensive patients at high cardiovascular risk treated with regimens based on valsartan or amlodipine: the VALUE randomised trial. Lancet. 2004;363:2022–31.
12. European Society of Hypertension-European Society of Cardiology Guidelines Committee. 2003 European Society of Hypertension-European Society of Cardiology guidelines for the management of arterial hypertension. J Hypertens. 2003;21:1011–53.
13. Mancia G, De Backer G, Dominiczak A, Cifkova R, Fagard R, Germano G, et al. 2007 Guidelines for the Management of Arterial Hypertension: The Task Force for the Management of Arterial Hypertension of the European Society of Hypertension (ESH) and of the European Society of Cardiology (ESC). J Hypertens. 2007;25:1105–87.
14. Mancia G, Laurent S, Agabiti-Rosei E, Ambrosioni E, Burnier M, Caulfield MJ, et al. Re-appraisal of European guidelines on hypertension management: a European Society of Hypertension Task Force document. J Hypertens. 2009;27:2121–58.

15. Mancia G, Fagard R, Narkiewicz K, Redón J, Zanchetti A, Böhm M, Christiaens T, Cifkova R, De Backer G, Dominiczak A, Galderisi M, Grobbee DE, Jaarsma T, Kirchhof P, Kjeldsen SE, Laurent S, Manolis AJ, Nilsson PM, Ruilope LM, Schmieder RE, Sirnes PA, Sleight P, Viigimaa M, Waeber B, Zannad F, Task Force Members. 2013 ESH/ESC guidelines for the management of arterial hypertension. J Hypertens. 2013;31:1281–357.
16. Szlachcic J, Hirsch AT, Tubau JF, Vollmer C, Henderson S, Massie BM. Diltiazem versus propranolol in essential hypertension: responses of rest and exercise blood pressure and effects on exercise capacity. Am J Cardiol. 1987;59:393–9.
17. Tigerstedt R, Bergman PG. Niere unt Kreislauf. Scand Arch Physiol. 1898;8:223–71.
18. Goldblatt JH, Lynch RF, Hanzal RF, et al. Studies on experimental hypertension. Production of persistent elevation of systolic blood pressure by means of renal ischemia. J Exp Med. 1934;59:347–79.
19. Skeggs LT, Marsh WH, Kahn JR, Shumway NP. The existence of two forms of hypertension. J Exp Med. 1954;99:275–82.
20. Laragh JH. Interrelationships between angiotensin, norepinephrine, epinephrine, aldosterone secretion, and electrolyte metabolism in men. Circulation. 1962;25:203–11.
21. Laragh JH, Ulick S, Januszewicz V, Deming QB, Kelly WG, Lieberman S. Aldosterone secretion and primary and malignant hypertension. J Clin Invest. 1960;39:1091–106.
22. Laragh JH, Ulick S, Januszewicz V, Kelly WG, Lieberman S. Electrolyte metabolism and aldosterone secretion in benign and malignant hypertension. Ann Intern Med. 1960;53:259–72.
23. Laragh JH, Angers M, Kelly WG, Lieberman S. Hypotensive agents and pressor substances. The effect of epinephrine, norepinephrine, angiotensin II and others on the secretory rate of aldosterone in man. JAMA. 1960;174:234–40.
24. Laragh JH. The role of aldosterone in man: evidence for regulation of electrolyte balance and arterial pressure by renal-adrenal system which may be involved in malignant hypertension. JAMA. 1960;174:293–5.
25. Conn JW. Primary aldosteronism, a new clinical syndrome. J Lab Clin Med. 1955;45:6–17.
26. Conn JW. The evolution of primary aldosteronism: 1954–1967. Harvey Lect. 1966–67;62:257–91.
27. Brunner HR, Laragh JH, Baer L, et al. Essential hypertension: renin and aldosterone, heart attack and stroke. N Engl J Med. 1972;286:441–9.
28. Sealey JE, Blumenfeld JD, Bell GM, et al. On the renal basis for essential hypertension: nephron heterogeneity with discordant renin secretion and sodium excretion causing a hypertensive vasoconstriction volume relationship. J Hypertens. 1988;6:763–7.
29. Blumenfeld JD, Mann SJ, Laragh JH. Clinical evaluation and differential diagnosis of the individual hypertensive patient. In: Laragh JH, Brenner BM, editors. Hypertension. New York: Raven; 1995. p. 1897–912.
30. Buhler FR, Laragh JH, Vaughan ED, et al. Antihypertensive action of propranolol. Specific antirenin responses in high and normal renin forms of essential, renal, renovascular and malignant hypertension. Am J Cardiol. 1973;32:511–22.
31. Pettinger WA, Mitchell HC. Renin release, saralasin and the vasodilator-beta-blocker drug interaction in men. N Engl J Med. 1975;292:1214–7.
32. Hollifield JW, Sherman K, Zwagg RV, Shand DG. Proposed mechanisms of propranolol's antihypertensive effect in essential hypertension. N Engl J Med. 1976;295:68–73.
33. Stumpe KO, Kolloch R, Vetter H, et al. Acute and long-term studies of the mechanisms of action of beta-blocking drugs in lowering blood pressure. Am J Med. 1976;60:853–65.
34. Menard J, Bertagna X, Nguyen PT, et al. Rapid identification of patients with essential hypertension sensitive to acebutolol. Am J Med. 1976;60:886–90.
35. Moore SB, Goodwin FJ. Effect of beta adrenergic blockade on plasma renin activity and intractable hypertension in patients receiving regular dialysis treatment. Lancet. 1976;2:67–70.
36. Crane MG, Hams JJ, Johns VJ. Hyporeninemic hypertension. Am J Med. 1972;52:457–66.

37. Vaughan ED, Laragh JH, Gavras I, et al. Volume factor in low and normal renin essential hypertension. Treatment with either spironolactone or chlorthalidone. Am J Cardiol. 1973;32:523–32.
38. Carey RM, Douglas JG, Liddle GW. The syndrome of essential hypertension and suppressed plasma renin activity. Normalization of blood pressure with spironolactone. Arch Intern Med. 1972;130:849–54.
39. Adlin EV, Marks AD, Channick BJ. Spironolactone and hydrochlorothiazide in essential hypertension. Blood pressure response and plasma renin activity. Arch Intern Med. 1972;130:855–8.
40. Crane MG, Harris JJ. Effect of spironolactone in hypertensive patients. Am J Med Sci. 1970;260:311–30.
41. Douglas JG, Hollifield JW, Liddle GW. Treatment of low-renin essential hypertension. Comparison of spironolactone and a hydrochlorothiazide-triamterene combination. JAMA. 1974;227:518–21.
42. Karlberg BE, Kagedal B, tegler L, et al. A crossover study with special reference to initial plasma renin activity. Am J Cardiol. 1976;37:642–9.
43. Baer L, Parra JZ, Williams GS. Detection of renovascular hypertension with angiotensin II blockade. Ann Intern Med. 1977;86:257–60.
44. Drayer JI, Keim HJ, Weber MA, Case DB, Laragh JH. Unexpected pressor responses to propranolol in essential hypertension. An interaction between renin, aldosterone and sympathetic activity. Am J Med. 1976;60:897–903.
45. Blumenfeld JD, Laragh JH. Renin system analysis: a rational method for the diagnosis and treatment of the individual patient with hypertension. Am J Hypertens. 1998;11:894–6.
46. Egan B, Basile J, Rehman S, Davis P, Grob III C, Riehle J, Walters C, Lackland D, Merali C, Sealey J, Laragh J. Plasma renin test–guided drug treatment algorithm for correcting patients with treated but uncontrolled hypertension: a randomized controlled trial. Am J Hypertens. 2009;22:792–801.
47. Williams B, MacDonald TM, Morant S, et al. Spiromolactone vs placebo, bisoprolol and doxazosin to determine the optimal treatment for drug resistant hypertension (PATHWAY-2): a randomized, double-blind, crossover trial. Lancet. 2015;386:2059–68.
48. Moser M. Stepped-care approach to hypertension: is it still useful? Prim Cardiol. 1985;11:186–98.
49. Freis ED, Materson BJ, Flamenhaum V. Comparison of propranolol or hydrochlorothiazide alone for treatment of hypertension. III. Evaluation of the renin-angiotensin system. Am J Med. 1983;74:1029–41.
50. Esler M, Zweifler A, Randall O, Julius S, DeQuattro V. The determinants of plasma-renin activity in essential hypertension. Ann Intern Med. 1978;88:746–52.
51. Holland OB, Gomez-Sanchez C, Fairchild C, Kaplan NM. Role of renin classification for diuretic treatment of black hypertensive patients. Arch Intern Med. 1979;139:1365–70.
52. Preibsz JJ, Sealey JE, Aceto RM, Laragh J. Renin. Clinical aspects of essential hypertension. Cardiovasc Rev Rep. 1982;3:787–804.
53. Woods JW, Pittman AW, Pulliam CC, Werf Jr EE, Walder W, Allen CA. Renin profiling in hypertension and its use in treatment with propranolol and chlorthalidone. N Engl J Med. 1976;294:1137–43.
54. Lund-Johansen P. The hemodynamics of essential hypertension. In: Robertson JIS, editor. Handbook of hypertension, vol. 1. 3rd ed. New York: Elsevier Scientific Publications; 1983. p. 151–72.
55. Julius S, Pascual AV, Sannerstedt R, Mitchell C. Relationship between cardiac output and peripheral resistance in borderline hypertension. Circulation. 1971;43:382–90.
56. Julius S, Esler M. Autonomic nervous cardiovascular regulation in borderline hypertension. Am J Cardiol. 1975;36:685–96.
57. Tarazi RC. Hemodynamic role of extracellular fluid in hypertension. Circ Res. 1976;38 Suppl 2:73–83.
58. Messerli FH, Frohlich ED, Suarez DH, et al. Borderline hypertension: relationship between age, hemodynamics and circulating catecholamines. Circulation. 1981;64:760–4.

59. Mehta SK, Walsh JT, Goldberg AD, Topham WS. Increasing daytime vascular resistance with progressive hypertension in ambulant patients. Am Heart J. 1987;113:156–62.
60. Letcher RL, Chien S, Laragh JH. Changes in blood viscosity accompanying the response to prazosin in patients with essential hypertension. J Cardiovasc Pharmacol. 1979;1 Suppl 6:S8–20.
61. Lund-Johansen P. Advances in medicine: selective α blockade for managing hypertension. Secaucus: Advanced Therapeutics Communications, Inc.; 1984.
62. Hansen J. Hydrochlorothiazide in the treatment of hypertension. The effects on blood volume, exchangeable sodium and blood pressure. Acta Med Scand. 1968;183:317–21.
63. Leth A. Changes in plasma and extracellular fluid volumes in patients with essential hypertension during long-term treatment with hydrochlorothiazide. Circulation. 1970;42:479–85.
64. Conway J, Lauwers P. Hemodynamic and hypotensive effects of long-term therapy with chlorothiazide. Circulation. 1960;21:21–7.
65. Lund-Johansen P. Hemodynamic changes in long-term diuretic therapy of essential hypertension. A comparative study of chlorthalidone, polythiazide and hydrochlorothiazide. Acta Med Scand. 1970;187:509–18.
66. DeLeeuw PW, Wester A, Stienstra R. Hemodynamic and endocrinological studies with prazosin in essential hypertension. In: Lund-Johansen P, Mason DT, editors. Recent advances in hypertension and congestive heart failure—prazosin. Amsterdam: Excerpta Medica; 1978. p. 11–23.
67. Lowenthal DT. Hypertension and exercise physiology: clinical and therapeutic applications. In: Lowenthal DT, Bharadwaja K, Oaks WW, editors. Therapeutics through exercise. New York: Grune & Stratton, Inc; 1979.
68. Trap-Jensen J, Clausen JP, Noer I, Larsen OA, Krogsgaard AR, Christensen NJ. The effects of beta-adrenoceptor blockers on cardiac output, liver blood flow and skeletal muscle blood flow in hypertensive patients. Acta Physiol Scand. 1976;440:30–9.
69. Smith IS, Fernandes M, Kim KE, et al. A three-phase clinical evaluation of prazosin. Postgrad Med. 1975; Special No:53–60.
70. Lund-Johansen P. Central haemodynamic effects of beta blockers in hypertension. A comparison between atenolol, metoprolol, timolol, penbutolol, alprenolol, pindolol and bunitrolol. Eur Heart J. 1983;4(Suppl D):1–12.
71. Okun R. Effectiveness of prazosin as initial antihypertensive therapy. Am J Cardiol. 1983;51:644–50.
72. Itskovitz HD. Hemodynamic effects of antihypertensive drugs. Am Fam Physician. 1983;27:137–42.
73. Tarazi RC, Dustan HP, Frohlich E. Long-term thiazide therapy in essential hypertension. Circulation. 1970;41:709–17.
74. Ventura H, Taler SJ, Strobeck J. Hypertension as a hemodynamic disease: the role of impedance cardiography in diagnostic, prognostic, and therapeutic decision making. Am J Hypertens. 2005;18:26S–43.
75. Buell JC. A practical, cost effective, noninvasive system for cardiac output and hemodynamic analysis. Am Heart J. 1988;116:657–66.
76. Verhoeve PE, Cadwell CA, Tsadok S. Reproducibility of noninvasive bioimpedance measurements of cardiac function. J Card Fail. 1998;4:S53–4.
77. Treister N, Wagner K, Jansen P. Reproducibility of impedance cardiography parameters in outpatients with clinically stable coronary artery disease. Am J Hypertens. 2005;18:S44–50.
78. Fuller HD. The validity of cardiac output measurement by thoracic impedance: a meta-analysis. Clin Invest Med. 1992;15:103–12.
79. Van de Water JM, Miller TW, Vogel RL, et al. Impedance cardiography: the next vital sign technology? Chest. 2003;123:2028–33.
80. Taler SJ, Textor SC, Augustine JE. Resistant hypertension: comparing hemodynamic management to specialist care. Hypertension. 2002;39:982–8.
81. Smith R, Levy P, Ferrario C, Consideration of Noninvasive Hemodynamic Monitoring to Target Reduction of Blood Pressure Levels Study Group. Value of noninvasive hemodynamics to achieve blood pressure control in hypertensive subjects. Hypertension. 2006;47:771–7.

82. Krzesiński P, Gielerak G, Kowal J. A "patient-tailored" treatment of hypertension with use of impedance cardiography: a randomized, prospective and controlled trial. Med Sci Monit. 2013;19:242–50.
83. Ferrario C, Flack J, Strobeck J, Smits G, Peters C. Individualizing hypertension treatment with impedance cardiography: a meta-analysis of published trials. Ther Adv Cardiovasc Dis. 2010;4:5–16.
84. Arnett DK, Boerwinkle E, Davis BR, Eckfeldt J, Ford CE, Black H. Pharmacogenetic approaches to hypertension therapy: design and rationale for the Genetics of Hypertension Associated Treatment (GenHAT) study. Pharmacogenomics J. 2002;2:309–17.
85. Conn JN, Limas CJ, Guiha NH. Hypertension and the heart. Arch Intern Med. 1974; 133:969–79.
86. Lund-Johansen P. Hemodynamics of essential hypertension. Clin Sci. 1980;59:343s–54.
87. Messerli FH, Ventura HO, Glaze LB, Sundgaard-Riise K, Dunn G, Frohlich ED. Essential hypertension in the elderly: hemodynamics, intravascular volume, plasma renin activity and circulating catecholamine levels. Lancet. 1983;2:983–8.
88. Simon AC, Levenson JA, Safar ME. Systolic hypertension: differences of mechanism according to age and possible application of treatment. Eur Heart J. 1982;3(Suppl c):65–9.
89. Meade TW, Imerson JD, Gordon D, Peart WS. The epidemiology of plasma renin. Clin Sci. 1983;64:273–80.
90. Buehler FR, Bolli P, Kiowski W, Erne P, Hulthen UL, Block LH. Renin profiling to select antihypertensive drugs. Am J Med. 1984;77(Suppl 2A):36–42.
91. Kiowski W, Buehler FR, Fadayomi MO, Erne P, Muller FB, Hulthen UL, Bolli P. Age, race, blood pressure and renin: predictors for antihypertensive treatment with calcium antagonists. Am J Cardiol. 1985;56:81H–5.
92. European Working Party on High Blood Pressure in the Elderly. Efficacy of antihypertensive drug treatment according to age, sex, blood pressure, and previous cardiovascular disease in patients over the age of sixty. Lancet. 1986;2:589–92.
93. Brennan PJ, Greenberg G, Miall WE, Thompson SG. Seasonal variation in arterial blood pressure. Br Med J. 1982;285:919–23.
94. Buehler FR, Burkart F, Luetold BE, Kueng M, Marbet G, Pfisterer M. Antihypertensive beta-blocking action as related to renin and age: a pharmacological tool to identify pathogenic mechanisms in essential hypertension. Am J Cardiol. 1975;36:653–69.
95. Case DB, Atlas SA, Laragh JH, Sealy JE, Sullivan PA, Mckinstry DW. Clinical experience with blockade of the renin-angiotensin aldosterone system by an oral converting enzyme inhibitor (SQ14, 225, captopril) in hypertensive patients. Prog Cardiovasc Dis. 1978;21: 195–206.
96. Buhler FR, Burkart F, Lutold BE, Kung M, Marbet G, Pfisterer M. Antihypertensive beta blocking action as related to renin and age: a pharmacologic tool to identify pathogenic mechanisms in essential hypertension. Am J Cardiol. 1975;36:653–69.
97. Davies RO, Irvin JD, Kramsch GK, Walker JF, Moncloa F. Enalapril world-wide experience. Am J Med. 1984;77(Suppl 2A):23–35.
98. Dickerson JE, Hingorani AD, Ashby MJ, Palmer CR, Brown MJ. Optimisation of antihypertensive treatment by cross-over rotation of four major classes. Lancet. 1999;353:2008–13.
99. Deary AJ, Schumann AL, Murfet H, Haydock SF, Foo RS-Y, Brown MJ. Double-blind, placebo-controlled crossover comparison of five classes of antihypertensive drugs. J Hypertens. 2002;20:771–7.
100. Gueyffier F, Subtil F, Bejan-Angoulvant T, et al. Can we identify response markers to antihypertensive drugs? First results from the IDEAL trial. J Hum Hypertens. 2015;29:22–7.
101. Brown MJ, Cruickshank JK, Dominczak AF, MacGregor G, Poulter NR, Russell GI, Thom S, Williams B. Better blood pressure control: how to combine drugs. J Hum Hypertens. 2003;17:81–6.
102. National Institute for Health and Clinical Excellence (NICE) Hypertension: the clinical management of primary hypertension in adults. Br J Gen Pract. 2012;62(596):163–164.

103. Dahlof B, Devereux RB, Kjeldsen SE, Julius S, Beevers G, de Faire U, et al; LIFE Study Group. Cardiovascular morbidity and mortality in the Losartan Intervention For Endpoint reduction in hypertension study (LIFE): a randomised trial against atenolol. Lancet. 2002;359:995–1003.
104. Dahlof B, Sever PS, Poulter NR, et al. Prevention of cardiovascular events with an antihypertensive regimen of amlodipine adding perindopril as required versus atenolol adding bendroflumethiazide as required in the ASCOT-BPLA: a multicenter randomised controlled trial. Lancet. 2005;366:895–906.
105. Messerli FH, Bangalore S, Julius S. Risk/benefit assessment of beta blockers and diuretics precludes their use for first-line therapy in hypertension. Circulation. 2008;117:2706–15.
106. Lindholm LH, Carlberg B, Samuelsson O. Should beta blockers remain first choice in the treatment of primary hypertension? A meta-analysis. Lancet. 2005;366:1545–53.
107. Niarchos AP, Laragh JH. Renin dependency of blood pressure in isolated systolic hypertension. Am J Med. 1984;77:407–14.
108. Niarchos AP, Weinstein DL, Laragh JH. Comparison of the effects of diuretic therapy and low sodium intake in isolated systolic hypertension. Am J Med. 1984;77:1061–8.
109. Beckett NS, Peters R, Fletcher AE, Staessen JA, Liu L, Dumitrascu D, et al. Treatment of hypertension in patients 80 years of age or older. N Engl J Med. 2008;358:1887–98.
110. SHEP Co-operative Research Group. Prevention of stroke by antihypertensive drug treatment in older persons with isolated systolic hypertension. Final results of the Systolic Hypertension in the Elderly Program (SHEP). JAMA. 1991;265:3255–64.
111. Dahlof B, Lindholm LH, Hansson L, Schersten B, Ekbom T, Wester PO. Morbidity and mortality in the Swedish Trial in Old Patients with Hypertension (STOP-Hypertension). Lancet. 1991;338:1281–5.
112. Amery A, Birkenhager W, Brixko P, Bulpitt C, Clement D, Deruyttere M, et al. Mortality and morbidity results from the European Working Party on High Blood Pressure in the Elderly trial. Lancet. 1985;1:1349–54.
113. Medical Research Council trial of treatment of hypertension in older adults: principal results. MRC Working Party. BMJ. 1992;304:405–12.
114. Staessen JA, Fagard R, Thijs L, Celis H, Arabidze GG, Birkenhager WH, et al. Randomised double-blind comparison of placebo and active treatment for older patients with isolated systolic hypertension. The Systolic Hypertension in Europe (Syst-Eur) Trial Investigators. Lancet. 1997;350:757–64.
115. Liu L, Wang JG, Gong L, Liu G, Staessen JA. Comparison of active treatment and placebo in older Chinese patients with isolated systolic hypertension. Systolic Hypertension in China (Syst-China) Collaborative Group. J Hypertens. 1998;16:1823–9.
116. Hansson L, Lindholm LH, Ekbom T, Dahlof B, Lanke J, Schersten B, et al. Randomised trial of old and new antihypertensive drugs in elderly patients: cardiovascular mortality and morbidity the Swedish Trial in Old Patients with Hypertension-2 study. Lancet. 1999;354:1751–6.
117. Coope J, Warrender TS. Randomised trial of treatment of hypertension in elderly patients in primary care. BMJ. 1986;293:1145–51.
118. Lithell H, Hansson L, Skoog I, Elmfeldt D, Hofman A, Olofsson B, et al. The Study on Cognition and Prognosis in the Elderly (SCOPE): principal results of a randomized double-blind intervention trial. J Hypertens. 2003;21:875–86.
119. Blood Pressure Lowering Treatment Trialists' Collaboration. Effects of different regimens to lower blood pressure on major cardiovascular events in older and younger adults: meta-analysis of randomised trials. BMJ. 2008;336:1121–3.
120. SPRINT Research Group. A randomized trial of intensive versus standard blood pressure control. N Engl J Med. 2015;373:2103–16.
121. Chrysant SG, Danisa K, Kern DC, Dillard BL, Smith WJ, Frohlich ED. Racial differences in pressure, volume and renin interrelationships in essential hypertension. Hypertension. 1979;1:136–41.

122. Luft FC, Rankin LI, Eloch R, Weyman AE, Willif LR, Murray RH, Grin CE, Weinberger MH. Cardiovascular and humoral responses to extremes of sodium intake in normal responses to extremes of sodium intake in normal black and white men. Circulation. 1979;60:697–706.
123. Sever PS, Peart WS, Meade TW, Davies IB, Gordon D. Ethnic differences in blood pressure with observations on noradrenaline and renin, 1. A working population. Clin Exp Hypertens. 1979;1:733–44.
124. Kaplan NM, Kern DC, Holland OB, Kramer NJ, Higgins J, Gomez-Sanchez C. The intravenous furosemide test: a simple way to evaluate renin responsiveness. Ann Intern Med. 1976;84:639–45.
125. Lilley JJ, Hsu L, Stone RA. Racial disparity of plasma volume in hypertension. Ann Intern Med. 1976;84:707–8.
126. Hollifield JW, Slaton PE, Liddle GW. Some biochemical consequences of diuretic therapy of low renin essential hypertension. In: Sambhi MP, editor. Systemic effects of antihypertensive agents, Florida, 1975. 3rd ed. New York: Stratton Intercontinential Medical Books Corp; 1979. p. 131–49.
127. Mitas II JA, Holle R, Levy SB, Stone RA. Racial analysis of the volume-renin relationship in human hypertension. Arch Intern Med. 1979;139:157–60.
128. Messerli FH. Using divergent pathophysiological aspects as clues to the initial antihypertensive agent in essential hypertension. Pract Cardiol. 1984;10:55–67.
129. Humphreys GS, Delvin DG. Ineffectiveness of propranolol in hypertensive Jamacains. Br Med J. 1968;2:601–3.
130. Veterans Administration Cooperative Study Group on Antihypertensive Agents. Comparison of propranolol and hydrochlorothiazide for the initial treatment of hypertension. 1. Results of short-term titration with emphasis on racial differences in response. JAMA. 1982;248:1996–2003.
131. Holland OB, Fairchild C. Renin classification for diuretic and beta-blocker for treatment of black hypertensive patients. J Chronic Dis. 1982;35:179–82.
132. Weber MA, Priest RT, Ricci BA, Eltorai MI, Brewer DD. Low-dose diuretic and beta-adrenoreceptor blocker in essential hypertension. Clin Pharmacol Ther. 1980;28:149–58.
133. Seedat YK. Trial of atenolol and chlorthalidone for hypertension in black South Africans. Br Med J. 1980;281:1241–3.
134. Grell GAC, Forrester TE, Alleyne GAO. Comparison of the effectiveness of a beta-blocker (atenolol) and a diuretic (chlorthalidone) in black hypertensive patients. South Med J. 1984;77:1524–9.
135. Ganguly A, Weinberger MH. Low renin hypertension. A current review of definitions and controversies. Am Heart J. 1979;98:642–52.
136. Moser M, Lunn J. Comparative effects of pindolol and hydrochlorothiazide in black hypertensive patients. Angiology. 1981;32:561–6.
137. Humphreys GS, Delvin DG. Ineffectiveness of propranolol in hypertensive Jamaicans. Br Med J. 1968;1:601–3.
138. Freis EP. Choice of initial treatment. J Cardiovasc Pharmacol. 1985;7 Suppl 1:S112–6.
139. Hollifield JW, Slaton P. Demographic approach to initiation of antihypertensive therapy: handbook of hypertension. In: Miami: Symposium Specialists Inc; 1981. pp. 51–8.
140. Goodman C, Rosendorff C, Coull A. Comparison of the antihypertensive effect of enalapril and propranolol in black South Africans. S Afr Med J. 1982;67:672–6.
141. Moser M, Lunn J. Responses to captopril and hydrochlorothiazide in black patients with hypertension. Clin Pharmacol Ther. 1982;32:307–12.
142. Weinberger MH. Blood pressure and metabolic responses to hydrochlorothiazide, captopril and the combination in black and white mild-to-moderate hypertensive patients. J Cardiovasc Pharmacol. 1985;7:S52–5.
143. Frishman WH, Zawada ET, Smith LK, Sowers J, Swartz SL, Kirkendall W, Lunn J, McCarron D, Moser M, Schnaper H. Comparison of hydrochlorothiazide and sustained-release diltiazem for mild-to-moderate systemic hypertension. Am J Cardiol. 1987;59:615–23.

144. Massie BM, MacCarthy EP, Ramanathan KB, Weiss RJ, Anderson M, Eidelson BA, Kondos GT, Labreche GG, Tubau JF, Ulep D. Diltiazem and propranolol in mild to moderate essential hypertension as monotherapy or with hydrochlorothiazide. Ann Intern Med. 1987;107:150–7.
145. Moser M, Lunn J, Matterson BJ. Comparative effects of diltiazem and hydrochlorothiazide in blacks with systemic hypertension. Am J Cardiol. 1985;56:101H–4.
146. Bühler FR, Bolli P, Kiowski W, Erne P, Hulthén UL, Block LH. Renin profiling to select antihypertensive baseline drugs. Renin inhibitors for high-renin and calcium entry blockers for low-renin patients. Am J Med. 1984;77:36–42.
147. Kannel WB, Schwartz MJ, McNamara PM. Blood pressure and risk of cardiovascular disease: the Framingham Heart Study. Chest. 1969;56:43–51.
148. Go A, Mozaffarian D, Roger V, et al. Heart disease and stroke statistics – 2013 update: a report from the American Heart Association. Circulation. 2013;127:e77–86.
149. Doumas M, Papademetriou V, Faselis C, Kokkinos P. Gender differences in hypertension: myths and reality. Curr Hypertens Rep. 2013;15:321–30.
150. Orshal JM, Khalil RA. Gender, sex hormones, and vascular tone. Am J Physiol Regul Integr Comp Physiol. 2004;286:R233–49.
151. Cheng S, Xanthakis V, Sullivan L, Vasan R. Blood pressure tracking over the adult life course. Hypertension. 2012;60:1393–9.
152. Kloner R, Sowers J, DiBona G, et al. Sex- and age-related antihypertensive effects of amlodipine. The Amlodipine Cardiovascular Community Trial Study Group. Am J Cardiol. 1996;77:713–22.
153. Saunders E, Cable G, Neutel J. Predictors of blood pressure response to angiotensin receptor blocker/diuretic combination therapy: a secondary analysis of the irbesartan/hydrochlorothiazide blood pressure reductions in diverse patient populations (INCLUSIVE) study. J Clin Hypertens (Greenwich). 2008;10:27–33.
154. Everett BM, Glynn RJ, Danielson E, Ridker PM. Combination therapy versus monotherapy as initial treatment for stage 2 hypertension: a prespecified subgroup analysis of a community-based, randomized, open-label trial. Clin Ther. 2008;30:661–72.
155. ALLHAT Officers and Coordinators for the ALLHAT Collaborative Research Group. Major outcomes in high-risk hypertensive patients randomized to angiotensin-converting enzyme inhibitor or calcium channel blocker vs diuretic: the Antihypertensive and Lipid-Lowering Treatment to Prevent Heart Attack Trial (ALLHAT). JAMA. 2002;288:2981–97.
156. Zanchetti A, Julius S, Kjeldsen S, et al. Outcomes in subgroups of hypertensive patients treated with regimens based on valsartan and amlodipine: an analysis of findings from the VALUE trial. J Hypertens. 2006;24:2163–8.
157. b-Blocker Heart Attack Trial Research Group. A randomized trial of propranolol in patients with acute myocardial infarction. I. Mortality results. JAMA. 1982;247:1707–14.
158. Fletcher A, Beevers DG, Bulpitt C, et al. Beta adrenoceptor blockade is associated with increased survival in male but not female hypertensive patients: a report from the DHSS Hypertension Care Computing Project (DHCCP). J Hum Hypertens. 1988;2:219–27.
159. Wing L, Reid C, Ryan P, et al. A comparison of outcomes with angiotensin-converting-enzyme inhibitors and diuretics for hypertension in the elderly. N Engl J Med. 2003;348:583–92.
160. Turnbull F, Woodward M, Neal B, et al. Do men and women respond differently to blood pressure-lowering treatment? Results of prospectively designed overviews of randomized trials. Eur Heart J. 2008;29:2669–80.
161. Landsberg L, Aronne LJ, Beilin LJ, et al. Obesity-related hypertension: pathogenesis, cardiovascular risk, and treatment. A position paper of the Obesity Society and the American Society of Hypertension. J Clin Hypertens. 2013;15:14–33.
162. Weber MA, Neutel JM, Smith DH. Contrasting clinical properties and exercise responses in obese and lean hypertensive patients. J Am Coll Cardiol. 2001;37:169–74.
163. Blood Pressure Lowering Treatment Trialists' Collaboration. Effects of blood pressure lowering on cardiovascular risk according to baseline body-mass index: a meta-analysis of randomized trials. Lancet. 2015;385:867–74.

164. Weber MA, Jamerson K, Bakris GL, et al. Effects of body size and hypertension treatments on cardiovascular event rates: subanalysis of the ACCOMPLISH randomised controlled trial. Lancet. 2013;381:537–45.
165. Wassertheil-Smoller S, Fann C, Allman RM, et al. Relation of low body mass to death and stroke in the systolic hypertension in the elderly program. Arch Intern Med. 2000;160:494–500.
166. Verdecchia P, Angeli F, Borgioni C, Gattobigio R, de Simone G, Devereux RB, Porcellati C. Changes in cardiovascular risk by reduction of left ventricular mass in hypertension: a meta-analysis. Am J Hypertens. 2003;16:895–9.
167. Muiesan ML, Salvetti M, Rizzoni D, Castellano M, Donato F, Agabiti Rosei E. Association of change in left ventricular mass with prognosis during long-term antihypertensive treatment. J Hypertens. 1995;13:1091–5.
168. Koren MJ, Ulin RJ, Koren AT, Laragh JH, Devereux RB. Left ventricular mass change during treatment and outcome in patients with essential hypertension. Am J Hypertens. 2002;15:1021–8.
169. Agabiti-Rosei E, Trimarco B, Muiesan ML, Reid J, Salvetti A, Tang R, Hennig M, Baurecht H, Parati G, Mancia G, Zanchetti A, ELSA Echocardiographic Substudy Group. Cardiac structural and functional changes during long-term antihypertensive treatment with lacidipine and atenolol in the European Lacidipine Study on Atherosclerosis (ELSA). J Hypertens. 2005;23:1091–8.
170. Devereux RB, Dahlof B, Gerdts E, Boman K, Nieminen MS, Papademetriou V, Rokkedal J, Harris KE, Edelman JM, Wachtell K. Regression of hypertensive left ventricular hypertrophy by losartan compared with atenolol: the Losartan Intervention for Endpoint Reduction in Hypertension (LIFE) trial. Circulation. 2004;110:1456–62.
171. Devereux RB, Wachtell K, Gerdts E, Boman K, Nieminen MS, Papademetriou V, Rokkedal J, Harris K, Aurup P, Dahlof B. Prognostic significance of left ventricular mass change during treatment of hypertension. JAMA. 2004;292:2350–6.
172. Klingbeil AU, Schneider M, Martus P, Messerli FH, Schmieder RE. A meta-analysis of the effects of treatment on left ventricular mass in essential hypertension. Am J Med. 2003;115:41–6.
173. Terpstra WF, May JF, Smit AJ, de Graeff PA, Havinga TK, van den Veur E, Schuurman FH, Meyboom-de Jong B, Crijns HJ. Long-term effects of amlodipine and lisinopril on left ventricular mass and diastolic function in elderly, previously untreated hypertensive patients: the ELVERA trial. J Hypertens. 2001;19:303–9.
174. Devereux RB, Palmieri V, Sharpe N, De Quattro V, Bella JN, de Simone G, Walker JF, Hahn RT, Dahlof B. Effects of once-daily angiotensin-converting enzyme inhibition and calcium channel blockade-based antihypertensive treatment regimens on left ventricular hypertrophy and diastolic filling in hypertension. The Prospective Randomized Enalapril Study Evaluating Regression of Ventricular Enlargement (PRESERVE) trial. Circulation. 2001;104:1248–54.
175. Zanchetti A, Ruilope LM, Cuspidi C, Macca G, Verschuren J, Kerselaers W. Comparative effects of the ACE inhibitor fosinopril and the calcium antagonist amlodipine on left ventricular hypertrophy and urinary albumin excretion in hypertensive patients. Results of FOAM, a multicenter European study. J Hypertens. 2001;19 Suppl 2:S92 (abstract).
176. Cuspidi C, Muiesan ML, Valagussa L, Salvetti M, Di Biagio C, Agabiti-Rosei E, Magnani B, Zanchetti A, CATCH investigators. Comparative effects of candesartan and enalapril on left ventricular hypertrophy in patients with essential hypertension: the Candesartan Assessment in the Treatment of Cardiac Hypertrophy (CATCH) study. J Hypertens. 2002;20:2293–300.
177. Thurmann PA, Kenedi P, Schmidt A, Harder S, Rietbrock N. Influence of the angiotensin II antagonist valsartan on left ventricular hypertrophy in patients with essential hypertension. Circulation. 1998;98:2037–42.
178. Malmqvist K, Kahan T, Edner M, Held C, Hagg A, Lind L, Muller-Brunotte R, Nystrom F, Ohman KP, Osbakken MD, Ostergern J. Regression of left ventricular hypertrophy in human hypertension with irbesartan. J Hypertens. 2001;19:1167–76.

179. Dahlof B, Zanchetti A, Diez J, Nicholls MG, Yu CM, Barrios V, Aurup P, Smith RD, Johansson M, REGAAL Study Investigators. Effects of losartan and atenolol on left ventricular mass and neurohormonal profile in patients with essential hypertension and left ventricular hypertrophy. J Hypertens. 2002;20:1855–64.
180. Galzerano D, Tammaro P, del Viscovo L, Lama D, Galzerano A, Breglio R, Tuccillo B, Paolisso G, Capogrosso P. Three-dimensional echocardiographic and magnetic resonance assessment of the effect of telmisartan compared with carvedilol on left ventricular mass a multicenter, randomized, longitudinal study. Am J Hypertens. 2005;18:1563–9.
181. Papademetriou V, Katsiki N, Doumas M, Faselis C. Halting arterial aging in patients with cardiovascular disease: hypolipidemic and antihypertensive therapy. Curr Pharm Des. 2014;20:6339–49.
182. Tziomalos K, Athyros V, Doumas M. Do we have effective means to treat arterial stiffness and high central aortic blood pressure in patients with and without hypertension? Open Hypertens J. 2013;5:56–7.
183. Doumas M, Papademetriou V, Athyros V, Karagiannis A. Arterial stiffness and emerging biomarkers: still a long journey to go. Angiology. 2015;66:901–13.
184. Ong KT, Delerme S, Pannier B, Safar ME, Benetos A, Laurent S, Boutouyrie P. Aortic stiffness is reduced beyond blood pressure lowering by short-term and long-term antihypertensive treatment: a meta-analysis of individual data in 294 patients. J Hypertens. 2011;29:1034–42.
185. Shahin Y, Khan JA, Chetter I. Angiotensin converting enzyme inhibitors effect on arterial stiffness and wave reflections: a meta-analysis and meta-regression of randomised controlled trials. Atherosclerosis. 2012;221:18–33.
186. Karalliedde J, Smith A, De Angelis L, Mirenda V, Kandra A, Botha J, Ferber P, Viberti G. Valsartan improves arterial stiffness in type 2 diabetes independently of blood pressure lowering. Hypertension. 2008;51:1617–23.
187. Achouba A, Trunet P, Laurent S. Amlodipine-valsartan combination decreases central systolic blood pressure more effectively than the amlodipine-atenolol combination: the EXPLOR study. Hypertension. 2010;55:1314–22.
188. Doumas M, Gkaliagkousi E, Katsiki N, Reklou A, Lazaridis A, Karagiannis A. The effect of antihypertensive drugs on arterial stiffness and central hemodynamics: not all fingers are made the same. Open Hypertens J. 2013;5:75–81.
189. Mancia G, Schumacher H, Redon J, Verdecchia P, Schmieder R, Jennings G, et al. Blood pressure targets recommended by guidelines and incidence of cardiovascular and renal events in the Ongoing Telmisartan Alone and in Combination With Ramipril Global Endpoint Trial (ONTARGET). Circulation. 2011;124:1727–36.
190. Schmieder RE, Hilgers KF, Schlaich MP, Schmidt BM. Renin-angiotensin system and cardiovascular risk. Lancet. 2007;369:1208–19.
191. UKPDS Group. Tight blood pressure control and risk of macrovascular and microvascular complications in type 2 diabetes: UKPDS 38. UK Prospective Diabetes Study Group. BMJ. 1998;317:703–13.
192. Blood Pressure Lowering Treatment Trialists' Collaboration. Effects of different blood pressure-lowering regimens on major cardiovascular events in individuals with and without diabetes mellitus: results of prospectively designed overviews of randomized trials. Arch Intern Med. 2005;165:1410–9.
193. Parving HH, Brenner BM, McMurray JJV, de Zeeuw D, Haffer SM, Solomon SD. Cardiorenal endpoints in a trial of aliskiren for type 2 diabetes. N Engl J Med. 2012;367:2204–13.
194. ONTARGET Investigators. Telmisartan, ramipril, or both in patients at high risk for vascular events. N Engl J Med. 2008;358:1547–59.
195. Weber MA, Bakris GL, Jamerson K, et al. Cardiovascular events during differing hypertension therapies in patients with diabetes. J Am Coll Cardiol. 2010;56:77–85.
196. Alberti KG, Eckel RH, Grundy SM, Zimmet PZ, Cleeman JI, Donato KA, et al. Harmonizing the metabolic syndrome: a joint interim statement of the International Diabetes Federation

Task Force on Epidemiology and Prevention; National Heart, Lung and Blood Institute; American Heart Association; World Heart Federation; International Atherosclerosis Society; and International Association for the Study of Obesity. Circulation. 2009;120:1640–5.

197. Benetos A, Thomas F, Pannier B, Bean K, Jego B, Guize L. All-cause and cardiovascular mortality using the different definitions of metabolic syndrome. Am J Cardiol. 2008;102:188–91.
198. Nilsson PM, Engstrom G, Hedblad B. The metabolic syndrome and incidence of cardiovascular disease in nondiabetic subjects: a population-based study comparing three different definitions. Diabet Med. 2007;24:464–72.
199. Bakris GL, Fonseca V, Katholi RE, McGill JB, Messerli FH, Phillips RA, et al. Metabolic effects of carvedilol vs metoprolol in patients with type 2 diabetes mellitus and hypertension: a randomized controlled trial. JAMA. 2004;292:2227–36.
200. Celik T, Iyisoy A, Kursaklioglu H, Kardesoglu E, Kilic S, Turhan H, et al. Comparative effects of nebivolol and metoprolol on oxidative stress, insulin resistance, plasma adiponectin and soluble P-selectin levels in hypertensive patients. J Hypertens. 2006;24:591–6.
201. Stears AJ, Woods SH, Watts MM, Burton TJ, Graggaber J, Mir FA, Brown MJ. A double-blind, placebo-controlled, crossover trial comparing the effects of amiloride and hydrochlorothiazide on glucose tolerance in patients with essential hypertension. Hypertension. 2012;59:934–42.
202. Shafi T, Appel LJ, Miller 3rd ER, Klag MJ, Parekh RS. Changes in serum potassium mediate thiazide-induced diabetes. Hypertension. 2008;52:1022–9.
203. Gueyffier F, Boissel JP, Boutitie F, Pocock S, Coope J, Cutler J, et al. Effect of antihypertensive treatment in patients having already suffered from stroke. Gathering the evidence. The INDANA (INdividual Data ANalysis of Antihypertensive intervention trials) Project Collaborators. Stroke. 1997;28:2557–62.
204. Law MR, Morris JK, Wald NJ. Use of blood pressure lowering drugs in the prevention of cardiovascular disease: meta-analysis of 147 randomised trials in the context of expectations from prospective epidemiological studies. BMJ. 2009;338:b1665.
205. Blood Pressure Lowering Treatment Trialists' Collaboration. Effects of different blood-pressure-lowering regimens on major cardiovascular events: results of prospectively-designed overviews of randomised trials. Lancet. 2003;362:1527–35.
206. Verdecchia P, Reboldi G, Angeli F, Gattobigio R, Bentivoglio M, Thijs L, et al. Angiotensin-converting enzyme inhibitors and calcium channel blockers for coronary heart disease and stroke prevention. Hypertension. 2005;46:386–92.
207. Papademetriou V, Doumas M. Treatment strategies to prevent stroke: focus on optimal lipid and blood pressure control. Expert Opin Pharmacother. 2009;10:955–66.
208. PATS Collaborating Group. Poststroke antihypertensive treatment study. A preliminary result. Chin Med J (Engl). 1995;108:710–7.
209. PROGRESS Collaborative Group. Randomised trial of a perindopril-based blood-pressure-lowering regimen among 6105 individuals with previous stroke or transient ischaemic attack. Lancet. 2001;358:1033–41.
210. Schrader J, Luders S, Kulschewski A, Hammersen F, Plate K, Berger J, et al; MOSES Study Group. Morbidity and mortality after stroke, eprosartan compared with nitrendipine for secondary prevention: principal results of a prospective randomized controlled study (MOSES). Stroke. 2005;36:1218–26.
211. Reboldi G, Angeli F, Cavallini C, Gentile G, Mancia G, Verdecchia P. Comparison between angiotensin-converting enzyme inhibitors and angiotensin receptor blockers on the risk of myocardial infarction, stroke and death: a meta-analysis. J Hypertens. 2008;26:1282–9.
212. Yusuf S, Hawken S, Ounpuu S, Dans T, Avezum A, Lanas F, et al; INTERHEART Study Investigators. Effect of potentially modifiable risk factors associated with myocardial infarction in 52 countries (the INTERHEART study): case–control study. Lancet. 2004;364:937–52.
213. Borghi C, Bacchelli S, Degli Esposti D, Bignamini A, Magnani B, Ambrosioni E. Effects of the administration of an angiotensin converting enzyme inhibitor during the acute phase of myocardial infarction in patients with arterial hypertension. SMILE Study Investigators. Survival of Myocardial Infarction Long Term Evaluation. Am J Hypertens. 1999;12:665–72.

214. Gustafsson F, Kober L, Torp-Pedersen C, Hildebrand P, Ottesen MM, Sonne B, Carlsen J. Long-term prognosis after acute myocardial infarction in patients with a history of arterial hypertension. Eur Heart J. 1998;4:588–94.
215. Telmisartan Randomized Assessment Study in ACE intolerant subjects with cardiovascular disease (TRANSCEND) Investigators. Effects of the angiotensin-receptor blocker telmisartan on cardiovascular events in high-risk patients intolerant to angiotensin-converting enzyme inhibitors: a randomised controlled trial. Lancet. 2008;372:1174–83.
216. Yusuf S, Diener HC, Sacco RL, Cotton D, Ounpuu S, Lawton WA, et al. Telmisartan to prevent recurrent stroke and cardiovascular events. N Engl J Med. 2008;359:1225–37.
217. Massie BM, Carson PE, McMurray JJ, Komajda M, McKelvie R, Zile MR, et al. Irbesartan in patients with heart failure and preserved ejection fraction. N Engl J Med. 2008;359:2456–67.
218. Manolis A, Doumas M, Poulimenos L, Kallistratos M, Mancia G. The unappreciated importance of blood pressure in recent and older atrial fibrillation trials. J Hypertens. 2013;31:2109–17.
219. Camm AJ, Lip GY, De Caterina R, Savelieva I, Atar D, Hohnloser SH, et al. 2012 focused update of the ESC Guidelines for the management of atrial fibrillation: an update of the 2010 ESC Guidelines for the management of atrial fibrillation. Eur Heart J. 2012;33:2719–3274.
220. Wachtell K, Lehto M, Gerdts E, Olsen MH, Hornestam B, Dahlof B, et al. Angiotensin II receptor blockade reduces new-onset atrial fibrillation and subsequent stroke compared with atenolol: the Losartan Intervention For End Point Reduction in Hypertension (LIFE) study. J Am Coll Cardiol. 2005;45:712–9.
221. Schmieder RE, Kjeldsen SE, Julius S, McInnes GT, Zanchetti A, Hua TA. Reduced incidence of new-onset atrial fibrillation with angiotensin II receptor blockade: the VALUE trial. J Hypertens. 2008;26:403–11.
222. Cohn JN, Tognoni G. A randomized trial of the angiotensin-receptor blocker valsartan in chronic heart failure. N Engl J Med. 2001;345:1667–75.
223. Vermes E, Tardif JC, Bourassa MG, Racine N, Levesque S, White M, et al. Enalapril decreases the incidence of atrial fibrillation in patients with left ventricular dysfunction: insight from the Studies Of Left Ventricular Dysfunction (SOLVD) trials. Circulation. 2003;107: 2926–31.
224. Ducharme A, Swedberg K, Pfeffer MA, Cohen-Solal A, Granger CB, Maggioni AP, et al. Prevention of atrial fibrillation in patients with symptomatic chronic heart failure by candesartan in the Candesartan in Heart failure: assessment of Reduction in Mortality and morbidity(CHARM) program. Am Heart J. 2006;152:86–92.
225. Tveit A, Grundvold I, Olufsen M, Seljeflot I, Abdelnoor M, Arnesen H, Smith P. Candesartan in the prevention of relapsing atrial fibrillation. Int J Cardiol. 2007;120:85–91.
226. The GISSI-AF Investigators. Valsartan for prevention of recurrent atrial fibrillation. N Engl J Med. 2009;360:1606–17.
227. Goette A, Schon N, Kirchhof P, Breithardt G, Fetsch T, Hausler KG, et al. Angiotensin II-antagonist in paroxysmal atrial fibrillation (ANTIPAF) trial. Circ Arrhythm Electrophysiol. 2012;5:43–51.
228. The Active I Investigators. Irbesartan in patients with atrial fibrillation. N Engl J Med. 2011;364:928–38.
229. Schaer BA, Schneider C, Jick SS, Conen D, Osswald S, Meier CR. Risk for incident atrial fibrillation in patients who receive antihypertensive drugs: a nested case–control study. Ann Intern Med. 2010;152:78–84.
230. Nasr IA, Bouzamondo A, Hulot JS, Dubourg O, Le Heuzey JY, Lechat P. Prevention of atrial fibrillation onset by beta-blocker treatment in heart failure: a meta-analysis. Eur Heart J. 2007;28:457–62.
231. Swedberg K, Zannad F, McMurray JJ, Krum H, van Veldhuisen DJ, Shi H, et al; EMPHASIS-HF Study Investigators. Eplerenone and atrial fibrillation in mild systolic heart failure: results from the EMPHASIS-HF (Eplerenone in Mild Patients Hospitalization And Surv Ival Study in Heart Failure) study. J Am Coll Cardiol. 2012;59:1598–603.

Chapter 16
The J-Curve Phenomenon in Hypertension

Yuan-Yuan Kang and Ji-Guang Wang

Introduction

Almost immediately after antihypertensive therapy was proven effective in preventing cardiovascular complications [1, 2], the J-curve discussion emerged to warn the risks of low or too low blood pressure either as a physiologic or pathologic state or consequence of antihypertensive drug treatment [3, 4]. In theory, there must be a turning point of blood pressure, below which the risk of cardiovascular events increases (Fig. 16.1), because blood pressure is essential for blood perfusion of all organs, such as the brain, heart and kidneys. In the research setting, there is strong evidence that the relationship between blood pressure and cardiovascular risk is direct and strong from 115/70 mmHg of systolic/diastolic blood pressure upwards [5]. Nonetheless, studies repeatedly demonstrated a J-curve relationship between blood pressure and cardiovascular risk in various populations [6–14]. Clinical trialists attempted to address this question by randomized controlled trials [15]. Some believe that a three-group trial should be designed to prove or refute the J-curve hypothesis [16]. However, such a trial is difficult to conduct, because blood pressure separation between groups can be small and insufficient. Others designed trials to compare intensive with less intensive or the so-called standard blood pressure lowering, with [17–20] or without goals of blood pressure control [21, 22]. Such trials

Y.-Y. Kang, Ph.D.
Centre for Epidemiological Studies and Clinical Trials, Shanghai Key Laboratory of Hypertension, The Shanghai Institute of Hypertension, Ruijin Hospital, Shanghai Jiaotong University School of Medicine, Shanghai, China

J.-G. Wang, M.D., Ph.D. (✉)
Centre for Epidemiological Studies and Clinical Trials, Shanghai Key Laboratory of Hypertension, The Shanghai Institute of Hypertension, Ruijin Hospital, Shanghai Jiaotong University School of Medicine, Shanghai, China

The Shanghai Institute of Hypertension, Ruijin 2nd Road 197, Shanghai 200025, China
e-mail: jiguangwang@aim.com

E.A. Andreadis (ed.), *Hypertension and Cardiovascular Disease*,
DOI 10.1007/978-3-319-39599-9_16

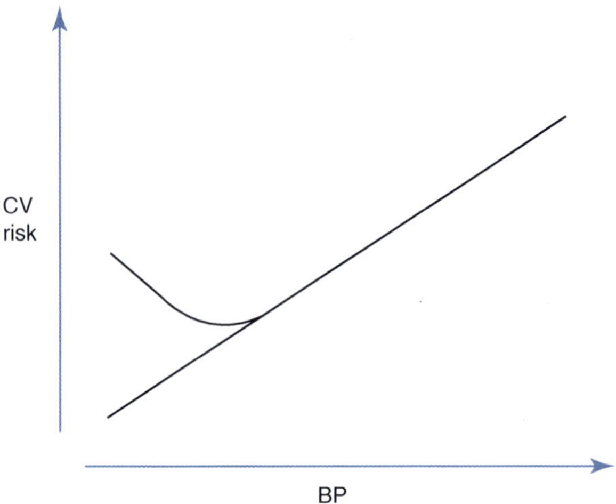

Fig. 16.1 Scheme of the J-curve phenomenon in the relationship between blood pressure (*BP*) and cardiovascular (*CV*) risk

do not help at all in answering the question "whether there is a J-curve", regardless of the results. For instance, the recently published Systolic Blood Pressure Intervention Trial (SPRINT) demonstrated benefit in the group of 120 mmHg systolic in comparison with the group of 140 mmHg [20]. However, the size of benefit was only 12 %, if heart failure would be excluded from the primary endpoint [20]. The trial cannot entirely exclude the possibility that blood pressure levels in between, for instance, 130 mmHg systolic, may offer an even greater benefit than 120 mmHg.

Until now, the J-curve issue apparently remains unresolved [16]. It is possible that the issue cannot be resolved, because the optimal blood pressure may vary between individuals, across organs, and with many conditions. Blood pressure changes over time, even within every single cardiac cycle from systole to diastole and over arteries from the central aorta to the peripheral arteries. Experts on blood pressure monitoring suggest that the wise thing to do is to measure blood pressure accurately and comprehensively by performing blood pressure monitoring in and outside the clinic and on various arterial sites. These suggestions point to future research on blood pressure lowering treatment including the J-curve issue.

In this chapter, we review the literature on the J-curve phenomenon in hypertension, discuss the concept, mechanisms and evidence and put forward current conclusions and future research.

The Concept of J-Curve Phenomenon

Although Stewart first reported higher risks of myocardial infarction in patients who achieved a diastolic blood pressure below 90 mmHg than those with a blood pressure in the range of 100–109 mmHg more than 30 years ago [3], it was Cruickshank who described the J-curve phenomenon on the incidence of myocardial infarction and on-treatment diastolic blood pressure, with the lowest incidence at diastolic blood pressure levels 85–90 mmHg [4]. The J-curve phenomenon was started with myocardial infarction for diastolic blood pressure in treated hypertension [3, 4], but expanded to total and cardiovascular mortality [12], dementia [23], stroke [24, 25], etc., to systolic blood pressure [12, 25] and to other patient [7, 13, 24, 25] or general populations [23]. However, it is clinically relevant only with treated hypertension or the use of drugs with antihypertensive action on other clinical conditions. Low blood pressure because of frailty, failing left ventricle (systolic pressure) or stiffened arteries (diastolic pressure) may be detrimental but is not really relevant for cardiovascular prevention, and hence should not be confused with the J-curve issue in the treatment of hypertension.

Plausible Mechanisms of the J-Curve Phenomenon

One general simple mechanism for the J-curve phenomenon in treated hypertension could be that the treated blood pressure is too low to perfuse sufficient amount of blood into critical organs, such as the heart, brain and kidneys. However, the threshold below which the blood perfusion decreases differs not only between individuals but also between organs within an individual. Several factors may have significant influence on the J-curve phenomenon.

First, atherosclerotic plaques may cause arterial stenosis, and decrease blood perfusion in vessels distal to the plaques. If the blood pressure is too low, the perfusion pressure in the distal arteries would be even lower, which will cause ischemia in tissues. On chronic conditions, ischemia will cause structural and functional remodeling and dysfunction. On acute conditions, for instance, ischaemia induced by abrupt blood pressure drop, ischaemic events will occur in critical organs. In the Randomized Olmesartan and Diabetes Microalbuminuria Prevention (ROADMAP) trial, although blood pressure lowering with olmesartan 40 mg daily significantly reduced the risk of microalbuminuria, it significantly increased the risk of cardiovascular mortality [22]. This increase in the risk of fatal events was mainly observed in patients with coronary heart disease and lower blood pressure at baseline [22]. This observation strongly suggests the importance of arterial stenosis in the J-curve phenomenon.

Second, the J-curve phenomenon may also depend on the feature of regional circulation. Coronary circulation is different from cerebral and renal circulation in blood flow regulation. On both cerebral and renal circulation, there is autoregulation mainly by adjusting the size of vessel diameter, but not resistance, because the peripheral resistance is generally low. However, coronary circulation has high peripheral resistance. When blood pressure is low, coronary circulation is more susceptible for the reduced perfusion pressure, especially in the presence of plaques and impaired flow reserve (Fig. 16.2) [4]. Several blood pressure lowering trials demonstrated divergent results on coronary and cerebral prevention [19, 26]. In the

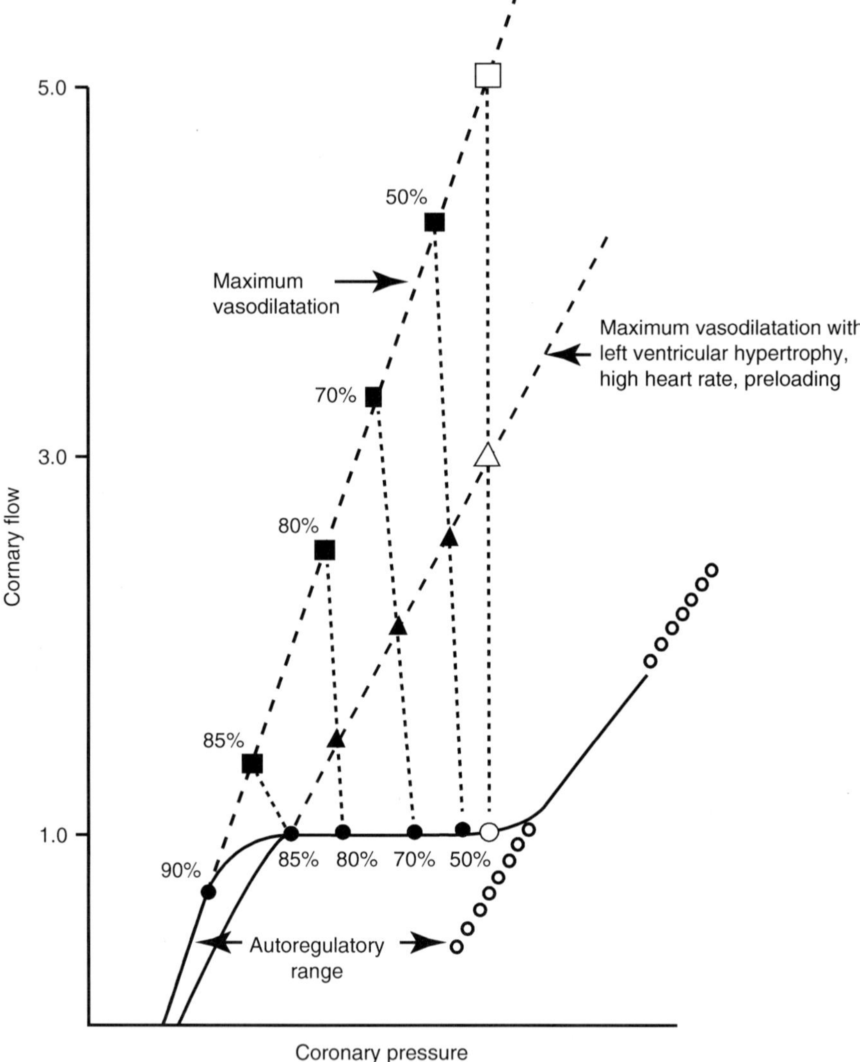

Fig. 16.2 Relationship between coronary flow and pressure at various clinical conditions (Reproduced with permission from Cruickshank et al. [4])

Action to Control Cardiovascular Risk in Diabetes (ACCORD) trial, intensive blood pressure lowering to 120 mmHg systolic, compared with 140 mmHg, significantly reduced the risk of fatal and nonfatal stroke (–41 %), but did not influence the risk of coronary events (–6 %) [19]. Similar results were observed in the Nateglinide and Valsartan in Impaired Glucose Tolerance Outcomes Research (NAVIGATOR) trial (–21 % and –3 %, respectively) [26].

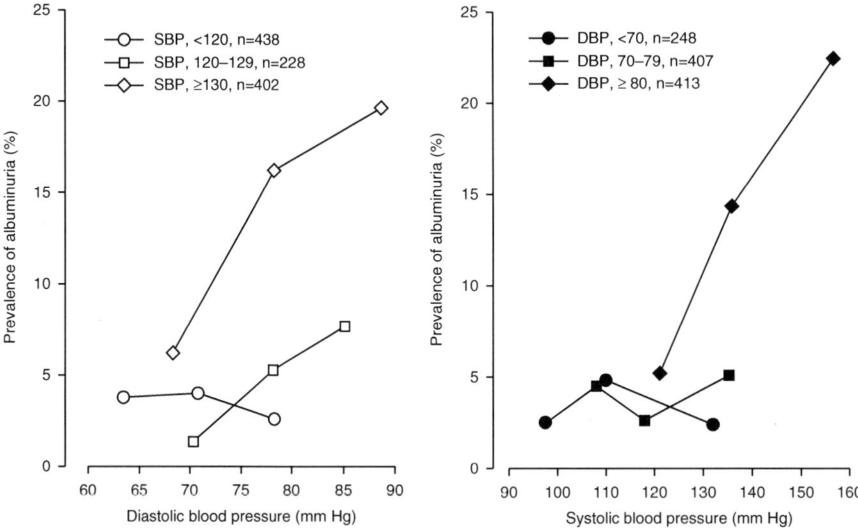

Fig. 16.3 Prevalence of albuminuria in relation to the joint effect of systolic (*SBP*) and diastolic blood pressures (*DBP*) (Reproduced with permission from Sheng et al. [27])

Third, the J-curve phenomenon may be dependent on the joint effect of systolic and diastolic pressure. Although we measure within a cardiac cycle, the highest systolic and lowest diastolic blood pressure using the current techniques, pressure changes from systole to diastole gradually and continuously. It is therefore not appropriate to discuss J curve for systolic and diastolic pressure separately. In a recent study, we investigated the single and joint effect of systolic and diastolic pressure on the risk of albuminuria [27]. We found that there was no J-curve for systolic blood pressure whenever diastolic pressure was 80 mmHg or higher, and for diastolic blood pressure whenever systolic blood pressure was 120 mmHg or higher (Fig. 16.3) [27].

Fourth, blood pressure variability may influence the J-curve phenomenon. For the diagnosis of hypertension and evaluation of antihypertensive treatment, several blood pressure readings on several occasions are averaged. However, blood pressure changes overtime (Fig. 16.4). Increased blood pressure variability can be attributable to the high as well as the low pressure values. The extreme low pressure values may induce ischaemia and ischaemic events. This phenomenon may become prominent in patients with critical diseases, such as stroke. In our recently published Intensive Blood Pressure Reduction Trial 2 (INTERACT2), intensive blood pressure lowering had modest beneficial effect on clinical outcomes in patients with acute primary intracerebral haemorrhage [28]. However, blood pressure variability was significantly associated with clinical outcomes [29], indicating an effect of not only high extreme values, but also low extreme values. Too low blood pressure might be detrimental in these critically ill patients.

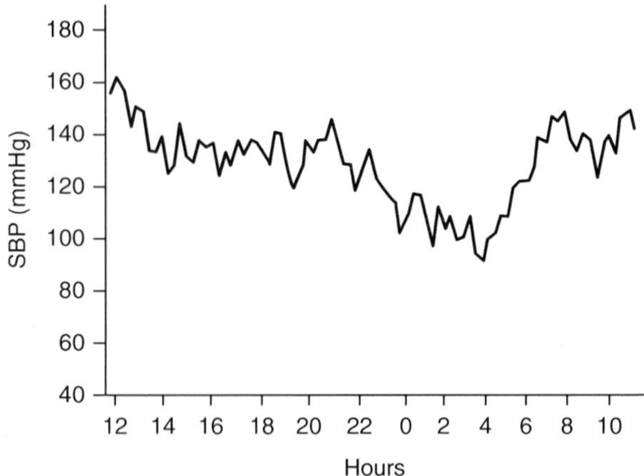

Fig. 16.4 Twenty-four-hour ambulatory blood pressure (*SBP*) profile

The Evidence of the J-Curve Phenomenon

Evidence from Randomized Controlled Trials

There is very little clinical trial evidence on the J-curve phenomenon. Nevertheless, the Hypertension Optimal Treatment (HOT) trial compared three levels of diastolic blood pressures, <90, <85 and <80 mmHg, respectively [15], and the ongoing Systolic Hypertension Optimal Trial (SHOT) trial is investigating three levels of systolic blood pressures, <145, <135 and <125 mmHg, respectively [16].

The HOT trial was published in 1998 [15]. Difference in blood pressure reduction between the three groups was small and around 2.2/2.0 mmHg between <90 and <85 mmHg groups, and 1.9/2.0 mmHg between <85 and <80 mmHg groups. For the comparisons between the three groups, statistical significance for clinical outcomes was achieved for myocardial infarction in diabetic subgroup of patients, but not in the overall study population or non-diabetic subgroup of patients or for other clinical outcomes, eg, stroke [15]. The HOT investigators had to perform post-hoc analysis to investigate the nadir level of blood pressure based on the non-randomized observational data. This post-hoc analysis demonstrated that the nadir was 138.5 mmHg systolic and 82.6 mmHg diastolic (Fig. 16.5) [15].

The SHOT trial is conducted in patients with a recent history of stroke [16]. The SHOT investigators plan to recruit 7500 patients. The recruitment is ongoing in China and European countries. It is hoped that the SHOT trial provide evidence on whether or not there is a J-curve relationship between the level of systolic blood pressure and risk of stroke in the systolic blood pressure range from 125 to 145 mmHg.

Several trials compared two levels of blood pressures, according to predefined target blood pressure [17–20] or two different treatments that led to a difference in

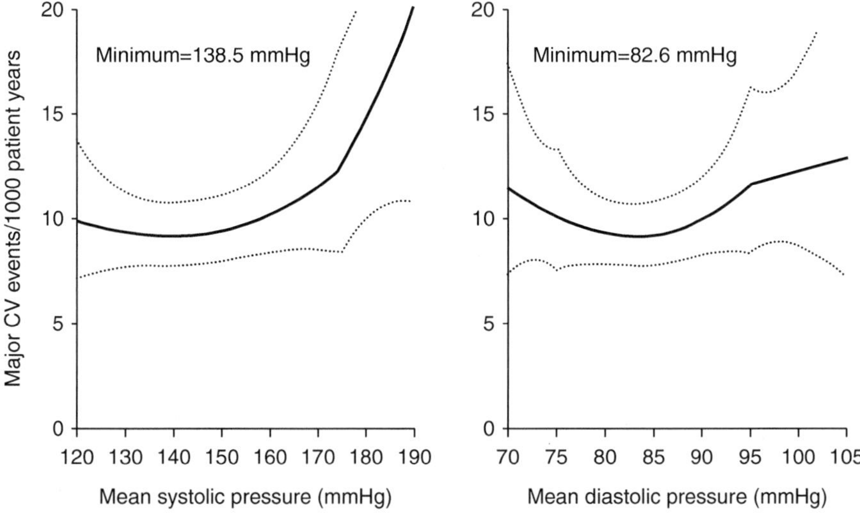

Fig. 16.5 Post-hoc analysis on the nadir level of blood pressure in the Hypertension Optimal blood pressure Trial (HOT) for major cardiovascular (*CV*) events (Reproduced with permission from Hanssen et al. [15])

blood pressure [21, 22]. However, these trials did not provide any trial evidence on the J-curve phenomenon, regardless of the results. At least three levels of blood pressures are required to show a J-curve relationship.

Evidence from Observational Studies

The J-curve phenomenon was initiated from observational studies [3, 4]. Since then, numerous studies have investigated the relationship between blood pressure and clinical outcomes. The prospective studies collaboration included 61 prospective observational studies worldwide, with 12,000 stroke deaths and 34,000 coronary deaths during 12.7 million person years of follow-up, the investigators concluded that blood pressure was strongly and directly related to vascular mortality without any evidence of a threshold down to at least 115/75 mmHg [5]. However, if the figure depicting the relationship between blood pressure and stroke and coronary deaths were scrutinized, there was indeed a J-curve relationship, especially for diastolic blood pressure. When diastolic pressure was in the lowest subgroup, the risk of stroke and coronary deaths tended to be similar as the adjacent higher blood pressure subgroup and showed a shallow J-shaped relationship [5].

Several studies did show strong J-curve phenomenon in elderly population [30] or in patients with coronary heart disease [14], diabetes mellitus [31] or chronic kidney disease [32]. The results of these studies were often confounded by reverse causality and other factors. For instance, several studies demonstrated that low blood pressure was associated with dementia [23, 33]. It is probably because demented patients have malnutrition and then low pressure. Similar mechanism may explain the J-curve relationship between blood pressure and heart failure mortality [34]. This reverse causality issue largely invalidates observational studies in the investigation of the J-curve issue [35, 36].

Observational Evidence from Antihypertensive Treatment Trials

Although this kind of analyses are still observational in nature, there are several advantages over observational studies. First, blood pressure level was mainly, though not entirely, achieved by antihypertensive treatment. Such blood pressure could be considered as treatment-induced and therefore is clinically relevant for the J-curve issue in antihypertensive therapy. Second, blood pressure was usually measured regularly and carefully. Blood pressure fluctuates substantially over time and across conditions. The more measurements obtained, the closer to the true pressure values and more precise in blood pressure evaluation. Third, the collection of information on clinical outcomes is accurate and complete. Patients enrolled in a trial were followed-up regularly. The occurrence of an event could be identified timely and the data collection could then be done within a shorter period of occurrence. Fourth, antihypertensive treatment was usually homogeneous. This excludes, to some extent, the possibility that the difference on outcomes was actually the consequence of different treatments.

Early trials included patients with high blood pressure at entry and high goal pressure during treatment. Data from these trials therefore provides very little evidence on the J-curve issue in the blood pressure ranges from 120 to 140 mmHg systolic and from 80 to 90 mmHg diastolic. Recent studies included patients with mildly elevated blood pressure or even high normal blood pressure [9, 22, 26, 37] or defined a tight goal of blood pressure control (<130/85 mmHg in the presence of diabetes mellitus or renal impairment) [8, 10, 38]. The investigators from two clinical trials performed analyses on the relationship between achieved blood pressure and clinical outcomes [8–10].

The Telmisartan Alone and in combination with Ramipril Global Endpoint Trial (ONTARGET) included 25,588 patients with coronary, peripheral, or cerebrovascular disease or diabetes mellitus [37]. Patients were treated with either telmisartan or ramipril alone or in combination from a mean systolic/diastolic blood pressure of 141.8/82.132 mmHg at baseline to approximately 132–135/76–78 mmHg during follow-up [37]. In a post-hoc analysis, patients were categorized into quartiles of systolic and diastolic blood pressure at baseline and within each quartile further into tertiles of the changes in systolic blood pressure from baseline [9]. In adjusted analyses, a J-shaped relationship was noticed in the lowest quartile of systolic blood pressure at entry (<130 mmHg) for total and cardiovascular mortality. Patients with a systolic blood pressure decrease had a significantly higher risk of total and cardiovascular morality than those with a blood pressure increase of at least 10 mmHg from baseline. In further analysis according to decile distributions of on-treatment systolic blood pressure, a J-curved relationship was seen for total and cardiovascular mortality and coronary events with a nadir level around 130 mmHg, but not for fatal and nonfatal stroke.

The International Verapamil-Trandolapril Study (INVEST) compared two antihypertensive regimens based on verapamil or atenolol, respectively, in patients with coronary heart disease [38]. The goal of blood pressure control was 140/90 mmHg or 130/85 mmHg in the absence or presence of diabetes mellitus or renal impairment. Post-hoc analyses were performed to compare clinical outcomes according to systolic blood pressure during follow-up (<130, 130–139 and ≥140 mmHg) [8, 10]. In adjusted analysis in all subjects, a J-shaped relationship was observed for all clinical outcomes except stroke, particularly for diastolic blood pressure, with a nadir at 119/84 mmHg [8]. In the subgroup of patients with diabetes mellitus, compared with patients whose systolic blood pressure during follow-up was 140 mmHg or higher, patients who achieved a lower systolic blood pressure (<140 mmHg) had significantly improved clinical outcomes. However, further lowering systolic blood pressure to a level below 130 mmHg did not provide additional health benefit [10].

Similar analyses were performed for many other antihypertensive treatment trials [39, 40]. The results of these analyses were similar, indicating a nadir level of approximately 130 mmHg systolic and 80 mmHg diastolic. Further reducing blood pressure to an even lower level either had no further benefit or increased the risks of clinical outcomes.

Conclusions and Future Perspectives

Although there is very little clinical trial evidence on the J-curve issue, there is abundant observational evidence indicating a nadir level of blood pressure below which blood pressure lowering might be detrimental. The currently ongoing SHOT trial might provide more evidence on this issue for fatal and nonfatal stroke, and probably also for other clinical outcomes. However, the optimal blood pressure might be different between individuals and across outcomes. Indeed, 120 mmHg of systolic pressure compared with 140 mmHg might prevent stroke in diabetic patients and heart failure in non-diabetic patients. However, it is probably too naive to attempt to find a universal optimal blood pressure level for all patients. Nonetheless, it is probably possible to find a universal beneficial blood pressure level for most hypertensive patients. If we would continue defining hypertension as a blood pressure of at least 140 mmHg systolic and 90 mmHg diastolic, 130/80 mmHg might be beneficial to most patients. This hypothesis should be investigated in future randomized controlled trials that compares 130 mmHg with 140 mmHg of systolic pressure with the use of modern blood pressure measuring techniques, such as ambulatory and home blood pressure monitoring.

References

1. Veterans Administration Cooperative Study Group on Antihypertensive Agents. Effects of treatment on morbidity in hypertension. Results in patients with diastolic blood pressures averaging 115 through 129 mm Hg. JAMA. 1967;202:1028–34.
2. Veterans Administration Cooperative Study Group on Antihypertensive Agents. Effects of treatment on morbidity in hypertension. II. Results in patients with diastolic blood pressure averaging 90 through 114 mm Hg. JAMA. 1970;213:1143–52.
3. Stewart IMG. Relation of reduction in pressure to first myocardial infarction in patients receiving treatment for severe hypertension. Lancet. 1979;313:861–5.
4. Cruickshank J, Thorp J, Zacharias FJ. Benefits and potential harm of lowering high blood pressure. Lancet. 1987;329:581–4.
5. Prospective Studies Collaboration. Age-specific relevance of usual blood pressure to vascular-mortality: a meta-analysis of individual data for one million adults in 61 prospective studies. Lancet. 2002;360:1903–13.
6. D'Agostino RB, Belanger AJ, Kannel WB, Cruickshank JM. Relation of low diastolic blood pressure to coronary heart disease death in presence of myocardial infarction: the Framingham Study. BMJ. 1991;303:385–9.
7. Boutitie F, Gueyffier F, Pocock S, Fagard R, Boissel JP. J-shaped relationship between blood pressure and mortality in hypertensive patients: new insights from a meta-analysis of individual-patient data. Ann Intern Med. 2002;136:438–48.
8. Messerli FH, Mancia G, Conti CR, Hewkin AC, Kupfer S, Champion A, Kolloch R, Benetos A, Pepine CJ. Dogma disputed: can aggressively lowering blood pressure in hypertensive patients with coronary artery disease be dangerous? Ann Intern Med. 2006;144:884–93.
9. Sleight P, Redon J, Verdecchia P, Mancia G, Gao P, Fagard R, Schumacher H, Weber M, Bohm M, Williams B, Pogue J, Koon T, Yusuf S. Prognostic value of blood pressure in patients with high vascular risk in the Ongoing Telmisartan Alone and in combination with Ramipril Global Endpoint Trial study. J Hypertens. 2009;27:1360–9.
10. Cooper-DeHoff RM, Gong Y, Handberg EM, Bavry AA, Denardo SJ, Bakris GL, Pepine CJ. Tight blood pressure control and cardiovascular outcomes among hypertensive patients with diabetes and coronary artery disease. JAMA. 2010;304:61–8.
11. Bangalore S, Qin J, Sloan S, Murphy SA, Cannon CP. What is the optimal blood pressure in patients after acute coronary syndromes? Relationship of blood pressure and cardiovascular events in the Pravastatin or Atorvastatin Evaluation and Infection Therapy-Thrombolysis in Myocardial Infarction (PROVE IT-TIMI) 22 Trial. Circulation. 2010;122:2142–51.
12. Bangalore S, Messerli FH, Wun CC, Zuckerman AL, DeMicco D, Kostis JB, LaRosa JC. J-curve revisited: an analysis of blood pressure and cardiovascular events in the Treating to New Targets (TNT) Trial. Eur Heart J. 2010;31:2897–908.
13. Anderson RJ, Bahn GD, Moritz TE, Kaufman D, Abraira C, Duckworth W. Blood pressure and cardiovascular disease risk in the Veterans Affairs Diabetes Trial. Diabetes Care. 2011;34:34–8.
14. Dorresteijn JA, van der Graaf Y, Spiering W, Grobbee DE, Bots ML, Visseren FL, Secondary Manifestations of Arterial Disease Study Group. Relation between blood pressure and vascular events and mortality in patients with manifest vascular disease: J-curve revisited. Hypertension. 2012;59:14–21.
15. Hansson L, Zanchetti A, Carruthers SG, Dahlof B, Elmfeldt D, Julius S, Ménard J, Rahn KH, Wedel H, Westerling S. Effects of intensive blood-pressure lowering and low-dose aspirin in patients with hypertension: principal results of the Hypertension Optimal Treatment (HOT) randomised trial. Lancet. 1998;351:1755–62.
16. Zanchetti A, Liu L, Mancia G, Parati G, Grassi G, Stramba-Badiale M, Silani V, Bilo G, Corrao G, Zambon A, Scotti L, Zhang X, Wang H, Zhang Y, Zhang X, Guan TR, Berge E, Redon J, Narkiewicz K, Dominiczak A, Nilsson P, Viigimaa M, Laurent S, Agabiti-Rosei E, Wu Z, Zhu D, Rodicio JL, Ruilope LM, Martell-Claros N, Pinto F, Schmieder RE, Burnier M, Banach M,

Cifkova R, Farsang C, Konradi A, Lazareva I, Sirenko Y, Dorobantu M, Postadzhiyan A, Accetto R, Jelakovic B, Lovic D, Manolis AJ, Stylianou P, Erdine S, Dicker D, Wei G, Xu C, Xie H, Coca A, O'Brien J, Ford G. Blood pressure and LDL-cholesterol targets for prevention of recurrent strokes and cognitive decline in the hypertensive patient: design of the European Society of Hypertension-Chinese Hypertension League Stroke in Hypertension Optimal Treatment randomized trial. J Hypertens. 2014;32:1888–97.

17. The JATOS Study Group. Principal results of the Japanese Trial to Assess Optimal Systolic Blood Pressure in Elderly Hypertensive Patients (JATOS). Hypertens Res. 2008;31:2115–27.
18. Ogihara T, Saruta T, Rakugi H, Matsuoka H, Shimamoto K, Shimada K, Imai Y, Kikuchi K, Ito S, Eto T, Kimura G, Imaizumi T, Takishita S, Ueshima H, Valsartan in Elderly Isolated Systolic Hypertension Study Group. Target blood pressure for treatment of isolated systolic hypertension in the elderly: valsartan in elderly isolated systolic hypertension study. Hypertension. 2010;56:196–202.
19. The ACCORD Study Group. Effects of intensive blood-pressure control in type 2 diabetes mellitus. N Engl J Med. 2010;362:1575–85.
20. The SPRINT Research Group. A randomized trial of intensive versus standard blood-pressure control. N Engl J Med. 2015;373:2103–16.
21. The ADVANCE Collaborative Group. Effects of a fixed combination of perindopril and indapamide on macrovascular and microvascular outcomes in patients with type 2 diabetes mellitus (the ADVANCE trial): a randomized controlled trial. Lancet. 2007;370:829–40.
22. Haller H, Ito S, Izzo Jr JL, Januszewicz A, Katayama S, Menne J, Mimran A, Rabelink TJ, Ritz E, Ruilope LM, Rump LC, Viberti G, ROADMAP Trial Investigators. Olmesartan for the delay or prevention of microalbuminuria in type 2 diabetes. N Engl J Med. 2011;364:907–17.
23. Guo Z, Viitanen M, Fratiglioni L, Winblad B. Low blood pressure and dementia in elderly people: the Kungsholmen project. BMJ. 1996;312:805–8.
24. Irie K, Yamaguchi T, Minematsu K, Omae T. The J-curve phenomenon in stroke recurrence. Stroke. 1993;24:1844–9.
25. Rothwell PM, Howard SC, Spence JD, Carotid Endarterectomy Trialists' Collaboration. Relationship between blood pressure and stroke risk in patients with symptomatic carotid occlusive disease. Stroke. 2003;34:2583–90.
26. The NAVIGATOR Study Group. Effect of valsartan on the incidence of diabetes and cardiovascular events. N Engl J Med. 2010;362:1477–90.
27. Sheng CS, Liu M, Zou J, Huang QF, Li Y, Wang JG. Albuminuria in relation to the single and combined effects of systolic and diastolic blood pressure in Chinese. Blood Press. 2013;22:158–64.
28. Anderson CS, Heeley E, Huang Y, Wang J, Stapf C, Delcourt C, Lindley R, Robinson T, Lavados P, Neal B, Hata J, Arima H, Parsons M, Li Y, Wang J, Heritier S, Li Q, Woodward M, Simes RJ, Davis SM, Chalmers J, the INTERACT2 Investigators. Rapid blood-pressure lowering in patients with acute intracerebral hemorrhage. N Engl J Med. 2013;368:2355–65.
29. Manning L, Hirakawa Y, Arima H, Wang X, Chalmers J, Wang J, Lindley R, Heeley E, Delcourt C, Neal B, Lavados P, Davis SM, Tzourio C, Huang Y, Stapf C, Woodward M, Rothwell PM, Robinson TG, Anderson CS, INTERACT2 Investigators. Blood pressure variability and outcome after acute intracerebral haemorrhage: a post-hoc analysis of INTERACT2, a randomised controlled trial. Lancet Neurol. 2014;13:364–73.
30. Tervahauta M, Pekkanen J, Enlund H, Nissinen A. Change in blood pressure and 5-year risk of coronary heart disease among elderly men: the Finnish cohorts of the Seven Countries Study. J Hypertens. 1994;12:1183–9.
31. Sundström J, Sheikhi R, Ostgren CJ, Svennblad B, Bodegård J, Nilsson PM, Johansson G. Blood pressure levels and risk of cardiovascular events and mortality in type-2 diabetes: cohort study of 34 009 primary care patients. J Hypertens. 2013;31:1603–10.
32. Kovesdy CP, Lu JL, Molnar MZ, Ma JZ, Canada RB, Streja E, Kalantar-Zadeh K, Bleyer AJ. Observational modeling of strict vs. conventional blood pressure control in patients with chronic kidney disease. JAMA Intern Med. 2014;174:1442–9.

33. Razay G, Williams J, King E, Smith AD, Wilcock G. Blood pressure, dementia and Alzheimer's disease: the OPTIMA longitudinal study. Dement Geriatr Cogn Disord. 2009;28:70–4.
34. Lee DS, Ghosh N, Floras JS, Newton GE, Austin PC, Wang X, Liu PP, Stukel TA, Tu JV. Association of blood pressure at hospital discharge with mortality in patients diagnosed with heart failure. Circ Heart Fail. 2009;2:616–23.
35. Witteman JC, Grobbee DE, Valkenburg HA, van Hemert AM, Stijnen T, Burger H, Hofman A. J-shaped relation between change in diastolic blood pressure and progression of aortic atherosclerosis. Lancet. 1994;343:504–7.
36. Flack JM, Neaton J, Grimm Jr R, Shih J, Cutler J, Ensrud K, MacMahon S. Blood pressure and mortality among men with prior myocardial infarction: Multiple Risk Factor Intervention Trial Research Group. Circulation. 1995;92:2437–45.
37. The ONTARGET Investigators. Telmisartan, ramipril, or both in patients at high risk for vascular events. N Engl J Med. 2008;358:1547–59.
38. Pepine CJ, Handberg EM, Cooper-DeHoff RM, Marks RG, Kowey P, Messerli FH, Mancia G, Cangiano JL, Garcia-Barreto D, Keltai M, Erdine S, Bristol HA, Kolb HR, Bakris GL, Cohen JD, Parmley WW. A calcium antagonist versus a non-calcium antagonist hypertension treatment strategy for patients with coronary artery disease. The International Verapamil-Trandolapril Study (INVEST): a randomized controlled trial. JAMA. 2003;290:2805–16.
39. Mancia G, Kjeldsen SE, Zappe DH, Holzhauer B, Hua TA, Zanchetti A, Julius S, Weber MA. Cardiovascular outcomes at different on-treatment blood pressures in the hypertensive patients of the VALUE trial. Eur Heart J. 2016;37:955–64. pii: ehv633.
40. Okin PM, Hille DA, Kjeldsen SE, Dahlöf B, Devereux RB. Impact of lower achieved blood pressure on outcomes in hypertensive patients. J Hypertens. 2012;30:802–10.

Chapter 17
Follow-Up of the Hypertensive Patients with Cardiovascular Disease

Carmine Morisco, Bruno Trimarco, and Giovanni de Simone

Arterial hypertension is one of the most important independent risk factor for cardiovascular (CV) diseases [1]. Subjects with hypertension are exposed to high risk of coronary artery disease (CHD), stroke, peripheral artery disease, heart failure, kidney disease and a number of "soft" adverse manifestation of CV disease, including transitory ischemic attack, atrial fibrillation and other supraventricular arrhythmias [2, 3].

The occurrence of CV events in hypertensive patients is directly related to the hemodynamic burden, due to the increased pressure overload, but also depends on neuro-hormonal and metabolic abnormalities that are associated with hypertension, favoring development and evolution of the arteriosclerotic disease [4]. The progression of arterial hypertension toward the most severe stages of CV disease, terminating with major CV events, occurs through an intermediate step, which is the time when target organ damage develops in a condition in which the hypertensive patient is clinically silent, except for high blood pressure (BP). This step can be defined "preclinical CV disease" [5] and is of strategic importance to reduce the burden of the clinically-overt hypertension-related CV disease (Fig. 17.1).

This progression involves early alterations in CV structure and function, including asymptomatic atherosclerosis, vascular hypertrophy and thickening, development of left ventricular (LV) geometric changes, with or without increase in LV mass, and chronic kidney disease (microalbuminuria and reduced glomerular filtration rate). High BP promotes the acceleration of age-related CV remodeling, favoring development of concentric LV remodeling or hypertrophy [6] and stiffening of conductance arteries [7].

The structural phenotype of hypertensive heart disease includes many different LV geometric patterns and several vascular abnormalities, all longitudinally associated with major CV events [8–13].

C. Morisco, M.D. • B. Trimarco, M.D. • G. de Simone, M.D., FESC, FACC, FAHA (✉)
Hypertension Research Center, FEDERICO II University Naples, Naples, Italy
e-mail: simogi@unina.it

E.A. Andreadis (ed.), *Hypertension and Cardiovascular Disease*,
DOI 10.1007/978-3-319-39599-9_17

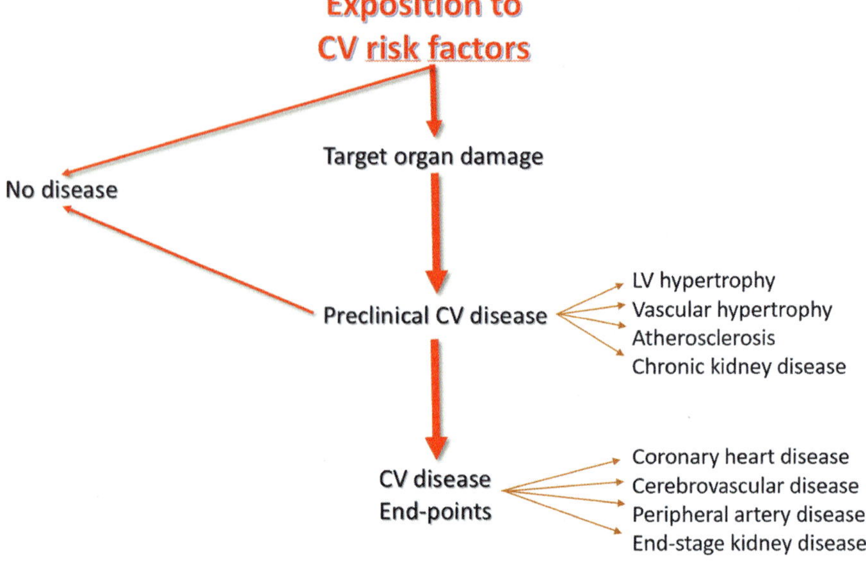

Fig. 17.1 Time course of the natural history of cardiovascular disease from exposition to CV risk factors to the end-points. Thickness of the *arrows* expresses the probability of evolution (From EACVI guidelines (These guidelines should be published by the end of 2016 and should be added to the references, if timing will be consistent), adapted from Ref. [5])

The diagnostic and therapeutic strategies in hypertensive patients must consider all determinants of CV risk, such as the severity of hypertension, the presence and the number of the other conventional cardiovascular (CV) risk factors, target organ damage, as well as prevalent CV disease, the presence of metabolic syndrome, diabetes and/or chronic kidney disease.

In this chapter, we will examine the hemodynamic and circulating markers of CV risk, focusing on secondary prevention. More detailed suggestions will also be given for specific major CV events, with indications on the most appropriate way to implement good secondary prevention programs. Most indications are presumed from current recommendations and guidelines [14–16], but also empirical, albeit reasonable suggestions are given.

General Parameters to Monitor for Follow-Up

In contrast with the goal of primary prevention, hypertensive patients with prevalent CV disease are at high risk of new major CV events and do not require direct risk stratification by the current risk-scores [17]. They require aggressive treatment, to achieve optimal control of both BP and associated markers of CV risk. Thus, follow-up of hypertensive patients with prevalent CV disease should be articulated in three directions:

1. Optimal control of blood pressure;
2. Reduction of impact of associated CV risk factors, with special emphasis on obesity.
3. Regression (or reduction) of target organ damage.

These goals can be achieved by careful clinical monitoring of management effect (including therapy and life style modifications) and using both CV imaging technologies and circulating biomarkers [18, 19].

BP Control

Uncontrolled arterial hypertension worsens the prognosis of prevalent CV disease [20]. There is little specific recommendation for the control of BP after a major CV event. The traditional indication to reduce systolic BP below 140 mmHg and diastolic BP below 90 mmHg has been changed in the most recent guidelines, which suggest forcing BP below 130/80 mmHg in some circumstances [14–16, 21]. This recommendation is now reinforced by the evidence that a tight BP control to values below 130/80 mmHg might be a better strategy also for primary prevention [22, 23]. Although there is not yet general agreement on this strategy, following the results of the SPRINT trial [23], the most recent AHA/ACC/ASH Scientific Statement [24], report that reducing "< 130/80 mm Hg may be appropriate, especially in patients with a history of a previous myocardial infarction or stroke, or at high risk for developing either". As suggested, most of these results extracted from clinical trials need also "external validation" [25], by observational reports on large-scale registries in real-world contexts, to definitively force these new optimal limits to get into clinical practice [26].

Given the importance of BP control in the context of secondary prevention, procedures additional to the office BP recording are particularly needed. The most practical way to achieve this goal is the home-measurement of BP, possibly performed early in the morning, to capture the BP morning surge [27], using automated and validated arm-devices, which are less prone to method errors than the usual aneroid sphygmomanometers [28, 29]. Although the meaning of morning surge might change in relation to age and biological conditions [30], when there is significant discrepancy between home and office BP measurement, 24 h ambulatory blood pressure monitoring might be required [31]. Development of innovative technologies allows the remote control of BP, throughout electronic communication (SMS, e-mail, or direct automated telecommunication). New technologies can allow a better management of hypertension especially in high-risk patients. If physician's counseling and patient's reporting are effective, BP measurement in the outpatient clinic becomes much less important than in the past, and should be programmed based on the major CV clinical condition.

Reduction of Impact of Associated CV Risk Factors

Arterial hypertension is most often combined with other CV risk factors. More than 80 % of hypertensive patients present with additional comorbidities, including glucose intolerance, hyperinsulinemia, lipid disorders (reduced HDL-cholesterol and increased LDL-cholesterol and triglycerides), obesity and metabolic syndrome [32–35], which are associated with increased CV morbidity and mortality. More than 50 % of hypertensive patients present at least two of these comorbidities and, generally, one of those is obesity [35]. Obesity is an important risk factor also for incident hypertension, especially in women [36, 37]. When combined with arterial hypertension, obesity exponentially increases the chance of harmful LV modifications: the probability of LVH sharply raises when hypertension is associated with obesity [38, 39], and is independently related to central fat distribution (Fig. 17.2).

In the presence of obesity, control of BP is particularly difficult [40, 41], and, even worse, regression of LV hypertrophy (LVH) is obtained with more difficulty, even when BP is controlled [42, 43]. Obesity also tracks insulin resistance, high risk of diabetes and inflammatory status, all factors that substantially worsen prognosis of patients with prevalent CV disease.

Obesity is, therefore, a critical condition to manage especially when CV risk is already very high, as in patients with prevalent CV disease. Appropriate counseling and diet should be integral part of management of arterial hypertension and physical exercise programs should be implemented, whenever possible. Attention should also be paid to type of therapy, as suggested in observational studies [41], as discussed in the next sections.

Regression (or Reduction) of Target Organ Damage

There are three "windows" through which the status of target organ can be monitored during follow-up: kidney, left ventricle and conduit arteries [5].

Microalbuminuria

Microalbuminuria assessment, either as albumin excretion in a 24-h urine collection or albumin-to-creatinine ratio in a random spot urine collection [44], was introduced as a predictor of impaired renal function among diabetic patients, but is also a potent marker of hypertensive target organ damage, associated with increased CV morbidity and mortality [45–47]. Prevalence of microalbuminuria in non-diabetic

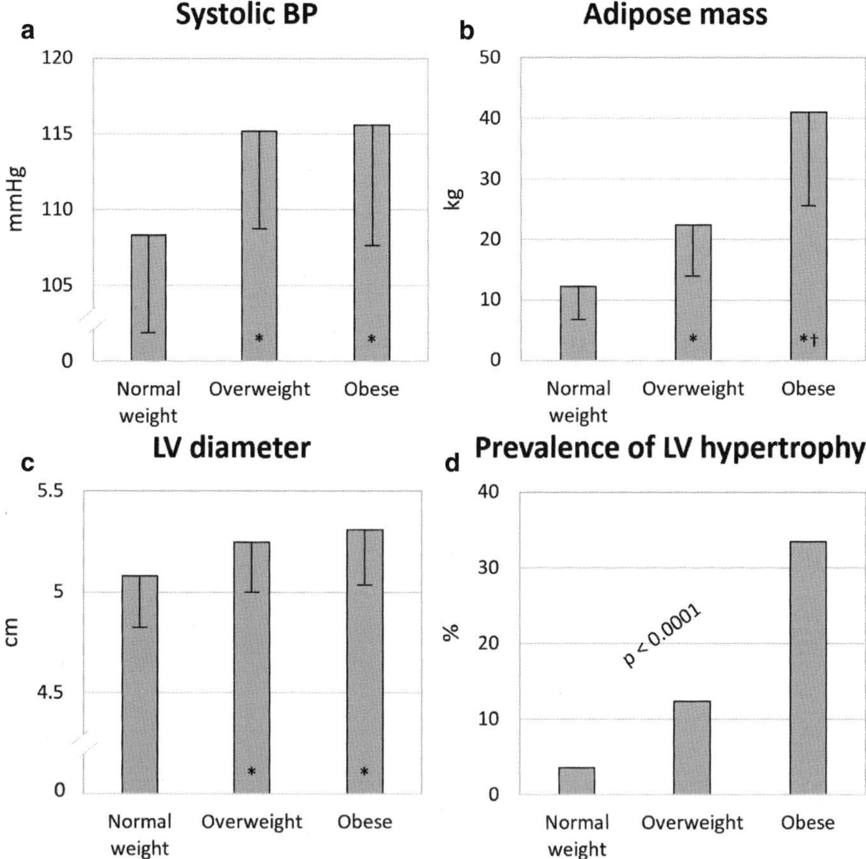

Fig. 17.2 Systolic blood pressure (BP, Panel **a**), adipose mass (Panel **b**), left ventricular (LV) diastolic diameter (Panel **c**) and prevalence of LVH (Panel **d**) in normal weight (n = 114), overweight (n = 113) and obese adolescents (n = 223). Note that prevalence of LVH follows the excess of adipose mass, more than BP or LV chamber dimension (Adapted from Ref. [38])

patients with hypertension is in general 8–15 %, but this prevalence varies in the literature, according to both differences in the methods used to detect it and the heterogeneity of the patients included in the different studies [45]. Similar to ECG, detection of microalbuminuria is cheap and widely available, and should be part of the first-line tools for the stratification of CV risk in patients with essential hypertension [45]. Given its sensitivity to BP, assessment of microalbuminuria might be particularly helpful in the context of high-risk patients, to monitor the effects of anti-hypertensive therapy on target organ. In addition microalbuminuria is also associated with a number of other markers of increased CV risk, including endothelial dysfunction, insulin resistance, vascular inflammation, hypercoagulability, and mechanical stress [48, 49], though not necessarily these associations fully explain the increased rate of microalbuminuria-associated CV event. It is reasonable to infer that microalbuminuria is expression of different degrees of CV damage. Given the cheap cost of evaluation of the albumin-to-creatinine ratio in a random spot urine sample [44], assessment of microalbuminuria can be scheduled frequently in high-risk patients.

LV Mass

LV mass is the most potent predictor of adverse outcome in arterial hypertension, an evidence especially due to conventional 2D echocardiography, and more recently confirmed with more accurate technologies [8, 9]. Assessment of LVH and other markers of target organ damage significantly improves risk stratification produced by conventional risk factors [10, 11], even in the context of secondary prevention [50]. Assessment of LV mass is profitably associated with evaluation of LV geometry by computation of relative wall thickness (or LV mass/volume ratio) and LV end-diastolic volume [8, 9].

Despite the intrinsic limits of 2D echocardiography, LV mass can be measured and monitored in the single patient, pending a critical evaluation of the test-retest changes [51].

Together with information on LV geometry, echocardiographic follow-up also provides data on left atrial volume (or dimension), LV systolic and diastolic function, all parameters variably associated with adverse prognosis, though not necessarily independent of the magnitude of estimated LV mass [52]. However, in specific context of secondary prevention, these additional parameters might have substantial importance as will be detailed in the next sections.

Carotid Intima-Media Thickness (CIMT)

Carotid intima-media thickness (CIMT) is another critical marker of target organ damage. Increased CIMT and, to a greater extend, evidence of carotid plaque are associated with increased risk of CV events, independently of risk factors [53, 54]. Similar to LVH, carotid plaque significantly improves risk stratification produced by conventional risk factors [11, 54]. Whether evaluation of carotid artery adds to models of risk, including assessment of LV geometry is unclear. However, not necessarily patients with high LV mass have increased carotid intima-media thickness (and vice-versa), and there is evidence that CV risk increases with increasing number of target organ damages. Accordingly, multi-organ evaluation is recommended to improve risk stratification.

With appropriate imaging technique, the plaque progression or regression can be documented [55, 56], and follow-up scheduled according to the clinical needs. However, because treatment-induced changes in left ventricular mass and carotid artery wall thickness are slow, guidelines suggest to perform these examinations not before than 1 year intervals [21].

Specific Strategies for Secondary Prevention

In this section, we will examine the major manifestations of CV disease occurring during the natural history of arterial hypertension: myocardial infarction (coronary heart disease), heart failure and stroke, which require specific attention during follow-up.

Hypertension and Coronary Heart Disease (CHD)

Follow-up of patients with CHD is more difficult in the presence of hypertension. The final goal of a correct follow-up is prevention of new CHD episodes. To achieve this goal, management of hypertension and associated conditions (obesity, dyslipidemia, glucose intolerance) should be sufficiently aggressive to obtain adequate risk factors control.

In patients with previous myocardial infarction or unstable angina, new episodes of ischemia might be silent, with impact on outcome [57], though an extensive evaluation in patients without symptomatic modifications of their clinical status is not recommended [58]. Controls with more sensitive techniques beyond the routine resting ECG may be scheduled, whenever the clinical conditions suggest that some change could have occurred, including symptoms that might be considered as equivalent to angina, such as shortness of breath, dizziness, palpitations, or even tiredness in unusual contexts.

In the context of arterial hypertension, discrimination of silent ischemia by simple exercise-ECG might be even more difficult, due to high possibility of false positive results due to the coexistence of LVH [58, 59].

However, in the presence of arterial hypertension and LVH, a negative exercise-ECG has a very high negative predictive value. Therefore, a negative maximal exercise-ECG can exclude with substantial margin of confidence the presence of residual ischemia and perform as the first step in a more extensive diagnostic protocol, whenever possible for the conditions of the patients.

When doubts remain, due to ambiguous or positive exercise ECG, in the absence of angina, CV imaging techniques are extremely useful and important. If the clinical conditions suggest a screening more extensive than with ECG and exercise ECG, exercise or pharmacological stress echocardiography may be indicated, especially in elderly women in whom the possibility of false positive is higher even independently of the presence of LVH [58, 60]. Stress-echocardiography exhibit substantially higher specificity than exercise ECG in hypertensive patients with LVH for the identification of coronary epicardial lesions [59, 61], though coronary microvascular disease might be better identified by radionuclide single photon emission computed tomography (SPECT) [62, 63]. Coronary microvascular lesions might be also identified by performing high-dose dipyridamole challenge and recording of Doppler-signal of the left anterior descending artery for evaluation of coronary blood flow reserve [64, 65], in the absence of epicardial lesions. However, this technique is not widely available and requires highly skilled echocardiography laboratories.

In general, the limitation of the stress-echocardiography procedures is the high operator dependency, though the new technologies of strain imaging (Speckle Tracking Echocardiography) are likely to attenuate the inter-observer variability. Thus, the choice of imaging method depends on indications, type of available facility, and the experience of the laboratories.

Sometimes, when the indication for a new coronary angiography is borderline [66], 64-layer-computed tomography (CT) of the coronary arteries has specificity and sensitivity ≈ 90 % in the diagnosis of coronary artery atheroma in all coronary segments, except for the circumflex coronary artery and the distal segments of the vessels. The positive and negative predictive value are very high, 91–93 % and 96–100 %, respectively. This method also allows visualization of the vessel wall and the presence of calcifications. However, the emission of ionizing radiation and the high cost limit its use as a screening method, and indication needs to be very strict [67].

Hypertension and Heart Failure (HF)

In hypertensive patients, the definition of HF needs particular attention. Most patients are chronically in stage B HF, but many of them may be classified in stage C or even D, independently of their clinical symptoms [68]. According to the AHA/ACC classification [68], all hypertensive patients with LVH are at least in class C and may be classified as "chronic HF", or LV dysfunction. LV dysfunction may be, therefore, assimilated to a condition of compensated HF. Decompensation can occur in the presence of reduced (HFrEF) or preserved ejection fraction (HFpEF). In either condition, the common characteristic is the elevation of LV filling pressure and end-diastolic wall stress, needed to sustain stroke volume.

Hypertension is the most prevalent major risk factor among individuals who move from asymptomatic LV dysfunction to decompensated HF [69]. Such a high incidence occurs because of both the direct hemodynamic burden imposed by hypertension and the evolution of hypertension toward HF, which can follow two different pathways, either through CHD or directly without the intermediate step of CHD (Fig. 17.3). Prevention of episodes of decompensated HF requires optimal management of CV risk factors, including optimal BP control [68], and a clear focus on the objectives to achieve, also in relation to the phenotypical presentation of HF, as shown in Fig. 17.3.

Figure 17.3 also provides a pathophysiologic explanation of why does the coexistence of hypertension and CHD increase risk of HF. Neuro-hormonal activation and promotion of early ventricular remodeling are at the basis of mechanisms of evolution from hypertension to HF. The relation between hypertension and HFrEF is usually mediated by CHD. More interesting is the evidence that hypertension plays a key direct role in the incidence of HFpEF. The prevalence of HFpEF is rap-

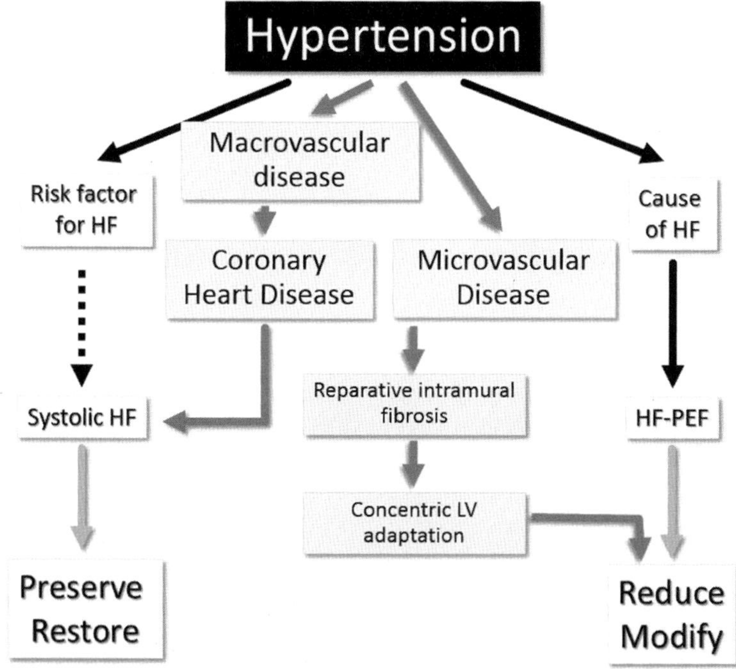

Fig. 17.3 Pathway of the progression of hypertension toward heart failure (HF). The *black arrows* indicate the two main pathways; the *dark grey arrows* indicate mechanisms; the *light gray arrows* indicate the strategies of management in relation to vital myocardium

idly rising [70], paralleling the decline of HFrEF, substantially related to the increase of the procedures of rescue revascularization after acute myocardial infarction [71]. HFpEF exhibit morbidity, mortality, hospitalizations and healthcare costs at least comparable to, and perhaps greater than HFrEF [72]. Unfortunately, while prevention of decompensation is effective in the presence of HFrEF, the results on HFpEF are still doubtful [73, 74].

HFpEF occurs in elderly, predominantly female hypertensive patients, with small-chamber hypertrophied hearts and a high prevalence of type 2 diabetes mellitus, and atrial fibrillation. The association between essential hypertension and LV dysfunction has been described in observational studies since 1950. Although the pathophysiologic abnormalities present in HFpEF include many specific features, Table 17.1 shows that the diagnosis of HFpEF might be difficult. Even more than with HFrEF, HFpEF requires clinical criteria, but echocardiography is of great importance for the ability to detect all abnormalities characteristic of this syndrome and focus attention on specific morphologic and/or functional alterations that might require careful monitoring. In the absence of specific indication to prevent decompensation, effective hypertension control remains the hallmark of the management of every presentation of HF, which has received supportive evidence over the past decades [73, 75–77].

Table 17.1 Pathophysiology of HFpEF and measurable abnormalities

Pathophysiology	Measurable abnormality
Diastolic dysfunction	↑LV filling pressure
Abnormal vascular-ventricular coupling	↑Effective arterial elastance
LV systolic dysfunction	↓Midwall shortening ↓Longitudinal strain
Chronotropic incompetence	↓Exercise cardiac output
Impaired vasodilator reserve	↓Coronary blood flow reserve
Reduced left atrial function	↓Left atrial systolic force
Volume overload	↑Stroke volume

Thus, echocardiographic monitoring of specific hemodynamic and functional abnormalities might be particularly useful in HFpEF, because no specific therapy is available to prevent decompensation [68]. Characteristics of hemodynamic loading conditions, LV geometry and filling pressure may force to a more aggressive management with specific classes of medications [8]. For instance, evidence of a rising LV filling pressure, even in the absence of dyspnea might suggest use of small doses of loop-diuretics and/or mineralocorticoid receptor antagonists, to prevent clinically overt decompensation. Timing of the echocardiographic follow-up needs to be established based on the clinical conditions of the single patients and requires experience and ability to produce pathophysiologic inference to guide management.

Patients with early-stage HFpEF can have symptoms of exertional intolerance in the absence of increased LV filling pressure in resting conditions. These patients might still develop sharp elevations of LV filling pressure during exercise. In these patients, the diagnosis of HFpEF can be favored by hemodynamic evaluation during stress-echocardiography, allowing checking the characteristics reported in Table 17.2.

Another potentially useful strategy that might be used for the follow-up of hypertensive patients with stage B HF is monitoring circulating markers. Circulating brain natriuretic peptide (BNP) or N-terminal fragment (NT) of the BNP prohormone (NT-proBNP) are related to increased wall stress due to either volume or pressure overload and are emerging as clinically useful biomarkers to monitor compensation of stage B HF [78], a strategy that might be economically convenient to better identify the timing for echocardiographic controls [79]. Interestingly, though NT-proBNP natriuretic peptides are useful in both phenotypic presentations of HF, HFrEF and HFpEF [80–82], their circulating values can be normal for diastolic dysfunction characterized by abnormal LV relaxation and/or mild-to moderate degrees of increased LV filling pressure. Thus more than to the absolute value, attention should be paid to the changes over time.

Hypertension and Stroke

Hypertension is a common problem in secondary prevention of stroke, being involved in nearly 70 % of all stroke cases [83]. The hypertension-related stroke is today mostly ischemic and results from artery-to-artery embolization or embolization from heart [84]. Risk of recurrent stroke decreases when BP is optimally controlled at least to the conventional level (<140/90 mmHg) [85]. Although doubts persist about the advantage of aggressive BP control for secondary prevention of stroke [86], there is increasing evidence that forcing BP beyond the conventional limits might be convenient [87]. It is reasonable to tailor therapy taking into account the general conditions and risk profile of patients.

The other important condition substantially related to risk of recurrent stroke is atrial fibrillation (AF). AF is the most common sustained arrhythmia not only in the context of arterial hypertension. Its prevalence and incidence increase in patients with arterial hypertension [88]. Although the relative risk of AF is relatively modest (<2), the very high prevalence of arterial hypertension produces a very high population-attributable risk of AF [89], recalling for a substantial health system burden.

In a recent epidemiologic study [90], the hazard of AF in a registry of hypertensive patients increases with increasing LV mass, left atrial dimensions and carotid intima-media thickness, independently of sex and age and accounting for preceding CV events that could have influenced the incidence of AF (Fig. 17.4). Thus, also for the secondary prevention of stroke, non-invasive CV imaging can provide important information to modulate the strength of therapy and management.

One important pitfall in the evaluation of risk of stroke associated with AF is the impossibility to capture clinically silent episode of AF that might have high impact

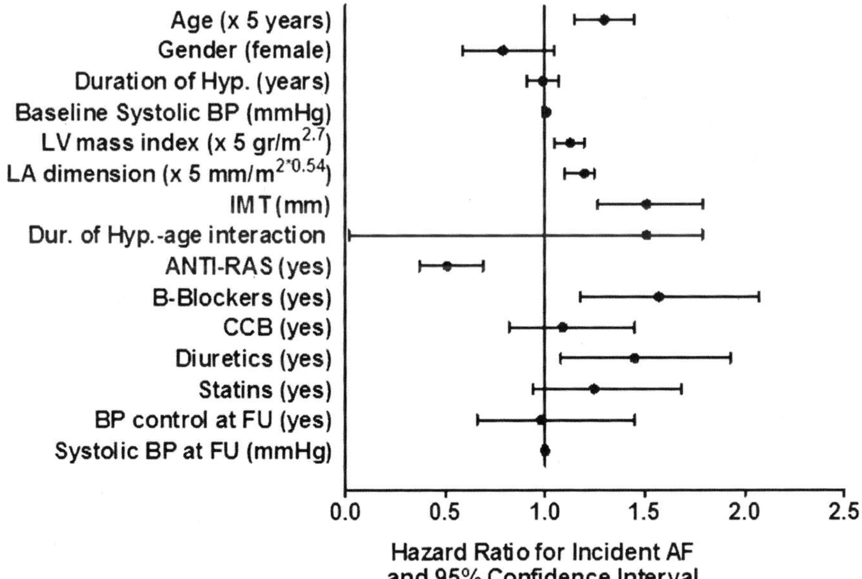

Fig. 17.4 Hazard of incident AF in a registry of 7062 hypertensive patients. The model takes into account the possibility that CV events could precede the occurrence of AF (competing risk event analysis). *BP* blood pressure, *CCB* Ca-channel blockers, *Dur* duration, *Hyp* hypertension, *IMT* intimal medial thickness, *LA* left atrial, *LV* left ventricular (From Ref. [90])

on the risk of stroke. This possibility might be especially relevant in patients with arterial hypertension and LV hypertrophy, who exhibit a negligible left atrial contribution to LV filling, due to increased chamber stiffness (restrictive or pseudo-normal filling pattern). Because LV filling occurs efficiently during early relaxation, in these patients, the abrupt fall of atrial contribution does not reduces stroke volume to a level that can cause symptoms, as it might happen when LV filling pattern is characterized by abnormal LV relaxation, requiring a substantial atrial contribution to filling. Thus, in patients with intermittent symptoms attributable to episodes of AF or a high-risk profile (elderly males with LVH, left atrial dilatation and/or high carotid intima-media thickness, as shown in Fig. 17.4), the use of Holter monitoring, event recorders or implantable loop recorders may be worth to identify silent episodes.

Therapy

Therapy and management in hypertensive patients with prevalent CV disease should be primarily addressed to control effectively BP, as well as any other major risk factor. Thus, any class of antihypertensive medication should be used to decrease BP at least to <140/90 mmHg. Some class of medications might be more indicated than others are.

In addition to be the most effective in reducing LV mass [91], medications inhibiting the renin-angiotensin system, namely ACE-inhibitors, are particularly recommended also for stroke prevention [84, 92]. Mineralocorticoid receptor inhibitors can be conveniently used to achieve control of BP and to optimize therapy also in Class II NYHA HF [77].

For patients in sinus rhythm, anti-platelet therapy should be continued for secondary prevention of CHD, or even reinforced, for stroke prevention. Anticoagulation is indicated for patients in AF and in those with CHA2DS2-VASc score ≥ 2. Although the CHA2DS2-Vasc was initially conceived for patients with AF, it has been shown to be useful also in patients in sinus rhythm [93].

References

1. Kannel WB. Blood pressure as a cardiovascular risk factor: prevention and treatment. JAMA. 1996;275(20):1571–6.
2. The effect of antihypertensive drug treatment on mortality in the presence of resting electrocardiographic abnormalities at baseline: the HDFP experience. The Hypertension Detection and Follow-up Program Cooperative Research Group. Circulation. 1984;70(6):996–1003.
3. Major outcomes in moderately hypercholesterolemic, hypertensive patients randomized to pravastatin vs usual care: the Antihypertensive and Lipid-Lowering Treatment to Prevent Heart Attack Trial (ALLHAT-LLT). JAMA. 2002;288(23):2998–3007.
4. Fagard R. Hypertensive heart disease: pathophysiology and clinical and prognostic consequences. J Cardiovasc Pharmacol. 1992;19 Suppl 5:S59–66.

5. Devereux RB, Alderman MH. Role of preclinical cardiovascular disease in the evolution from risk factor exposure to development of morbid events. Circulation. 1993;88(4 Pt 1):1444–55.
6. de Simone G, Daniels SR, Kimball TR, Roman MJ, Romano C, Chinali M, et al. Evaluation of concentric left ventricular geometry in humans: evidence for age-related systematic underestimation. Hypertension. 2005;45(1):64–8.
7. Casalnuovo G, Gerdts E, de Simone G, Izzo R, De Marco M, Giudice R, et al. Arterial stiffness is associated with carotid atherosclerosis in hypertensive patients (The Campania Salute Network). Am J Hypertens. 2012;25(7):739–45.
8. de Simone G, Izzo R, Aurigemma GP, De Marco M, Rozza F, Trimarco V, et al. Cardiovascular risk in relation to a new classification of hypertensive left ventricular geometric abnormalities. J Hypertens. 2015;33(4):745–54.
9. Tsao CW, Gona PN, Salton CJ, Chuang ML, Levy D, Manning WJ, et al. Left ventricular structure and risk of cardiovascular events: a Framingham Heart Study Cardiac Magnetic Resonance Study. J Am Heart Assoc. 2015;4(9):e002188.
10. Armstrong AC, Jacobs Jr DR, Gidding SS, Colangelo LA, Gjesdal O, Lewis CE, et al. Framingham score and LV mass predict events in young adults: CARDIA study. Int J Cardiol. 2014;172(2):350–5.
11. Sehestedt T, Jeppesen J, Hansen TW, Wachtell K, Ibsen H, Torp-Pedersen C, et al. Risk prediction is improved by adding markers of subclinical organ damage to SCORE. Eur Heart J. 2010;31(7):883–91.
12. Khouri MG, Peshock RM, Ayers CR, de Lemos JA, Drazner MH. A 4-tiered classification of left ventricular hypertrophy based on left ventricular geometry: the Dallas heart study. Circ Cardiovasc Imaging. 2010;3(2):164–71.
13. Zile MR, Gaasch WH, Patel K, Aban IB, Ahmed A. Adverse left ventricular remodeling in community-dwelling older adults predicts incident heart failure and mortality. JACC Heart Fail. 2014;2(5):512–22.
14. Mancia G, Laurent S, Agabiti-Rosei E, Ambrosioni E, Burnier M, Caulfield MJ, et al. Reappraisal of European guidelines on hypertension management: a European Society of Hypertension Task Force document. J Hypertens. 2009;27(11):2121–58.
15. Weber MA, Schiffrin EL, White WB, Mann S, Lindholm LH, Kenerson JG, et al. Clinical practice guidelines for the management of hypertension in the community: a statement by the American Society of Hypertension and the International Society of Hypertension. J Clin Hypertens (Greenwich). 2014;16(1):14–26.
16. James PA, Oparil S, Carter BL, Cushman WC, Dennison-Himmelfarb C, Handler J, et al. 2014 evidence-based guideline for the management of high blood pressure in adults: report from the panel members appointed to the Eighth Joint National Committee (JNC 8). JAMA. 2014;311(5):507–20.
17. WHO. Prevention of cardiovascular disease (CVDs): pocket guidelines for assessment and management of CVD risk. WHO library Cataloguing-in-Publication Data, editor. Geneva; 2007.
18. van Holten TC, Waanders LF, de Groot PG, Vissers J, Hoefer IE, Pasterkamp G, et al. Circulating biomarkers for predicting cardiovascular disease risk; a systematic review and comprehensive overview of meta-analyses. PLoS One. 2013;8(4):e62080.
19. Tzoulaki I, Siontis KC, Ioannidis JP. Prognostic effect size of cardiovascular biomarkers in datasets from observational studies versus randomised trials: meta-epidemiology study. BMJ. 2011;343:d6829.
20. Miller J, Kinni H, Lewandowski C, Nowak R, Levy P. Management of hypertension in stroke. Ann Emerg Med. 2014;64(3):248–55.
21. Mancia G, De Backer G, Dominiczak A, Cifkova R, Fagard R, Germano G, et al. 2007 guidelines for the management of arterial hypertension: the task force for the management of arterial hypertension of the European Society of Hypertension (ESH) and of the European Society of Cardiology (ESC). J Hypertens. 2007;25(6):1105–87.

22. Verdecchia P, Staessen JA, Angeli F, de Simone G, Achilli A, Ganau A, et al. Usual versus tight control of systolic blood pressure in non-diabetic patients with hypertension (Cardio-Sis): an open-label randomised trial. Lancet. 2009;374(9689):525–33.
23. Wright Jr JT, Williamson JD, Whelton PK, Snyder JK, Sink KM, Rocco MV, et al. A randomized trial of intensive versus standard blood-pressure control. N Engl J Med. 2015;373(22):2103–16.
24. Rosendorff C. Treatment of hypertension in patients with coronary artery disease. A case-based summary of the 2015 AHA/ACC/ASH scientific statement. Am J Med. 2015;(15):10.
25. de Simone G, Izzo R, Verdecchia P. Are observational studies more informative than randomized controlled trials in hypertension? Pro side of the argument. Hypertension. 2013;62(3):463–9.
26. Patsopoulos NA. A pragmatic view on pragmatic trials. Dialogues Clin Neurosci. 2011;13(2):217–24.
27. Kaplan NM. Morning surge in blood pressure. Circulation. 2003;107(10):1347.
28. Coleman AJ, Steel SD, Ashworth M, Vowler SL, Shennan A. Accuracy of the pressure scale of sphygmomanometers in clinical use within primary care. Blood Press Monit. 2005;10(4):181–8.
29. Beevers G, Lip GY, O'Brien E. ABC of hypertension. Blood pressure measurement. Part I-sphygmomanometry: factors common to all techniques. BMJ. 2001;322(7292):981–5.
30. Ohkubo T, Metoki H, Imai Y. Prognostic significance of morning surge in blood pressure: which definition, which outcome? Blood Press Monit. 2008;13(3):161–2.
31. White WB, Giles T, Bakris GL, Neutel JM, Davidai G, Weber MA. Measuring the efficacy of antihypertensive therapy by ambulatory blood pressure monitoring in the primary care setting. Am Heart J. 2006;151(1):176–84.
32. National Cholesterol Education Program (NCEP) Expert Panel on Detection, Evaluation, and Treatment of High Blood Cholesterol in Adults (Adult Treatment Panel III). Third Report of the National Cholesterol Education Program (NCEP) Expert Panel on Detection, Evaluation, and Treatment of High Blood Cholesterol in Adults (Adult Treatment Panel III) final report. Circulation. 2002;106(25):3143–421.
33. Kannel WB, Brand N, Skinner Jr JJ, Dawber TR, McNamara PM. The relation of adiposity to blood pressure and development of hypertension. The Framingham study. Ann Intern Med. 1967;67(1):48–59.
34. Landsberg L, Aronne LJ, Beilin LJ, Burke V, Igel LI, Lloyd-Jones D, et al. Obesity-related hypertension: pathogenesis, cardiovascular risk, and treatment. J Clin Hypertens. 2013;15(1):14–33.
35. Kannel WB. Risk stratification in hypertension: new insights from the Framingham Study. Am J Hypertens. 2000;13(1 Pt 2):3S–10.
36. Fujita M, Hata A. Sex and age differences in the effect of obesity on incidence of hypertension in the Japanese population: a large historical cohort study. J Am Soc Hypertens. 2014;8(1):64–70.
37. de Simone G, Devereux RB, Chinali M, Roman MJ, Best LG, Welty TK, et al. Risk factors for arterial hypertension in adults with initial optimal blood pressure: the Strong Heart Study. Hypertension. 2006;47(2):162–7.
38. Chinali M, de Simone G, Roman MJ, Lee ET, Best LG, Howard BV, et al. Impact of obesity on cardiac geometry and function in a population of adolescents: the Strong Heart Study. J Am Coll Cardiol. 2006;47(11):2267–73.
39. de Simone G, Palmieri V, Bella JN, Celentano A, Hong Y, Oberman A, et al. Association of left ventricular hypertrophy with metabolic risk factors: the HyperGEN study. J Hypertens. 2002;20(2):323–31.
40. Arcucci O, de Simone G, Izzo R, Rozza F, Chinali M, Rao MA, et al. Association of suboptimal blood pressure control with body size and metabolic abnormalities. J Hypertens. 2007;25:2296–300.
41. De Marco M, de Simone G, Izzo R, Mancusi C, Sforza A, Giudice R, et al. Classes of antihypertensive medications and blood pressure control in relation to metabolic risk factors. J Hypertens. 2012;30(1):188–93.

42. de Simone G, Okin PM, Gerdts E, Olsen MH, Wachtell K, Hille DA, et al. Clustered metabolic abnormalities blunt regression of hypertensive left ventricular hypertrophy: the LIFE study. Nutr Metab Cardiovasc Dis. 2009;19(9):634–40.
43. de Simone G, Devereux RB, Izzo R, Girfoglio D, Lee ET, Howard BV, et al. Lack of reduction of left ventricular mass in treated hypertension: the strong heart study. J Am Heart Assoc. 2013;2(3):e000144.
44. Babazono T, Takahashi C, Iwamoto Y. Definition of microalbuminuria in first-morning and random spot urine in diabetic patients. Diabetes Care. 2004;27(7):1838–9.
45. Pontremoli R, Leoncini G, Ravera M, Viazzi F, Vettoretti S, Ratto E, et al. Microalbuminuria, cardiovascular, and renal risk in primary hypertension. J Am Soc Nephrol. 2002;13 Suppl 3:S169–72.
46. Jensen JS, Feldt-Rasmussen B, Strandgaard S, Schroll M, Borch-Johnsen K. Arterial hypertension, microalbuminuria, and risk of ischemic heart disease. Hypertension. 2000;35(4):898–903.
47. Gerstein HC, Mann JF, Yi Q, Zinman B, Dinneen SF, Hoogwerf B, et al. Albuminuria and risk of cardiovascular events, death, and heart failure in diabetic and nondiabetic individuals. JAMA. 2001;286(4):421–6.
48. Stuveling EM, Bakker SJ, Hillege HL, Burgerhof JG, de Jong PE, Gans RO, et al. C-reactive protein modifies the relationship between blood pressure and microalbuminuria. Hypertension. 2004;43(4):791–6.
49. Jager A, van Hinsbergh VW, Kostense PJ, Emeis JJ, Nijpels G, Dekker JM, et al. C-reactive protein and soluble vascular cell adhesion molecule-1 are associated with elevated urinary albumin excretion but do not explain its link with cardiovascular risk. Arterioscler Thromb Vasc Biol. 2002;22(4):593–8.
50. Liao Y, Cooper RS, McGee DL, Mensah GA, Ghali JK. The relative effects of left ventricular hypertrophy, coronary artery disease, and ventricular dysfunction on survival among black adults. JAMA. 1995;273(20):1592–7.
51. de Simone G, Muiesan ML, Ganau A, Longhini C, Verdecchia P, Palmieri V, et al. Reliability and limitations of echocardiographic measurement of left ventricular mass for risk stratification and follow-up in single patients: the RES trial. Working Group on Heart and Hypertension of the Italian Society of Hypertension. Reliability of M-mode Echocardiographic Studies. J Hypertens. 1999;17(12 Pt 2):1955–63.
52. de Simone G, Izzo R, Chinali M, De Marco M, Casalnuovo G, Rozza F, et al. Does information on systolic and diastolic function improve prediction of a cardiovascular event by left ventricular hypertrophy in arterial hypertension? Hypertension. 2010;56(1):99–104.
53. O'Leary DH, Polak JF, Kronmal RA, Manolio TA, Burke GL, Wolfson Jr SK. Carotid-artery intima and media thickness as a risk factor for myocardial infarction and stroke in older adults. Cardiovascular Health Study Collaborative Research Group. N Engl J Med. 1999;340(1):14–22.
54. Zanchetti A, Hennig M, Hollweck R, Bond G, Tang R, Cuspidi C, et al. Baseline values but not treatment-induced changes in carotid intima-media thickness predict incident cardiovascular events in treated hypertensive patients: findings in the European Lacidipine Study on Atherosclerosis (ELSA). Circulation. 2009;120(12):1084–90.
55. Moreno PR, Kini A. Resolution of inflammation, statins, and plaque regression. J Am Coll Cardiol Img. 2012;5(2):178–81.
56. Ibanez B, Vilahur G, Badimon JJ. Plaque progression and regression in atherothrombosis. J Thromb Haemost. 2007;5 Suppl 1:292–9.
57. Zellweger MJ, Weinbacher M, Zutter AW, Jeger RV, Mueller-Brand J, Kaiser C, et al. Long-term outcome of patients with silent versus symptomatic ischemia six months after percutaneous coronary intervention and stenting. J Am Coll Cardiol. 2003;42(1):33–40.
58. Gibbons RJ, Balady GJ, Beasley JW, Bricker JT, Duvernoy WF, Froelicher VF, et al. ACC/AHA Guidelines for Exercise Testing. A report of the American College of Cardiology/American Heart Association Task Force on Practice Guidelines (Committee on Exercise Testing). J Am Coll Cardiol. 1997;30(1):260–311.
59. Marwick TH, Torelli J, Harjai K, Haluska B, Pashkow FJ, Stewart WJ, et al. Influence of left ventricular hypertrophy on detection of coronary artery disease using exercise echocardiography. J Am Coll Cardiol. 1995;26(5):1180–6.

60. Gibbons RJ, Balady GJ, Bricker JT, Chaitman BR, Fletcher GF, Froelicher VF, et al. ACC/AHA 2002 guideline update for exercise testing: summary article: a report of the American College of Cardiology/American Heart Association Task Force on Practice Guidelines (Committee to Update the 1997 Exercise Testing Guidelines). Circulation. 2002;106(14):1883–92.
61. Marwick TH, Gillebert TC, Aurigemma G, Chirinos J, Derumeaux G, Galderisi M, et al. Recommendations on the use of echocardiography in adult hypertension: a report from the European Association of Cardiovascular Imaging (EACVI) and the American Society of Echocardiography (ASE)dagger. Eur Heart J Cardiovasc Imaging. 2015;16(6):577–605.
62. Pingitore A, Picano E, Varga A, Gigli G, Cortigiani L, Previtali M, et al. Prognostic value of pharmacological stress echocardiography in patients with known or suspected coronary artery disease: a prospective, large-scale, multicenter, head-to-head comparison between dipyridamole and dobutamine test. Echo-Persantine International Cooperative (EPIC) and Echo-Dobutamine International Cooperative (EDIC) Study Groups. J Am Coll Cardiol. 1999;34(6):1769–77.
63. de Simone G, Parati G. Imaging techniques for non-invasive assessment of coronary heart disease in hypertension: value of an integrated approach. J Hypertens. 2001;19(4):679–82.
64. Galderisi M, de Simone G, D'Errico A, Sidiropulos M, Viceconti R, Chinali M, et al. Independent association of coronary flow reserve with left ventricular relaxation and filling pressure in arterial hypertension. Am J Hypertens. 2008;21(9):1040–6.
65. Cortigiani L, Rigo F, Gherardi S, Sicari R, Galderisi M, Bovenzi F, et al. Additional prognostic value of coronary flow reserve in diabetic and nondiabetic patients with negative dipyridamole stress echocardiography by wall motion criteria. J Am Coll Cardiol. 2007;50(14):1354–61.
66. Fihn SD, Blankenship JC, Alexander KP, Bittl JA, Byrne JG, Fletcher BJ, et al. 2014 ACC/AHA/AATS/PCNA/SCAI/STS focused update of the guideline for the diagnosis and management of patients with stable ischemic heart disease: a report of the American College of Cardiology/American Heart Association Task Force on Practice Guidelines, and the American Association for Thoracic Surgery, Preventive Cardiovascular Nurses Association, Society for Cardiovascular Angiography and Interventions, and Society of Thoracic Surgeons. Circulation. 2014;130(19):1749–67.
67. Mark DB, Berman DS, Budoff MJ, Carr JJ, Gerber TC, Hecht HS, et al. ACCF/ACR/AHA/NASCI/SAIP/SCAI/SCCT 2010 expert consensus document on coronary computed tomographic angiography: a report of the American College of Cardiology Foundation Task Force on Expert Consensus Documents. Circulation. 2010;121(22):2509–43.
68. Yancy CW, Jessup M, Bozkurt B, Butler J, Casey Jr DE, Drazner MH, et al. 2013 ACCF/AHA guideline for the management of heart failure: executive summary: a report of the American College of Cardiology Foundation/American Heart Association Task Force on practice guidelines. Circulation. 2013;128(16):1810–52.
69. Levy D, Larson MG, Vasan RS, Kannel WB, Ho KK. The progression from hypertension to congestive heart failure. JAMA. 1996;275(20):1557–62.
70. Owan TE, Hodge DO, Herges RM, Jacobsen SJ, Roger VL, Redfield MM. Trends in prevalence and outcome of heart failure with preserved ejection fraction. N Engl J Med. 2006;355(3):251–9.
71. Roger VL, Go AS, Lloyd-Jones DM, Adams RJ, Berry JD, Brown TM, et al. Heart disease and stroke statistics--2011 update: a report from the American Heart Association. Circulation. 2011;123(4):e18–209.
72. Bhatia RS, Tu JV, Lee DS, Austin PC, Fang J, Haouzi A, et al. Outcome of heart failure with preserved ejection fraction in a population-based study. N Engl J Med. 2006;355(3):260–9.
73. Yusuf S, Pfeffer MA, Swedberg K, Granger CB, Held P, McMurray JJ, et al. Effects of candesartan in patients with chronic heart failure and preserved left-ventricular ejection fraction: the CHARM-Preserved Trial. Lancet. 2003;362(9386):777–81.
74. Zile MR, Gaasch WH, Anand IS, Haass M, Little WC, Miller AB, et al. Mode of death in patients with heart failure and a preserved ejection fraction: results from the Irbesartan in Heart Failure With Preserved Ejection Fraction Study (I-Preserve) trial. Circulation. 2010;121(12):1393–405.

75. Major outcomes in high-risk hypertensive patients randomized to angiotensin-converting enzyme inhibitor or calcium channel blocker vs diuretic: the Antihypertensive and Lipid-Lowering Treatment to Prevent Heart Attack Trial (ALLHAT). JAMA. 2002;288(23):2981–97.
76. Carson P, Tognoni G, Cohn JN. Effect of Valsartan on hospitalization: results from Val-HeFT. J Card Fail. 2003;9(3):164–71.
77. Boccanelli A, Mureddu GF, Cacciatore G, Clemenza F, Di Lenarda A, Gavazzi A, et al. Anti-remodelling effect of canrenone in patients with mild chronic heart failure (AREA IN-CHF study): final results. Eur J Heart Fail. 2009;11(1):68–76.
78. Felker GM, Hasselblad V, Hernandez AF, O'Connor CM. Biomarker-guided therapy in chronic heart failure: a meta-analysis of randomized controlled trials. Am Heart J. 2009;158(3):422–30.
79. Ferrandis MJ, Ryden I, Lindahl TL, Larsson A. Ruling out cardiac failure: cost-benefit analysis of a sequential testing strategy with NT-proBNP before echocardiography. Ups J Med Sci. 2013;118(2):75–9.
80. Mottram PM, Leano R, Marwick TH. Usefulness of B-type natriuretic peptide in hypertensive patients with exertional dyspnea and normal left ventricular ejection fraction and correlation with new echocardiographic indexes of systolic and diastolic function. Am J Cardiol. 2003;92(12):1434–8.
81. Tschope C, Kasner M, Westermann D, Gaub R, Poller WC, Schultheiss HP. The role of NT-proBNP in the diagnostics of isolated diastolic dysfunction: correlation with echocardiographic and invasive measurements. Eur Heart J. 2005;26(21):2277–84.
82. Dahlstrom U. Can natriuretic peptides be used for the diagnosis of diastolic heart failure? Eur J Heart Fail. 2004;6(3):281–7.
83. Staessen JA, Kuznetsova T, Stolarz K. Hypertension prevalence and stroke mortality across populations. JAMA. 2003;289(18):2420–2.
84. Esenwa C, Gutierrez J. Secondary stroke prevention: challenges and solutions. Vasc Health Risk Manag. 2015;11:437–50.
85. Kernan WN, Ovbiagele B, Black HR, Bravata DM, Chimowitz MI, Ezekowitz MD, et al. Guidelines for the prevention of stroke in patients with stroke and transient ischemic attack: a guideline for healthcare professionals from the American Heart Association/American Stroke Association. Stroke. 2014;45(7):2160–236.
86. Aiyagari V, Gorelick PB. Management of blood pressure for acute and recurrent stroke. Stroke. 2009;40(6):2251–6.
87. Benavente OR, Coffey CS, Conwit R, Hart RG, McClure LA, Pearce LA, et al. Blood-pressure targets in patients with recent lacunar stroke: the SPS3 randomised trial. Lancet. 2013;382(9891):507–15.
88. Benjamin EJ, Levy D, Vaziri SM, D'Agostino RB, Belanger AJ, Wolf PA. Independent risk factors for atrial fibrillation in a population-based cohort. The Framingham Heart Study. JAMA. 1994;271(11):840–4.
89. Huxley RR, Lopez FL, Folsom AR, Agarwal SK, Loehr LR, Soliman EZ, et al. Absolute and attributable risks of atrial fibrillation in relation to optimal and borderline risk factors: the Atherosclerosis Risk in Communities (ARIC) study. Circulation. 2011;123(14):1501–8.
90. Losi MA, Izzo R, De Marco M, Canciello G, Rapacciuolo A, Trimarco V, et al. Cardiovascular ultrasound exploration contributes to predict incident atrial fibrillation in arterial hypertension: the Campania Salute Network. Int J Cardiol. 2015;199:290–5.
91. Fagard RH, Celis H, Thijs L, Wouters S. Regression of left ventricular mass by antihypertensive treatment: a meta-analysis of randomized comparative studies. Hypertension. 2009;54(5):1084–91.
92. Randomised trial of a perindopril-based blood-pressure-lowering regimen among 6,105 individuals with previous stroke or transient ischaemic attack. Lancet. 2001;358(9287):1033–41.
93. Mitchell LB, Southern DA, Galbraith D, Ghali WA, Knudtson M, Wilton SB. Prediction of stroke or TIA in patients without atrial fibrillation using CHADS2 and CHA2DS2-VASc scores. Heart. 2014;100(19):1524–30.

Chapter 18
Hypertension and Sudden Cardiac Death

Mohammad Shenasa

Abbreviations

ACE	Angiotensin-converting enzyme
AF	Atrial fibrillation
APD	Action potential duration
ARB	Angiotensin-receptor blocker
CAD	Coronary artery disease
CCT	Cardiac computerized tomography
CHF	Congestive heart failure
DAD	Delayed afterdepolarization
EAD	Early afterdepolarization
ECG	Electrocardiogram
HCM	Hypertrophic cardiomyopathy
HF	Heart failure
HTN	Hypertension
LAD	Left anterior descending
LV	Left ventricle
LVH	Left ventricular hypertrophy
MI	Myocardial infarction
MRI	Magnetic resonance imaging
OSA	Obstructive sleep apnea
PET	Positron-emission tomography
PVC	Premature ventricular complex
SCD	Sudden cardiac death
SPECT	Single-photon emission computed tomography

M. Shenasa, M.D.
Heart and Rhythm Medical Group, Department of Cardiovascular Services, O'Connor Hospital, San Jose 95128, CA, USA
e-mail: Mohammad.shenasa@gmail.com

E.A. Andreadis (ed.), *Hypertension and Cardiovascular Disease*,
DOI 10.1007/978-3-319-39599-9_18

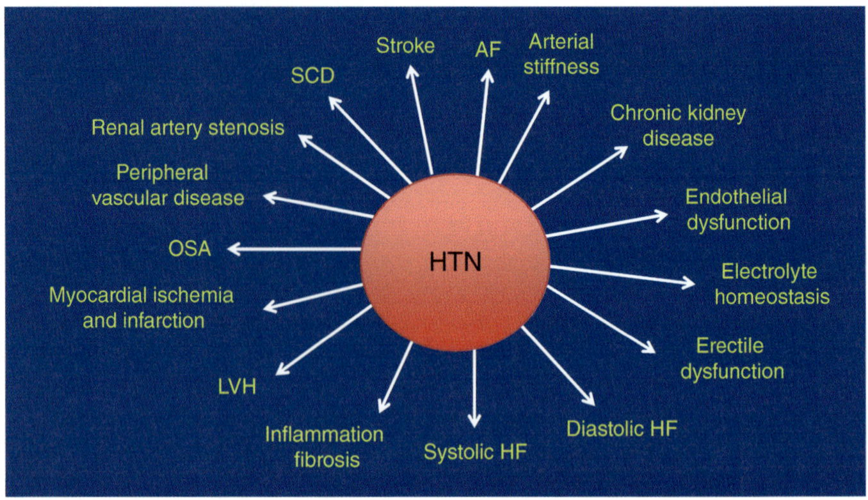

Fig. 18.1 Relationship of HTN to different pathologies. *Abbreviations*: *AF* atrial fibrillation, *HF* heart failure, *LVH* left ventricular hypertrophy, *OSA* obstructive sleep apnea, *SCD* sudden cardiac death

Introduction

Hypertension (HTN) is the most common chronic disease of the cardiovascular system [1]. The definition of normal, prehypertensive, and hypertensive blood pressure are as follows: (1) Normal < 120/80 mmHg, (2) Prehypertensive 120–139/80–89 mmHg, (3) Hypertensive > 140/90 mmHg, although the guidelines have recently changed based on the most latest epidemiologic data [2–7]. Currently, HTN affects 70 million Americans, and over one billion people worldwide. It is estimated that there will be an affected 1.5 billion people worldwide by the year 2025. A report from the national health and nutrition examination survey (NHAES), reported that in 2005–2006 an estimated 37 % of the United States population were prehypertensive [8, 9]. HTN is more common in blacks (40 %) compared to whites (25 %) and is the most common readily identifiable and reversible risk factor for myocardial infarction (MI), stroke, heart failure (HF) (both systolic and diastolic), atrial fibrillation (AF), ventricular arrhythmias, sudden cardiac death (SCD), kidney disease [10], peripheral vascular disease, renal artery stenosis [11], obstructive sleep apnea (OSA) [12], erectile dysfunction and many others as shown in Fig. 18.1. Indeed, HTN is the leading risk factor for global mortality and accounts for 13 % of all worldwide death in 2004, and far exceeds the cause of death by tobacco use (9 %), diabetes (6 %), physical inactivity (6 %), and obesity (5 %) [13, 14]. On the other hand, it is estimated that 36.2 % (13 million) people in the United States have undiagnosed HTN, i.e. they are not aware of their high blood pressure or are not taking their medication [15].

HTN has many diverse and complex etiologies and multiple pathways, which leads to diseases such as cardiac, central nervous system, baroreceptor, hormonal (renin angiotensin aldosterone pathway), vascular, renovascular, endothelial dysfunction, etc. These mechanisms will all lead to cardiovascular remodeling and fibrosis at the target organ. In the presenting scheme, HTN may be divided as preclinical, clinical manifestations of systolic and diastolic HTN, hypertensive state and hypertensive emergencies. Age wise, HTN may be present in children, adolescents, and the elderly, where etiologies and management significantly differs.

HTN increases the risk of stroke by 50 % [16, 17], AF by 40–50 % [18], and SCD significantly [19].

Genetic and environmental factors are important and are often underappreciated risk factors to HTN and its subsequent complications such as left ventricular hypertrophy (LVH), AF, stroke, HF, and SCD [20]. The pathophysiology of HTN is beyond the scope of this review; therefore, this review will focus on HTN, LVH, arrhythmias and SCD.

Hypertensive Heart Disease

Definition: Hypertensive heart disease is a result of long-standing HTN and is characterized by anatomical and functional changes in the myocardial structure and function in the absence of other primary cardiovascular abnormalities [21]. Hypertensive heart disease includes cardiovascular sequelae of HTN such as: LVH, left atrial enlargement, and functional mitral regurgitation that together make diastolic dysfunction.

LVH and diastolic dysfunction are common findings in patients with essential HTN, even in children and adolescents [22].

The clinical spectrum of hypertensive heart disease ranges from preclinical changes such as grade I diastolic dysfunction (impaired left ventricular (LV) relaxation) to manifest concentric LVH to eventually LV dilatation and congestive heart failure (CHF). LVH is not only a target organ response to increased afterload, but is also the most potent cardiovascular risk factor.

Thus, cardiovascular effects of HTN are summarized below;

- Cardiac hypertrophy
- Diastolic dysfunction [22]
- Systolic dysfunction
- Coronary atherosclerosis
- Microvascular dysfunction
- Atrial and ventricular arrhythmias
- Peripheral vascular disease
- Cerebrovascular disease
- Kidney disease

Figures 18.2 [23] and 18.3 describe pathways linking myocardial remodeling with clinical manifestations in hypertensive heart disease.

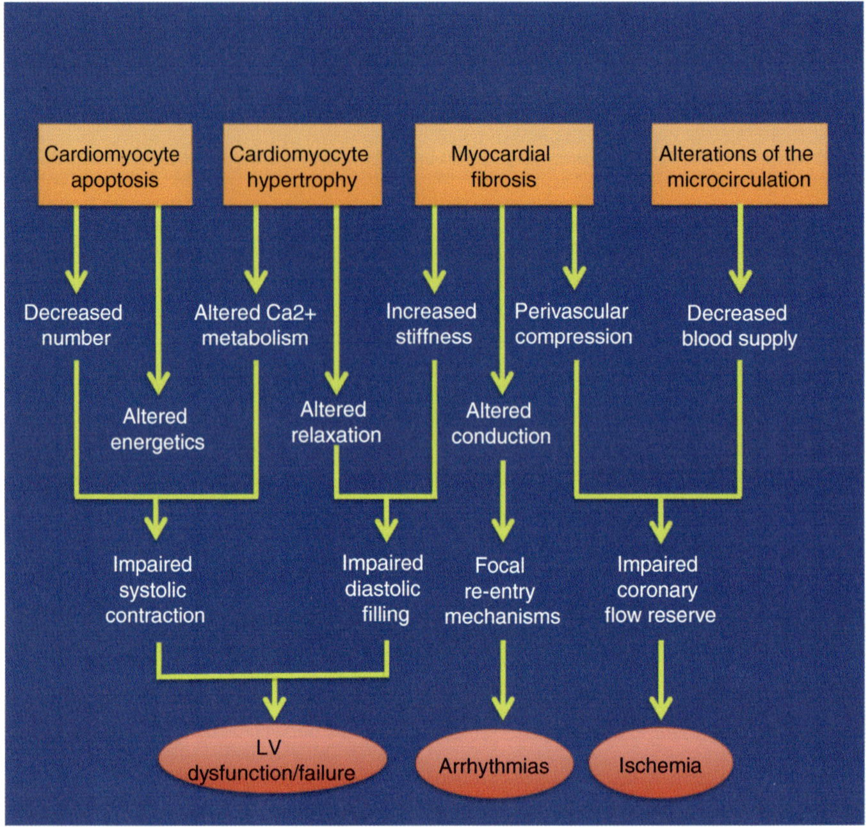

Fig. 18.2 Pathways linking myocardial remodeling with clinical manifestations in hypertensive heart disease. *Abbreviation*: *LV* left ventricular (From Diez and Frohlich [23])

Left Ventricular Hypertrophy

As stated by sir William Osler in 1892, "The course of any case of cardiac hypertrophy may be divided into three stages: The period of development which varies with the nature of the primary lesion… The period of full compensation in which the heart's vigor meets the requirements of the circulation… The period of broken compensation which…takes place slowly and results from degeneration and weakening of the heart muscle" [24, 25].

Definition: As said earlier, LVH is an adaptive to chronic afterload pressure, which results in pathological changes in structure and functional changes in the cardiovascular system. LVH is thus a powerful, independent predictor of cardiovascular adverse vents; however, it is reversible when its cause is corrected. As the result of increased workload, whether due to pressure overload or volume overload,

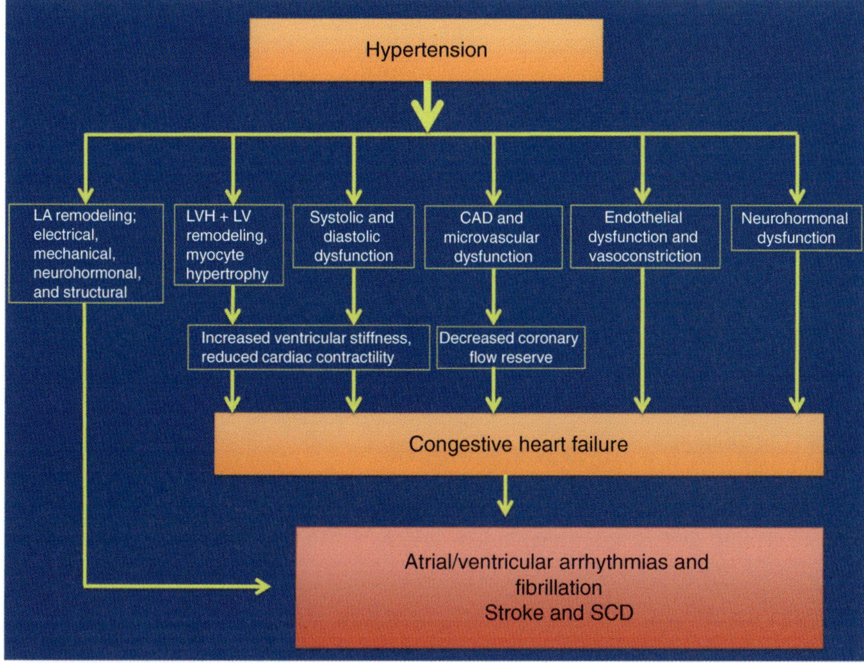

Fig. 18.3 Pathways leading from HTN, to hypertensive heart disease, to LVH, to CHF, to atrial/ventricular arrhythmias, stroke and SCD. *Abbreviations*: *CAD* coronary artery disease, *CHF* congestive heart failure, *HTN* hypertension, *LV* left ventricular, *LVH* left ventricular hypertrophy, *SCD* sudden cardiac death

there is an increase in cardiac myocyte size (myocyte hypertrophy) without any increase in the myocardial cell numbers. During the process of LVH there is also an increase in fibroblasts and interstitial collagen accumulation, leading to fibrosis which leads to diastolic dysfunction and the progression of HF [25–27]. This process results in remodeling of the myocardium, which also causes cellular electrophysiological abnormalities and arrhythmogenesis. In addition, microvascular changes and subendocardial ischemia contribute independently to arrhythmogenesis.

Geometric Patterns of LVH

LVH depends on LV geometry under normal and abnormal conditions and plays an important role in the pathogenesis of different forms of LVH. The LV geometry adaptation and response to HTN is heterogeneous and is affected by multiple factors including genetic predisposition [28]. Abnormal LV geometry predicts progression of LVH in HF [29].

Differential diagnosis of hypertensive LVH from other forms of LVH is important and outlined here: (Fig. 18.4)

1. Physiological LVH
2. Pathological LVH
3. Concentric LVH
4. Eccentric LVH

The most important differential includes:

1. LVH in hypertensive heart disease
2. LVH in hypertrophic cardiomyopathy (HCM), especially in early phases of the disease
3. LVH in athletes
4. Other myocardial infiltrative diseases such as cardiac amyloidosis, glycogen storage diseases, Fabry disease, etc. Several clinical, family history, genetic background and imaging techniques are useful in the differential diagnosis of different types of LVH.

In a broad etiology, LVH may be categorized as pressure and volume overload.

Pressure Overload

Causes concentric LVH and includes HTN, aortic stenosis, static exercise, and infiltrative myocardial disease (Fig. 18.5) [30, 31].

Volume Overload

Causes eccentric LVH and includes mitral and aortic insufficiency, anemia, dynamic exercise, HF, and obesity (Fig. 18.5) [30, 31].

Assessment of LV geometric pattern is crucial before and after the management of HTN in these patients [32].

Among the consequences of long-term HTN, three major adverse effects include stroke, LVH, and SCD.

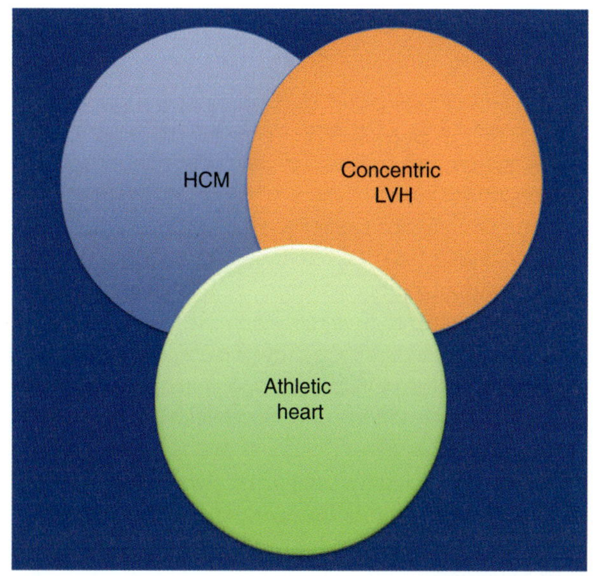

Fig. 18.4 Differential diagnosis of LVH. This figure illustrates the three important differential diagnosis of LVH. As it shows, there is some overlap between the three conditions, where other imaging technologies will be useful. *Abbreviations*: *HCM* hypertrophic cardiomyopathy, *LVH* left ventricular hypertrophy

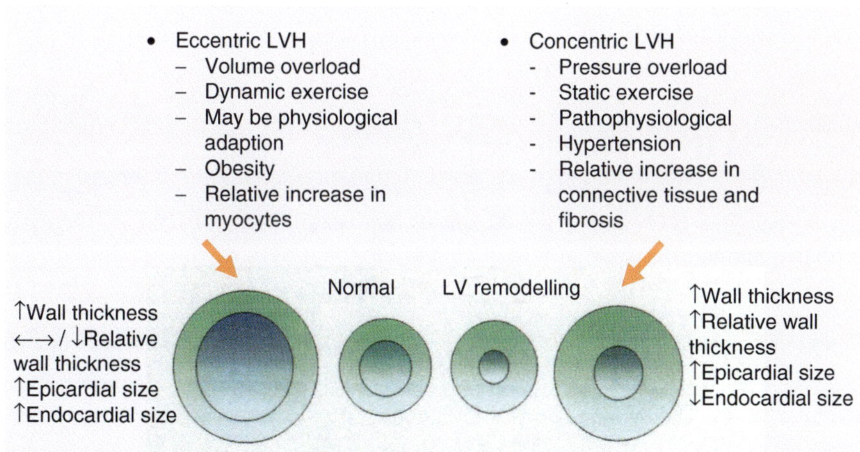

Fig. 18.5 LV geometry, HTN, and LVH (Adapted and modified from Kahan and Bergfeldt [30] and Marvao et al. [31]. With permission)

Hypertension and LVH

LVH is common sequelae of HTN (pressure overload) and is a compensatory mechanism; however, as LVH progresses in concentric geometry, eventually it progresses to LV dilatation and cardiac failure. More than 1/3 of patients who have HTN have electrocardiographic evidence of LVH. As LVH progresses, the risk of AF, ventricular arrhythmias, and SCD increases. New onset AF in patients with HTN and LVH significantly increases the risk of SCD and stroke independent of other risk factors. The disarrayed ventricular fiber structure in hypertensive patients with LVH predisposes to ventricular arrhythmias and SCD. Furthermore, AF, due to irregular R-R intervals, significantly predisposes the occurrence of malignant arrhythmias and SCD. In particular, the presence of irregular heart rate is an important trigger for malignant ventricular tachyarrhythmias. Short-long-short RR intervals during AF increases the likelihood of promoting ventricular arrhythmias and is a very dangerous combination. In addition, antiarrhythmic and antihypertensive therapy for AF rhythm control plays a significant risk factor for proarrhythmias and SCD. These issues are often underrecognized. Patients with HTN develop microvascular dysfunction and ischemia, which also promotes malignant arrhythmias and SCD. These patients also have normal epicardial coronary arteries; however, there is evidence of subendocardial ischemia, and they may often present with chest pain. Both clinical and experimental studies have demonstrated that induction ischemia in LVH increases the risk of ventricular tachyarrhythmias and SCD. See section Role of Myocardial Ischemia in Arrhythmogenesis in LVH.

Preclinical Hypertension and LVH

Even preclinical HTN and its consequences increases the risk of LVH, CHF, myocardial ischemia (decrease in microvascular circulation), arrhythmias, stroke, and SCD. Furthermore, HTN is often latent and is diagnosed randomly during physical examination or by patients themselves.

The natural history of HTN progresses from isolated high blood pressure to hypertensive heart disease that induces LVH. As compensatory hemodynamic mechanisms of HTN exhaust itself, subsequently, progress toward chamber enlargement and HF. Drivers of HTN and LVH include:

- Angiotensin II [33]
- Norepinephrine
- Epinephrine
- Increase peripheral and cardiac sympathetic drive [34]
- Endothelin
- Natriuretic peptides
- Adrenomedullin
- Leptin
- Other unknown factors

Diagnostic Modalities for the Diagnosis of LVH

Electrocardiogram (ECG) Criteria for the Diagnosis of LVH The two most commonly used criteria are as follows [35–39]:

1. The Sokolow-Lyon voltage criteria: S wave in lead V1 + R wave in lead V5 or V6 greater than or equal to 3.50 mV or R wave in lead V5 or V6 greater than 2.60 mV
2. The Cornell voltage criteria: For women, R wave in lead aVL + S wave in lead V3 greater than 2.00 mV. For men, R wave in lead aVL + S wave in lead V3 greater than 2.80 mV [39]

The diagnostic yield of ECG is only 2.4 % with specificity and sensitivity of 25–60 % [39].

ECG Changes in HTN Includes signs of LV chamber hypertrophy as above and ST-T wave abnormalities such as down sloping, convex ST-segment with inverted asymmetrical T-wave at the opposite direction of QRS axis in lead V5 or v6. Also, P-wave abnormalities are noticeable criteria of LVH. Aggressive HTN management may reverse and normalize some of these ECG changes [40].

ECG Manifestation of LVH [36, 41–45]:

1. Increased QRS voltage.
2. Increased QRS duration: This may be further complicated by the development of initially incomplete and finally complete left bundle branch block.
3. Left axis deviation.
4. Repolarization abnormalities.
5. Left atrial abnormalities.
6. QT prolongation [46, 47]. A further detailed analysis is shown in table 6.2 from ECG Handbook of Contemporary Challenges [40].

Echocardiographic Criteria for LVH

According to the data from Framingham Heart Study, LVH was defined as LV mass index ≥ 150 g/m^2 [43, 48–52].

The following echocardiographic indices are usually measured for diagnosis and evaluation of LVH:

- LV geometry
- LV wall thickness and motion
- LV systolic and diastolic function
- LV diastolic abnormalities such as Doppler transmitral flow
- LV strain patterns
- Stroke volume
- Evidence of ischemia during stress echocardiography

Echocardiogram is useful to differentiate normal geometry from concentric and eccentric LVH, respectively. As mentioned, it is important to differentiate physiological LVH (such as in athletes) from pathological LVH, hypertensive versus HCM [38, 40]. The LV mass is measured by echocardiographic measurements of LV mass (g) = 0.8{1.04[(IVS + LVID + PWT)^3–LVID^3]} + 0.6 g.[1] LV mass is also recognized as a surrogate for LVH and plays an important predictor as adverse events in patients with HTN [55–57].

Cardiac Computerized Tomography (CCT) Provides high resolution and accurate information of LV mass, volume and function. It can further provide additional information on the other related structural heart diseases. A major limitation of CCT is ionizing radiation exposure as well as contrast-use in patients with impaired renal function.

Cardiac Magnetic Resonance Imaging (MRI) MRI is currently considered the gold standard for measurement of LV mass and volume [58]. Cardiac MRI has several advantages including; (1) high spatial and temporal resolution, (2) multi-plane image acquisition. The disadvantages of CMR include (1) high cost, (2) availability, (3) artifact due to arrhythmias.

Single-Photon Emission Computed Tomography (SPECT) and Positron Emission Tomography (PET) SPECT imaging is useful where coronary artery disease (CAD) and ischemia is suspected. In this case, SPECT can also provide adequate information on LV mass, volume, and function. PET imaging remains investigational and is not used clinically.

Pathophysiological Mechanisms of Developing LVH in Hypertension

The pathogenesis of clinical HTN is well described by Singh et al. [59]. Long-standing HTN is the most common cause of LVH. LVH is also a preclinical surrogate of HTN and hypertensive heart disease. HTN increases afterload pressure, cardiac and vascular remodeling, myocardial compensatory mechanism to increase afterload pressure which leads to concentric LVH. As the result of myocyte enlargement, the interstitial component that in long-term leads to fibrosis and arrhythmias [60]. It is important to detect and measure the magnitude of fibrosis that is induced by HTN to be able to assess the risk of cardiovascular events and the reversibility of HTN-induced myocardial and hemodynamic changes [61]. Subsequently, these changes reduce LV compliance, increase atrial size and volume, constitute diastolic dysfunction and over time lead to LV dilatation and HF.

---

[1] IVS = diastolic interventricular septal thickness, LVID = diastolic LV internal dimension, PWT = diastolic posterior LV wall thickness [53, 54].

On the other hand, sodium retention in patients with HTN produce volume overload that through a separate mechanism increases LV mass. Altered endothelial function promotes arterial stiffness and vascular dysfunction, including peripheral vascular disease.

It is well established that both systolic and diastolic blood pressure are closely related to increased myocytes (cell size) and hypertrophy resulting in increased LV mass.

Neurohormonal factors including renin-angiotensin-aldosterone system also play an important role. There is an increase in sympathetic nervous system and myocardial sensitivity to these hormonal changes.

Independently, HTN promotes development of both microvascular abnormalities that leads to a reduction in coronary vasodilator reserve as well as large epicardial CAD.

Electrophysiologic changes that promote arrhythmogenesis are summarized in Fig. 18.6 [62] and are well discussed in a recent publication titled LVH and Arrhythmogenesis from our group [38].

Studies are now investigating the rule of specific genes that are involved in HTN-related LVH. These new findings will hopefully identify the subjects with HTN who may develop LVH and its subsequent adverse consequences such as AF, ventricular arrhythmias, and SCD [63].

Hypertension, Ventricular Arrhythmias, and SCD: LVH and Arrhythmogenesis

HTN and LVH are independent risk factors for increased morbidity and mortality including AF, ventricular arrhythmias, CAD, CHF and SCD. Other risk factors for arrhythmias in hypertensive patient include age, levels of diurnal and nocturnal systolic blood pressure during 24 h, left atrial dimension and volume, LV mass, maximum duration of dispersion in P-wave and QT interval on the ECG, alcohol and other risk factors [64, 65].

Large bodies of literature exist on relationship of HTN-LVH and ventricular arrhythmias (Table 18.1 [66]).

Several studies on clinical and experimental effects show the prevalence of ventricular arrhythmias in LVH. A recent meta-analysis reported that incidences of ventricular arrhythmias was 5.5 % in patients with LVH as compared to those without LVH [67, 68]. Furthermore, data from the Oregon Sudden Unexpected Death Study (Oregon SUDS) confirmed the association between LVH and SCD. LVH was identified as an independent risk factor for SCD [19, 67].

Clinical markers of an arrhythmic risk in LVH and their prognostic significance include:

- Premature ventricular complexes (PVCs), couplets, non-sustained VT, and VT
- Ventricular arrhythmias on Holter monitoring
- QT interval prolongation and dispersion

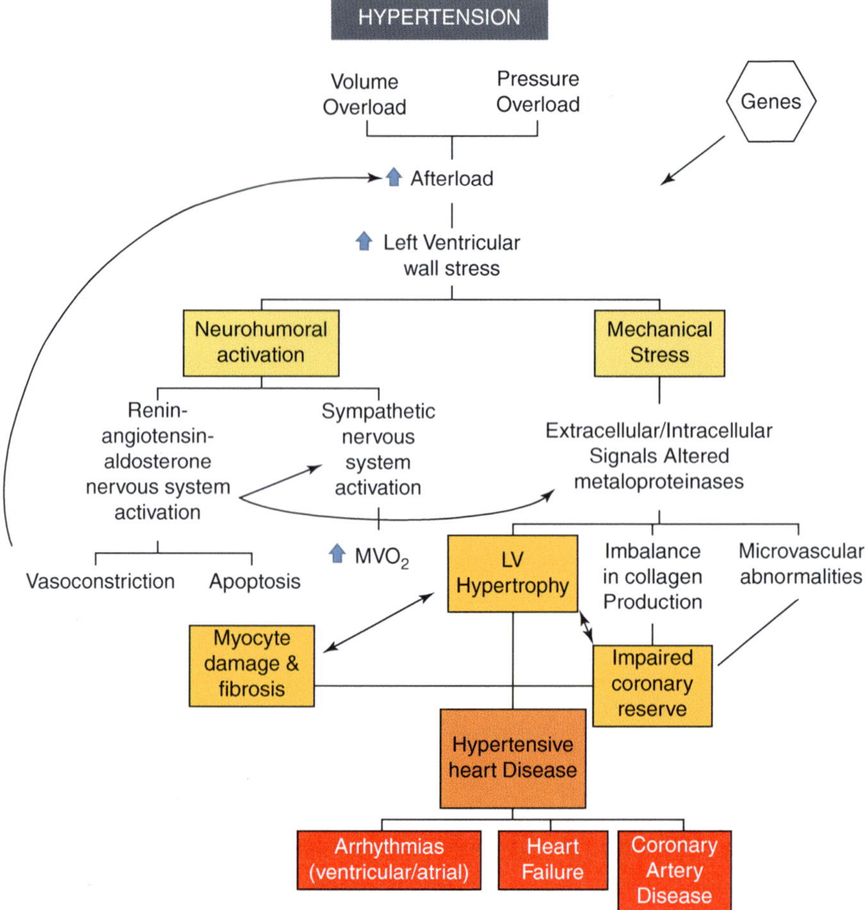

Fig. 18.6 Pathophysiologic pathways of hypertensive heart disease and LVH that lead to arrhythmias, heart failure, and coronary artery disease. *Abbreviations*: *LV* left ventricle, *MVO_2* mixed venous oxygen saturation (Adapted from Georgiopoulou et al. [62]. With permission)

- QRS duration
- Myocardial ischemia (in the absence of CAD)
- LV dysfunction
- Late potentials
- Fractionated electrograms
- Programmed electrical stimulation
- Heart rate variability

Other factors that contribute to arrhythmogenesis in LVH include genetic factors related to gap-junction remodeling, autonomic nervous activity, and increased sympathetic activation that enhances induction of ventricular tachyarrhythmias by

Table 18.1 Risk of ventricular arrhythmias in LVH by ECG and ECHO: result from the Framingham Study; age-adjusted relative odds

	Men		Women	
	ECG LVH	Echo-LVH	ECG LVH	Echo-LVH
PVCs	1.8*	1.5+	1.5 ns	1.4 ns
Complex or Frequent	1.9*	2.7+	1.5 ns	1.8=
Multiform	2.0*	3.2+	1.6 ns	1.9=
Couplet	3.2+	3.6=	2.2 ns	2.1 ns
VT	1.8+	4.1*		2.0 ns
R/T	5.6+	8.9+	3.9 ns	3.7 ns

Modified from Kannel and Cobb [66]. With permission

Abbreviations: *ECG* electrocardiogram, *Echo* echocardiogram, *LVH* left ventricular hypertrophy, *PVCs* premature ventricular complex, *ns* not significant

*$p<0.05$, + $p<0.01$, = $p<0.001$

inducing early and delayed afterdepolarizations (EADs and DADs). Cellular signaling pathways for cardiac hypertrophy and failure which are different specifically in pressure overload versus volume overload also play a significant role in the genesis of LVH to HF [69]. Mechanisms and electrophysiological effects of LVH include [70]:

- Myocardial Fibrosis
- Dispersion of Refractoriness
- Eccentric Hypertrophy
- Increase of action potential duration (APD)
- Decreased action potential upstroke velocity
- QT prolongation
- T-wave and/or repolarization alternans
- Increased sympathetic activity
- Electrolyte abnormalities
- Slowing of membrane repolarization or recovery manifest as an increase in QT interval duration. Similar to impulse conduction velocity, the recovery times within the myocardium may vary as a result of hypertrophy and fibrosis.
- The abnormalities in impulse conduction and myocardial repolarization dispersion that promotes reentry mechanisms, which are facilitated by the presence of interstitial fibrosis.

As mentioned above, ventricular arrhythmias in hypertensive patients with LVH include; PVCs, ventricular couplets, nonsustained and sustained ventricular tachycardia, ventricular fibrillation, and SCD. LVH produces cardiac (atrial and ventricular) remodeling at different levels such as;

1. Ion-channel remodeling [70, 71]
2. Gap-junction remodeling
3. Remodeling of the cytoskeleton, proteins, and calcium hemostasis
4. Depolarization and repolarization change/dispersion of refractoriness

5. Abnormal conduction
6. Electromechanical contraction disturbances

All of these factors lead to arrhythmias and pump failure.

Myocardial fibrosis and remodeling are the final common pathways that lead to ventricular tachycardia and fibrillation. The electrical changes that are posed by LVH include, in part, abnormalities of depolarization (QRS prolongation) and repolarization (QT prolongation). In addition, myocardial fibrosis also causes inhomogeneity of conduction and refractoriness.

All of these facilitate reentrant arrhythmias, such as VT and VF which leads to SCD. For detailed cellular and ionic mechanism of LVH-induced ventricular arrhythmias refer to the recent publication titled Left Ventricular Hypertrophy and Arrhythmogenesis by Shenasa, et al. [38].

Other mechanisms include upregulation of Na^{+} and Ca^{2+} exchange current and sarcoplasmic reticulum. Figure 18.7 demonstrates that LVH produced in a guinea pig model where transient ischemia due to left anterior descending (LAD) coronary artery occlusion causes ventricular tachyarrhythmias [38].

The enhanced EADs and DADs are triggers for sustained ventricular tachyarrhythmia [72].

Role of Myocardial Ischemia in Arrhythmogenesis in LVH

Significant evidence from experimental and clinical data demonstrate that either regional or global ischemia imposed on the hypertrophied myocardium creates a substrate for development of ventricular tachyarrhythmias.

Myocardial ischemia is a common finding in HTN with or without CAD. Silent ischemia is present in 90% of cases and is correlated with the presence of LVH. Myocardial ischemia was found to be an independent risk factor in most of the studies [73, 74]. Potential mechanisms of the relationship between HTN and myocardial ischemia are summarized as following:

- Increased coronary arteriolar resistance
- Impaired coronary flow reserve
- Endothelial dysfunction
- Epicardial coronary artery atherosclerosis
- Compression of coronary arterioles by muscle and fibrosis
- Arteriolar wall thickening
- Coronary artery size mismatch
- Increased blood viscosity

These changes result in increased LV end-diastolic blood pressure, peripheral vascular resistance, oxygen demand due to rise in wall tension, and decreased subendocardial blood flow and coronary reserve and chronic ischemia.

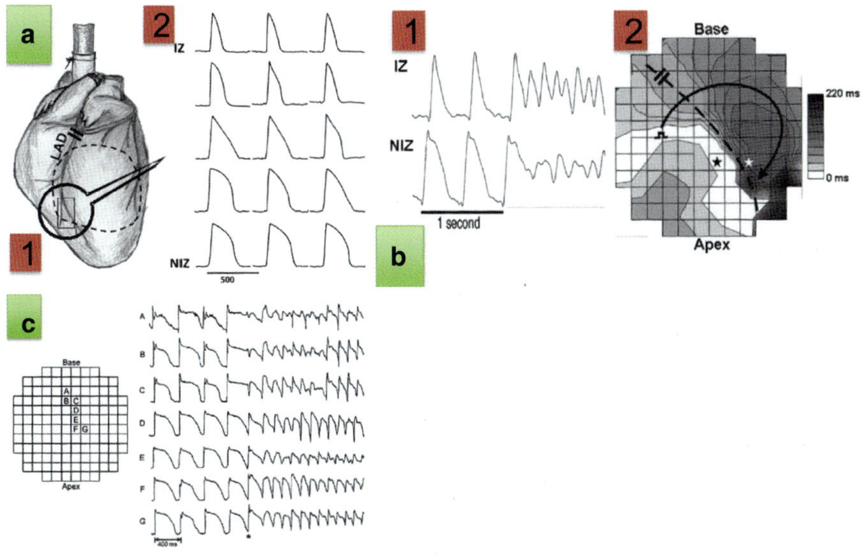

Fig. 18.7 (**a–c**) Optical recordings of membrane voltage obtained from a hypertrophied guinea pig heart. (**a**) Perfused Langendorff preparation. (1): The site of left anterior descending artery ligation marked by the double bar and the outline of the ischemic zone (*dotted line*). (2): Action potentials from 3 horizontal and 5 vertical contiguous pixels across the border between the ischemic zone and nonischemic zone (*highlighted*). The recordings were obtained after 5 min of ischemia during pacing at cycle length 400 ms. Note the development of varying degrees of shortening of APD in the ischemic zone (IZ) compared with the nonischemic zone (NIZ). (**b**) 10 min after left anterior descending artery occlusion illustrates the onset of ventricular tachyarrhythmia. (1): Action potential recordings from two sites 2 mm apart on each side of the border between the IZ and NIZ (*asterisks*). The first three action potentials are paced at a cycle length of 500 ms. Note the development of a 60-ms conduction delay between the two sites, the marked shortening of APD of the IZ site, and the onset of a non-self-terminating VT. (2): Epicardial isochronal activation map of the last paced beat before the onset of VT shows development of an arc of conduction block (represented by crowded isochrones) at the border between the IZ and NIZ. A wave front that started at the site of pacing in the right ventricle circulated around the arc of block in a pattern consistent with circus movement reentry. (**c**) After 8 min of ischemia. Seven action potential (AP) recordings labeled *A* to *G* are illustrated on the right, and their position on the epicardial surface of the ventricle is shown in the schematic photodiode array on the left. The first 4 APs at each recording represent paced APs at a cycle length of 400 ms. The fifth AP was a spontaneous premature beat (*asterisk*) that initiated a non-self-terminating VT. Recordings *A* to *C* were from contiguous sites close to the basal region of the ventricle and showed APD alternans with the first AP with short duration followed by an AP with long duration (ABAB sequence). Recordings *E* to *G* were from contiguous sites toward the apical region of the ventricle and showed APD alternans with the first AP with long duration (BABA sequence). Recording *D* was obtained from a site between the two groups of discordant alternans, and it showed no discernible APD alternans. Because of the spatially discordant alternans, the premature focal excitation failed to activate sites with prolonged APD (sites *A*, *B*, and *C* which only showed a subthreshold potential), whereas it activated sites with shorter APD (sites *E*, *F*, and *G*). This spatial heterogeneity of activation provided the substrate for reentrant excitation. *Abbreviations*: *IZ* ischemic zone, *NIZ* nonischemic zone (From Shenasa et al. [38]. With permission)

LVH inherently demonstrates inhomogeneity of conduction and repolarization. The addition of ischemia that shortens APD further increases this inhomogeneity and creates a suitable substrate for reentrant arrhythmias. Furthermore, regional ischemia increases the flow of K^+ current. This increases the susceptibility to ventricular tachyarrhythmias. El-Sherif, et al. recently demonstrated a guinea pig model of LVH with superimposed regional ischemia by LAD ligation [75]. Using optical mapping in these models, APD was measured in controlled LVH and LVH plus ischemia, which showed greater APD shortening and alterations in the LVH plus ischemia group. Similarly, those with a greater degree of dispersion of repolarization at the ischemic zone border created a substrate for development of ventricular arrhythmias (Fig. 18.7b) [38].

Hypertension, LVH and Atrial Fibrillation

This section is well described in Chap. 9 by Sverre Erik Kjeldsen, et al. However, we will focus on the relationship of HTN, LVH, and AF.

HTN is the most common cause of AF and is present in almost 70 % of patients with AF. Because of this close relationship, HTN is considered a major risk factor for AF and an integral part of any scoring system such as $CHADS_2$ and CHA_2DS_2-VASc [76, 77]. Several epidemiologic studies have already eluded to the close relationship between HTN and AF [78, 79]. The Atrial Fibrillation Registry for Ankle-brachial Index Prevalence Assessment (ARAPACIS) (multicenter, observational, prospective longitudinal study) showed that 52 % of patients with nonvalvular AF have a high prevalence of LVH [80]. LVH is also an important predictor of response to medical therapy for rhythm control, where the treatment algorithm uses antiarrhythmic agents that can potentially cause proarrhythmias in the presence of LVH [81]. Other predisposing risk factors include female gender, 'older' age, HTN, and previous MI [82]. These patients are therefore at high thromboembolic risk and aggressive screening and management is warranted.

The risk of AF in patients with HTN is independent from any other risk factors such as HF (systolic or diastolic), diabetes, CAD, etc. [83, 84]. Increase in LV mass due to HTN is also an independent risk factor for the development of AF [85, 86]. This data is certainly underestimated, as many patients with HTN, LVH, and AF remain asymptomatic. Combination of HTN and AF is present in 72 % of patients with stroke and 82 % of patients with chronic kidney disease. Figure 18.8 shows prevalence of HTN in different trials of AF. LVH also plays an independent risk factor for developing AF [79]. With increasing aging population, both HTN and AF as well as age related comorbidities such as diabetes and HF, the incidence is rising. HTN increases the risk of new onset AF and progression from paroxysmal to persistent AF by 1.8 fold and 1.5 fold, respectively.

AF in patients with HTN and LVH is an independent risk factor for SCD (Fig. 18.9 [87]) [87, 88].

Mechanisms by which HTN predisposes to development of AF is complex:

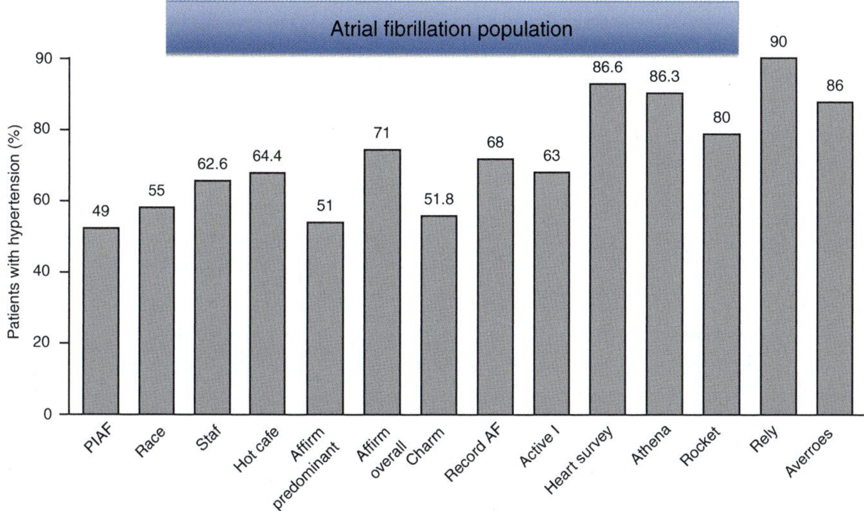

Fig. 18.8 Presence of hypertension in different trials of AF (Reproduced from Manolis et al. [83]. With permission)

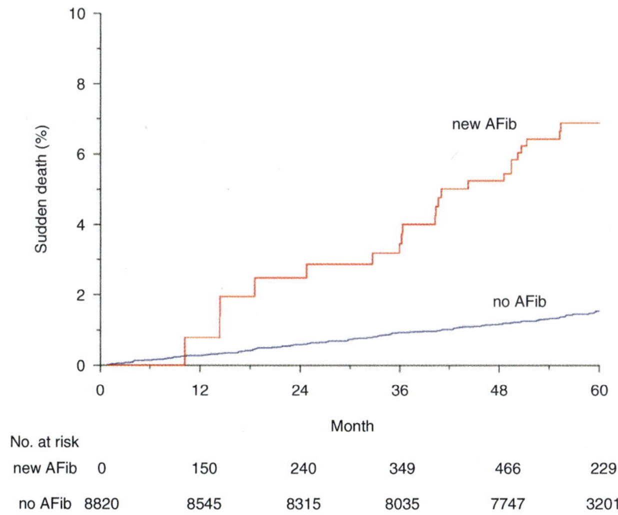

Fig. 18.9 Relationship of SCD to new-onset AF in hypertensive patients with LVH. Survival curves illustrating the rate of sudden cardiac death in relation to development of new-onset atrial fibrillation (AFib) over time (From Okin et al. [87]. With permission)

As shown in Fig. 18.3, HTN causes cardiovascular (atrial, ventricular, and vascular) remodeling via multiple mechanisms that include LVH, diastolic dysfunction, electrical, mechanical, neurohormonal, and structural remodeling in the left atrium. HTN causes left atrial hypertrophy and amyloidosis [89]. Some of these changes are summarized below:

1. It is assumed that angiotensin-converting enzyme (ACE) Inhibitor and angiotensin receptor blockers (ARBs) prevent or at least slow the progression of atrial fibrosis and remodeling. The association of HTN and AF is very high and the prevalence of HTN in patients with AF in some reported are up to 90%. Figure 18.8 [83] demonstrates the prevalence of HTN in multiple AF trials ranging from 50 to 90% [79, 83]. Beyond the close and direct association of HTN and AF, other cardiovascular comorbidities share common association with the two conditions including diabetes, CAD, kidney disease, which are discussed elsewhere in this review. (Fig. 18.1) Most importantly, HTN and AF are the most important risk factors for stroke and SCD. Theoretically, it is assumed that ACE inhibitors and ARBs reduced the incidence of AF in HTN patients by lowering the systolic blood pressure, sympathetic activity, reducing left atrial size and structural changes.
2. HTN causes an increase in LA size and volume, leading to electrical, mechanical, neurohormonal, and structural remolding of AF is well established (Fig. 18.3). In this regard, antihypertensive therapies may reduce, at least in part, the development and progression of AF. Needless to say, today no randomized controlled trials have shown that antihypertensive therapies have significantly reduced the incidence of AF. To date, most of the studies and randomized trials on ACE inhibitors and ARBs with the exception of one report did not report reduction in incident AF. The final common pathway that HTN leads to AF is related to inflammation and fibrosis that creates a substrate for focal triggers and reentrant AF [90].
3. Renin-angiotensin-aldosterone system (neurohormonal pathway) plays an important link to the development of AF. As it will be discussed later, HTN is among the few AF risk factors that can be modified to reduce the risk of AF. Other HTN as Mitchel, et al. reported a 20 mmHg increase in pulse pressure was associated with 24% increase in risk of AF over a 20-year follow-up [91].

Hypertension and Stroke

It is well established that HTN is linked to an increase risk of stroke [92, 93]. Data from the Framingham longitudinal studies and those of other communities like the Olmsted County, Minnesota confirmed the epidemiology and relationship of HTN to stroke that is beyond the scope of this review [94–96]. HTN alone and its consequences, especially AF and LVH, account as independent risk factor for stroke and AF [97, 98]. The yearly incidence of stroke in patients with nonvalvular AF is about 5%, which is five times higher than the match population without AF [99]. Stroke remains the most devastating complication of HTN and AF with significant social and economical burden. Stroke is the third common cause of death and number one cause of disability [92, 100]. HTN and stroke are a global problem [101]. Pathophysiology of stroke-related (secondary) HTN is complex and is not the focus of this review. HTN and stroke share many common risk factors such as CAD, structural heart disease (valvular heart disease), HF, HCM, myocarditis, pulmonary embolism, OSA, obesity, diabetes, metabolic syndrome, hyperthyroidism, and chronic kidney disease [12, 102, 103]. The combination of diabetes and HTN is considered a deadly duet that increases the risk of HF, stroke, and LVH [104]. Emdin C, et al. recently reported that blood pressure increased the risk of new-onset diabetes [105]. This conclusion was based on a meta-analysis of perspective studies in 4.1 million adults. This suggests a complex interplay of many factors that the two diseases share.

Briefly, HTN causes cardiac and vascular remodeling via complex pathways of oxidative stress, arterial baroreceptor, dysfunction and endothelial inflammation, fibrosis, genetic, and environmental factors. Ischemic (embolic) stroke remains the most common form of stroke accounting for about 70 % of all cases of stroke. Etiology of stroke is very diverse and can be divided into two major categories of non-modifiable risk factors such as age, gender, race, genetic profile, and modifiable risk factors such as HTN, diabetes [104], AF, obesity, CAD, dyslipidemia, smoking, HF, neurohormonal abnormalities, chronic kidney disease, contraceptive use, and many others. Aggressive blood pressure control certainly lowers the risk of stroke prevention [106]. Therefore, hypertensive therapy remains the most effective stroke prevention. Guidelines for the prevention of ischemic stroke have been well discussed elsewhere and are beyond the scope of this review [107]. It is also important to achieve adequate blood pressure control after stroke [108].

Hypertension, LVH, and Congestive Heart Failure

Besides diastolic dysfunction and HF, HTN and LVH are common cause of congestive HF, i.e. HF with reduced systolic function. As said earlier, the spectrum of HTN-LVH begins with preclinical course followed by LVH as compensatory mechanism and structural remodeling to pressure overload and vascular and cardiac remodeling that leads to cardiac chamber dilatation and end stage HF. Other factors and comorbidities that enhances progression of HTN-LVH to HF includes OSA [109], obesity, chronic kidney disease, and others. Furthermore, these uncontrolled comorbidities reduce the effectiveness of interventions on AF, such as lower success rate and higher recurrences of AF after catheter ablation [110].

Regression of LVH

Reversal of electrocardiographic and echocardiographic changes, lowers LVH and subsequently the incidence of arrhythmias, i.e. atrial, VT, SCD [111]. Furthermore, antihypertensive treatment with ACE inhibitors have significant effect both LVH and its electrophysiological consequences such as normalization of APD and refractoriness [112] Similarly, ARBs like losartan reduces LVH and arrhythmias in patients with preserved LV systolic function [113].

Okin, et al. and Deverueux, et al. have shown that regression of LVH by optimal management of antihypertensive therapy significantly reduces its consequences [114–117].

Similarly, the LIFE study has shown that absence of in-treatment ECG LVH is associated with reduced risk of SCD independently of treatment modality, blood pressure reduction, prevalent coronary heart disease, and other cardiovascular risk factors in hypertensive patients with LVH [118].

Another example of LVH regression is related to severe aortic stenosis. Lindman, et al. reported that transcatheter aortic valve replacement has been associated with early regression of severe LVH [119].

Blood pressure response during exercise that is often under recognized is quite important, as many patients may have abnormal or borderline resting blood pressure; however, they demonstrate an exaggerated response to dynamic exercise that will significantly increase the risk of stroke and has an independent prognostic value in the management of HTN and its complications [120]. Similarly, nocturnal blood pressure that is often missed during a daily office visit to physicians or healthcare facilities is underappreciated and has a close relationship between the occurrence of AF, obstructive sleep apnea (OSA), and SCD [121].

Prognostic Significance of LVH

LVH irrespective of its etiology and diagnostic methods poses an increased risk of all-cause and cardiovascular mortality in and overall increases mortality rate by 1.5–3.5 fold per year. As said earlier, LVH is considered a silent killer but it is a treatable and reversible condition.

Future Directions

Basic and clinical research will focus on better identification of genetic factors, risk profile, and imaging modalities for early (preclinical) diagnosis of LVH and its arrhythmogenic consequences. Identification of novel genes will hopefully lead to an improved understanding of etiology mechanisms and better management of HTN [122]. Biochemical markers and target therapies such as fibrosis and reverse remodeling will provide better evidence-based paradigm shift in target therapies. Improved electrocardiographic and echocardiographic markers of LVH and geometry may better identify patients at risk of SCD [123]. Non-invasive detection of fibrosis with cardiac MRI and measurement of late gadolinium enhancement has been reported to be useful in characterization of different forms of LVH and remodeling [124]. In the future, cardiac MRI will be used more often both as a screening and risk-stratification

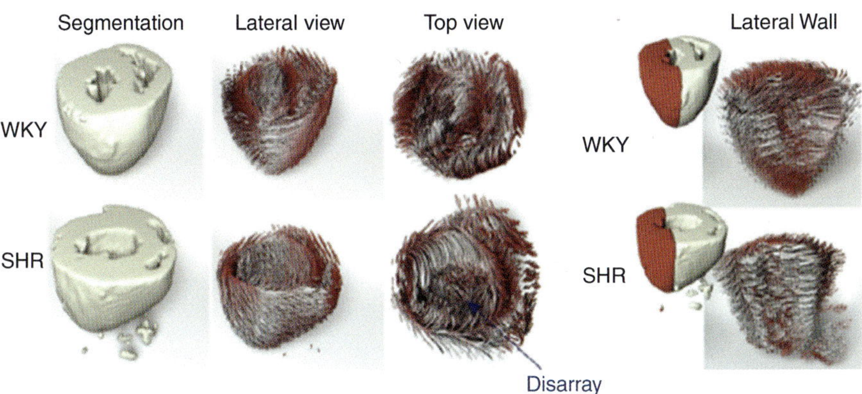

Fig. 18.10 Fiber tractography results from normal WKY (*top*) and diseased SHR (*bottom*) rats. First column: The MRI based segmented myocardia, where the hypertrophied cardiac wall of the SHR may be seen. Second and third columns: Two different views of the fiber tracking results of the entire wall. Seen from the top, there is marked myofiber disarray in the lateral region of the SHR, as opposed to the WKY. Last column: A close-up, focusing on the free wall region where the disarray in the SHR is more noticeable. *Abbreviations*: *MRI* magnetic resonance imaging, *SHR* spontaneously hypertensive rat, *WKY* Wistar-Kyoto rat heart (From Giannakidis et al. [126]. With permission) see video 1

technique in patients at risk of cardiovascular events [125]. Tissue characterization, by different imaging techniques such as fiber tracking and fiber orientation, will help us understand the progression of LVH in patients with HTN (Fig. 18.10 [126]; Video 1 [126]) [40]. Recently, novel approaches for resistant HTN regarding renal denervation has been reported to be effective for blood pressure control and lowers its complications such as LVH and atrial and ventricular arrhythmias; however, long-term follow-ups are currently pending [127–131]. HF and renal failure are the two important complications of long-standing HTN. Complex mechanisms interplay between HTN, HF, and chronic renal failure that is well discussed in the report by Damman, et al. that is beyond the scope of this discussion [132]. The readers are recommended to consider this excellent review. Large scale, landmark trials are on their way to provide guidelines for blood pressure in specific cohorts (i.e. race, gender, genetic profile, and geographic regions) and will provide better identification for high-risk patients [133]. For example, the recently published SPRINT trial suggested that a more aggressive blood pressure control compared to lenient management resulted in lower rates of fatal and non-fatal cardiovascular events and death [134].

Summary

1. HTN remains the most common (non-communicable) disease.
2. HTN is the most common cause of LVH. The natural history of LVH has a wide spectrum of preclinical to end stage HF.

3. HTN is also the most common cause of AF.
4. LVH is commonly associated with increased risk of AF, ventricular arrhythmias, and SCD. LVH is often underrecognized and is considered a silent killer; however, it is a treatable and reversible condition [60].
5. An important differential diagnosis of LVH is HCM and athletes heart, where appropriate imaging modalities are useful.
6. Aggressive and appropriate control of HTN may reverse LVH and its consequences, i.e. decrease the incidence of AF and ventricular arrhythmias.
7. LVH is a common yet underdiagnosed condition as its diagnosis depends on ECGs and other imaging methods.
8. HTN is a very heterogeneous disease with diverse etiologies; thus, the management should target towards a specific etiology and patient profile, i.e. age, gender, ethnicity, geographical region, family, background, genetic profile, etc.
9. LVH has a very heterogeneous etiology; however, the most common cause is long-term HTN and valvular heart disease.
10. LVH diagnosis is based on the ECG and other imaging modalities such as: Echocardiogram, Cardiac MRI, and Cardiac CT.
11. Atrial and ventricular arrhythmias are common in moderate to severe LVH, and are often underdiagnosed and require specific management based on the etiologies.
12. The mechanisms of atrial and ventricular arrhythmias in LVH are diverse and depend on specific causes, mostly related to dispersion of refractoriness that promotes reentry arrhythmias.
13. The appropriate management of specific causes of LVH such as HTN control and valvular heart disease may reverse LVH and its consequences.
14. HTN begets LVH and LVH begets arrhythmias (AF, VT, SCD).

Acknowledgements The author wishes to thank Mariah Smith for her support in preparation of this manuscript.

References

1. Dellsperger KC, Martins JB, Clothier JL, Marcus M. Incidence of sudden cardiac death associated with coronary artery occlusion in dogs with hypertension and left ventricular hypertrophy is reduced by chronic f3-adrenergic blockade. Circulation. 1990;82:941–50.
2. James PA, Oparil S, Carter BL, Cushman WC, Dennison-Himmelfarb C, Handler J, Lackland DT, LeFevre ML, MacKenzie TD, Ogedegbe O, Smith Jr SC, Svetkey LP, Taler SJ, Townsend RR, Wright Jr JT, Narva AS, Ortiz E. 2014 evidence-based guideline for the management of high blood pressure in adults: report from the panel members appointed to the Eighth Joint National Committee (JNC 8). JAMA. 2014;311(5):507–20. doi:10.1001/jama.2013.284427.
3. Mozaffarian D, Benjamin EJ, Arnett DK, Blaha MJ, Cushman M. Heart disease and stroke statistics—2015 update. A report from the American Heart Association. Circulation. 2015;131:e29–322.
4. Piper MA, Evans CV, Burda BU, Margolis KL, O'Connor E, Whitlock EP. Diagnostic and predictive accuracy of blood pressure screening methods with consideration of rescreening

intervals: a systematic review for the U.S. Preventive Services Task Force. Ann Intern Med. 2015;162(3):192–204. doi:10.7326/M14-1539.
5. Cloutier L, Daskalopoulou SS, Padwal RS, Lamarre-Cliche M, Bolli P, McLean D, Milot A, Tobe SW, Tremblay G, McKay DW, Townsend R, Campbell N, Gelfer M. A new algorithm for the diagnosis of hypertension in Canada. Can J Cardiol. 2015;31(5):620–30. doi:10.1016/j.cjca.2015.02.014.
6. Pickering T, Miller N, Ogedegbe G, Krakoff L, Artinian N, Goff D. Call to action on use and reimbursement for home blood pressure monitoring: a joint scientific statement from the American Heart Association, American Society of Hypertension, and Preventive Cardiovascular Nurses Association. J Am Soc Hypertens. 2008;2:192–202.
7. Chobanian A, Bakris G, Black H. Joint national committee on prevention, detection, evaluation, and treatment of high blood pressure, national heart, lung, and blood institute; national high blood pressure education program coordinating committee. Seventh report of the Joint National Committee on prevention, detection, evaluation, and treatment of high blood pressure. Hypertension. 2003;42:1206–52.
8. Ostchega Y, Yoon SS, Hughes J, Louis T. Hypertension awareness, treatment, and control-continued disparities in adults: United States, 2005–2006. 2008.
9. Wang Y, Wang JQ. The prevalence of prehypertension and hypertension among US adults according to the New Joint National Committee guidelines: new challenges of the old problem. Arch Intern Med. 2004;164:2126–34.
10. De Nicola L, Gabbai FB, Agarwal R, Chiodini P, Borrelli S, Bellizzi V, Nappi F, Conte G, Minutolo R. Prevalence and prognostic role of resistant hypertension in chronic kidney disease patients. J Am Coll Cardiol. 2013;61(24):2461–7. doi:10.1016/j.jacc.2012.12.061.
11. Protasiewicz M, Kadziela J, Poczatek K, Poreba R, Podgorski M, Derkacz A, Prejbisz A, Mysiak A, AJanuszewicz A, Witkowski A. Renal artery stenosis in patients with resistant hypetension. Am J Cardiol. 2013;112:1417–20.
12. Sanchez-de-la-Torre M, Khalyfa A, Sanchez-de-la-Torre A, Martinez-Alonso M, Martinez-Garcia MA, Barcelo A, Lloberes P, Campos-Rodriguez F, Capote F, Diaz-de-Atauri MJ, Somoza M, Gonzalez M, Masa JF, Gozal D, Barbe F, Spanish Sleep N. Precision medicine in patients with resistant hypertension and obstructive sleep apnea: blood pressure response to continuous positive airway pressure treatment. J Am Coll Cardiol. 2015;66(9):1023–32. doi:10.1016/j.jacc.2015.06.1315.
13. Mensah GA. Preface: hypertension and hypertensive heart disease. Cardiol Clin. 2010;28(4):xiii–xiv. doi:10.1016/j.ccl.2010.09.001.
14. World Health Organization. Global health risks: mortality and burden of disease attributable to selected major risks. Geneva: World Health Organization; 2009.
15. Wall H, Hannan J, Wright J. Patients with undiagnosed hypertension-hiding in plain sight. JAMA. 2014;312(19):1973–4.
16. World Heart Federation. Stroke and hypertension. 2016. http://www.world-heart-federation.org/cardiovascular-health/stroke/stroke-and-hypertension/. Accessed 20 Mar 2016.
17. Stroke Association. High Blood Pressure and Stroke. 2012.
18. Raman SV. The hypertensive heart. An integrated understanding informed by imaging. J Am Coll Cardiol. 2010;55(2):91–6. doi:10.1016/j.jacc.2009.07.059.
19. Messerli FH. Hypertension and sudden cardiac death. Am J Hypertens. 1999;12(12 Pt 3):181S–8.
20. Arnett DK, Li N, Tang W, Rao DC, Devereux RB, Claas SA, Kraemer R, Broeckel U. Genome-wide association study identifies single-nucleotide polymorphism in KCNB1 associated with left ventricular mass in humans: the HyperGEN Study. BMC Med Genet. 2009;10:43. doi:10.1186/1471-2350-10-43.
21. Prisant M. Hypertensive heart disease. J Clin Hypertens. 2005;7:231–8.
22. Lee H, Kong YH, Kim KH, Huh J, Kang IS, Song J. Left ventricular hypertrophy and diastolic function in children and adolescents with essential hypertension. J Clin Hypertens. 2015;21:21. doi:10.1186/s40885-015-0031-8.

23. Diez J, Frohlich ED. A translational approach to hypertensive heart disease. Hypertension. 2010;55(1):1–8. doi:10.1161/HYPERTENSIONAHA.109.141887.
24. Osler W. The principle and practice of medicine. New York: D. Appleton and Company; 1892. p. 628–35.
25. Gradman AH, Alfayoumi F. From left ventricular hypertrophy to congestive heart failure: management of hypertensive heart disease. Prog Cardiovasc Dis. 2006;48(5):326–41. doi:10.1016/j.pcad.2006.02.001.
26. Lopez B, Ravassa S, Gonzalez A, Zubillaga E, Bonavila C, Berges M, Echegaray K, Beaumont J, Moreno MU, San Jose G, Larman M, Querejeta R, Diez J. Myocardial collagen cross-linking is associated with heart failure hospitalization in patients with hypertensive heart failure. J Am Coll Cardiol. 2016;67(3):251–60. doi:10.1016/j.jacc.2015.10.063.
27. Moon JC, Treibel TA, Schelbert EB. Myocardial fibrosis in hypertensive heart failure: does quality rather than quantity matter? J Am Coll Cardiol. 2016;67(3):261–3. doi:10.1016/j.jacc.2015.10.070.
28. Ganau A, Devereux RB, Roman MJ, De Simone G, Pickering TG, Saba PS, Vargiu P, Simongini I, Laragh J. Patterns of left ventricular hypertrophy and geometric remodeling in essential hypertension. J Am Coll Cardiol. 1992;19(7):1550–8.
29. Lieb W, Gona P, Larson MG, Aragam J, Zile MR, Cheng S, Benjamin EJ, Vasan RS. The natural history of left ventricular geometry in the community: clinical correlates and prognostic significance of change in LV geometric pattern. JACC Cardiovasc Imaging. 2014;7(9):870–8. doi:10.1016/j.jcmg.2014.05.008.
30. Kahan T, Bergfeldt L. Left ventricular hypertrophy in hypertension: its arrhythmogenic potential. Heart. 2005;91(2):250–6. doi:10.1136/hrt.2004.042473.
31. de Marvao A, Dawes TJ, Shi W, Durighel G, Rueckert D, Cook SA, O'Regan DP. Precursors of hypertensive heart phenotype develop in healthy adults: a high-resolution 3D MRI study. JACC Cardiovasc Imaging. 2015;8(11):1260–9. doi:10.1016/j.jcmg.2015.08.007.
32. Muiesan ML, Salvetti M, Monteduro C, Bonzi B, Paini A, Viola S, Poisa P, Rizzoni D, Castellano M, Agabiti-Rosei E. Left ventricular concentric geometry during treatment adversely affects cardiovascular prognosis in hypertensive patients. Hypertension. 2004;43(4):731–8. doi:10.1161/01.HYP.0000121223.44837.de.
33. Dahlöf B. Left ventricular hypertrophy and angiotensin II antagonists. Am J Hypertens. 2001;14(2):174–82. doi:10.1016/s0895-7061(00)01257-7.
34. Schlaich MP, Kaye DM, Lambert E, Sommerville M, Socratous F, Esler MD. Relation between cardiac sympathetic activity and hypertensive left ventricular hypertrophy. Circulation. 2003;108(5):560–5. doi:10.1161/01.CIR.0000081775.72651.B6.
35. Sokolow M, Lyon TP. The ventricular complex in left ventricular hypertrophy as obtained by unipolar precordial and limb leads. Am Heart J. 1949;37(2):161–86. doi:10.1016/0002-8703(49)90562-1.
36. Romhilt D, Bove K, Norris F, Conyers E. A critical appraisal of the electrocardiographic criteria for the diagnosis of left ventricular hypertrophy. Circulation. 1969;40(2):185–95.
37. Mirvis D, Goldberger A. Electrocardiography. In: Braunwald's heart disease: a textbook of cardiovascular medicine, vol. 10. Philadelphia: Elsevier; 2015. p. 114–54.
38. Shenasa M, Shenasa H, El-Sherif N. Left ventricular hypertrophy and arrhythmogenesis. Card Electrophysiol Clin. 2015;7(2):207–20. doi:10.1016/j.ccep.2015.03.017.
39. Levy D, Labib S, Anderson K, Christinansen J, Kannel WB, Castelli WP. Determinants of sensitivity and specificity of electrocardiographic criteria for left ventricular hypertrophy. Circulation. 1990;81:815–20.
40. Shenasa M, Shenasa H. Electrocardiographic markers of sudden cardiac death in different substrates. In: Shenasa M, Josephson M, Estes M, editors. The ECG handbook of contemporary challenges. Minneapolis: Cardiotext Publishing; 2015.
41. Pewsner D, Juni P, Egger M, Battaglia M, Sundstrom J, Bachmann LM. Accuracy of electrocardiography in diagnosis of left ventricular hypertrophy in arterial hypertension: systematic review. BMJ. 2007;335(7622):711. doi:10.1136/bmj.39276.636354.AE.

42. Sundstrom J, Lind L, Arnlov J, Zethelius B, Andren B, Lithell HO. Echocardiographic and electrocardiographic diagnoses of left ventricular hypertrophy predict mortality independently of each other in a population of elderly men. Circulation. 2001;103(19):2346–51. doi:10.1161/01.cir.103.19.2346.
43. Levy D, Savage DD, Garrison RJ, Anderson KM, Kannel WB, Castelli WP. Echocardiographic criteria for left ventricular hypertrophy: the Framingham Heart Study. Am J Cardiol. 1987;59(9):956–60. doi:10.1016/0002-9149(87)91133-7.
44. Yuda S, Khoury V, Marwick T. Influence of wall stress and left ventricular geometry on the accuracy of dobutamine stress echocardiography. J Am Coll Cardiol. 2002;40:1311–9.
45. Rosenberg MA, Manning WJ. Diastolic dysfunction and risk of atrial fibrillation: a mechanistic appraisal. Circulation. 2012;126(19):2353–62. doi:10.1161/CIRCULATIONAHA.112.113233.
46. Soliman EZ, Shah AJ, Boerkircher A, Li Y, Rautaharju PM. Inter-relationship between electrocardiographic left ventricular hypertrophy and QT prolongation as predictors of increased risk of mortality in the general population. Circ Arrhythm Electrophysiol. 2014;7(3):400–6. doi:10.1161/CIRCEP.113.001396.
47. Haugaa KH, Bos JM, Borkenhagen EJ, Tarrell RF, Morlan BW, Caraballo PJ, Ackerman MJ. Impact of left ventricular hypertrophy on QT prolongation and associated mortality. Heart Rhythm. 2014;11(11):1957–65. doi:10.1016/j.hrthm.2014.06.025.
48. Lorenz CH, Walker E, Morgan V, Klei S, Graham T. Normal human right and left ventricular mass, systolic function, and gender differences by cine magnetic resonance imaging. J Cardiovasc Magn Reson. 1999;1:7–21.
49. Levy D, Murabito JM, Anderson K, Christiansen J. Echocardiographic left ventricular hypertrophy: clinical characteristics: the Framingham Heart Study. Clin Exp Hypertens. 1992;14:85–97.
50. Kannel WB, Gordon T, Castelli WP, Margolis JR. Electrocardiographic left ventricular hypertrophy and risk of coronary heart disease. The Framingham Study. Ann Intern Med. 1970;72(6):813–22. doi:10.7326/0003-4819-72-6-813.
51. Echocardiography. Braunwald's heart disease: a textbook of cardiovascular medicine. Philadelphia: Elsevier; 2015.
52. Levy D, Garrison RJ, Savage DD, Kannel WB, Castelli WP. Prognostic implications of echocardiographically determined left ventricular mass in the Framingham Heart Study. N Engl J Med. 1990;322(22):1561–6. doi:10.1056/NEJM199005313222203.
53. Lorell BH, Carabello BA. Left ventricular hypertrophy: pathogenesis, detection, and prognosis. Circulation. 2000;102:470–9.
54. Kerut E, Mcllwai E, Plotnick G. Handbook of Echo-Doppler interpretation. New York: Wiley-Blackwell; 2004.
55. Koren M, Deverux R, Casale P, Savage D, Laragh J. Relation of left ventricular mass and geometry to morbidity and mortality in uncomplicated essential hypertension. Ann Intern Med. 1991;114:345–52.
56. Schilaci G, Verdecchia P, Porcellati C, Cuccurullo O, Cosco C, Perticone F. Continuous relation between left ventricular mass and cardiovascular risk in essential hypertension. Hypertension. 2000;35:580–6.
57. Klingbeil AU, Schneider M, Martus P, Messerli FH, Schmieder RE. A meta-analysis of the effects of treatment on left ventricular mass in essential hypertension. Am J Med. 2003;115(1):41–6. doi:10.1016/S0002-9343(03)00158-X.
58. Shapiro E. Evaluation of left ventricular hypertrophy by magnetic resonance imaging. Am J Card Imaging. 1994;8:310–5.
59. Singh M, Mensah GA, Bakris G. Pathogenesis and clinical physiology of hypertension. Cardiol Clin. 2010;28(4):545–59. doi:10.1016/j.ccl.2010.07.001.
60. Bauml MA, Underwood DA. Left ventricular hypertrophy: an overlooked cardiovascular risk factor. Cleve Clin J Med. 2010;77(6):381–7. doi:10.3949/ccjm.77a.09158.
61. Kuruvilla S, Janardhanan R, Antkowiak P, Keeley EC, Adenaw N, Brooks J, Epstein FH, Kramer CM, Salerno M. Increased extracellular volume and altered mechanics are associated

with LVH in hypertensive heart disease, not hypertension alone. JACC Cardiovasc Imaging. 2015;8(2):172–80. doi:10.1016/j.jcmg.2014.09.020.

62. Georgiopoulou VV, Kalogeropoulos AP, Raggi P, Butler J. Prevention, diagnosis, and treatment of hypertensive heart disease. Cardiol Clin. 2010;28(4):675–91. doi:10.1016/j.ccl.2010.07.005.
63. Boon-Peng H, Mat Jusoh JA, Marshall CR, Majid F, Danuri N, Basir F, Thiruvahindrapuram B, Scherer SW, Yusoff K. Rare copy number variants identified suggest the regulating pathways in hypertension-related left ventricular hypertrophy. PLoS One. 2016;11(3):e0148755. doi:10.1371/journal.pone.0148755.
64. Hoit BD. Left atrial size and function: role in prognosis. J Am Coll Cardiol. 2014;63(6):493–505. doi:10.1016/j.jacc.2013.10.055.
65. Tin LL, Beevers DG, Lip GYH. Hypertension, left ventricular hypertrophy, and sudden death. Curr Cardiol Rep. 2002;4(6):449–57. doi:10.1007/s11886-002-0105-6.
66. Kannel WB, Cobb J. Left ventricular hypertrophy and mortality: results from the Framingham Study. Cardiology. 1992;81(4–5):291–8.
67. Stevens SM, Reinier K, Chugh SS. Increased left ventricular mass as a predictor of sudden cardiac death: is it time to put it to the test? Circ Arrhythm Electrophysiol. 2013;6(1):212–7. doi:10.1161/CIRCEP.112.974931.
68. Chatterjee S, Bavishi C, Sardar P, Agarwal V, Krishnamoorthy P, Grodzicki T, Messerli FH. Meta-analysis of left ventricular hypertrophy and sustained arrhythmias. Am J Cardiol. 2014;114(7):1049–52. doi:10.1016/j.amjcard.2014.07.015.
69. Hunter JJ, Chien KR. Signaling pathways for cardiac hypertrophy and failure. N Engl J Med. 1999;341(17):1276–83. doi:10.1056/NEJM199910213411706.
70. Kowey P, Friehling T, Sewter J, Wu Y, Sokil A, Paul J, Nocella J. Electrophysiological effects of left ventricular hypertrophy: effect of calcium and potassium channel blockers. Circulation. 1991;83:2067–75.
71. Marionneau C, Brunet S, Flagg TP, Pilgram TK, Demolombe S, Nerbonne JM. Distinct cellular and molecular mechanisms underlie functional remodeling of repolarizing K+ currents with left ventricular hypertrophy. Circ Res. 2008;102(11):1406–15. doi:10.1161/CIRCRESAHA.107.170050.
72. Antoons G, Oros A, Bito V, Sipido KR, Vos MA. Cellular basis for triggered ventricular arrhythmias that occur in the setting of compensated hypertrophy and heart failure: considerations for diagnosis and treatment. J Electrocardiol. 2007;40(6):S8–14. doi:10.1016/j.jelectrocard.2007.05.022.
73. Zehender M, Buchner C, Meinertz T, Just H. Prevalence, circumstances, mechanisms, and risk stratification of sudden cardiac death in unipolar single-chamber ventricular pacing. Circulation. 1992;85:596–605.
74. Pringle SD, Dunn FG, Macfarlane PW, McKillop JH, Lorimer AR, Cobbe SM. Significance of ventricular arrhythmias in systemic hypertension with left ventricular hypertrophy. Am J Cardiol. 1992;69(9):913–7. doi:10.1016/0002-9149(92)90792-W.
75. Koshevnikov DCE, El-Sherif N. Mechanisms of enhanced arrhythmogenecity of regional ischemia in the hypertrophied heart. Heart Rhythm. 2009;6:522–7.
76. Benjamin EJ, Levy D, Vaziri SM, D'Agostino RB, Belanger AJ, Wolf PA. Independent risk factors for atrial fibrillation in a population-based cohort: the Framingham Heart Study. JAMA. 1994;271(11):840–4. doi:10.1001/jama.1994.03510350050036.
77. Grundvold I, Skretteberg PT, Liestol K, Erikssen G, Kjeldsen SE, Arnesen H, Erikssen J, Bodegard J. Upper normal blood pressures predict incident atrial fibrillation in healthy middle-aged men: a 35-year follow-up study. Hypertension. 2012;59(2):198–204. doi:10.1161/HYPERTENSIONAHA.111.179713.
78. Lau YF, Yiu KH, Siu CW, Tse HF. Hypertension and atrial fibrillation: epidemiology, pathophysiology, and therapeutic implications. J Hum Hypertens. 2012;26:563–9.
79. Shenasa M, Shenasa H, Rouhani S. Atrial fibrillation in different clinical substrates. In: Shenasa M, Camm AJ, editors. Management of atrial fibrillation. Oxford University Press; Great Clarendon Street, Oxford, OX2 6DP, United Kingdom: 2015. p. 39.

80. Violi F, DavÏ G, Proietti M, Pastori D, Hiatt WR, Corazza GR, Perticone F, Pignatelli P, Farcomeni A, Vestri AR, Lip GYH, Basili S, Investigators oBoTA. Ankle-Brachial Index and cardiovascular events in atrial fibrillation. The ARAPACIS Study. Thrombosis and haemostasis. 2016. doi:10.1160/TH15-07-0612.
81. Badheka AO, Shah N, Grover PM, Patel N, Chothani A, Mehta K, Singh V, Deshmukh A, Savani GT, Rathod A, Panaich SS, Patel N, Arora SB, Coffey JO, Mitrani RD, Halperin JL, Viles-Gonzalez JF. Outcomes in atrial fibrillation patients with and without left ventricular hypertrophy when treated with a lenient rate-control or rhythm-control strategy. Am J Cardiol. 2014;113:1159–65.
82. Proietti M, Marra AM, Tassone EJ, De Vuono S, Corrao S, Gobbi P, Perticone F, Corazza GR, Basili S, Lip GY, Violi F, Raparelli V, Investigators AS, Group GIS . Frequency of left ventricular hypertrophy in non-valvular atrial fibrillation. Am J Cardiol. 2015;116(6):877–82. doi:10.1016/j.amjcard.2015.05.060.
83. Manolis AJ, Rosei EA, Coca A, Cifkova R, Erdine SE, Kjeldsen S, Lip GY, Narkiewicz K, Parati G, Redon J, Schmieder R, Tsioufis C, Mancia G. Hypertension and atrial fibrillation: diagnostic approach, prevention and treatment. Position paper of the Working Group 'Hypertension Arrhythmias and Thrombosis' of the European Society of Hypertension. J Hypertens. 2012;30(2):239–52. doi:10.1097/HJH.0b013e32834f03bf.
84. Conti A, Alesi A, Trausi F, Scorpiniti M, Angeli E, Bigiarini S, Bianchi S, Donnini C, Lazzeretti D, Padeletti L. Hypertension and atrial fibrillation: prognostic aspects of troponin elevations in clinical practice. Crit Pathw Cardiol. 2014;13:141–6.
85. Tedrow U, Conen D, Ridker PM, Cook NR, Koplan B, Manson JE. The long-and short-term impact of elevated body mass index on the risk of new atrial fibrillation: the WHS (Women's Health Study). J Am Coll Cardiol. 2010;55:2319–27.
86. Lloyd-Jones DM, Wang TJ, Leip EP, Larson MG, Levy D, Vasan RS, D'Agostino RB, Massaro JM, Beiser A, Wolf PA, Benjamin EJ. Lifetime risk for development of atrial fibrillation: the Framingham Heart Study. Circulation. 2004;110(9):1042–6. doi:10.1161/01.CIR.0000140263.20897.42.
87. Okin PM, Bang CN, Wachtell K, Hille DA, Kjeldsen SE, Dahlof B, Devereux RB. Relationship of sudden cardiac death to new-onset atrial fibrillation in hypertensive patients with left ventricular hypertrophy. Circ Arrhythm Electrophysiol. 2013;6(2):243–51. doi:10.1161/CIRCEP.112.977777.
88. Reinier K, Marijon E, Uy-Evanado A, Teodorescu C, Narayanan K, Chugh H, Gunson K, Jui J, Chugh SS. The association between atrial fibrillation and sudden cardiac death: the relevance of heart failure. JACC Heart Fail. 2014;2(3):221–7. doi:10.1016/j.jchf.2013.12.006.
89. Sidorova TN, Mace LC, Wells KS, Yermalitskaya LV, Su PF, Shyr Y, Atkinson JB, Fogo AB, Prinsen JK, Byrne JG, Petracek MR, Greelish JP, Hoff SJ, Ball SK, Glabe CG, Brown NJ, Barnett JV, Murray KT. Hypertension is associated with preamyloid oligomers in human atrium: a missing link in atrial pathophysiology? J Am Heart Assoc. 2014;3(6):e001384. doi:10.1161/JAHA.114.001384.
90. Shenasa M, Shenasa H, Soleimanieh M. Update on atrial fibrillation. Egypt Heart J. 2014;66(3):193–216. doi:10.1016/j.ehj.2014.03.004.
91. Mitchell GF, Vasan RS, Keyes MJ, Parise H, Wang T, Larson MG, D'Agostino R, Kannel WB, Levy D, Benjamin EJ. Pulse pressure and risk of new-onset atrial fibrillation. JAMA. 2007;297:709–15.
92. Yu JG, Zhou RR, Cai GJ. From hypertension to stroke: mechanisms and potential prevention strategies. CNS Neurosci Ther. 2011;17(5):577–84. doi:10.1111/j.1755-5949.2011.00264.x.
93. Ravenni R, Jabre JF, Casiglia E, Mazza A. Primary stroke prevention and hypertension treatment: which is the first-line strategy? Neurol Int. 2011;3(2):e12. doi:10.4081/ni.2011.e12.
94. Miyasaka Y, Barnes ME, Gersh BJ, Cha SS, Seward JB, Bailey KR, Iwasaka T, Tsang TS. Time trends of ischemic stroke incidence and mortality in patients diagnosed with first atrial fibrillation in 1980 to 2000: report of a community-based study. Stroke. 2005;36(11):2362–6. doi:10.1161/01.STR.0000185927.63746.23.

95. Miyasaka Y, Barnes ME, Gersh BJ, Cha SS, Bailey KR, Abhayaratna WP, Seward JB, Tsang TS. Secular trends in incidence of atrial fibrillation in Olmsted County, Minnesota, 1980 to 2000, and implications on the projections for future prevalence. Circulation. 2006;114(2):119–25. doi:10.1161/CIRCULATIONAHA.105.595140.
96. Meissner I, Whisnant J, Garraway W. Hypertension management and stroke recurrence in a community. Stroke. 1988;19:459.
97. Di Tullio MR, Zwas DR, Sacco RL, Sciacca RR, Homma S. Left ventricular mass and geometry and the risk of ischemic stroke. Stroke. 2003;34(10):2380–4. doi:10.1161/01.STR.0000089680.77236.60.
98. Fustinoni O. Left ventricular hypertrophy: an unseemly risk factor for stroke? Stroke. 2003;34:2385–6.
99. Wolf PA, Abbott RD, Kannel WB. Atrial fibrillation: a major contributor to stroke in the elderly: the Framingham Study. Arch Intern Med. 1987;147(9):1561–4. doi:10.1001/archinte.1987.00370090041008.
100. Cressman M, Gifford R. Hypertension and stroke. J Am Coll Cardiol. 1983;1(2):521–7.
101. Singh RB, Suh IL, Singh VP, Chaithiraphan S, Laothavorn P, Sy RG, Babilonia NA, Rahman ARA, Sheikh S, Tomlinson B, Sarraf-Zadigan N. Hypertension and stroke in Asia: prevalence, control and strategies in developing countries for prevention. J Hum Hypertens. 2000;14(10/11):749–63. doi:10.1038/sj.jhh.1001057.
102. Williams PT, Franklin BA. Incident diabetes mellitus, hypertension, and cardiovascular disease risk in exercising hypercholesterolemic patients. Am J Cardiol. 2015;116(10):1516–20. doi:10.1016/j.amjcard.2015.08.011.
103. Long AN, Dagogo-Jack S. Comorbidities of diabetes and hypertension: mechanisms and approach to target organ protection. J Clin Hypertens. 2011;13(4):244–51. doi:10.1111/j.1751-7176.2011.00434.x.
104. McFarlane S, Sica D, Sowers J, McFarlane SI, Sica DA, Sowers JR. Stroke in patients with diabetes and hypertension. J Clin Hypertens. 2005;7:286–92.
105. Emdin CA, Anderson SG, Woodward M, Rahimi K. Usual blood pressure and risk of new-onset diabetes: evidence from 4.1 million adults and a meta-analysis of prospective studies. J Am Coll Cardiol. 2015;66(14):1552–62. doi:10.1016/j.jacc.2015.07.059.
106. Howard G, Banach M, Cushman M, Goff DC, Howard VJ, Lackland DT, McVay J, Meschia JF, Muntner P, Oparil S, Rightmyer M, Taylor HA. Is blood pressure control for stroke prevention the correct goal? The lost opportunity of preventing hypertension. Stroke. 2015;46(6):1595–600. doi:10.1161/STROKEAHA.115.009128.
107. Kernan WN, Ovbiagele B, Black HR, Bravata DM, Chimowitz MI, Ezekowitz MD, Fang MC, Fisher M, Furie KL, Heck DV, Johnston SC, Kasner SE, Kittner SJ, Mitchell PH, Rich MW, Richardson D, Schwamm LH, Wilson JA, American Heart Association Stroke Council CoC, Stroke Nursing CoCC, Council on Peripheral Vascular D. Guidelines for the prevention of stroke in patients with stroke and transient ischemic attack: a guideline for healthcare professionals from the American Heart Association/American Stroke Association. Stroke. 2014;45(7):2160–236. doi:10.1161/STR.0000000000000024.
108. Okin PM, Kjeldsen SE, Devereux RB. Systolic blood pressure control and mortality after stroke in hypertensive patients. Stroke. 2015;46(8):2113–8. doi:10.1161/STROKEAHA.115.009592.
109. Shukla A, Aizer A, Holmes D, Fowler S, Park DS, Bernstein S, Bernstein N, Chinitz L. Effect of obstructive sleep apnea treatment on atrial fibrillation recurrence. JACC. 2015;1(1–2):41–51. doi:10.1016/j.jacep.2015.02.014.
110. Santoro F, Di Biase L, Trivedi C, Burkhardt JD, Paoletti Perini A, Sanchez J, Horton R, Mohanty P, Mohanty S, Bai R, Santangeli P, Lakkireddy D, Reddy M, Elayi CS, Hongo R, Beheiry S, Hao S, Schweikert RA, Viles-Gonzalez J, Fassini G, Casella M, Dello Russo A, Tondo C, Natale A. Impact of uncontrolled hypertension on atrial fibrillation ablation outcome. JACC. 2015;1(3):164–73. doi:10.1016/j.jacep.2015.04.002.
111. Moser A, Herbert PR. Prevention of disease progression, left ventricular hypertrophy and congestive heart failure in hypertension treatment trials. J Am Coll Cardiol. 1996;27:5.

112. Rials S, Wu Y, Xu X, Filart R, Marinchak R, Kowey P. Regression of left ventricular hypertrophy with captopril restores normal ventricular action potential duration, dispersion of refractoriness, and vulnerability to inducible ventricular fibrillation. Circulation. 1997;96:1330–6.
113. Zakynthinos E, Pierrutsakos C, Daniil Z, Papadogiannis D. Losartan controlled blood pressure and reduced left ventricular hypertrophy but did not alter arrhythmias in hypertensive men with preserved systolic function. Angiology. 2005;56(4):439–49. doi:10.1177/000331970505600412.
114. Okin PM, Wachtell K, Devereux RB, Harris KE, Jern S, Julius S, Lindholm LH, Nielminen MS, Edelman JM, Hille DA, Dahlo B. Regression of electrocardiographic left ventricular hypertrophy and decreased incidence of new-onset atrial fibrillation in patients with hypertension. JAMA. 2006;296:1242–8.
115. Devereux RB. Prognostic significance of left ventricular mass change during treatment of hypertension. JAMA. 2004;292:2350–6.
116. Malmqvist K, Kahan T, Edner M, Held C, Hägg A, Lind L, Müller-Brunotte R, Nyström F, Öhman KP, Osbakken MD, Östergren J, investigators obot. Regression of left ventricular hypertrophy in human hypertension with irbesartan. J Hypertens. 2001;19(6):1167–76.
117. Gosse P, Dubourg O, Gueret P. Regression of left ventricular hypertrophy with echocardiography: some lession from the LIVE study. J Hypertens. 2003;21:217–21.
118. Wachtell K, Okin PM, Olsen MH, Dahlof B, Devereux RB, Ibsen H, Kjeldsen SE, Lindholm LH, Nieminen MS, Thygesen K. Regression of electrocardiographic left ventricular hypertrophy during antihypertensive therapy and reduction in sudden cardiac death: the LIFE Study. Circulation. 2007;116(7):700–5. doi:10.1161/CIRCULATIONAHA.106.666594.
119. Lindman BR, Stewart WJ, Pibarot P, Hahn RT, Otto CM, Xu K, Devereux RB, Weissman NJ, Enriquez-Sarano M, Szeto WY, Makkar R, Miller DC, Lerakis S, Kapadia S, Bowers B, Greason KL, McAndrew TC, Lei Y, Leon MB, Douglas PS. Early regression of severe left ventricular hypertrophy after transcatheter aortic valve replacement is associated with decreased hospitalizations. JACC Cardiovasc Interv. 2014;7(6):662–73. doi:10.1016/j.jcin.2014.02.011.
120. Le VV, Mitiku T, Sungar G, Myers J, Froelicher V. The blood pressure response to dynamic exercise testing: a systematic review. Prog Cardiovasc Dis. 2008;51(2):135–60. doi:10.1016/j.pcad.2008.07.001.
121. Drawz P, Alper A, Anderson AH, Brecklin C, Charleston J, Chen J, Deo R, Fischer M, He J, Hsu C, Huan Y, Keane M, Kusek JW, Makos GK, Miller ER, Soliman E, Steigerwalt SP, Taliercio JJ, Townsend RR, Weird M, Wright Jr J, Xie D, Rahman M. Masked hypertension and elevated nighttime blood pressure in CKD: prevalence and association with target organ damage. Clin J Am Soc Nephrol. 2016;11(4):642–52.
122. Arora P, Newton-Cheh C. Blood pressure and human genetic variation in the general population. Curr Opin Cardiol. 2010;25(3):229–37. doi:10.1097/HCO.0b013e3283383e2c.
123. Narayanan K, Reinier K, Teodorescu C, Uy-Evanado A, Chugh H, Gunson K, Jui J, Chugh SS. Electrocardiographic versus echocardiographic left ventricular hypertrophy and sudden cardiac arrest in the community. Heart Rhythm. 2014;11(6):1040–6. doi:10.1016/j.hrthm.2014.03.023.
124. Rudolph A, Abdel-Aty H, Bohi S, Philipp B, Zagrosek A, Dietz R, Schulz-Menger J. Noninvasive detection of fibrosis applying contrast-enhanced cardiac magnetic resonance in different forms of left ventricular hypertrophy. J Am Coll Cardiol. 2009;53:284–91. doi:10.1016/j.jacc.2008.08.064.
125. Kawel N, Turkbey EB, Carr JJ, Eng J, Gomes AS, Hundley WG, Johnson C, Masri SC, Prince MR, van der Geest RJ, Lima JA, Bluemke DA. Normal left ventricular myocardial thickness for middle-aged and older subjects with steady-state free precession cardiac magnetic resonance: the multi-ethnic study of atherosclerosis. Circ Cardiovasc Imaging. 2012;5(4):500–8. doi:10.1161/CIRCIMAGING.112.973560.
126. Giannakidis A, Rohmer D, Veress A, Gullberg GT. Diffusion tensor magnetic resonance imaging-derived myocardial fiber disarray in hypertensive left ventricular hypertrophy: visualization,

quantification and the effect on mechanical function. In: Shenasa M, Hindricks G, Borggrefe M, Breithardt G, Josephson M, editors. Cardiac mapping. 4th ed. New York: Wiley-Blackwell; 2013. p. 579.

127. Bertog SC, Sobotka PA, Sievert H. Renal denervation for hypertension. JACC Cardiovasc Interv. 2012;5(3):249–58. doi:10.1016/j.jcin.2011.12.011.
128. Thukkani AK, Bhatt DL. Renal denervation therapy for hypertension. Circulation. 2013;128(20):2251–4. doi:10.1161/CIRCULATIONAHA.113.004660.
129. Ott C, Mahfoud F, Schmid A, Ditting T, Sobotka PA, Veelken R, Spies A, Ukena C, Laufs U, Uder M, Bohm M, Schmieder RE. Renal denervation in moderate treatment-resistant hypertension. J Am Coll Cardiol. 2013;62(20):1880–6. doi:10.1016/j.jacc.2013.06.023.
130. Rocha-Singh KJ, Katholi RE. Renal sympathetic denervation for treatment-resistant hypertension…in moderation. J Am Coll Cardiol. 2013;62(20):1887–9. doi:10.1016/j.jacc.2013.06.020.
131. Schirmer SH, Sayed MM, Reil JC, Lavall D, Ukena C, Linz D, Mahfoud F, Bohm M. Atrial remodeling following catheter-based renal denervation occurs in a blood pressure- and heart rate-independent manner. JACC Cardiovasc Interv. 2015;8(7):972–80. doi:10.1016/j.jcin.2015.02.014.
132. Damman K, Tang WH, Felker GM, Lassus J, Zannad F, Krum H, McMurray JJ. Current evidence on treatment of patients with chronic systolic heart failure and renal insufficiency: practical considerations from published data. J Am Coll Cardiol. 2014;63(9):853–71. doi:10.1016/j.jacc.2013.11.031.
133. Lobo MD. Hypertension landmark trials 2015: a European perspective of the practicing clinician. J Am Coll Cardiol. 2016;67(11):1372–4. doi:10.1016/j.jacc.2016.01.027.
134. SPRINT Research Group. A randomized trial of intensive versus standard blood-pressure control. N Engl J Med. 2015;373:2103.

Chapter 19
Approach to Erectile Dysfunction in Patients with Hypertension and Coronary Artery Disease

Chrysoula Boutari, Michael Doumas, and Athanasios J. Manolis

Introductory Text

Undoubtedly, arterial hypertension is a major public health problem, which affects >25 % of the general population. Hypertensive patients are not only under major cardiovascular risk, but experience a lower health quality. Erectile dysfunction (ED) is considered to be one of the most important quality-of-life complications of hypertension and coronary artery disease (CAD) [1]. Given the fact that high blood pressure affects all the vessels of the body, it is not surprising that several structural and functional alterations in the penile vasculature are induced by hypertension [2–5].

This chapter aims to summarize the epidemiology and pathophysiology of ED in patients with hypertension and CAD, to discuss the management of ED in untreated and treated hypertensive patients as well as in patients with CAD, to present ED as an early indicator of asymptomatic CAD, and finally to highlight the role of sexual counseling in CAD patients.

C. Boutari, M.D.
2nd Propedeutic Department of Internal Medicine, Aristotle University,
126, Vas. Olgas Street, Thessaloniki 54645, Greece

M. Doumas, M.D., Ph.D. (✉)
Department of Medicine, Veteran Affairs Medical Center and George Washington University, Washington, DC, USA

2nd Propedeutic Department of Internal Medicine, Aristotle University,
126, Vas. Olgas Street, Thessaloniki 54645, Greece
e-mail: michalisdoumas@yahoo.co.uk

A.J. Manolis, M.D., FESC, FACC, FAHA
Cardiology Department, Asklepeion General Hospital, Athens, Greece

E.A. Andreadis (ed.), *Hypertension and Cardiovascular Disease*,
DOI 10.1007/978-3-319-39599-9_19

Epidemiology of Erectile Dysfunction in Hypertension and in Coronary Artery Disease

The elements about the risk for ED when hypertension occurs come either from small clinical studies or large studies that include subgroups of hypertensive men. Specifically, Derby et al. [6] used a single question for self assessed ED in the population-based sample of Massachusetts Male Aging Study (MMAS) and they found that hypertensive patients aged 40–70 years had an 80 % greater risk for ED. Braun et al. [7] performed the Cologne Male Survey aiming to evaluate the epidemiology of male sexuality in Germany. The group of hypertensives aged 30–80 years had a 58 % increased risk for ED. A similar proportion was reported by Martin Morales et al. [8] who estimated the prevalence for ED in Spain in a cross-sectional study, using the International Index of Erectile Function (IIEF) questionnaire. Marumo et al. [9] used the same questionnaire (IIEF) and found a 48 % prevalence of sexual dysfunction in the hypertensive men included in the study. A cross-national study [10] of the prevalence of ED in community-based populations in Brazil, Italy, Japan and Malaysia showed that among a random sample of 540 hypertensive men aged 40–70 years the odds ratio for ED was 1.45 (95 % confidence intervals 1.15–1.84). Mirone et al. [11] examined the determinants of ED in men who asked for a free of charge urologic or andrologic consultation. They suggested a 30 % increased risk of ED in men with hypertension (odds ratio 1.30, 95 % confidence intervals 1.10–1.40). Ponholzer et al. [12] used the IIEF-5, too. They assessed the prevalence and risk factors for ED in 2869 men aged 20–80 years in the area of Vienna. They examined hypertension as a risk factor for ED and estimated an odds ratio of 2.05 (95 % confidence intervals 1.61–2.60). One year later, Saigal et al. [13] analyzed data from the 2001–2002 National Health and Nutrition Examination Study in order to evaluate the prevalence of ED in a population of 3,506 men, 20 years and older. They found that ED affected almost 20 % of participants and hypertension was one of the modifiable risk factors which were independently associated with ED (odds ratio 1.56). The Male Attitudes Regarding Sexual Health (MARS) study [14] was a cross-sectional, nationally representative probability survey, which included 1,955 men, ≥ 40 years old. Lauren et al. aimed to estimate by race/ethnicity in the United States, the prevalence of ED and the impact of socio-demographic, health, relationship, psychological and lifestyle variables. The probability for ED increased with hypertension about 60 %. Selvin et al. [15] carried out a cross-sectional analysis of data from adult male participants in the 2001–2002 National Health and Nutrition Examination Survey (NHANES) and they aimed to assess the prevalence of ED in the US adult male population. The prevalence of ED among men with hypertension was 44.1 %.

Several studies have, over the years, demonstrated that the prevalence of sexual dysfunction is almost twice as frequent and of higher severity in hypertensive individuals than in the normotensive population [16]. Furthermore, it has been reported, by Doumas et al., that hypertensive subjects have up to a seven fold higher incidence of sexual dysfunction than normotensive individuals, with a relative risk that ranges from 1.3 to 6.9 [2]. Bulpitt et al. observed a prevalence of 7 % of erectile dysfunction among normotensive men, versus 17 % and 25 % in men with untreated and treated hypertension, respectively [17].

In a sample of 594 men aged 30–75 years from primary health-care clinics (298 normotensive and 296 hypertensive participants), ED was reported by 24 % of normotensive subjects and 66 % of hypertensive patients [18]. Moreover, Cordero et al. demonstrated that the prevalence of ED increased linearly with age [19].

Erectile dysfunction and coronary artery disease (CAD) share several common risk factors. Aging, genetic susceptibility, hypertension, dyslipidemia, obesity, metabolic syndrome, hypertriglyceridemia, and diabetes mellitus contribute to the development of both CAD and ED [20–22].

Montorsi et al. showed that almost half of the 300 patients with CAD (49 %) had a history of ED [23]. Interestingly, ED symptoms appeared before CAD in 70 % of the patients by an average of approximately 3 years. Furthermore, Thompson et al. demonstrated that men with ED had 1.5 fold higher risk for cardiovascular events compared to them without ED [24].

In addition, a recent meta-analysis [25], which included about 90,000 patients, proved that after a follow-up period of about 6 years, patients with sexual disorders, compared with individuals without, had an increased risk for cardiovascular events by 44 %, for myocardial infarction 62 % and for all-cause mortality 25 %. A prior meta-analysis of 12 prospective cohort studies, involving 36,744 participants, suggested that ED increases the risk of coronary heart disease by 46 % and all-cause mortality by 19 % [26].

Pathophysiology of Erectile Dysfunction

There is a variety of factors that contribute to the normal erectile function. They are physiological, neurological, hormonal, vascular and cavernosal factors. Any abnormality or malfunction of these factors may provoke sexual dysfunction.

Neurogenic ED is defined as the inability to initiate and maintain a penile erection due to neurologic dysfunction. The causes of neurogenic ED can be central or peripheral neuropathies or a traumatic loss of neural function. The most common neurological disorders include stroke, spinal cord injury, multiple sclerosis, Parkinson's disease and radical pelvic surgeries [27].

High blood pressure impairs blood vessels. Male erectile is a vascular phenomenon. So the association between hypertension and ED is strong. Particularly, hypertension induces structural and functional abnormalities of the penile arteries. Atherosclerosis is the most principal structural abnormality which causes flow-limiting stenosis [28–30].

Montorsi et al. proposed the artery-size hypothesis. According to this and given the systemic nature of atherosclerosis, all vascular beds should be impaired. Penile arteries are smaller in diameter (1–2 mm) than coronary arteries (3–4 mm). Thus, larger coronary arteries better tolerate the same amount of plaque compared to the smaller penile arteries. According to this hypothesis ED occurs before coronary artery disease becomes symptomatic [31]. Other structural abnormalities occurring due to hypertension are the smooth muscle hypertrophy of the wall of the cavernous arteries and the increase in type III collagen fibers in the extracellular matrix [4]. The main functional abnormalities induced by high blood pressure are the defective nitric oxide-induced vasodilatory mechanism, due to decreased nitric oxide bioavailability [5] and the activation of the renin-angiotensin system, since angiotensin II causes vascular hypertrophy. Furthermore, angiotensin II acts on angiotensin type 1 receptors and causes the contraction of the corporeal smooth muscle [32].

There exists an important association of ED and hormonal alterations. Testosterone deficiency, hypogonadism or hyperprolactinemia have been shown to be associated with a higher risk of CAD and cardiac mortality [5, 33]. This relation is explained by the fact that low androgen levels might have proinflammatory and proapoptotic effects on endothelial tissue [34, 35]. Furthermore, androgens maintain the smooth muscle homeostasis, since they act on arterial tissues and vascular remodeling.

Diabetes mellitus (DM) type 2 is among the most common risk factors for ED. It may cause ED through a variety of alterations on psychology, endothelial cell function, central nervous system and peripheral nerve function. Except the neuronal and endothelial problems regarding the penis in diabetics, low testosterone is another factor, which exacerbates the sexual function [36]. The risk of ED is three fold higher among diabetic men (28 % vs 9.6 %). Moreover, ED in diabetics occurs at an earlier age (15 % at 30 years and 55 % at 60 years) [37].

Smoking is another parameter which contributes to the onset of ED through several mechanisms, such as hemodynamic alterations via nicotine, toxic agents which affect the vascular endothelium, hypercoagulability and increased platelet accumulation. It may impair penile erection by the deterioration of endothelium-dependent smooth muscle relaxation. Moreover, abnormal penile vascular findings and therefore ED are being significantly increased as risk factors, such as smoking, accumulate [38]. Interestingly, Jaffe et al. [39] showed that smoking may provoke ED by reducing high-density lipoprotein (HDL) and enhancing fibrinogen concentrations. It has been shown that the prevalence of erectile dysfunction was 40–70 % higher among smokers, compared to nonsmokers [40]. Also, smoking increases the age-adjusted risk of ED.

In addition, chronic renal failure and uremia have been associated with a high prevalence of ED (20–50 %) [41]. Psychological factors, hormonal alterations and atheromatous disease may be responsible for this association [42]. Uremia results in impaired nerve and endothelial-mediated relaxation of the smooth muscle of the corpus cavernosum [43].

Finally, specific antihypertensive drug categories, such as central acting drugs, beta-blockers and diuretics, impair the sexual function [16]. It has been demonstrated that the number of sexual intercourses per month was significantly lower with beta-blockers (both the first generation beta-blockers, such as atenolol, and the newer, such as carvedilol) than with placebo [44–46]. On the other hand, Croog et al [47] demonstrated that adding propranolol or methyldopa in mono therapy with a thiazide worsened the sexual symptoms, while this effect did not appear when patients were treated with captopril plus a diuretic. A large UK trial (MRC) divided hypertensives into four treatment groups: bendrofluazide, propranolol, or a placebo for either of these drugs. Twice as many participants taking bendrofluazide for treatment of mild hypertension reported ED compared to those taking propranolol or placebo [48]. In the Treatment of Mild Hypertension Study (TOMHS), the prevalence of sexual dysfunction in men taking low dose of chlorthalidone for 2 years was higher compared to placebo (17.1 % versus 8.1 %; $p=0.025$) [49].

Finally, many psychotropic drugs cause sexual dysfunction. The most important of them are antidepressants, such as the selective serotonin repute inhibitors and venlafaxine, and antipsychotics, such as risperidone and olanzapine [50].

Management of Erectile Dysfunction in Untreated Hypertensives

The primary step in the approach of hypertensive patients with erectile dysfunction who are not receiving antihypertensive treatment is the exclusion of other comorbidities or drugs. Indeed psychiatric, neurological, urologic and endocrine diseases should be excluded in order to establish the vasculogenic origin of the sexual dysfunction.

The next option a physician has approaching an untreated hypertensive is the lifestyle modification. As it has been mentioned above, the principal abnormality that occurs in ED is the endothelial dysfunction and thus risk factors like obesity, decreased physical activity, smoking, hypertension, diabetes mellitus and dyslipidemia have been linked with sexual dysfunction [1–5]. Derby et al. showed that moderate physical activity decreases the risk of ED up to 30 % compared to sedentary lifestyle [51]. Moreover, Chung et al. demonstrated that obesity increases the risk of ED up to 30 % and on the other hand physical activity was associated with a 30 % lower risk [52].

The next or parallel step when approaching a hypertensive patient with ED is to find the proper antihypertensive treatment, when it is indicated. Accumulating data indicate that antihypertensive drugs affect erectile function [53]. Beta blockers (like propranolol) and diuretics impair sexual function [53, 54]. However, nebivolol, which is a newer representative of its class, is considered to improve erectile function through increased nitric oxide bioavailability [55, 56].

On the other part, calcium antagonists and angiotensin converting enzyme inhibitors seem to have no effect on sexual function [57–59]. Nevertheless, angiotensin receptor blockers (ARBs) seem to ameliorate sexual function, since they block the vasoconstrictive action of angiotensin II, thus preventing termination of erection [44, 45].

In conclusion, ARBs, nebivolol, ACE-inhibitors and calcium antagonists are indicated for the treatment of untreated hypertensives with ED. ARBs and nebivolol are definitely the best choice towards this direction. On the other hand, diuretics and beta-blockers should be avoided, if possible.

Management of Erectile Dysfunction in Treated Hypertensives

What options do we have when encountering patients with ED who are already on antihypertensive treatment? In this case there is an important question: Is hypertension per se, antihypertensive medication or both, the factors causing erectile dysfunction?.

Doumas et al. demonstrated that the prevalence of sexual dysfunction in treated hypertensives is double than the prevalence in untreated patients (40.4 % versus 19.8 %) [16]. These findings indicate that antihypertensive therapy might be implicated in sexual dysfunction. Nevertheless, hypertensive patients, who are on antihypertensive medications, may have more severe hypertension, significant target organ damage or more comorbidities than untreated patients and perhaps these factors are responsible for sexual dysfunction.

It is true that medically induced erectile dysfunction is one of the major reasons for poor adherence and treatment discontinuation. This fact may have harmful effects on patients' cardiovascular profile [60, 61] and this is why we have to come up successfully against sexual dysfunction in patients who are already under antihypertensive therapy.

First of all, approaching this patient we should exclude other comorbidities, drugs and psychogenic factors that might contribute to sexual problems. Lifestyle modification such as weight loss, physical activity, should be recommended by the physicians [62].

If these steps fail to relieve erectile dysfunction, a change of antihypertensive drugs should be considered. Beta-blockers and diuretics should be the first categories to be changed, unless they are strictly indicated for the specific patient, due to other comorbidities. Beta-blockers have been associated with poor sexual desire and with erectile dysfunction [63–65]. Older drugs, such as central acting agents, diuretics and beta-blockers are associated with worse sexual function than newer drugs, such as angiotensin receptor blockers, angiotensin converting enzyme (ACE) inhibitors and calcium antagonists. Some small clinical trials [32, 66, 67] showed that not only the first-generation beta-blockers, such as atenolol, but also the newer, like carvedilol, have a negative effect on sexual function. On the other hand, angiotensin receptor blockers represent the mainstay of therapy [68], since they not only do not exert a detrimental role on sexual function, but they seem to have a beneficial role compared to placebo. The Ongoing Telmisartan Alone and in Combination with Ramipril Global Endpoint Trial (ONTARGET) and Telmisartan Randomized Assessment Study in Cardiovascular Disease (TRANSCEND) studies attempted to assess erectile function by using a validated questionnaire [69]. In the ONTARGET study, erectile function was not affected by the angiotensin-converting enzyme inhibitor ramipril, the angiotensin receptor blocker telmisartan, and their combination. In the TRANSCEND study there were no different effects in sexual function with telmisartan or placebo. The Nitric Oxide, Erectile Dysfunction and Beta-Blocker Treatment (MR-NOED) trial found that nebivolol improved sexual activity and avoided erectile dysfunction in male hypertensive patients on long-term beta-adrenoceptor antagonist therapy [70]. The influence of calcium channel antagonists on erectile function has not been assessed by any clinical trial, but they are considered to have no particular effect on sexual function [71].

To sum up, nebivolol and angiotensin II receptor antagonists are considered to have a beneficial effect on erectile function [72]. However, treating physicians should count in other comorbidities that may require the use of specific antihypertensive drugs, despite of its deleterious effects on sexual function, such as beta-blockers in heart failure patients. Nonetheless, even if sexual dysfunction carries on after modifying to one of the indicated drug categories, administration of phosphodiesterase type 5 (PDE-5) inhibitors is recommended for the treatment of sexual dysfunction.

Erectile Dysfunction as an Early Diagnostic Indicator of Asymptomatic Coronary Artery Disease

As has been mentioned above, erectile dysfunction and coronary artery disease share several common risk factors and they often coexist. The second Princeton Guidelines suggested that ED and CVD are both results of endothelial dysfunction and also ED should be considered as a cardiovascular risk marker [73].

This role of ED as an “early diagnostic window” for asymptomatic CAD can be explained by the “artery size hypothesis”. Both ED and CAD arise out of endothelial dysfunction and atherosclerosis. However, smaller arteries, such as penile arteries, are the first to be affected, prior to the larger ones, like coronary arteries, since the same size of plaque has a greater effect on blood flow through the penile arteries than through the coronary vessels.

Given the fact that an acute coronary syndrome often occurs as a result of the rupture of a subclinical plaque, ED may also be a warning sign of an acute coronary event [25]. It is interesting that ED occurs approximately 3 years before symptomatic CAD [74]. Several studies showed a temporal relationship between ED and CAD and they estimated that ED is presented about 2–5 years before a cardiovascular event. Hodges et al. [75] examined 207 patients with CVD attending cardiovascular rehabilitation programs and 165 age-matched controls from general practice in the UK. These patients completed four questionnaires. Fifty-six percent of the patients with CVD had symptoms of ED at the time of the study and they started about 5 ± 5.3 years ago. On the contrary, of the individuals in the control group 37 % had ED symptoms for about 6.6 ± 6.8 years. In the COBRA (AssoCiation Between eRectile dysfunction and coronary Artery disease) trial [76], 93 % of patients with a chronic coronary syndrome had ED symptoms for about 24 (range 12–36) months before the onset of angina. Furthermore, the time intervals for patients with one-, two-, and three- vessel disease were 12 (9.5–24), 24 (16.5–36) and 33 (21–47) months, respectively. Conclusively, there was a significant relationship between the number of vessels involved and the time intervals between ED and CAD onset ($p=0.016$).

The possibility of underlying coronary stenosis on a patient with vasculogenic ED has been estimated about 50 % and the possibility of asymptomatic CAD about 10 % [23, 77]. The large Prostate Cancer Prevention Trial proved that ED at entry or that developed later, during follow-up, predict any cardiac event with a hazard ratio of 1.45 ($p<0.001$, 95 % confidence interval: 1.25–1.69). Moreover, the cardiovascular risk associated with ED was at least as great as the risk associated with smoking, hypercholesteloremia, and family history of myocardial infarction [24]. A meta-analysis, including 36,744 participants, estimated that men with ED, compared with the reference group, had a risk of 48 % for cardiovascular disease, 46 % for coronary heart disease, 35 % for stroke and 19 % for all cause mortality, after adjustment for traditional cardiovascular risk factors [26].

Three studies, two meta-analyses and one systematic review, attempted to investigate the link between ED and the prediction of CVD [25, 26, 78, 79]. A population-based, longitudinal study included 1400 men aged 40–75 years, with no known CAD and with a follow-up of 10 years [79]. Men aged 40–49 years old with ED at baseline had a 50-fold greater cardiovascular risk than men who had normal erections (48.52 versus 0.94) and five-fold in the group 50–59 years. Chew et al. demonstrated that ED is not only significantly associated with, but also predictive of subsequent atherosclerotic CV events, in particular when ED occurs at a younger age [80]. Furthermore, a coronary angiographic study showed that men <60 years old with ED presented a higher risk of CAD (2.3 times) and more severe disease [81]. A meta-analysis of prospective cohort studies, including 36,744 men suggested that ED significantly increases the risk of CVD, CAD, stroke and all cause mortality and the increase was independent of conventional cardiovascular risk factors. Moreover, similar findings were reported by Vlachopoulos et al., who examined 14 studies in which were involved 92,757 men. Interestingly, the relative risk was higher at younger ages and intermediate-risk groups.

Since erectile dysfunction is linked with cardiovascular parameters, it could constitute a trustworthy tool for detecting asymptomatic cardiovascular disease. Therefore, sexual function should be incorporated into CVD risk assessment for all men and both cardiologists and general physicians should intervene with advice for lifestyle modification, weight loss, healthy diet and exercise.

Management of Erectile Dysfunction in Coronary Artery Disease Patients

Cardiovascular risk is defined as the risk of morbid events over a 3- to 5- year interval from the onset of ED [23, 75]. As it has been mentioned above, ED should be used as a trustworthy tool to evaluate CVD risk reduction. Several studies showed that ED is significantly associated with increased cardiovascular events. Araujo et al. estimated that ED was associated with hazard ratios (HRs) of 1.43 (95 % confidence intervals 1.00–2.05) for CVD mortality and they suggested that this HR is equivalent to HRs of some traditional CVD risk factors (such as age, smoking, hypertension, diabetes, dyslipidemia) [82]. Moreover, ED is predictive of asymptomatic CAD. The time interval among the onset of ED symptoms and the appearance of CAD symptoms is estimated at 2–5 years [23, 29, 75]. Furthermore, ED appears to be of more prognostic significance for CAD in younger men, aged 40–49 [79]. Also, Chew et al. showed that atherosclerotic cardiovascular events are seven times more likely in men <40 years old with ED [79]. Thus, ED may be reliable and useful in evaluating cardiovascular risk in younger patients. Also, as it has been reported above, a recent meta-analysis of 36,744 men, demonstrated that the more severe the ED is, the greater the cardiovascular risks are [26].

The Framingham Risk Score (FRS) is a powerful tool which estimates the 10 year cardiac event risk in patients and it is suggested by the 2010 ACCF/AHA guideline [83] for assessment of cardiovascular risk in asymptomatic adults. Nevertheless, it is doubtful whether the FRS estimates risk in younger patients suitably, in particular those with ED.

Although the Princeton III consensus recommendations for the management of erectile dysfunction and cardiovascular disease proposes the FRS as a method to assess subclinical atherosclerosis in men with ED, more CVD risk factors should be investigated in men with ED aged 30–60 years [84].

Lifestyle modification is recommended in order to improve the patients' cardiovascular health. Particularly, smoking cessation seems to reduce mortality in CAD by 36 % [85]. Physical activity is considered to reduce the occurrence of diabetes mellitus II and CAD by 30–50 % in physical active versus sedentary individuals [86–89]. Also, weight loss, healthy diet and moderate alcohol consumption can reduce CAD mortality by 36 % [90].

As regards the parameters in the context of laboratory testing, DM doubles the risk for CVD [91]. eGFR<60 ml/min and ratio of urinary albumin to creatinine >10 mg/g are associated with increased cardiovascular mortality [92, 93].

Testosterone measurement has become debatable in men without symptoms of low testosterone. Guay et al. found that 36 % of the patients in a medical endocrine-based center for male sexual dysfunction had hypogonadism [94]. This medical condition is a potential cause of ED [95, 96] and testosterone replacement therapy (TRT) is very effective [96].

A meta-analysis of 19 studies showed no association between endogenous total testosterone (TT) level and CVD risk in middle-aged men [97]. Another meta-analysis of 49 cross-sectional studies proved that lower TT levels and higher estradiol levels correlate with increased CVD risk [98]. On the other hand, the previous meta-analysis [97] showed that low TT levels predict increased risk for CVD in elderly men. It was also discussed that low TT may constitute a marker of poor health. Indeed, several studies demonstrated that androgen deficiency is associated with insulin resistance, DM II and metabolic syndrome [99–102]. In this direction, a meta-analysis of five randomized controlled trials showed that TRT was associated with a significant reduction of fasting plasma glucose, homeostatic model assessment index, triglycerides and waist circumference and an increase in HDL levels [103].

Testosterone levels should be measured in all men diagnosed with organic ED [84], especially for those who had no beneficial effects undergoing a PDE5 inhibitor therapy [83]. Consequently, males with TT levels <230 ng/dL seem to benefit from TRT. Men with TT levels between 231 and 346 ng/dL, with symptoms like decreased libido or ED and without contraindications should undergo TRT for 4–6 months, after extensive analysis of the potential risks and complications. The TRT should be continued more than 6 months only if there is a clinical profit [84].

High sensitivity C reactive protein (hsCRP) is an independent predictor of coronary events [83]. A meta-analysis of 54 long-term prospective studies and approximately 160,000 people without a history of vascular disease showed that high CRP concentration was associated with increased risk of CAD (37 %), ischemic stroke (27 %), vascular mortality (55 %) and nonvascular mortality (54 %).

Additionally, serum uric acid measurement is recommended, since high levels have been associated with increased cardiovascular risk [104]. Lipoprotein-associated phospholipase A2 levels seems to be independent predictors of CVD in healthy individuals after adjustment for hsCRP and traditional risk factors [105]. Moreover, glycated hemoglobin has been associated with risks of cardiovascular disease and it has been proved that the addition of glycated hemoglobin to prediction models of CAD improved CAD prediction in non diabetics without previous history of CAD [106].

Exercise stress testing is considered to be useful to evaluate CAD risk in patients with ED and DM II, since in patients with DM II, the rates of men with asymptomatic CAD and ED were seven times greater than the rates of participants with ED and without CAD (33.8 % versus 4.7 %) [107]. CIMT, CACS and ABI have been proposed by the 2010 ACCF/AHA guidelines state in the context of assessment of intermediate-risk patients [83]. Finally, endothelial dysfunction seems to be associated with higher cardiac death, myocardial infarction, revascularization and cardiac hospitalization in symptomatic outpatients during a 7 years follow-up [108].

As discussed previously, ED and CVD share several risk factors, and ED is an independent predictor of CVD. Therefore, the assessment of sexual function should be included into the initial evaluation of cardiovascular risk for all men [109, 110]. A meta-analysis of ten studies proved that episodic physical and sexual activity was associated with a high risk of acute cardiac events among individuals with high levels of habitual physical activity [111]. Thus, the physicians should estimate the cardiovascular risk associated with sexual activity in patients.

The PDE5 inhibitors (such as sildenafil, tadalafil, vardenafil, and avanafil) are used to treat ED. Analyses of placebo-controlled and postmarketing surveillance data have shown no new significant cardiovascular events [112, 113]. Additionally, several studies have demonstrated that PDE5 inhibitors have a possible role in the management of hypertension [114–116] and endothelial dysfunction [117–119] in patients at risk for CVD. Also, TRT should be performed for men with low or intermediate TT levels. Other approaches, like exercise, weight loss [120, 121], and partner and relationship factors [122–124], should be incorporated, too.

Furthermore, possible effects on erectile function of agents used to manage cardiovascular risk factors should be considered. The b-blocker nebivolol is less likely to cause ED than other b-blockers, since it has direct vasodilating properties [55, 125]. Angiotensin receptor blockers are considered to cause ED less likely than diuretics [66, 126]. Statins have been suggested to improve erectile function in men with and without PDE5 inhibitors [127–129].

Closing, it is clear that a careful and comprehensive approach to cardiovascular risk reduction will meliorate the overall health, and especially vascular health, including sexual function.

Sexual Counseling

Erectile dysfunction is a condition which affects and contributes significantly to the impaired life quality of both patients and their sexual partners. However, it is also under-reported, under-recognized and under-treated. Therefore, sexual counseling is a complex process on which the health-care professional should identify and manage patients with sexual dysfunction and also, determine, control and encounter factors limiting sexual activity [130, 131].

Some of the most common and considerable topics which should be discussed are the following: is sexual activity safe for a patient with CVD and when (after an acute event)?, which sexual position is suggested?, is sexual activity impaired by other drugs and comorbidities?, are PDE5 inhibitors safe?.

Although the advantages of regular exercise have been proved by several studies and it is considered that it reduces the risk for cardiovascular morbidity and mortality [132–138], some studies suggest that acute rigorous exercise may provoke an acute cardiac event [139–141]. Acute cardiac events occurring during or shortly after sexual intercourse are the so-called sexually-induced or coital acute cardiac events. However, coital angina is not very frequent and it represents less than 5 % of angina events [142].

A recent systematic review and meta-analysis assessed the effect of episodic physical and sexual activity on acute cardiac events. Episodic sexual activity was associated with an increased risk of acute myocardial infarction (relative risk = 2.70; 95 % CI: 1.48–4.91). However, the absolute rate of acute cardiac events is limited, since sexual activity is infrequent and its' effect is transient. The absolute rate of myocardial infarction is 2–3 per 10,000 person-years for every 1 h of additional sexual activity per week. Furthermore, the association between sexual activity and acute cardiac events depends on habitual physical activity. For every additional time per week an individual is involved in physical activity, the relative risk for myocardial infarction is reduced by 45 % [111].

Therefore, an individual who manages more than 3–5 METs during treadmill exercise test without developing symptoms like angina or dyspnea, ischemia at electrocardiogram, hypotension or arrhythmia, may engage in sexual intercourse without significant risk [143].

Unfortunately, there is a lack of evidence-based recommendations about the appropriate time after an acute event a patient should be exposed to sexual activity. Certainly, advice should be disease specific. After an acute MI, the interval of 1 week seems safe, provided that the patient did not have any serious complications (e.g., angina) during hospitalization, and mild-to-moderate physical activity does not trigger angina or dyspnea.

The intensity of sexual activity, which is a form of exercise, depends on the type and the duration of sexual activity. Boolean et al. demonstrated that non-coital sexual activities (non-coital stimulation of husband by wife and self-stimulation by husband) were associated with lower energy expenditures than coital activities [144]. It has also been shown that sexual activity provides modest physical stress, comparable with stage II of the Bruce treadmill protocol for men and Stage I for women. Moreover, the duration of treadmill exercise predicts the duration of sexual activity. Particularly, an increase of 2.3 min in sexual activity duration has been observed per each minute of treadmill duration [145].

Sexual problems are very common in patients with heart failure [146]. These patients often experience shortness of breath and fatigue [147]. Patients with advanced heart failure (classes III and IV according to New York Heart Association) should postpone sexual intercourse until their condition is improved.

When dyspnea or angina comes up with sexual activity, alternative types of sexual activity, convenient positioning and relaxation before and after activities may be very helpful. Sexual positions are considered to affect the energy expenditure during sexual activity. Bohlen et al., also, found that the man on top positioning requires more energy expenditure than the man on bottom positioning [144]. It is very helpful to recommend convenient and comfortable positions in patients with CVD.

A very significant factor which impairs sexual function is the concomitant medication a patient takes. In particular, patients with cardiovascular disease use drugs which may affect erectile function, such as diuretics and b-blockers [55, 148], as it has been reported previously. Therefore, the physician has to take into account both the beneficial and the negative effects and to replace drugs by others that have neutral effect or even actuate a reverse of erectile dysfunction.

PDE-5 inhibitors are vasorelaxing agents that block the activity of PDE-5 isoenzyme, which is localized throughout the smooth muscle cells of the vasculature. Thus, they increase the cyclic guanosine monophosphate (cGMP), exerting vasodilating properties. Given the fact that PDE-5 inhibitors are associated with few side effects, they can be safely administered in both hypertensive patients taking multiple antihypertensive regimes and patients with cardiovascular risk factors or cardiovascular disease [149, 150]. However, co-administration with organic nitrates is considered to be contraindicated, due to possible episodes of symptomatic hypotension [151]. Furthermore, precaution should be taken when PDE-5 inhibitors are combined with a-blockers, since there is a high risk of orthostatic hypotension effect. Thus, lower starting doses should be recommended in patients receiving a-blockers [53], and of course, close patient monitoring.

References

1. Manolis A, Doumas M. Sexual dysfunction: the 'prima ballerina' of hypertension-related quality-of-life complications. J Hypertens. 2008;26:2074–84.
2. Manolis AJ, Doumas M, Viigimaa M, Narkiewitz K. Hypertension and sexual dysfunction. European Society of Hypertension Scientific Newsletter: Update on Hypertension Management. Eur Soc Hyp. 2011;32:1–2.
3. Manolis A, Doumas M. Hypertension and sexual dysfunction. Arch Med Sci. 2009;5:S337–50.
4. Doumas M, Douma S. Sexual dysfunction in essential hypertension: myth or reality? J Clin Hypertens. 2006;8:269–74.
5. Viigimaa M, Doumas M, Vlachopoulos C, et al.; European Society of Hypertension Working Group on Sexual Dysfunction. Hypertension and sexual dysfunction: time to act. J Hypertens. 2011;29:403–7.
6. Derby CA, Araujo AB, Johannes CB, et al. Measurement of erectile dysfunction in population-based studies: the use of a single question self-assessment in the Massachusetts Male Aging. Int J Impot Res. 2000;12:197–204.
7. Braun M, Wassmer G, Klotz T, et al. Epidemiology of erectile dysfunction: results of the "Cologne Male Survey.". Int J Impot Res. 2000;12:305–11.
8. Martin-Morales A, Sanchez-Cruz JJ, Saenz de Tejada I, et al. Prevalence and independent risk factors for erectile dysfunction in Spain: results of the Epidemiologia de la Disfunction Erectil Masculina Study. J Urol. 2001;166:569–75.
9. Marumo K, Nakashima J, Murai M. Age-related prevalence of erectile dysfunction to Japan: assessment by the International Index of Erectile Function. Int J Urol. 2000;8:53–9.
10. Nicolosi A, Moreira Jr ED, Shirai M, et al. Epidemiology of erectile dysfunction in four countries: cross-national study of the prevalence and correlates of erectile dysfunction. Urology. 2003;61:201–6.
11. Mirone V, Ricci E, Gentile V, et al. Determinants of erectile dysfunction risk in a large series of Italian men attending andrology clinics. Eur Urol. 2004;45:87–91.
12. Ponholzer A, Temml C, Mock K, et al. Prevalence and risk factors for erectile dysfunction in 2869 men using a validated questionnaire. Eur Urol. 2005;47:80–6.
13. Saigal CS, Wessels H, Pace J, et al.; Urologic Diseases in America Project. Predictors and prevalence of erectile dysfunction in a racially diverse population. Arch Intern Med. 2006;166:207–12.
14. Laumann EO, West S, Glasser D, et al. Prevalence and correlates of erectile dysfunction by race and ethnicity among men aged 40 or older in the United States: from the male attitudes regarding sexual health survey. J Sex Med. 2007;4:57–65.
15. Selvin E, Burnett AL, Platz EA. Prevalence and risk factors for erectile dysfunction in the US. Am J Med. 2007;120:151–7.
16. Doumas M, Tsakiris A, Douma S, et al. Factors affecting the increased prevalence of erectile dysfunction in Greek hypertensive compared with normotensive subjects. J Androl. 2006;27(3):469–77.
17. Bulpitt CJ, Dollery CT, Carne S. Changes in symptoms in hypertensive patients after referral to hospital clinic. Br Heart J. 1976;38:121–8.
18. Bener A, Al-Ansari A, Al-Hamaq AO, et al. Prevalence of erectile dysfunction among hypertensive and nonhypertensive Qatari men. Medicina. 2007;43:870–8.
19. Cordero A, Bertomeu-Martinez V, Mazon P, Facila L, et al. Erectile dysfunction in high-risk hypertensive patients treated with beta-blockade agents. Cardiovasc Ther. 2010;28:15–22.
20. Fung MM, Bettencourt R, Barrett-Connor E. Heart disease risk factors predict erectile dysfunction 25 years later: the Rancho Bernardo study. J Am Coll Cardiol. 2004;43(8):1405–11.
21. Alberti L, Torlasco C, Lauretta L, et al. Erectile dysfunction in heart failure patients: a critical reappraisal. Andrology. 2013;1(2):177–91.
22. Ianni M, Callegari S, Rizzo A, et al. Pro-inflammatory genetic profile and familiarity of acute myocardial infarction. Immun Ageing. 2012;9(1):14.

23. Montorsi F, Briganti A, Salonia A, et al. Erectile dysfunction prevalence, time of onset and association with risk factors in 300 consecutive patients with acute chest pain and angiographically documented coronary artery disease. Eur Urol. 2003;44(3):360–4; discussion 4–5. Epub 2003/08/23.
24. Thompson IM, Tangen CM, Goodman PJ, et al. Erectile dysfunction and subsequent cardiovascular disease. JAMA. 2005;294(23):2996–3002.
25. Vlachopoulos CV, Terentes-Printzios DG, Ioakeimidis NK, et al. Prediction of cardiovascular events and all-cause mortality with erectile dysfunction: a systematic review and meta-analysis of cohort studies. Circ Cardiovasc Qual Outcomes. 2013;6(1):99–109.
26. Dong JY, Zhang YH, Qin LQ. Erectile dysfunction and risk of cardiovascular disease: meta-analysis of prospective cohort studies. J Am Coll Cardiol. 2011;58(13):1378–85.
27. Siddiqui MA, Peng B, Shanmugam N, et al. Erectile dysfunction in young surgically treated patients with lumbar spine disease: a prospective follow-up study. Spine (Phila Pa 1976). 2012;37:797–801.
28. Solomon H, Man JW, Jackson G. Erectile dysfunction and the cardiovascular patient: endothelial dysfunction is the common denominator. Heart. 2003;89(3):251–3. Epub 2003/02/20.
29. Montorsi P, Ravagnani PM, Galli S, et al. Association between erectile dysfunction and coronary artery disease: matching the right target with the right test in the right patient. Eur Urol. 2006;50(4):721–31. Epub 2006/08/12.
30. Montorsi P, Ravagnani PM, Galli S, et al. Common grounds for erectile dysfunction and coronary artery disease. Curr Opin Urol. 2004;14(6):361–5. Epub 2005/01/01.
31. Burchardt M, Burchardt T, Baer L, et al. Hypertension is associated with severe erectile dysfunction. J Urol. 2000;164:1188–91.
32. Becker AJ, Uckert S, Stief CG, et al. Possible role of bradykinin and angiotensin II in the regulation of penile erection and detumescence. Urology. 2001;57:193–8.
33. Hale TM, Okabe H, Bushfield TL. Recovery of erectile function after brief aggressive antihypertensive therapy. J Urol. 2002;168:348–54.
34. Mirone V, Imbimbo C, Fusco F, et al. Androgens and morphologic remodeling at penile and cardiovascular levels: a common piece in complicated puzzles? Eur Urol. 2009;56(2):309–16. Epub 2009/01/17.
35. Vlachopoulos C, Aznaouridis K, Ioakeimidis N, et al. Unfavorable endothelial and inflammatory state in erectile dysfunction patients with or without coronary artery disease. Eur Heart J. 2006;27(22):2640–8. Epub 2006/10/24.
36. Morelli A, Corona G, Filippi S, et al. Which patients with sexual dysfunction are suitable for testosterone replacement therapy. J Endocrinol Invest. 2007;30(10):880–8.
37. Koldny RC, Kahn CB, Goldstein HH. Sexual function in diabetic men. Diabetes. 1973;23:306–9.
38. Shabsigh R, Mulvany MJ. The myogenic response: established facts and attractive hypotheses. Clin Sci (Lond). 1999;96:313–26.
39. Jaffe A, Chen Y, Kisch ES, et al. Erectile dysfunction in hypertensive subjects: assessment of potential determinants. Hypertension. 1996;28:859–62.
40. Salonia A. Blackwell Publishing Ltd. Int J Androl. 2003;26:129–36.
41. Papadopoulou E, Varouktsi A, Lazaridis A, et al. Erectile dysfunction in chronic kidney disease: from pathophysiology to management. World J Nephrol. 2015;4:379–87.
42. Rosas SE, Joffe M, Franklin E, et al. Prevalence and determinants of erectile dysfunction in haemodialysis patients. Kidney Int. 2001;59:2259–66.
43. Saenz de Tejada I, Goldstein I, Azadzoi K, et al. Impaired neurogenic and endothelium-mediated relaxation of penile smooth muscle from diabetic men with impotence. N Engl J Med. 1989;320:1025–30.
44. Fogari R, Zoppi A, Poletti L, et al. Sexual activity in hypertensive men treated with valsartan or carvedilol: a crossover study. Am J Hypertens. 2001;14:27–31.
45. Fogari R, PretI P, Derosa G, et al. Effect of antihypertensive treatment with valsartan or atenolol on sexual activity and plasma testosterone in hypertensive men. Eur J Clin Pharmacol. 2002;58:177–80.

46. Douma S, Doumas M, Petidis K, et al. Beta blockers and sexual dysfunction: bad guys – good guys. In: Momoka E, Narami M, editors. Beta blockers: new research. New York: Nova Science Publishers Inc; 2008. p. 1–13.
47. Croog SH, Levine S, Sudilovsky A, et al. Sexual symptoms in hypertensive patients. A clinical trial of antihypertensive medications. Arch Intern Med. 1988;148:788–94.
48. Medical Research Council Working Party on Mild to Moderate Hypertension. Adverse reactions to bendrofluazide and propranolol for the treatment of mild hypertension. Lancet. 1981;2:539–43.
49. Grimm Jr RH, Grandits GA, Prineas RJ, et al. Long term effects on sexual function of five antihypertensive drugs and nutritional hygienic treatment in hypertensive men and women: treatment of mild hypertension study (TOMHS). Hypertension. 1997;29:8–14.
50. Seretti A, Chiesa A. A meta-analysis of sexual dysfunction in psychiatric patients taking antipsychotics. Int Clin Psychopharmacol. 2011;26:130–40.
51. Derby CA, Mohr BA, Goldstein I, et al. Modifiable risk factors and erectile dysfunction: can lifestyle changes modify risk? Urology. 2000;56:302–6.
52. Chung WS, Sohn JH, Park YY. Is obesity an underlying factor in erectile dysfunction? Eur Urol. 1999;36(1):68–70.
53. Manolis A, Douma M. Antihypertensive treatment and sexual dysfunction. Curr Hypertens Rep. 2012;14:285–92.
54. Douma S, Doumas M, Tsakiris A, Zamboulis C. Male and female sexual dysfunction: is hypertension an innocent bystander or a major contributor? Rev Bras Hypertens. 2007;14: 139–47.
55. Doumas M, Tsakiris A, Douma S, et al. Beneficial effects of switching from beta-blockers to nebivolol on the erectile function of hypertensive patients. Asian J Androl. 2006;8:177–82.
56. Brixius K, Middeke M, Lichtental A, et al. Nitric oxide, erectile dysfunction and beta-blocker treatment (MR NOED study): benefit of nebivolol versus metoprolol in hypertensive men. Clin Exp Pharmacol Physiol. 2007;34:327–31.
57. Viigimaa M, Vlachopoulos C, Lazaridis A, Doumas M. Management of erectile dysfunction in hypertension: tips and tricks. World J Cardiol. 2014;6:908–15.
58. Viigimaa M, Lazaridis A, Doumas M. Management of sexual dysfunction in hypertensive patients. Cardiol Clin Practice. 2012;4:53–60.
59. Doumas M, Viigimaa M, Papademetriou V. Combined antihypertensive therapy and sexual dysfunction: terra incognita. Cardiology. 2013;125:232–4.
60. Svensson S, Kjellgren KI, Ahler J. Reasons for adherence with antihypertensive medication. Int J Cardiol. 2000;76:157–63.
61. Lowentritt BH, Sklar GN. The effect of erectile dysfunction on patient medication compliance. J Urol. 2004;171:231–5.
62. Esposito K, Giugliano D. Lifestyle/dietary recommendations for erectile dysfunction and female sexual dysfunction. Urol Clin North Am. 2011;38(3):293–301.
63. Doumas M, Anyfanti P, Triantafyllou A. Management of erectile dysfunction: do not forget hypertension. Arch Intern Med. 2012;192(7):597–8.
64. Baumhakel M, Schlimmer N, Kratz M, et al. Cardiovascular risk, drugs and erectile function – a systematic analysis. Int J Clin Pract. 2011;65:289–98.
65. Silvestri A, Galetta P, Cerquetani E, et al. Report of erectile dysfunction after therapy with beta-blockers is related to patient knowledge of side-effects and is reversed by placebo. Eur Heart J. 2003;24:1928–32.
66. Llisterri JL, Lozano Vidal JV, Aznar Vicente J, et al. Sexual dysfunction in hypertensive patients treated with losartan. Am J Med Sci. 2001;321(5):336–41.
67. Dusing R. Effect of the angiotensin II antagonist valsartan on sexual function in hypertensive men. Blood Press Suppl. 2003;2:29–34.
68. Doumas M, Douma S. The effect of antihypertensive drugs on erectile function: a proposed management algorithm. J Clin Hypertens (Greenwich). 2006;8(5):359–64.
69. Jackson G, Benjamin N, Jackson N, et al. Effects of sildenafil citrate on human hemodynamics. Am J Cardiol. 1999;83(5A):13C–20.

70. Montague DK, Jarow JP, Broderick GA, et al.; Erectile Dysfunction Guideline Update Panel. The management dysfunction: an AUA update. J Urol. 2005;174:230–9.
71. Lauman EO, Paik A, Rosen RC. Sexual dysfunction in the United States: prevalence and predictors. JAMA. 1999;281(6):537–44.
72. Mancia G, Fagard R, Narckiewicz K, et al. 2013 ESH/ESC guidelines for the management of arterial hypertension: the task force for the management of arterial hypertension of the European Society of Hypertension (ESH) and of the European Society of Cardiology (ESC). Eur Heart J. 2013;34(28):2159–219.
73. Jackson G, Rosen RC, Kloner RA, et al. The second Princeton consensus on sexual dysfunction and cardiac risk: new guidelines for sexual medicine. J Sex Med. 2006;3:28–36.
74. Vlachopoulos C, Rokkas K, Ioakeimidis N, et al. Inflammation, metabolic syndrome, erectile dysfunction, and coronary artery disease: common links. Eur Urol. 2007;52(6):1590–600.
75. Hodges LD, Kirby M, Solanky J, et al. The temporal relationship between erectile dysfunction and cardiovascular disease. Int J Clin Pract. 2007;61:2019–25.
76. Montorsi P, Ravagnani PM, Galli S, et al. Association between erectile dysfunction and coronary artery disease. Role of coronary clinical presentation and extent of coronary vessels involvement: the COBRA trial. Eur Heart J. 2006;27:2632–9.
77. Vlachopoulos C, Rokkas K, Ioakeimidis N, et al. Prevalence of asymptomatic coronary artery disease in men with vasculogenic erectile dysfunction: a prospective angiographic study. Eur Urol. 2005;48(6):996–1002.
78. Gandaglia G, Briganti A, Jacjson G, et al. A systematic review of the association between erectile dysfunction and cardiovascular disease. Eur Urol. 2014;65:968–78.
79. Inman BA, Sauver JL, Jacobson DJ, et al. A population-based, longitudinal study of erectile dysfunction and future coronary artery disease. Mayo Clin Proc. 2009;84:108–13.
80. Chew KK, Finn J, Stuckey B, et al. Erectile dysfunction as a predictor for subsequent atherosclerotic cardiovascular events: findings from a linked-data study. J Sex Med. 2010;7:192–202.
81. Riedner CE, Rhoden EL, Fuchs SC, et al. Erectile dysfunction and coronary artery disease: an association of higher risk in younger men. J Sex Med. 2011;8:1445–53.
82. Araujo AB, Travison TG, Ganz P, et al. Erectile dysfunction and mortality. J Sex Med. 2009;6(9):2445–54.
83. Greenland P, Alpert JS, Beller GA, et al. 2010 ACCF/AHA guideline foe assessment of cardiovascular risk in asymptomatic adults: a report of the American College of Cardiology Foundation/American Heart Association Task Force on practice guidelines. Circulation. 2010;122(25):e584–636.
84. Nehra A, Jackson G, Miner M, et al. The Princeton III consensus recommendations for the management of erectile dysfunction and cardiovascular disease. Mayo Clin Proc. 2012;87(8):766–78.
85. Critchley JA, Capewell S. Mortality risk reduction associated with smoking cessation in patients with coronary heart disease: a systematic review. JAMA. 2003;290(1):86–97.
86. Thompson PD, Buchner D, Pina IL, et al. Exercise and physical activity in the prevention and treatment of atherosclerotic cardiovascular disease: a statement from the Council of Clinical Cardiology (Subcommittee on Exercise, Rehabilitation, and Prevention) and the Council on Nutrition, Physical Activity, and Metabolism (Subcommittee on Physical Activity). Circulation. 2003;107(24):3109–16.
87. Netz Y, Wu MJ, Becker BJ, et al. Physical activity and psychological well-being in advanced age: a meta-analysis of intervention studies. Psychol Aging. 2005;20(2):272–84.
88. Bassuk SS, Manson JE. Epidemiological evidence for the role of physical activity in reducing risk of type 2 diabetes and cardiovascular disease. J Appl Physiol. 2005;99(3):1193–204.
89. Mozaffarian D, Wilson PW, Kannel WB. Beyond established and novel risk factors: lifestyle risk factors for cardiovascular disease. Circulation. 2008;117(23):3031–8.
90. Cloutier M, Adamson E. The Mediterranean diet – newly revised and updated. HarperCollins Publishers, New York, New York, USA; 2004.
91. Sarwar N, Gao P, Seshasai SR, et al. Diabetes mellitus, fasting blood glucose concentration, and risk of vascular disease: a collaborative meta-analysis of 102 prospective studies. Lancet. 2010;375(9733):2215–22.

92. van der Velde M, Matsushita K, Coresh J, et al. Lower estimated glomerular filtration rate and higher albuminuria are associated with all-cause and cardiovascular mortality: a collaborative meta-analysis of high-risk population cohorts. Kidney Int. 2011;79(12):1341–52.
93. Matsushita K, van der Velde M, Astor BC, et al. Association of estimated glomerular filtration rate and albuminuria with all-cause and cardiovascular mortality in general population cohorts: a collaborative meta-analysis. Lancet. 2010;375(9731):2073–81.
94. Guay AT, Velasquez E, Perez JB. Characterization of patients in a medical endocrine-based center for male sexual dysfunction. Endocr Pract. 1999;5(6):314–21.
95. Blute M, Hakimian P, Kashanian J, et al. Erectile dysfunction and testosterone deficiency. Front Horm Res. 2009;37:108–22.
96. Buvat J, Montorsi F, Maggi M, et al. Hypogonadal men non-responders to the PDE-5 inhibitor tadalafil benefit from normalization of testosterone levels with a 1 % hydroalcoholic testosterone gel in the treatment of erectile dysfunction (TADTEST study). J Sex Med. 2011;8(1):284–93.
97. Ruige JB, Mahmoud AM, De Bacquer D, et al. Endogenous testosterone and cardiovascular disease in healthy men: a meta-analysis. Heart. 2011;97(11):870–5.
98. Corona G, Monami M, Boddi V, et al. Low testosterone is associated with an increased risk of MACE lethality in subjects with erectile dysfunction. J Sex Med. 2010;7(4):1557–64.
99. Grossmann M, Thomas MC, Panagiotopoulos S, et al. Low testosterone levels are common and associated with insulin resistance in male with diabetes. J Clin Endocrinol Metab. 2008;93(5):1834–40.
100. Laaksonen DE, Niskanen N, Punnonen K, et al. Sex hormones, inflammation and the metabolic syndrome: a population-based study. Eur J Endocrinol. 2003;149(6):601–8.
101. Osuna JA, Gomez-Perez R, Arata-Bellabarba G, et al. Relationship between BMI, total testosterone, sex hormone – binding-globulin, leptin, insulin and insulin resistance in obese men. Arch Androl. 2006;52(5):355–61.
102. Kapoor D, Aldred H, Clark S, et al. Clinical and biochemical assessment of hypogonadism in men with type 2 diabetes: correlations with bioavailable testosterone and visceral adiposity. Diabetes Care. 2007;30(4):911–7.
103. Corona G, Monami M, Rastrelli G, et al. Testosterone and metabolic syndrome: a meta-analysis study. J Sex Med. 2011;8(1):272–83.
104. Krishnan E, Sokolove J. Uric acid in heart disease: a new C-reactive protein? Curr Opin Rheumatol. 2011;23(2):174–7.
105. Koenig W, Khuseyinova N, Lowel H, et al. Lipoprotein-associated phospholipase A2 adds to risk prediction of incident coronary events by C-reactive protein in apparently healthy middle-aged men from the general population: results from the 14-year follow-up of a large cohort from southern Germany. Circulation. 2004;110(14):1903–8.
106. Selvin E, Steffes MW, Zhu H, et al. Glycated hemoglobin, diabetes and cardiovascular risk in diabetic adults. N Engl J Med. 2010;362(9):800–11.
107. Gazzaruso C, Giordanetti S, De Amici E, et al. Relationship between erectile dysfunction and silent myocardial ischemia in apparently uncomplicated type 2 diabetic patients. Circulation. 2004;110(1):22–6.
108. Rubinshtein R, Kuvin JT, Soffler M, et al. Assessment of endothelial function by noninvasive peripheral arterial tonometry predicts late cardiovascular adverse events. Eur Heart J. 2010;31(9):1142–8.
109. DeBusk R, Drory E, Goldstein E, et al. Management of sexual dysfunction in patients with cardiovascular disease: recommendations of The Princeton Consensus Panel. Am J Cardiol. 2000;86(2):175–81.
110. Kostis JB, Jackson G, Rosen R, et al. Sexual dysfunction and cardiac risk (the Second Princeton Consensus Conference). Am J Cardiol. 2005;96(2):313–21.
111. Dahabreh IJ, Paulus JK. Association of episodic physical and sexual activity with triggering of acute cardiac events: systematic review and meta-analysis. JAMA. 2011;305(12):1225–33.
112. Giuliano F, Jackson J, Montorsi F, et al. Safety of sildenafil citrate: review of 67 double-blind placebo-controlled trials and the postmarketing safety database. Int J Clin Pract. 2010;64(2):240–55.

113. Kloner RA, Jackson G, Hutter AM, et al. Cardiovascular safety update of tadalafil: retrospective analysis of data from placebo-controlled and open-label clinical trials of tadalafil with as needed, three times-per-week or once-a-day dosing. Am J Cardiol. 2006;97(12):1778–84.
114. Doumas M, Lazaridis A, Katsiki N, Athyros V. PDE-5 inhibitors: clinical points. Curr Drug Targets. 2015;16(5):420–6.
115. Scranton RE, Lawler E, Botteman M, et al. Effect of treating erectile dysfunction on management of systolic hypertension. Am J Cardiol. 2007;100(3):459–63.
116. Oliver JJ, Melville VP, Webb DJ. Effect of regular phosphodiesterase type 5 inhibition in hypertension. Hypertension. 2006;48(4):622–7.
117. Kimura M, Higashi Y, Hara K, et al. PDE5 inhibitor sildenafil citrate augments endothelium-dependent vasodilation in smokers. Hypertension. 2003;41(5):1106–10.
118. Gillies HC, Robin D, Jackson G. Coronary and systemic hemodynamic effects of sildenafil citrate: from basic science to clinical studies in patients with cardiovascular disease. Int J Cardiol. 2002;86(2–3):131–41.
119. Katz SD, Balidemaj K, Homma S, et al. Acute type 5-phosphodiesterase inhibition with sildenafil enhances flow mediated vasodilation in patients with chronic heart failure. J Am Coll Cardiol. 2000;36(3):845–51.
120. Esposito K, Giugliano F, Di Palo C, et al. Effect of lifestyle changes on erectile dysfunction in obese men: a randomized controlled trial. JAMA. 2004;291(24):2978–84.
121. Wing RR, Rosen RC, Fava JL, et al. Effects of weight loss intervention on erectile function in older men with type 2 diabetes in the Look AHEAD trial. J Sex Med. 2010;7(1):156–65.
122. Fisher WA, Eardley I, McCabe M, et al. Erectile dysfunction (ED) is a shared sexual concern of couples II: association of female partner characteristics with male partner ED treatment seeking and phosphodiesterase type 5 inhibitor utilization. J Sex Med. 2009;6(11):3111–24.
123. Riley A. The role of the partner in erectile dysfunction and its treatment. Int J Impot Res. 2002;14 suppl 1:S105–9.
124. Riley A. When treating erectile dysfunction, do not forget the partner. Int J Clin Pract. 2008;62(1):6–8.
125. Boydak B, Naltbangil S, Fici F, et al. A randomized comparison of the effects of nebivolol and atenolol with and without chlorothalidone on the sexual function of hypertensive men. Clin Drug Investig. 2005;25(6):409–16.
126. Baumhakel M, Schlimmer N, Bohm M, DO-IT Investigators. Effect of irbesartan on erectile function in patients with hypertension and metabolic syndrome. Int J Impot Res. 2008;20(5):493–500.
127. Bank AJ, Kelly AS, Kaiser DR. The effects of quinapril and atorvastatin on the responsiveness to sildenafil in men with erectile dysfunction. Vasc Med. 2006;11(4):251–7.
128. Saltzman EA, Guay AT, Jacobson J. Improvement in erectile function in men with organic erectile dysfunction by correction of elevated cholesterol levels: a clinical observation. J Urol. 2004;172(1):255–8.
129. Dadkhah F, Safarinejad MR, Asgari MA, et al. Atorvastatin improves the response to sildenafil in hypercholesterolemic men with erectile dysfunction not initially responsive to sildenafil. Int J Impot Res. 2010;22(1):51–60.
130. Nikolai MPJ, Both S, Liem SS, et al. Discussing sexual function in the cardiology practice. Clin Res Cardiol. 2013;102:329–36.
131. O'Donovan K. Addressing the taboos: resuming sexual activity after myocardial infarction. Br J Card Nurs. 2007;2:165–75.
132. Kokkinos P, Myers J, Kokkinos JP, et al. Exercise capacity and mortality in black and white men. Circulation. 2008;117:614–22.
133. Kokkinos P, Manolis A, Pittaras A, et al. Exercise capacity and mortality in hypertensive men with and without additional risk factors. Hypertension. 2009;53:494–9.
134. Blair SN, Kampert JB, Kohl III HW, et al. Influences of cardiorespiratory fitness and other precursors on cardiovascular disease and all-cause mortality in men and women. JAMA. 1996;276:205–10.

135. Kokkinos P, Myers J, Doumas M, et al. Exercise capacity and all-cause mortality in prehypertensive men. Am J Hypertens. 2009;22:735–41.
136. Kokkinos P, Doumas M, Myers J, et al. A graded association of exercise capacity and all-cause mortality in males with high-normal blood pressure. Blood Press. 2009;18:261–7.
137. Kokkinos P, Myers J, Faselis C, et al. Exercise capacity and mortality in older men: a 20-year follow-up study. Circulation. 2010;122:790–7.
138. Faselis C, Doumas M, Kokkinos JP, et al. Exercise capacity and progression from prehypertension to hypertension. Hypertension. 2012;60:333–8.
139. Gunby P. Snow falls; ischemic heart deaths rise. JAMA. 1979;241:1987.
140. Glass RI, Zack Jr MM. Increase in deaths from ischemic heart disease after blizzards. Lancet. 1979;8114:485–7.
141. Trichopoulos D, Katsouyanni K, Zavitsanos X, et al. Psychological stress and fatal heart attack: the Athens (1981) earthquake natural experiment. Lancet. 1983;8322:441–4.
142. DeBusk RF. Sexual activity in patients with angina. JAMA. 2003;290:3129–32.
143. Drory Y. Sexual activity and cardiovascular risk. Eur Heart J Suppl. 2002;4:H13–8.
144. Bohlen JG, Held JP, Sanderson MO, et al. Heart-rate, rate-pressure product, and oxygen uptake during four sexual activities. Arch Intern Med. 1984;144:1745–8.
145. Palmeri ST, Kostis JB, Casazza L, et al. Heart rate and blood pressure response in adult men and women during exercise and sexual activity. Am J Cardiol. 2007;100(12):1795–801.
146. Hoekstra T, Jaarsma T, Sanderman R, et al. Perceived sexual difficulties and associated factors in patients with heart failure. Am Heart J. 2012;163:246–51.
147. Hoekstra T, Lesman-Leegte E, Luttik ML, et al. Sexual problems in elderly male and female patients with heart failure. Heart. 2012;98:1647–52.
148. Dusing R. Effect of the angiotensin II antagonist valsartan on sexual function in hypertensive men. Blood Press. 2003;12:S29–34.
149. Pickering TG, Shpherd AM, Puddey I, et al. Sildenafil citrate for erectile dysfunction in men receiving multiple antihypertensive agents: a randomized controlled trial. Am J Hypertens. 2004;17:1135–42.
150. Kloner RA, Sadovsky R, Johnson EG, et al. Efficacy of tadalafil in the treatment of erectile dysfunction in hypertensive men on concomitant thiazide diuretic therapy. Int J Impot Res. 2005;17:450–4.
151. Webb DJ, Muirhead GJ, Wulff M, et al. Sildenafil citrate potentiates the hypotensive effects of nitric oxide donor drugs in male patients with stable angina. J Am Coll Cardiol. 2000;36:25–31.

Chapter 20
Postmenopausal Hypertension and Coronary Artery Disease Risk

Panagiota Pietri and Charalambos Vlachopoulos

Introduction

Cardiovascular disease is the leading cause of death in women worldwide [1, 2]. Female hormones, particularly estrogens, exert a protective role on the cardiac and vascular function through many pathophysiological mechanisms. However, this beneficial effect is abolished after menopause; loss of protection is associated with an increase in the incidence of hypertension [3], diabetes mellitus, dyslipidemia and, consequently, cardiovascular disease. Indeed, the large burden of cardiovascular disease in women is noted around the age of 50, coinciding with menopause [4]. However, although endogenous estrogens are cardioprotective, the results concerning the potential beneficial effect of hormone replacement therapy in postmenopausal women are contradictory.

In this chapter, the mechanisms underlying the association of hypertension with menopause will be presented and the pathways that lead from this association to the risk of coronary artery disease will be explored. Finally, the potential role of hormone replacement for the reduction of this risk will be discussed.

P. Pietri, M.D.
Hypertension Unit, Athens Heart Center, Athens Medical Center, Athens, Greece

C. Vlachopoulos, M.D., FESC (✉)
First Cardiology Department, Athens University School of Medicine, Hippokration Hospital, Athens, Greece
e-mail: cvlachop@otenet.gr

E.A. Andreadis (ed.), *Hypertension and Cardiovascular Disease*,
DOI 10.1007/978-3-319-39599-9_20

Postmenopausal Hypertension and CAD Risk: Common Pathophysiological Links

Menopause and Endothelial Function

Endothelial dysfunction has a pivotal role in the pathogenesis of hypertension and atherosclerosis and as such, may serve as a potential mechanism through which the decreased levels of female hormones may promote hypertension and coronary heart disease. Estrogen receptors are found in myocardial cells, vascular smooth muscle cells (VSMCs) and endothelial cells [5, 6]. There is ample evidence that estrogens exert vasodilatory effects either indirectly, by stimulating the production of nitric oxide (NO), or directly, by promoting VSMCs relaxation. Indeed, 17β-estradiol (E_2) through its binding to estrogen receptor *a* (ERa), causes an acute activation of endothelial NO synthase (eNOS), an effect that is inhibited by ERa antagonists [7]. Moreover, the inhibition of mitogen-activated protein (MAP) kinase prevents the activation of eNOS by E_2, while E_2 causes ER-dependent activation of MAP kinase implying that the effect of E_2 on the production of NO and the consequent vasodilation is modulated through the path of MAP kinase [7]. The beneficial effect of estrogens on endothelial function has also been highlighted by experimental data showing that E_2 up-regulates mitochondrial superoxide dismutase (SOD2) in mice and in vitro in human aortic endothelial cells [8]. The SOD2 is an antioxidant enzyme with vasculoprotective effects and its deficiency is related to an excessive generation of reactive oxygen species (ROS).

The role of female hormone loss on endothelial function is supported by an experimental study in rats showing that ovariectomized animals present abnormal endothelial responses to acetylcholine (Ach), including decreased Ach induced endothelium-dependent relaxation, decreased endothelium-dependent relaxation factor (EDRF) and increased endothelium-dependent contracting factor (EDCF) [9]. Moreover, ovariectomy was related to an increase in reactive oxygen species (ROS), a mechanism that mediated the abnormal response of endothelium to Ach, i.e. vasoconstriction instead of vasodilation [9]. Furthermore, in postmenopausal women, the endothelial vasodilator response to *β*-adrenergic receptor agonist isoproterenol is blunted compared to young premenopausal women, implying endothelial dysfunction and increased risk of hypertension given the evidence that this abnormal response is prevalent in hypertensive patients [10, 11]. This notion is reinforced by a prospective study in a large cohort of healthy postmenopausal women showing that, with each unit decrease of flow-mediated dilatation (FMD, a noninvasive index of endothelial function), there was a significant increase in the relative risk of hypertension after mean follow-up of 3.6 years [12]. In addition, other investigators demonstrated a beneficial effect of estrogen replacement therapy on endothelial function in postmenopausal hypertensive women [13].

Taken all these data into consideration, it might be argued that the lack of estrogens at post-menopause induces a state of endothelial dysfunction which may, in part, contribute to the increased prevalence of hypertension and coronary artery disease.

Menopause and Renin-Angiotensin-Aldosterone System

The activation of the renin-angiotensin-aldosterone system (RAAS) plays a fundamental role in the increase of blood pressure (BP), mainly through two pathophysiological mechanisms; the vasoconstrictive effect of angiotensin II (AT) (via stimulation of AT 1 receptors) and the aldosterone-induced sodium retention. While AT 1 receptors promote vasoconstriction, AT 2 receptors exert vasodilatory effects, thus reducing BP.

There is evidence that RAAS activity is positively modulated by androgens, while female hormones antagonize it. Indeed, data have shown that plasma renin activity (PRA) is 27 % higher in men than in women of normotensive population [14, 15]. Moreover, treatment with estrogen replacement therapy in postmenopausal women was related to lower renin levels compared to untreated postmenopausal women, reinforcing the potential inhibitory effects of estrogens on RAAS [16]. Other investigators have shown that hormone replacement therapy with estrogen/progestogen combination resulted in a 20 % decrease of serum angiotensin converting enzyme (ACE), an effect that was more pronounced in women with higher baseline ACE levels [17]. Further, estrogen upregulates renal AT 2 receptors, while it decreases the expression of AT 1 receptors, thus enhancing vasodilation and lowering of BP [18, 19].

The pressure-natriuresis relationship, which is highly modulated by RAAS, refers to the physiologic phenomenon of the increased excretion of sodium as a result of increased BP. This relationship is abnormal in hypertension with a rightward shift of the pressure-natriuresis relation curve. Previous experimental study demonstrated that, at 12 weeks of age, BP was higher in male, spontaneous, hypertensive rats (SHR) compared to females, a finding that was related to a blunted pressure-natriuresis relationship in male SHR compared to females [20]. Recently, investigators showed that renal expression of the AT 2 receptors is four-fold greater in wild-type female mice than males and these receptors modulate the chronic pressure-natriuresis curve, which is shifted leftward in female mice, an effect that was lost with age [21]. Additionally, there is evidence that the female hormone, progesterone, induces natriuresis exerting an anti-mineralocorticoid effect by inhibition of aldosterone binding to renal mineralocorticoid receptors [22].

To conclude on the role of RAAS at menopausal hypertensive women, it may be suggested that endogenous female hormones contribute to BP regulation through inhibition of RAAS but this effect is abolished after menopause, thus promoting BP increase and augmenting cardiovascular risk.

Finally, salt sensitivity (the acute increase in BP after increased sodium intake) seems to be regulated, at least in part, by estrogens. A previous study in normotensive women who were subject to surgical menopause showed that the prevalence of salt sensitivity was almost doubled after 4 months from the procedure, although all women remained normotensive [23]. Given that arterial hypertension may not occur until 5 or 10 years after menopause [24], authors suggested that increased salt sensitivity may be a masked predisposing factor for incident hypertension and subsequent increased cardiovascular risk in postmenopausal women [25].

Menopause and Low-Grade Inflammation

Arterial hypertension and low-grade inflammation are closely related through a bidirectional cause-and-effect relationship [26]. A large prospective study that established, for the first time, a possible causal relationship between low-grade inflammation and hypertension was conducted in over 20,000 normotensive females. These women were followed for a mean duration of 8 years and researchers demonstrated an increased risk of developing arterial hypertension among females with higher levels of high sensitivity C-reactive protein (hsCRP) [27].

Viscelar adiposity, which is increased in postmenopausal women [28], may contribute to low-grade inflammatory activation, which may, in turn, contribute to increased BP levels. Indeed, a previous study conducted in women who were followed from the premenopausal to postmenopausal state showed a significant increase in inflammatory biomarkers, including serum amyloid A (SAA), monocyte-chemotactic protein-1 and adiponectin, a change that was associated with an increase in abdominal adiposity either positively (SAA) or negatively (adiponectin) [29]. Similar results were obtained from a cross-sectional study, which showed that hsCRP levels were higher in postmenopausal compared to premenopausal women, while menopausal status and waist circumference were independent predictors of high hsCRP levels [30]. Moreover, postmenopausal women have higher levels of interleukin-8 (IL-8), which are found increased in both the adipose tissue and peripheral circulation [31].

Interestingly, in postmenopausal women, estradiol (E_2) is independently and significantly associated with CRP [32]. Considering that after menopause, the larger proportion of estradiol is produced from the adipose tissue after aromatization from testosterone and given that CRP and inflammatory cytokines are stimulators of aromatase [33], it might be suggested that adipose tissue regulates the relationship between estradiol and low-grade inflammation after menopause. Whether estradiol may also serve as an inflammatory marker in postmenopausal women, thus indicating a further increase of the risk for developing hypertension, is a hypothesis that warrants further investigation.

Data also support the stimulation of low-grade vascular inflammation elicited by estrogen depletion, both in postmenopausal women and in ovariectomized animals. Particularly, leukocytes from healthy postmenopausal women were more adhesive to the arterial endothelium than those from premenopausal women, while similar significant increases in arteriolar leukocyte adhesion and cell adhesion molecular expression were observed in overiectomized rats [34]. Interestingly, arterial inflammation was attenuated after chronic treatment with low-dose 17β-estradiol and after inhibition of renin-angiotensin system with losartan or benazepril [34].

Inflammatory biomarkers, such as CRP and fibrinogen, emerged as the only significant predictors, along with the age, of subclinical carotid atherosclerosis and clinical events in a small cohort of postmenopausal hypertensive women [35]. Given the predictive role of low-grade inflammation for future cardiovascular events in women [36, 37] (Fig. 20.1), it might be suggested that inflammatory activation may

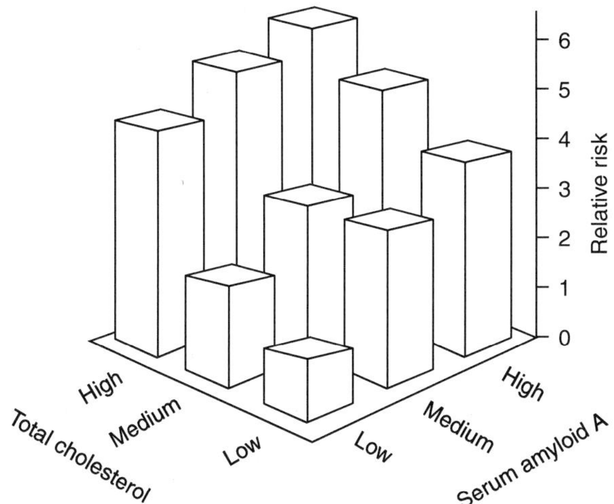

Fig. 20.1 Relative risk of cardiovascular events among 28,263 healthy postmenopausal women according to baseline levels of total cholesterol and markers of inflammation: hsCRP (*upper panel*), serum amyloid A (*lower panel*). The risk was highest among women with high total cholesterol levels and high levels of inflammatory markers. However, even among women with low total cholesterol levels, the risk was higher among those with high levels of hsCRP and serum amyloid A than among those with low levels of these markers, thus highlighting the strong predictive role of inflammatory biomarkers (Reprinted from Ridker et al. [37])

serve as an underlying mechanism for the increased risk of coronary artery disease after menopause. Whether this risk is further enhanced by the associated increased burden of arterial hypertension induced by subclinical inflammation, or it is the vascular inflammation *per se* the driving force for the incidence of both arterial hypertension and coronary artery disease, is a question that remains to be answered.

Menopause and Insulin Resistance

Insulin resistance, which increases with aging, promotes an adverse metabolic profile including a high incidence of arterial hypertension and diabetes mellitus [38]. As with low-grade inflammation, insulin resistance and arterial hypertension are closely related in a bidirectional way. Indeed, hypertensive patients exhibit higher levels of insulin compared to normotensive subjects [39]. Conversely, genetically determined hypertensive rats have insulin resistance and hyperinsulinemia [40, 41] suggesting either a causal relationship between insulin resistance and hypertension or a common pathogenetic predisposition of the two entities. The endothelial dysfunction (induced by insulin resistance), the inhibitory effect of AT II on insulin signaling, as well as the activation of inflammatory and prothrombotic state are some of the mechanisms linking insulin resistance and arterial hypertension. Whatever the underlying pathophysiological mechanisms are, insulin resistance and arterial hypertension are frequent comorbidities and both increase cardiovascular risk. In postmenopausal women, visceral adiposity and high insulin resistance have been shown to be the most detrimental combination for an unfavorable cardiometabolic health characterized by high levels of systolic and diastolic BP, increased levels of fasting glucose, triglycerides, inflammatory markers and decreased levels of HDL cholesterol [42]. Estrogens increase hepatic insulin sensitivity by decreasing gluconeogenesis and glycogenolysis [43], while they increase insulin secretion [44] and improve insulin function. Thus, estrogen deficiency has the opposite results by increasing insulin resistance [45]. Noteworthy, in middle-aged women, insulin resistance was associated with increased left ventricular mass and wall thickness, thus implying a pronouncing effect of insulin resistance to cardiac organ damage and the subsequent cardiovascular risk [46].

Previous data have demonstrated an independent prognostic role of metabolic syndrome (MS) in the incidence of coronary artery disease and the 3-year risk of death in postmenopausal women [47]. Considering the adverse prognostic role of MS in hypertensive patients [48] and given its increased incident rate in postmenopausal women [49], it may be argued that MS mediates, at least in part, the increased cardiovascular risk associated with hypertension in postmenopausal women. Indeed, the unfavorable effect of MS in the cardiometabolic health of hypertensive postmenopausal women has been demonstrated by a previous study which showed that there are two different forms of hypertension after menopause: an isolated one and another which is associated with MS and is related to a more severe risk profile and a less favorable response to antihypertensive treatment [50], thus predisposing to a higher cardiovascular risk. In an experimental study, the postmenopausal metabolic syndrome was characterized by enhanced AT II-induced contractile responses and impaired endothelial dependent vasodilatation, changes that were associated with increased protein expression of AT1 receptors in the aorta and the heart [51]. These changes were, partially, suppressed by administration of 17β estradiol (E_2) thus, reinforcing the beneficial effect of estrogens on the prevention of cardiovascular dysfunction in postmenopausal metabolic syndrome [51].

Target Organ Damage in Postmenopausal Hypertensive Women: A Mediator of Increased CAD Risk?

Postmenopausal Hypertension and Aortic Stiffness

Aortic stiffening is considered a vascular organ damage and the measurement of pulse wave velocity (PWV), a direct, non-invasive marker of aortic stiffness, is recommended for risk stratification in hypertensive patients [52]. The independent predictive value of PWV for future cardiovascular events has been highlighted by numerous studies in several populations, including hypertensive patients [53, 54]. Arterial stiffness is, principally, determined by age and BP [55]. Moreover, increased arterial stiffness is the main mechanism for the elevation of systolic and pulse pressure after middle age [55]. Noteworthy, the increase in systolic and pulse pressure after the age 50 is much greater in women than in men [56, 57]. Indeed, investigators have shown that, although aortic PWV rises similarly with aging in both genders, PWV has greater influence on pulse pressure in women than in men [58].

Whether menopause aggravates aortic stiffness in women after 50 or it is the aging *per se* that has the most detrimental effect on their aortic wall function and structure, is an issue of debate. A previous study showed that, in women between the ages of 45 and 56 years, those who experienced menopause for at least 6 years, had the highest risk for increased PWV independently of age or other cardiovascular risk factors, such as hypertension, diabetes, hyperlipidemia and smoking, suggesting that menopause augments the age-related increase in aortic stiffness during the early postmenopausal period [59]. Other investigators have shown that aortic distensibility (the inverse of aortic stiffness) is declining across time at all menopausal states but it is faster in the menopausal transition (defined as the change from premenopausal to perimenopausal or to postmenopausal stage) [60]. Furthermore, obstructive sleep apnea, which is common in perimenopausal women, has been independently associated with increased BP and aortic stiffness [61].

There is evidence that in postmenopausal women with angiographically confirmed CAD, increased levels of baseline pulse pressure, a crude index of arterial stiffness, is associated with subsequent progression of coronary atherosclerosis and, interestingly, no detectable effect on pulse pressure is observed after hormone replacement therapy [62]. The adverse prognostic role of pulse pressure in postmenopausal women has also been highlighted by other investigators who showed that for each 10 mmHg increase in 24 h ambulatory pulse pressure there was a 73 % higher risk for cardiovascular events after 7 years of follow-up [63] (Fig. 20.2).

The pathophysiological mechanisms that are implicated in the increased prevalence of hypertension after menopause may also contribute to the rise in aortic stiffness and, actually, the latter may be the main causal factor leading to hypertension. Indeed, low grade-inflammatory activation in postmenopausal hypertensive women [29–31] may enhance aortic stiffness given the evidence of an independent association of inflammatory biomarkers with PWV in hypertensive patients [64, 65]. The role of inflammation on vascular damage after menopause is reinforced by experimental data showing that aspirin, as an anti-inflammatory agent, improved the antioxidant capacity, endothelial dysfunction and arterial stiffness in aged ovariectomized rats [66].

Several dietary and pharmaceutical interventions are beneficial for the reduction of aortic stiffness in postmenopausal women. Indeed, moderate alcohol consumption is inversely associated with PWV among postmenopausal women, suggesting a possible cardioprotective effect [67]. Moreover, sodium restriction has shown to reduce 24 h systolic and pulse pressure in postmenopausal women, a benefit that was related to a decrease in aortic stiffness [68]. Similar favorable effects have been demonstrated for aerobic exercise [69, 70]. Regarding the effect of antihypertensive drugs on aortic stiffness, all agents may lower PWV, mainly through BP reduction, and, to date, no superiority of one class over the other has been established, even among postmenopausal women [71, 72].

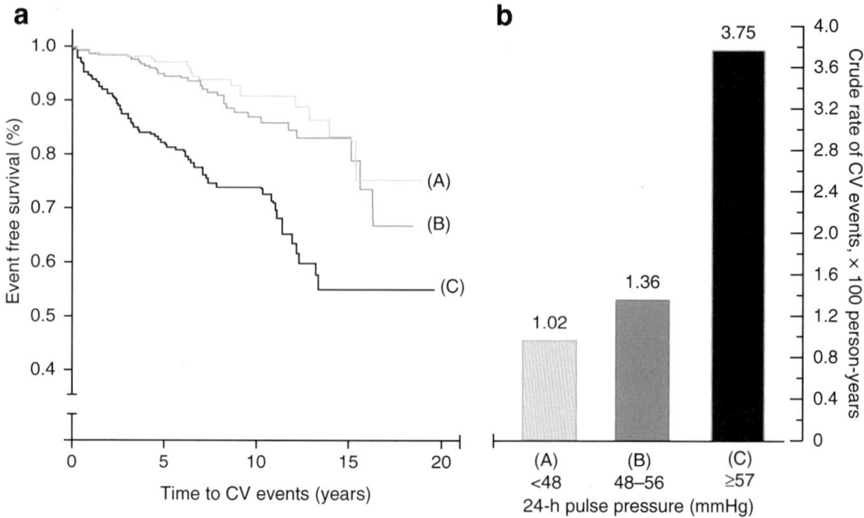

Fig. 20.2 (**a**) Event-free survival curves for cardiovascular (CV) events, including new-onset CAD, in postmenopausal hypertensive women according to tertriles of 24 h pulse pressure. (**b**) The rate of major CV events was significantly higher in women with 24 h pulse pressure ≥57 mmHg (Reprinted from Angeli et al. [63])

Finally, a beneficial effect on aortic stiffness has been demonstrated after hormonal therapy. A study conducted from our Department showed, for the first time, that intravenous administration of 17β-estradiol improved the elasticity of the aorta in postmenopausal women with or without coronary artery disease [73]. Moreover, a previous study showed that hormone replacement therapy decreased aortic stiffness in postmenopausal women, an effect that was independent of BP reduction [74]. The favorable effect of hormone therapy has also been shown for women in the menopausal transition who exhibited better arterial distensibility compared to women under no therapy [60].

The documented increased aortic stiffness in postmenopausal women may mediate part of their increased risk for CAD given that aortic stiffness determines left ventricular afterload and induces hypertrophy, thus potentiating the risk for myocardial ischemia [75]. Extending this knowledge, it might be speculated that dietary [76] and pharmaceutical interventions that lower aortic stiffness may improve cardiovascular risk in postmenopausal women, although, so far, such a hypothesis has been confirmed only for patients with end-stage renal disease [77].

Postmenopausal Hypertension and Left Ventricular Hypertrophy

Left ventricular hypertrophy (LVH) is considered a cardiac organ damage in hypertension and it is associated with increased risk of cardiovascular disease, including CAD [78, 79]. The screening for echocardiographically determined LVH is recommended by the ESH guidelines to improve risk stratification in hypertensive patients [52]. The results concerning the difference in prevalence of LVH between the two genders are controversial. Indeed, studies have shown that LVH is higher in men compared to women at premenopausal age [80, 81], whereas the opposite has also been documented [82]. Irrespective of the fact that the mechanisms underlying this gender discrepancy are not thoroughly investigated, there is evidence that, in middle-aged women, insulin resistance has a more pronounced effect on LVH compared to men, an effect that is largely accounted for by obesity [46]. In line with the above results, other investigators highlighted the strong influence of obesity on LVH in postmenopausal women with metabolic syndrome [83]. Moreover, high plasma levels of leptin, the hormone that is released from adipose tissue and regulates body weight and energy balance, are protective against LV hypertrophy in overweight sedentary postmenopausal women [84]. Blood pressure and other components of metabolic syndrome have also been elicited as independent predictors of LVH in a large sample of postmenopausal women [85]. Extrapolating, it might be suggested that menopause may aggravate LVH, apart from the increased BP *per se*, also through the increased rate of obesity and insulin resistance that accompany postmenopausal state [42–45]. Moreover, obesity may be implicated in the adverse prognosis of postmenopausal women with CAD given the evidence that it is among the nine predictors of heart failure in this group of patients [86].

Experimental study in ovariectomized hypertensive rats showed that estrogen deficiency is associated with increased myocardial inflammation and fibrosis, another possible mechanism for diastolic dysfunction and LVH [87]. Hemodynamic changes that take place in menopause have also been attributed to the grater LVH observed in postmenopausal compared to premenopausal women. In particular, postmenopausal women have higher peripheral resistance, less nocturnal BP fall and higher levels of hematocrit compared to premenopausal women; this greater hemodynamic load is associated with early concentric left ventricular remodeling [88].

Given the adverse prognostic role of LVH [78, 79] it might be suggested that its existence or the lack of its regression after antihypertensive treatment [89] contribute to the increased CAD risk in hypertensive postmenopausal women. A previous study in postmenopausal women with or at increased risk of CAD showed that among hypertensive women, 35 % had evidence of electrocardiographic LVH [90], thus implying a possible detrimental effect of LVH on the CAD risk in hypertensive women at menopause.

There are ample literature data on the role of hormone replacement therapy (HRT) on LVH, most of which conclude to a beneficial effect. Use of transdermal 17β-estradiol, on top of antihypertensive treatment, induced a greater reduction of LV mass, compared to controls, in postmenopausal women with mild or moderate arterial hypertension [91]. Furthermore, HRT led to a reduction in LV mass index, an effect that was not related to the reduction in serum angiotensin converting enzyme (ACE) activity and plasma aldosterone concentration induced by the hormonal therapy [92]. Other investigators demonstrated a significant reduction in LV mass after 6 month HRT, which was associated with a decrease in serum ACE activity, but only in postmenopausal women under treatment lacking RAAS inhibitors, thus indicating that HRT may exert a beneficial effect on LVH if RAAS is activated

[93]. Further evidence supports the favorable effect of estrogens and progesterone on the hemodynamic load of postmenopausal women by decreasing LV mass index, relative wall thickness and plasma norepinephrine levels, while increasing the stroke volume and cardiac index after 6-month therapy [94].

Considering that LVH is an independent risk factor of cardiovascular disease [78, 79] and its regression is associated with lower cardiovascular morbidity and mortality in hypertensive patients [95] it might be suggested that its reduction with HRT may improve CAD risk in postmenopausal women. Nevertheless, to date, such a hypothesis has not been confirmed.

Postmenopausal Hypertension and Microalbuminuria

Microalbuminuria is a manifestation of subclinical organ damage and is frequent in arterial hypertension and diabetes mellitus. Moreover, albumin excretion is predictive of incident hypertension, even when it is within upper normal limits [96]. Presence of microalbuminuria confers an increased risk of ischemic heart disease in hypertensive patients, independently of classic CV risk factors [97]. Furthermore, microalbuminuria has emerged as an independent predictor of cardiovascular mortality, especially among hypertensive individuals [98, 99]. The close relationship between microalbuminuria and CAD is, partly, attributed to the assumption that albumin excretion reflects a generalized endothelial dysfunction and hence, may be associated with the atherosclerotic disease [100, 101]. Furthermore, increased aortic stiffness and pulse pressure may also, pathophysiologically, link CAD and microalbuminuria. Indeed, aortic stiffness is an independent predictor of CAD in hypertensive patients [102]. Increased aortic stiffness leads to increased pulsatile stress on the small arteries of the kidney, thus promoting endothelial damage and finally leading to albumin excretion from the glomerulus [103, 104].

Data on the prevalence and prognostic role of microalbuminuria in postmenopausal women are scarce, albeit robust. In a study of over 12,000 postmenopausal women, urinary albumin levels were strong predictors of future myocardial infarction and cardiovascular mortality [105] (Fig. 20.3). In this cohort, the percentage of hypertension was higher among women in the highest quintile of albumin excretion; however, the increased cardiovascular risk associated with the higher levels of microalbuminuria was independent of the presence of hypertension or diabetes, further reinforcing the role of microalbuminuria as a distinct marker of vascular damage, even among postmenopausal women [105].

Results regarding the effect of HRT on urinary albumin excretion are contradictory. Experimental study in ovariectomized rats with nephrectomy showed that estradiol replacement was protective for the remnant kidney function by reducing albuminuria and diminishing glomerular injury [106]. In line with the experimental data, HRT was associated with a decrease in albumin excretion in postmenopausal women after 6 years of therapy [107]. Supporting data demonstrated a

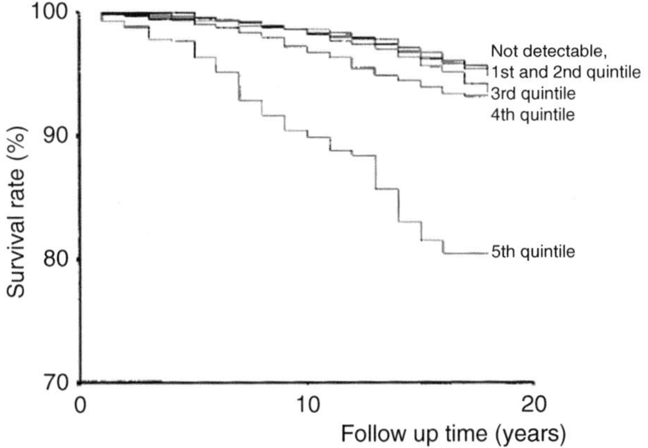

Fig. 20.3 Survival curves for cardiovascular mortality in relation to urinary albumin excretion in 12,239 postmenopausal women. Women in the highest quintile of urine albumin levels had the highest cardiovascular mortality rate (Reprinted from Roest et al. [105])

19 % reduction in albumin-creatinin-ratio (ACR) after a 5-year follow-up in postmenopausal women under HRT [108]. The role of estrogens as inhibitors of the activated RAAS system [16] and their beneficial effects on glomerular endothelial function, mainly through renal NO formation [109], have been proposed as potential mechanisms for the reduction of albuminuria induced by HRT. However, other investigators do not argue in favor of hormone replacement therapy for albumin reduction, establishing either neutral or negative results. In a small study of healthy postmenopausal women, daily use of 1 mg of 17β-estradiol had no significant effect on microalbuminuria after 6 months, an effect that may be attributed to the short period of treatment [110]. In a case–control study conducted in 4301 females, oral contraceptive use and HRT was associated with increased risk of having microalbuminuria [111]. However, this study has few limitations; first, it was not a prospective study and second, the participants were females from the general population and not just postmenopausal women. Thus, no definite results on the effect of HRT on albumin reduction can be assumed. Future studies should address whether the possible beneficial effects of HRT on the regression of microalbuminuria in hypertensive postmenopausal women will be translated to a reduction in their CAD risk.

Coronary Artery Disease Risk in Postmenopausal Hypertensive Women

The Effect of Classic Risk Factors

The increased risk of CAD among postmenopausal women may be largely ascribed to arterial hypertension. Indeed, results from the Women's Health Initiative substudy, in a large cohort of postmenopausal women, showed that the combination of an elevated systolic BP and resting heart rate were significant predictors of calcified CAD in postmenopausal, hysterectomized women [112]. Nevertheless, other classic risk factors that accompany hypertension after menopause may also be implicated.

Interestingly, in a previous study that compared the contribution of hypertension and other risk factors to the development in pre- and postmenopausal women, elevated systolic and pulse pressure emerged as risk factors for CAD only in premenopausal women, despite their significantly lower BP levels compared to postmenopausal women [113]. Consistent with these observations, data have shown that, among postmenopausal women, significant determinants of increased coronary calcium score (a predictor of CAD) were age, diabetes mellitus and lack of exercise but not hypertension, smoking or hyperlipidemia [114]. Other investigators have highlighted the predictive role of lipid abnormalities in the risk of CAD among postmenopausal women. Indeed, lipoprotein a (Lpa) and triglycerides were indicative of obstructive CAD, independently of other risk factors, including hypertension, in postmenopausal women who underwent coronary arteriography for chest pain [115]. Finally, a case–control study showed that smoking and early postmenopausal stage (<3 years) were the most important determinants of premature CAD in women less than 55 years old [116].

In conclusion, it might be suggested that, apart from arterial hypertension *per se*, other classic risk factors such as age, diabetes, smoking, hyperlipidemia and obesity that are accumulating and may be aggravated after menopause are strong predictors of CAD in postmenopausal hypertensive women.

The Effect of Menopause

Whether the estrogen depletion *per se* may constitute a predictor of CAD in postmenopausal women, independently of classic risk factors, is still not well clarified. Data from 651 postmenopausal women followed-up for 19 years, showed no association between baseline estrogen levels and CAD risk [117]. Similar results for an absent relationship between estrogens and CAD risk were demonstrated from the case–control Women's Health Study (WHS), conducted in postmenopausal women [118]. In these women, higher levels of free androgen index and lower levels of sex hormone binding globulin (SHBG) were noted among women who developed cardiovascular events but, still, this was not independent of body mass index (BMI) or other classic risk factors [118]. Recent data from approximately 100 postmenopausal women of WHS conclude to an association between CAD and estradiol but this disappears after adjustment for hypertension, BMI and cholesterol [119]. In a small prospective study in postmenopausal women with known CAD or at high risk of CAD, low estrone levels were associated with increased total mortality after adjustment for diabetes, obesity, dyslipidemia and family history; however, when age and hypertension were included in the analysis, these risk factors emerged as the only significant predictors of total mortality, while estrogens were excluded [120].

Hormonal changes, other than estrogen depletion *per se*, that accompany menopause have also been implicated to the increased CAD risk. Indeed, recent data in over 4,000 women from the Copenhagen City Heart Study followed up for ≤30 years showed that, women with the lowest levels of estradiol, as well as women with the highest testosterone concentrations exhibited higher risk of ischemic heart disease compared to women with higher estrogen or lower testosterone levels, respectively [120]. Moreover, the adverse effect of the extreme hormonal concentrations on classic cardiovascular risk factors, including hypertension, was more robust for testosterone levels compared to estradiol levels, suggesting that low estradiol is directly associated to increased CAD risk, while the risk from high levels of testosterone is mediated through other risk factors. Interestingly, the results were similar for postmenopausal women, who consisted the 70 % of the study population and to whom the lower levels of estradiol were observed, thus indicating that the extreme hormonal changes after menopause may unfavorably alter cardiovascular health [121].

Interpretation of existing evidence leads to the assumption that hormonal status in menopause, characterized by, either low levels of estrogens or high levels of androgens, are independent determinants of CAD. Future, prospective studies in postmenopausal hypertensive women need to elucidate the exact role of estrogen depletion *per se* on the incidence of CAD.

The Role of Hormone Replacement Therapy for Risk Reduction of Coronary Artery Disease

Despite the beneficial effects of endogenous estrogens on cardiovascular system [8, 9, 19, 20], results regarding the role of HRT on the reduction of coronary artery events are controversial. Study characteristics, such as the design (observational, case–control or randomized trials), the population (healthy postmenopausal women – primary prevention, or postmenopausal women with CAD – secondary prevention), the type of the studied hormone therapy (estrogens or estrogens plus progestin), the dosage or route administration, as well as the duration of treatment, are all features that may, at least in part, explain the different findings.

A large, randomized trial in over 16,000 healthy postmenopausal women followed-up for 5 years, demonstrated an increased risk of CAD with combined hormone therapy (conjugated equine estrogens plus medroxyprogesterone acetate), mostly evident at the first year of treatment [122]. Surprisingly, women assigned on HRT had greater reductions in total cholesterol, glucose and insulin levels and greater increases in triglycerides and high-density lipoprotein [122].

Systolic BP was 1–2 mmHg higher in women at HRT compared to placebo at follow-up, but the presence of hypertension did not modify the CAD risk among women on HRT [122]. On the other hand, in postmenopausal women with CAD, a randomized, placebo-controlled study (HERS), did not find significant difference in the CAD events between the combined therapy (estrogens plus progestin) and the placebo groups after 4 years of follow-up [123]. However, post-hoc analyses showed a statistically significant time trend, with more CAD events in the hormone group at 1 year and fewer events after 3 years, speculating that this early increased risk may be due to prothrombotic or pro-ischemic effect of treatment that is gradually outweighed by a beneficial effect on atherosclerotic risk factors and particularly, the lowering of low-density lipoprotein cholesterol levels [123].

Opposite to the above results, a randomized study in 1,006 postmenopausal women, concluded to a significant reduced risk of myocardial infarction and heart failure after 10 years of follow-up in women allocated to HRT (synthetic 17β estradiol ± norethisterone) early after menopause, compared to placebo [124]. In an attempt to explain the positive findings, authors suggested that the type of estrogens, the younger age of the participants and the early randomization to HRT (shortly after menopause) might have attributed to the beneficial effects of HRT and the divergence from previous studies. Regarding classic risk factors, the baseline mean BP and glucose levels were within normal limits with a slight increase in total cholesterol and LDL levels, but without any difference between women on HRT and placebo therapy; moreover, the percentage of smokers was similar between the two groups.

Whether a favorable cardiovascular risk profile early after menopause may serve as a substrate for the beneficial effects of HRT remains an unresolved issue with important clinical implications, if confirmed. By extrapolating available evidence, it might be suggested that a well-controlled BP in postmenopausal women may lead to reduced risk of CAD with HRT and vice versa, a lack of normalization of hypertension after HRT may induce increased CAD risk. Future, prospective studies on postmenopausal hypertensive women will address the role of BP regulation in the reduction of the CAD risk in women under HRT.

Conclusions

The prevalence of CAD is increased among postmenopausal hypertensive women. Possible pathophysiological mechanisms that may link arterial hypertension and coronary artery disease include endothelial dysfunction, RAAS activation, low-grade inflammation and insulin resistance (Fig. 20.4). Target organ damage may serve as mediator of the increased risk. Classic risk factors that accompany arterial hypertension after menopause are also strong predictors. Results concerning the effect of HRT on the risk reduction are contradictory and randomized trials in postmenopausal hypertensive women are needed to elucidate the precise role of blood pressure regulation on the outcomes after HRT.

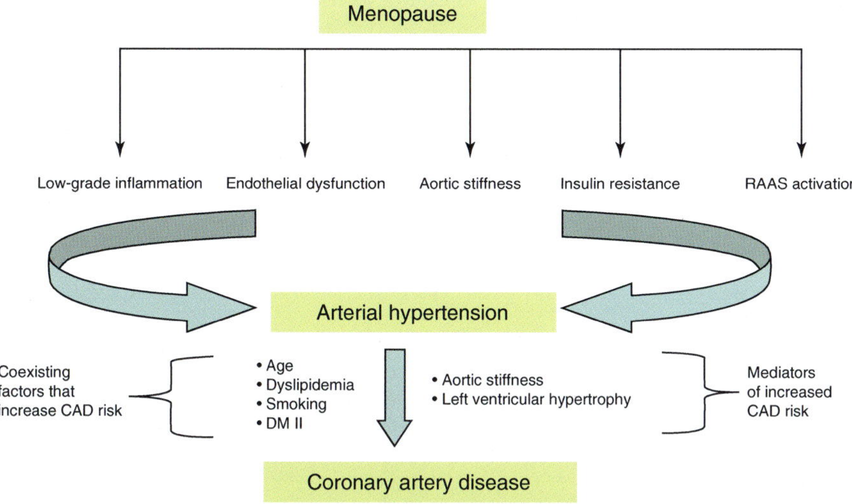

Fig. 20.4 Possible pathophysiological mechanisms linking postmenopausal hypertension with coronary artery disease (CAD) risk. Low-grade inflammatory activation, endothelial dysfunction, increased aortic stiffness, insulin resistance and activation of renin-angiotensin-aldosterone system (RAAS) are among the main mechanisms that increase the incidence of arterial hypertension in postmenopausal women. Arterial hypertension, either through the increased hemodynamic load per se or through the above-mentioned mechanisms, but also through the gathering of other classic risk factors, such as age, dyslipidemia, smoking and diabetes mellitus II (DM II) contribute to increased CAD risk. Target organ damage, including aortic stiffness and left ventricular hypertrophy, may serve as mediator of the increased CAD risk

References

1. Executive Summary: Heart Disease and Stroke Statistics-2014 update. A report from the American Heart Association. Circulation. 2014;129:399–410.
2. Nichols M, Townsend N, Scarborough P, Rayner M. European Cardiovascular Disease Statistics 2012 edition. Published by European Heart Network, Belgium and European Society of Cardiology, France.
3. Staessen J, Bulpitt CJ, Fagard R, Lijnen P, Amery A. The influence of menopause on blood pressure. J Hum Hypertens. 1989;3:427–33.
4. Barrett-Connor E, Bush TL. Estrogen and coronary heart disease in women. JAMA. 1991;265:1861–7.
5. Colburn P, Buonassissi V. Estrogen-binding sites in endothelial cell cultures. Science. 1978;201:817–9.
6. Nakao J, Chang WC, Murota SI, Orimo H. Estradiol-binding sites in rat aortic smooth muscle cells in culture. Atherosclerosis. 1981;38:75–80.
7. Chen Z, Yuhanna I, Galcheva-Gargova Z, Karas R, Mendelsohn M, Shaul P. Estrogen receptor a mediates the nongenomic activation of endothelial nitric oxide synthase by estrogen. J Clin Invest. 1999;103:401–6.
8. Liu Z, Gou Y, Zhang H, Zuo H, Zhang H, Liu Z, Yao D. Estradiol improves cardiovascular function through up-regulation of SOD2 on vascular wall. Redox Biol. 2014;3:88–99.
9. Wang D, Wang C, Wu X, Zheng W, Sandberg K, Ji H, Welch W, Wilcox C. Endothelial dysfunction and enhanced contractility in microvessels from ovariectomised rats: roles of oxidative stress and perivascular adipose tissue. Hypertension. 2014;63:1063–9.

10. Harvey R, Barnes J, Charkoudian N, Curry T, Eisenach J, Hart E, Joyner M. Forearm vasodilator responses to a β-adrenergic receptor agonist in premenopausal and postmenopausal women. Physiol Rep. 2014;2, e12032.
11. Stein CM, Nelson R, Deegan R, He H, Wood M, Wood AJ. Forearm beta adrenergic receptor-mediated vasodilatation is impaired, without alteration of forearm norepinephrine spillover, in borderline hypertension. J Clin Invest. 1995;96:579–85.
12. Rossi R, Chiurlia E, Nuzzo A, Cioni E, Origliani G, Modena MG. Flow-mediated vasodilation and risk of developing hypertenion in healthy postmenopausal women. J Am Coll Cardiol. 2004;44:1636–40.
13. Higashi Y, Sanada M, Sasaki S, Nakagawa K, Goto C, Matsuura H, Ohama K, Chayama K, Oshima T. Effect of estrogen replacement therapy on endothelial function in peripheral resistance arteries in normotensive and hypertensive postmenopausal women. Hypertension. 2001;37(2 Pt 2):651–7.
14. James GD, Sealey JE, Muller F, Alderman M, Madhavan S, Laragh JH. Renin relationship to sex, race and age in normotensive population. J Hypertens. 1986;4 Suppl 5:S387–9.
15. Kaplan NM, Kem DC, Holland OB. The intravenous furosemide test: a simple way to evaluate renin responsiveness. Ann Intern Med. 1976;4:639–45.
16. Schunkert H, Danser AH, Hense H-W, Derkx FH, Kurzinger S, Riegger GAJ. Effects of estrogen replacement therapy on the renin-angiotensin system in post-menopausal women. Circulation. 1997;95:39–45.
17. Proudler AJ, Ahmed AH, Crook D, Fogelman I, Rymer JM, Stevenson JC. Hormone replacement therapy and serum angiotensin-enzyme activity in postmenopausal women. Lancet. 1995;346:89–90.
18. Armando I, Jezova M, Juorio AV, Terron JA, Falcon-Neri A, Semino-Mora C, Imboden H, Saavedra JM. Estrogen up-regulates renal angiotensin II AT 2 receptors. Am J Physiol Renal Physiol. 2002;283:F934–43.
19. Brown RD, Hilliard LM, Head GA, Jones ES, Widdop RE, Denton KM. Sex differences in the pressor and tubuloglomerular feedback response to angiotensin II. Hypertension. 2012;59:129–35.
20. Reckelhoff J, Zhang H, Granger J. Testosterone exacerbates hypertension and reduces pressure-natriuresis in male spontaneously hypertensive rats. Hypertension. 1998;31:435–9.
21. Mirabito K, Hilliard L, Kett M, Brown R, Booth S, Widdop R, Moritz K, Evans R, Denton K. Sex- and age-related differences in the chronic pressure-natriuresis relationship: role of the angiotensin type 2 receptor. Am J Physiol Renal Physiol. 2014;307:F901–7.
22. Wambach G, Higgins J. Antimineralocorticoid action of progesterone in the rat: correlation of the effect on electrolyte excretion and interaction with renal mineralocorticoid receptors. Endocrinology. 1978;102:1686–93.
23. Schulman I, Aranda P, Raij L, Veronesi M, Aranda F, Martin R. Surgical menopause increases salt sensitivity of blood pressure. Hypertension. 2006;47:1168–74.
24. Dubey RK, Imthurn B, Zacharia LC, Jackson EK. Hormone replacement therapy and cardiovascular disease: what went wrong and where do we go from here? Hypertension. 2004;44:789–95.
25. Morimoto A, Uzu T, Fujii T, Nishimura M, Kuroda S, Nakamura S, Inenaga T, Kimura G. Sodium sensitivity and cardiovascular events in patients with essential hypertension. Lancet. 1997;350:1734–7.
26. Pietri P, Vlachopoulos C, Tousoulis D. Arterial hypertension and inflammation: from pathophysiological links to risk prediction. Curr Med Chem. 2015;22:2754–61.
27. Sesso H, Buring JE, Rifai N, Blake GJ, Gaziano JM, Ridker PM. C-reactive protein and the risk of developing hypertension. JAMA. 2003;290:2945–51.
28. Tchernof A, Desmeules A, Richard C, Laberge P, Daris M, Mailloux J, Rheaume C, Dupont P. Ovarian hormone status and abdominal visceral adipose tissue metabolism. J Clin Endocrinol Metab. 2004;89:3425–30.
29. Lee C, Carr M, Murdoch S, Mitchell E, Woods N, Wener M, Chandler W, Boyko E, Brunzell J. Adipokines, inflammation and visceral adiposity across the menopausal transition: a prospective study. J Clin Endocrinol Metab. 2009;94:1104–10.

30. Silva DC, Costa LO, Vasconcelos AA, Cerqueira JC, Fantato D, Torres DC, Santos AC, Costa HF. Waist circumference and menopausal status are independent predictors of endothelial low-grade inflammation. Endocr Res. 2014;39:22–5.
31. Alvehus M, Simonyte K, Andersson T, Söderström I, Burén J, Rask E, Mattsson C, Olsson T. Adipose tissue IL-8 is increased in normal weight women after menopause and reduced after gastric bypass surgery in obese women. Clin Endocrinol. 2012;77:684–90.
32. Maggio M, Ceda GP, Lauretani F, Bandinelli S, Corsi AM, Giallauria F, Guralnik J, Zuliani G, Cattabiani C, Parrino S, Ablondi F, Dall'Aglio E, Ceresini G, Basaria S, Ferrucci L. SHBG, sex hormones, and inflammatory markers in older women. J Clin Endocrinol Metabol. 2011;96:1053–9.
33. Purohit A, Reed MJ. Regulation of estrogen synthesis in postmenopausal women. Steroids. 2002;67:979–83.
34. Abu-Taha M, Rius C, Hermenegildo C, Noguera I, Cerda-Nicolas J-M, Issekutz M, Jose P, Cortijo J, Morcillo E, Sanz M-J. Menopause and ovariectomy cause a low grade inflammation that may be prevented by chronic treatment with low doses of estrogen or losartan. J Immunol. 2009;183:1393–402.
35. Rizzo M, Corrado E, Coppola G, Muratori I, Novo G, Novo S. Markers of inflammation are strong predictors of subclinical and clinical atherosclerosis in women with hypertension. Coron Artery Dis. 2009;20:15–20.
36. Johnson BD, Kip KE, Marroquin OC, Ridker PM, Kelsey SF, Shaw LJ, Pepine CJ, Sharaf B, Bairey Merz CN, Sopko G, Olson MB, Reis SE, National Heart, Lung, and Blood Institute. Serum amyloid A as a predictor of coronary artery disease and cardiovascular outcome in women: the National Heart, Lung, and Blood Institute-Sponsored Women's Ischemia Syndrome Evaluation (WISE). Circulation. 2004;109:726–32.
37. Ridker PM, Hennekens CH, Buring JE, Rifai N. C-reactive protein and other markers of inflammation in the prediction of cardiovascular disease in women. N Engl J Med. 2000;342:836–43.
38. Reaven GM. Blanting lecture 1988. Role of insulin resistance in human disease. Diabetes. 1988;37:1595–607.
39. Shen DC, Shieh SM, Wu DA, Reaven GM. Resistance to insulin stimulated glucose uptake in patients with hypertension. J Clin Endocrinol Metab. 1988;66:580–3.
40. Kotchen TA, Zhang HY, Covelli M, Blehschmidt N. Insulin resistance and blood pressure in Dahl rats and in one-kidney, one-clip hypertensive rats. Am J Physiol. 1991;261:E692–7.
41. Reaven GM, Chang H. Relationship between blood pressure, plasma insulin and triglyceride concentration, and insulin action in SHR and WKY rats. Am J Hypertens. 1991;4:34–8.
42. Piché M, Weisnagel J, Corneau L, Nadeau A, Bergeron J, Lemieux S. Contribution of abdominal visceral obesity and insulin resistance to the cardiovascular risk profile of postmenopausal women. Diabetes. 2005;54:770–7.
43. Ahmed-Sorour H, Bailey CJ. Role of ovarian hormones in the long-term control of glucose homeostasis, glycogen formation and gluconeogenesis. Ann Nutr Metab. 1981;25:208–12.
44. Godsland IF. Oestrogens and insulin secretion. Diabetologia. 2005;48:2213–20.
45. Bailey CJ, Ahmed-Sorour H. Role of ovarian hormones in the long-term control of glucose homeostasis. Effects of insulin secretion. Diabetologia. 1980;19:475–81.
46. Rutter M, Parise E, Benjamin E, Levy D, Larson M, Meigs J, Nesto R, Wilson P, Vasan R. Impact of glucose intolerance and insulin resistance on cardiac structure and function. Sex-related differences in the Framingham Heart Study. Circulation. 2003;107:448–54.
47. Kip K, Marroquin O, Kelley D, Johnson D, Kelsey S, Shaw L, Rogers W, Reis S. Clinical importance of obesity versus the metabolic syndrome in cardiovascular risk in women. A Report from the Women's Ischemia Syndrome Evaluation (WISE) Study. Circulation. 2004;109:706–13.
48. Schillaci G, Pirro M, Vaudo G, Gemelli F, Marchesi S, Porcellati C, Mannarino E. Prognostic value of the metabolic syndrome in essential hypertension. J Am Coll Cardiol. 2004;43:1817–22.

49. Park YW, Zhu S, Palaniappan L, Heshka S, Carnethon MR, Heymsfield SB. The metabolic syndrome: prevalence and associated risk factor findings in the US population from the Third National Health and Nutrition Examination Survey, 1988–1994. Arch Intern Med. 2003;163:427–36.
50. Rossi R, Nuzzo A, Origliani G, Modena MG. Metabolic syndrome affects cardiovascular risk profile and response to treatment in hypertensive postmenopausal women. Hypertension. 2008;52:865–72.
51. Bendale DS, Karpe PA, Chabra R, Shete SP, Shah H, Tikoo K. 17-β oestradiol prevents cardiovascular dysfunction in post-menopausal metabolic syndrome by affecting SIRT1/AMPK/H3 acetylation. Br J Pharmacol. 2013;170:779–95.
52. 2013 ESH/ESC Guidelines for the management of arterial hypertension. The Task Force for the management of arterial hypertension of the European Society of Hypertension (ESH) and of the European Society of Cardiology (ESC). J Hypertens. 2013;31:1281–357.
53. Vlachopoulos C, Aznaouridis K, Stefanadis C. Prediction of cardiovascular events and all-cause mortality with arterial stiffness: a systematic review and meta-analysis. J Am Coll Cardiol. 2010;55:1318–27.
54. Ben-Shlomo Y, Spears M, Boustred C, May M, Anderson SG, Benjamin EJ, Boutouyrie P, Cameron J, Chen CH, Cruickshank JK, Hwang SJ, Lakatta EG, Laurent S, Maldonado J, Mitchell GF, Najjar SS, Newman AB, Ohishi M, Pannier B, Pereira T, Vasan RS, Shokawa T, Sutton-Tyrell K, Verbeke F, Wang KL, Webb DJ, Willum Hansen T, Zoungas S, McEniery CM, Cockcroft JR, Wilkinson IB. Aortic pulse wave velocity improves cardiovascular event prediction: an individual participant meta-analysis of prospective observational data from 17,635 subjects. J Am Coll Cardiol. 2014;63:636–46.
55. Nichols W, O'Rourke M, Vlachopoulos C. McDonald's blood flow in arteries. 6th ed. NW: CRC Press, Taylor & Francis Group; 2011. pp 411–67.
56. Vokonas PS, Kannel WB, Cupples LA. Epidemiology and risk of hypertension in the elderly: the Framingham Study. J Hypertens. 1988;6:S3–9.
57. Schoenberger JA. Epidemiology of systolic and diastolic systemic blood pressure elevation in the elderly. Am J Cardiol. 1986;57:45C–51.
58. Smulyan H, Asmar R, Rudnicki A, London G, Safar M. Comparative effects of aging in men and women on the properties of the arterial tree. J Am Coll Cardiol. 2001;37:1374–80.
59. Zaydun G, Tomiyama H, Hashimoto H, Arai T, Koji Y, Yambe M, Motobe K, Hori S, Yamashina A. Menopause is an independent factor augmenting the age-related increase in arterial stiffness in the early postmenopausal phase. Atherosclerosis. 2006;184:137–42.
60. Shufelt C, Elboudwarej O, Johnson BD, Mehta P, Bittner V, Braunstein G, Berga S, Stanczyk F, Dwyer K, Merz CN. Carotid artery distensibility and hormone therapy and menopause: the Los Angeles Atherosclerosis Study. Menopause. 2015;464(1):360–6.
61. Pedrosa R, Barros I, Drager L, Bittencourt M, Medeiros AK, Carvalho L, Lustosa T, Carvalho M, Ferreira M, Lorenzi-Filho G, Costa L. OSA is common and independently associated with hypertension and increased arterial stiffness in consecutive perimenopausal women. Chest. 2014;146:66–72.
62. Nair G, Waters D, Rogers W, Kowalchuk G, Stuckey T, Herrington D. Pulse pressure and coronary atherosclerosis progression in postmenopausal women. Hypertension. 2005;45:53–7.
63. Angeli F, Angeli E, Ambrosio G, Mazzotta G, Cavallini C, Reboldi G, Verdecchia P. Neutrophil count and ambulatory pulse pressure as predictors of cardiovascular adverse events in postmenopausal women with hypertension. Am J Hypertens. 2011;24:591–8.
64. Pietri P, Vyssoulis G, Vlachopoulos C, Zervoudaki A, Gialernios T, Aznaouridis K, Stefanadis C. Relationship between low-grade inflammation and arterial stiffness in patients with essential hypertension. J Hypertens. 2006;24:2231–8.
65. Vlachopoulos C, Pietri P, Aznaouridis K, Vyssoulis G, Vasiliadou C, Bratsas A, Tousoulis D, Xaplanteris P, Stefanadi E, Stefanadis C. Relationship of fibrinogen with arterial stiffness and wave reflections. J Hypertens. 2007;25:2110–6.
66. Dermeci B, Demir O, Dost T, Birincioglu M. Antioxidative effect of aspirin on vascular function of aged ovariectomized rats. Age. 2014;36:223–9.

67. Sierksma A, Lebrun C, van der Schouw Y, Grobbee D, Lamberts S, Hendriks H, Bots M. Alcohol consumption in relation to aortic stiffness and aortic wave reflections: a cross-sectional study in healthy postmenopausal women. Arterioscler Thromb Vasc Biol. 2004;24:342–8.
68. Seals D, Tanaka H, Clevenger C, Monahan K, Reiling MJ, Hiatt W, Davy K, DeSouza C. Blood pressure reductions with exercise and sodium restriction in postmenopausal women with elevated systolic blood pressure: role of arterial stiffness. J Am Coll Cardiol. 2001;38:506–13.
69. Matsubara T, Miyaki A, Akazawa N, Choi Y, Ra S-G, Tanahashi K, Kumagai H, Oikawa S, Maeda S. Aerobic exercise training increases plasma Klotho levels and reduces arterial stiffness in postmenopausal women. Am J Physiol Heart Circ Physiol. 2014;306:H348–55.
70. Tanahashi K, Akazawa N, Miyaki A, Choi Y, Ra SG, Matsubara T, Kumagai H, Oikawa S, Maeda S. Aerobic exercise training decreases plasma asymmetric dimethylarginine concentrations with increase in arterial compliance in postmenopausal women. Am J Hypertens. 2014;27:415–21.
71. Shahin Y, Khan JA, Chetter I. Angiotensin converting enzyme inhibitors effect on arterial stiffness and wave reflections: a meta-analysis and meta-regression of randomized controlled trials. Atherosclerosis. 2012;221:18–33.
72. Hayoz D, Zappe D, Meyer M, Baek IY, Kandra A, Joly M, Mazzolai L, Haesler E, Periard D. Changes in aortic pulse wave velocity in hypertensive postmenopausal women: comparison between a calcium channel blocker vs angiotensin receptor blocker regimen. J Clin Hypertens. 2012;14:773–8.
73. Stefanadis C, Tsiamis E, Dernellis J, Toutouzas P. Effect of estrogen on aortic function in postmenopausal women. Am J Physiol. 1999;276:H658–62.
74. da Costa LS, de Oliviera MA, Rubim VS, Wajngarten M, Aldrighi JM, Rosano GM, Neto CD, Gebara OC. Effects of hormone replacement therapy or raloxifene on ambulatory blood pressure and arterial stiffness in treated hypertensive postmenopausal women. Am J Cardiol. 2004;94:1453–6.
75. Nichols W, O'Rourke M, Vlachopoulos C. McDonald's blood flow in arteries. 6th ed. NW: CRC Press, Taylor & Francis Group; 2011. pp 461–3
76. Vlachopoulos C, Pietri P, Tousoulis D. Pharmacologic and environmental factors: coffee, smoking, and sodium. In: Berbari A, Mancia G, editors. Arterial disorders. Definition, clinical manifestations, mechanisms and therapeutic approaches. Switzerland: Springer International Publishing; 2015. p. 175–86.
77. Guerin A, Blacher J, Pannier B, Marchais S, Safar M, London G. Impact of aortic stiffness attenuation on survival of patients in end-stage renal failure. Circulation. 2001;103:987–92.
78. Koren MJ, Devereux RB, Casale PN, Savage DD, Laragh JH. Relation of left ventricular mass and geometry to morbidity and mortality in uncomplicated essential hypertension. Ann Intern Med. 1991;114:345–52.
79. Verdecchia P, Carini G, Circo A, Dovellini E, Giovannini E, Lombardo M, Solinas P, Gorini M, Maggioni AP, the MAVI Study Group. Left ventricular mass and cardiovascular morbidity in essential hypertension: the MAVI Study. J Am Coll Cardiol. 2001;38:1829–18357.
80. Gardin J, Wagenknecht L, Anton-Culver H, Flack J, Gidding S, Kurosaki T, Wong N, Manolio T. Relationship of cardiovascular risk factors to echocardiographic left ventricular mass in healthy young black and white adult men and women. CARDIA Study Circul. 1995;92:380–7.
81. Marcus R, Krause L, Weber AB, Dominguez-Meja A, Schork NJ, Julius S. Sex-specific determinants of increased left ventricular mass in the Tecumseh Blood Pressure Study. Circulation. 1994;90:928–36.
82. Palatini P, Mos L, Santonastaso M, Saladini F, Benetti E, Mormino P, Bortolazzi A, Cozzio S. Premenopausal women have increased risk of hypertensive target organ damage compared with men of similar age. J Womens Health. 2011;20:1175–81.
83. Olszanecka A, Dragan A, Kawecka-Jaszcz K, Czarnecka D. Influence of metabolic syndrome and its components on subclinical organ damage in hypertensive perimenopausal women. Adv Med Sci. 2014;59:232–9.

84. Di Blasio A, Di Donato F, De Stefano A, Gallina S, Granieri M, Napolitano G, Petrella V, Riccardi I, Santarelli F, Valentini P, Ripari P. Left ventricle wall thickness and plasma leptin levels: baseline relationships and effects of 4 months of walking training in healthy overweight postmenopausal women. Menopause. 2011;18:77–84.
85. Oberman A, Prineas RJ, Larson JC, LaCroix A, Lasser NL. Prevalence and determinants of electrocardiographic left ventricular hypertrophy among a multiethnic population of postmenopausal women (The Women's Health Initiative). Am J Cardiol. 2006;97:512–9.
86. Bibbins-Domingo K, Lin F, Vittinghoff E, Barrett-Connor E, Hulley SB, Grady D, Shlipak MG. Predictors of heart failure among women with coronary disease. Circulation. 2004;110:1424–30.
87. Mori T, Kai H, Kajimoto H, Koga M, Kudo H, Takayama N, Yasuoka S, Anegawa T, Kai M, Imaizumi T. Enhanced cardiac inflammation and fibrosis in ovariectomized hypertensive rats: a possible mechanism for diastolic dysfunction in postmenopausal women. Hypertens Res. 2011;34:496–502.
88. Hinderliter AL, Sherwood A, Blumenthal JA, Light KC, Girdler SS, McFertidge J, Johnson K, Waugh R. Changes in hemodynamics and left ventricular structure after menopause. Am J Cardiol. 2002;89:830–3.
89. Muiesan ML, Salvetti M, Rizzoni D, Castellano M, Donato F, Agabiti-Rosei E. Association of change in left ventricular mass with prognosis during long-term antihypertensive treatment. J Hypertens. 1995;13:1091–5.
90. Wenger NK, Mischke JM, Schroeder K, Collins P, Grady D, Kornitzer M, Mosca L, Barrett-Connor E. Electrocardiograms of menopausal women with coronary heart disease or at increased risk for its occurrence. Am J Cardiol. 2010;106:1580–7.
91. Modena MG, Muia Jr N, Aveta P, Molinari R, Rossi R. Anatomy and performance in hypertensive women. Hypertension. 1999;34:1041–6.
92. Miya Y, Sumino H, Ichikawa S, Nakamura T, Kanda T, Kumakura H, Takayama Y, Mizunuma H, Sakamaki T, Kurabayashi M. Effects of hormone replacement therapy on left ventricular and growth-promoting factors in hypertensive postmenopausal women. Hypertens Res. 2002;25:153–9.
93. Manhem K, Ghanoum B, Johansson M, Milsom I, Gustafsson H. Influence of chronic hormone replacement therapy on left ventricular mass and serum-ACE activity. Blood Press. 2010;19:295–300.
94. Light KC, Hinderliter AL, West SG, Grewen KM, Steege JF, Sherwood A, Girdler SS. Hormone replacement improves hemodynamic profile and left ventricular geometry in hypertensive and normotensive postmenopausal women. J Hypertens. 2001;19:269–78.
95. Bang CN, Devereux RB, Okin PM. Regression of electrocardiographic left ventricular hypertrophy or strain is associated with lower incidence of cardiovascular morbidity and mortality independent of blood pressure reduction- A LIFE review. J Electrocardiol. 2014;47:630–5.
96. Forman JP, Fisher ND, Schopick EL, et al. Higher levels of albuminuria within the normal range predict incident hypertension. J Am Soc Nephrol. 2008;19:1983–8.
97. Jensen JS, Feldt-Rasmussen B, Strandgaard S, Schroll M, Borch-Johnsen K. Arterial hypertension, microalbuminuria, and risk of ischemic heart disease. Hypertension. 2000;35:898–903.
98. Jager A, Kostense P, Ruhé H, Heine R, Nijpels G, Dekker J, Bouter L, Stehouwer C. Microalbuminuria and peripheral arterial disease are independent predictors of cardiovascular and all-cause mortality, especially among hypertensive subjects. Arterioscler Thromb Vasc Biol. 1999;19:617–24.
99. Bigazzi R, Bianchi S, Baldari D, Campese VM. Microalbuminiuria predicts cardiovascular events and renal insufficiency in patients with essential hypertension. J Hypertens. 1998;16:1325–33.
100. Deckert T, Feldt-Rasmussen B, Borch-Johnsen K, Jensen T, Kofoed Enevoldsen A. Albuminuria reflects widespread vascular damage. The Steno hypothesis. Diabetologia. 1989;32:219–26.
101. Stehouwer CDA, Nauta JJP, Zeldenrust GC, Hackeng WHL, Donker AJM, den Ottolander GJH. Urinary albumin excretion, cardiovascular disease, and endothelial dysfunction in non-insulin-dependent diabetes mellitus. Lancet. 1992;340:319–23.

102. Boutouyrie P, Tropeano AI, Asmar R, Gautier I, Benetos A, Lacolley P, Laurent S. Aortic stiffness is an independent predictor of primary coronary events in hypertensive patients: a longitudinal study. Hypertension. 2002;39:10–5.
103. O'Rourke M, Safar M. Relationship between aortic stiffening and microvascular disease in brain and kidney: cause and logic of therapy. Hypertension. 2005;46:200–4.
104. Hashimoto J, Ito S. Central pulse pressure and aortic stiffness determine renal hemodynamics: pathophysiological implication for microalbuminuria in hypertension. Hypertension. 2011;58:839–46.
105. Roest M, Banga JD, Janssen W, Grobbee D, Sixma J, de Jong P, de Zeeuw D, van der Schouw Y. Excessive urinary albumin levels are associated with future cardiovascular mortality in postmenopausal women. Circulation. 2001;103:3057–61.
106. Antus B, Hamar P, Kokeny G, Szollosi Z, Mucsi I, Nemes Z, Rosivall L. Estradiol is nephroprotective in the rat remnant kidney. Nephrol Dial Transplant. 2003;18:54–61.
107. Schopick E, Fisher N, Lin J, Forman J, Curhan G. Post-menopausal hormone use and albuminuria. Nephrol Dial Transplant. 2009;24:3739–44.
108. Agarwal M, Selvan V, Freedman B, Liu Y, Wagenknecht L. The relationship between albuminuria and hormone therapy in postmenopausal women. Am J Kidney Dis. 2005;45: 1019–25.
109. Xiao S, Gillespie DG, Baylis C, Jackson E, Dubey R. Effects of estradiol and its metabolites on glomerular endothelial nitric oxide synthesis and mesangial cell growth. Hypertension. 2001;37(Part 2):645–50.
110. Machado RB, Careta MF, Balducci GP, Araujo TS, Bernardes CR. Effects of estrogen therapy on microalbuminuria in healthy post-menopausal women. Gynecol Endocrinol. 2008;24:681–5.
111. Monster T, Janssen W, de Jong P, de Jong-van den Berg L, Prevention of Renal and Vascular End Stage Disease Study Group. Oral contraceptive use and hormone replacement therapy are associated with microalbuminuria. Arch Intern Med. 2001;161:2000–5.
112. Allison MA, Manson JE, Aragaki A, Eaton CB, Hsai J, Phillips L, Kuller L, Trevisan M. Resting heart rate and coronary artery calcium in postmenopausal women. J Womens Health (Larchmt). 2011;20:661–9.
113. Gierach GL, Johnson BD, Bairey Merz CN, Kelsey SF, Bittner V, Olson MB, Shaw LJ, Mankad S, Pepine CJ, Reis SE, Rogers WJ, Sharaf BL, Sopko G, WISE Study Group. Hypertension, menopause, and coronary artery disease risk in the Women's Ischemia Syndrome Evaluation (WISE) Study. J Am Coll Cardiol. 2006;47(3 Suppl):S50–8.
114. Khurana C, Rosenbaum CG, Howard BV, Adams-Campbell LL, Detrano RC, Klouj A, Hsia J. Coronary artery calcification in black women and white women. Am Heart J. 2003;145:724–9.
115. Sposito AC, Mansur AP, Maranhão RC, Martinez TR, Aldrighi JM, Ramires JA. Triglycerides and lipoprotein (a) are markers of coronary artery disease severity among postmenopausal women. Maturitas. 2001;39:203–8.
116. Lubiszewska B, Kruk M, Broda G, Ksiezycka E, Piotrowski W, Kurjata P, Zielinski T, Ploski R. The impact of early menopause on risk of coronary artery disease (PREmature Coronary Artery Disease In Women–PRECADIW case–control study). Eur J Prev Cardiol. 2012;19:95–101.
117. Barrett-Connor E, Goodman-Gruen D. Prospective study of endogenous sex hormones and fatal cardiovascular disease in postmenopausal women. BMJ. 1995;311(7014):1193–6.
118. Rexrode K, Manson J, Lee I, Ridker P, Sluss P, Cook N, Buring J. Sex hormone levels and risk of cardiovascular events in postmenopausal women. Circulation. 2003;108:1688–93.
119. Chen Y, Zeleniuch-Jacquotte A, Arslan A, Wojcik O, Toniolo P, Shore R, Levitz M, Koenig K. Endogenous hormones and coronary heart disease in postmenopausal women. Atherosclerosis. 2011;216:414–9.
120. de Padua Mansur A, Silva TC, Takada JY, Avakian SD, Strunz CM, Machado César LA, Mendes Aldrighi J, Ramires JA. Long-term prospective study of the influence of estrone levels on events in postmenopausal women with or at high risk for coronary artery disease. ScientificWorldJournal. 2012;2012:363595.

121. Benn M, Voss SS, Holmegard HN, Jensen GB, Tybjaerg-Hansen A, Nordestgaard BG. Extreme concentrations of endogenous sex hormones, ischemic heart disease, and death in women. Arterioscler Thromb Vasc Biol. 2015;35:471–7.
122. Manson J, Hsia J, Johnson K, Rossouw J, Assaf A, Lasser N, Trevisan M, Black H, Heckbert S, Detrano R, Strickland O, Wong N, Crouse J, Stein E, Cushman M, Women's Health Initiative Investigators. Estrogen plus progestin and the risk of coronary heart disease. N Engl J Med. 2003;349:523–34.
123. Hulley S, Grady D, Bush T, Furberg C, Herrington D, Riggs B, Vittinghoff E, Heart and Estrogen/progestin Replacement Study (HERS) Research Group. Randomized trial of estrogen plus progestin for secondary prevention of coronary heart disease in postmenopausal women. JAMA. 1998;280:605–13.
124. Schierbeck L, Rejnmark L, Landbo Tofteng C, Stilgren L, Eiken P, Mosekilde L, Køber L, Beck Jensen J-E. Effect of hormone replacement therapy on cardiovascular events in recently postmenopausal women: randomised trial. BMJ. 2012;345:e6409.

Chapter 21
"The Economic Burden of Hypertension"

Amelie F. Constant, Eleni V. Geladari, and Charalampia V. Geladari

Introduction

Hypertension (HTN) represents a growing health and economic burden, worldwide. It can strike indiscriminately at any age and affect people from all walks of life. More than a quarter of the world's adult population, equaling approximately 972 million, had HTN in 2000. Out of them, 333 million adults come from economically developed countries and 639 million from economically developing countries [1]. This prevalence has been estimated to increase to a total of 1.56 billion adults, by 2025 [1]. HTN has become a major contributor to cerebrovascular stroke, heart attack, and chronic renal disease, and may be responsible for up to seven million deaths annually worldwide [2]. Early detection, treatment and self-care of HTN has significant benefits on the prevention and control of high blood

A.F. Constant, Ph.D. (✉)
Department of Economics, Migration Economics, United Nations University, UNU-MERIT, Maastricht, The Netherlands

Society of Government Economists SGE, Washington, DC, USA

IZA, Bonn, Germany

Temple University, Philadelphia, PA, USA
e-mail: Afconstant299@gmail.com

E.V. Geladari, M.D.
4th Department of Internal Medicine, "Evangelismos" State General Hospital, Athens, Greece

Division of Cardiology, Department of Medicine, Beth Israel Deaconess Medical Center, Harvard Medical School, Boston, MA, USA

C.V. Geladari, M.D.
Division of Cardiology, Department of Medicine, Beth Israel Deaconess Medical Center, Harvard Medical School, Boston, MA, USA

4th Department of Internal Medicine, Hypertension and Cardiovascular Disease Prevention Outpatient Center, Evangelismos General Hospital, Athens, Greece

E.A. Andreadis (ed.), *Hypertension and Cardiovascular Disease*,
DOI 10.1007/978-3-319-39599-9_21

pressure (BP) levels, thus minimizing the increased cardiovascular risk generated by their deleterious consequences to the heart, brain, and kidneys [3].

In recent decades, several studies aimed to contribute to a better understanding of the economic burden of HTN across countries, to inform and raise awareness about the potential impacts of preventive policies. However, their great limitation is their failure to assess the gaps of information regarding direct costs of care for hypertensive patients when financial records are incomplete or absent. Even so, most of the studies agree that integrated programs must be established at the primary care level for control of HTN on the part of governments and public health policy-makers, since it has been demonstrated that in most countries this is the weakest level of the health system. Only this concerted effort could lead to reduced rates of health care costs and better HTN management [3].

HTN is a quite stealthy condition because it can go undetected for years (patients may not have symptoms), while it still damages blood vessels and renders patients incapacitated if not detected early [4]. Prevention and early detection can save lives and reduce public health care costs [4]. Moreover, the reduced quality of life of the affected individuals has detrimental effects on the wellbeing of their families creating tensions, frictions and an overall anxiety for the future. Thus, there is also a social burden as HTN imposes a toll on communities. Some striking statistics for the US from CDC indicate that 1 in 2 Americans suffer from this chronic condition [5]. Public policy is extremely important for both the prevention and treatment of HTN. It can influence preventive health care by direct spending on prevention or by encouraging public sector programs on patient education and awareness on HTN [6].

Costs of Hypertension Across the Continents

The Americas

Analysis of pooled data from the National Health and Nutrition Examination Survey demonstrates that the age-adjusted prevalence of HTN among US adults aged 18 and over was 29.1 % in 2011–2012; while it was similar for men and women it increased with age [5, 7]. Wang et al. aimed to examine the HTN-associated hospitalizations and costs from 1979 to 2006 [8]. Researchers concluded that the proportions of hospitalizations that were associated with HTN (with HTN being either a primary or secondary diagnosis) increased over the period. In addition, they observed that in 2008 US dollars, the annual costs for HTN-related hospitalizations nearly tripled over the past 28 years, reaching approximately US$ 113 billion during 2003–2006 [8]. The much higher costs observed were attributed to the fact that many patients were hospitalized due to other conditions, including coronary artery disease or stroke, having HTN as a secondary diagnosis [8]. Importantly, the implementation of effective interventions to prevent HTN and its complications would be an important step toward reducing the high costs of the US healthcare system (Table 21.1) [8].

Table 21.1 Suggested policies to reduce hypertension costs

1. Effective implementation of a primary health care system.
Reliable equipment for HTN diagnosis.
Trained and educated healthcare workforce.
Easier access to appropriate outpatient treatment of HTN.
2. Adoption of a healthier lifestyle (i.e., low-salt diet, smoking cessation, increased physical activity).
3. Public awareness campaigns and educational programs on arterial HTN and its sequelae.
4. Strict physician adherence to evidence-based HTN guidelines for treatment initiation and HTN management.
5. Absolute CVD risk reduction (elimination of all major CVD risk factors, including atherosclerosis, smoking, obesity, and physical inactivity).
6. Circulating biomarkers may be used for early detection of HTN, which may improve health care costs.

In contrast to the Wang et al. study, which indicated that the in-hospital mortality for patients with HTN declined, Ayala et al., reported that the death rate attributed to HTN in the US increased from 1980 to 1998. Specifically, the death rate increased with patient age and the Charlson Comorbidity Index (CCI) [9]. The latter measures the likelihood of death or serious disability in the subsequent year. In 2010, Wang and coworkers, showed that the average annual hospitalization costs associated with HTN as a secondary diagnosis among insured adults aged 18–64 were $2,734 out of a total of $21,094, per patient [10]. Clearly, hospitalizations with HTN as a secondary diagnosis are expected to increase in the future as the US population ages, since the elderly usually suffer from multiple chronic conditions [10].

A cross-sectional analysis conducted on a US nationally representative random sample of 1.217.103 Medicare fee-for-service beneficiaries aged 65 and over, who were enrolled in both Medicare Part A and Medicare Part B in 1999, showed that per capita Medicare expenditures increased with the number of types of chronic conditions. They went from $211 among beneficiaries without a chronic condition to $13,973 among beneficiaries with four or more types of chronic conditions [11]. Another study, revealed that as much as $108.8 billion in health care spending in the US was attributed to HTN. The study proposed lifestyle modification and medical intervention as important preventive measures to reduce national health care expenditures [12]. In the meanwhile, Balu et al., indicated that the total incremental annual direct expenditures for HTN patients were estimated to be more than US$ 54.0 billion in 2001 after adjusting for demographics and comorbidities; the mean incremental annual direct expenditures for an individual with HTN was found to be $1,131. Prescription medicines, inpatient visits, and outpatient visits constituted more than 90% of the overall incremental expenditures [13].

In 2004, researchers from Massachusetts tried to investigate the economic impact that would result from better adherence to evidence-based therapeutic guidelines for managing HTN in patients older than 65. The study enrolled a total of 133,624 patients being treated for HTN. More than 2.05 million prescriptions for antihypertensive medications were filled in 2001, with 815.316 having a more appropriate alternative regimen according to evidence-based recommendations. These findings suggest that the costs to payers in 2001 would have been reduced by $11.6 million if physicians had followed the evidence-based guidelines for the treatment of HTN [14]. In a special article published recently in the *New England Journal of Medicine* (*NEJM*) it was reported that the full implementation of the new hypertension guidelines would result in approximately 56,000 fewer cardiovascular events and 13,000 fewer deaths from cardiovascular causes annually, which would result in overall cost savings [15]. The population enrolled included previously untreated adults between the ages of 35 and 74 [16]. From an employer perspective, Goetzel et al., demonstrated that the estimated annual cost of HTN was about $150 per employee, whereas the annual cost of absenteeism due to HTN was $77 per employee. In addition, the HTN-associated expenditures due to presenteeism (on-the-job productivity losses) were estimated at $406 per employee [17, 18].

In Canada, the hypertension-attributable costs are estimated to rise from $13.9 billion in 2010, to $20.5 billion by the year 2020, due to demographic changes, increasing HTN prevalence, and increasing per-patient costs [19]. To avoid HTN complications and therefore reduce its associated costs, the Canadian HTN Society has led the development of programs for the prevention of HTN, improvement of HTN knowledge and awareness among Canadians, and improvement of HTN treatment and control by healthcare professionals [20].

Similarly, the prevalence of HTN is following an increasing trend in Latin America [21]. HTN often goes undetected in Brazil, where the annual direct cost of treating HTN is about US$ 671.6 million, based on 2005 data, representing 0.08 % of the GDP for that year [22]. Public awareness campaigns and educational programs on arterial HTN are desperately needed to build public understanding of HTN and its deleterious consequences [22]. In Mexico, in 2011, the total cost of HTN amounted to US$ 5,733,350,291 [23]. A revision in the planning, organization, and allocation of resources, particularly programs for health promotion and prevention of HTN may be important preventive measures to reduce the catastrophic costs due to HTN.

Europe

On the other side of the Atlantic and based on pooled data from the European Healthcare Access Panel, it is expected that while the total population of the five largest European Union member countries (Germany, the UK, France, Italy, and Spain) will grow only by 5.7 %. The number of people living with HTN will, however, triple increasing by 15.3 % [24]. This implies that much greater costs will be imposed on the European healthcare systems and societies. Studying these same five countries, a group of researchers estimated the direct cost associated with hypertension to be € 51.1 billion. Germany ranked the highest with € 17.8 billion, followed by Spain with € 12.2, France with € 8.8, Italy with € 8.1, and England with € 4.1 billion. The authors went a step further to examine the counterfactual of what the economic impact on the national health systems will be if the countries were to increase adherence to antihypertensive therapy. Interestingly, they found that increasing adherence to antihypertensive therapy to 70% would save a total of € 323.7 million [25].

An Italian Study, known as the Pandora Project, showed that the main chunk of HTN-associated costs in Italy came from antihypertensive drugs (42.7 % of the total cost). Next was hospitalization with 28.4% (including hospitalizations for arterial HTN, acute myocardial infarction, coronary artery disease, heart failure, and stroke), followed by visits to general practitioners (15.1%) and laboratory tests (10.6%) [26]. The same study found that the annual direct medical costs associated with HTN were almost 40% lower in new hypertensive incident cases than in prevalent cases [26].

In 2014, Greek researchers conducted a cost-effectiveness analysis of HTN treatment versus a hypothetical no-treatment strategy focusing on clinical endpoints and retaining a 1-year time horizon [27]. The results of the analysis indicated (i) that the incremental cost for a patient to achieve blood pressure control is € 603.1, on average, varying according to disease severity (higher for the severely ill), and (ii) that the incremental cost required for a 1 mmHg reduction in systolic blood pressure (SBP) is €13.7, on average, also heavily influenced by baseline blood pressure [27]. Thus, the results from this study indicate that severely ill patients could be a priority group in terms of treatment administration [27]. Recall that Greece entered a severe financial crisis in 2008, which largely affected all healthcare services and patients suffering from chronic conditions, such as HTN [28]. It is clear that austerity measures and reduction of public health expenditures by the state have led to high out-of-pocket expenditures and to unavoidable insurance coverage loss for primary care services [28].

Asia

Indeed, the 2008 global economic crisis further increased the prevalence of HTN as well as stress perception even in countries in Asia [29]. Recently, Shin et al., investigated the effect of the 2008 global economic crisis on health indicators in Korea. [29] Their results indicated that Gross Domestic Product (GDP) growth rates, as a macroeconomic indicator, are inversely associated with HTN prevalence with a 1-year lag, and inversely associated with stress perception with no year lag [29].

Furthermore, in Vietnam, HTN has been one of the main contributors to the overall burden of disease [30, 31]. It is estimated that its prevalence among adults ranges from 20 to 30% [32]. As such, HTN, imposes high costs to society. More specifically, since there is no ambulatory BP monitoring service available in the community, patients must be admitted to a hospital for diagnosis and initiation of treatment [33]. The required hospitalization to diagnose primary or secondary HTN, generates high costs compared to annual medication treatment at a community health station for HTN and total health expenditure per capita in Vietnam [34].

Indeed, the dangerous complications that occur if HTN is not detected and/or treated early increase the number of inpatient days making the need for the Vietnamese health-care sector to invest in effective interventions to control high BP, imperative [34].

In the Philippines, the main reason for costly inpatient admissions to treat HTN and its sequelae, is the lack of access to outpatient antihypertensive medications [35]. Therefore, the Philippine Health Insurance Corporation (PhilHealth), could improve the quality of care of hypertensive patients by facilitating access to appropriate outpatient treatment of HTN [35]. In Nepal, another Asian country, the healthcare system is totally unprepared to deal with the increasing prevalence rates of HTN observed by scientists, which demands urgent implementation of new policies for effective prevention and control of HTN [36]. The country's healthcare workforce should be equipped with basic essential tools such as reliable blood pressure measuring devices, and trained on how to use them properly. Of equal importance in preventing, controlling and lowering HTN is the education of its population. The promotion of a healthier lifestyle, such as following a low-salt diet, smoking cessation, and physical activity, is critical for reducing HTN associated risks [36]. The total cost of HTN in rural south-west China was estimated to be $231.7 million, with the direct costs, representing the largest component of the economic cost. [37] Notably, the same study found that age and sex were powerful determinants of the cost of HTN, with the costs being higher among males compared to women [37].

An interesting paradigm that no country can escape the plight of HTN is Japan, a country with universal health care for more than 50 years that has achieved the highest life expectancy in the world. Hypertension is so prevalent that affects approximately 40 million Japanese. Studying 314,622 beneficiaries of the medical insurance system in Japan, aged 40–69 years without a history of cardiovascular, cerebrovascular, or end-stage renal disease, Nakamura et al. (2013) found that the economic burden of HTN was the highest for younger men followed by older men. Inpatient medical expenditures attributable to overall hypertension was 7.2 % of the total medical expenditure for the 40–54 year old men and 6.9 % for the 55–69 year old. Comparable numbers for Japanese women were 2.8 % and 3.8 %, respectively [38].

Africa

Cardiovascular disease (CVD) is one of the leading causes of global morbidity and mortality, and represents a major economic burden on health care systems [37]. The absolute CVD risk (estimated on the basis of the number and severity of all major risk factors) reduction and the blood pressure level-approach (based on a single cutoff point to define HTN and initiate treatment) are the two suggested approaches to the primary prevention of CVD, internationally [39–41]. To examine which of the two approaches suggested by the international guidelines is beneficial in terms of costs to the healthcare systems, researchers from Massachusetts, conducted a cost-effectiveness analysis of blood pressure level- and absolute risk-based HTN guidelines in persons without known CVD or target organ damage (TOD) [42]. Whereas in South Africa a BP-level approach is followed in HTN guidelines currently, they concluded that a different strategy based on the absolute risk reduction of CVD is more effective at saving lives and less costly for this developing country [42]. The results of this study could be generalized to other developing countries with multiethnic populations [42].

With the ever increasing migration from less developed to more developed countries we expect to observe a lot more cases of HTN. The stress of migrating and different cultural lifestyles can definitely contribute to the increased prevalence of HTN and other cardiovascular diseases. Health care professional should therefore consider the ethnic diversity and different genetics of the population so as to make the best diagnosis [43].

Summary: Future Perspectives

The resulting economic burden of HTN and its sequelae is enormous, and already threatens fragile health care systems globally. Early detection and appropriate treatment of HTN are crucial for the prevention of costly CVD. In addition, the effectiveness of patient education should not be diminished. An approach toward the development of a primary healthcare system able to deliver effective and affordable care to hypertensives should be adopted. Selection of cheaper, generic drugs whenever no clear benefit exists over the selection of expensive ones, and strict physician adherence to HTN guidelines for initiation of treatment taking into account the absolute CVD risk, are some of the suggested strategies to overcome the economic hurdles generated by this devastating disease. Indeed, therapeutic inertia, partly because of unfamiliarity with clinical guidelines and clinical uncertainty, has been well documented as a contributing factor to lack of BP control, which may be a harbinger for increased health care spending [44]. Therefore, the adoption and use of standardized, evidence-based protocols is of crucial importance [44].

While organizations such as the World Health Organization (WHO) have issued guidelines to prevent and control HTN, we want to point out that cultural and genetic differences among individuals in different countries demand a fine-tuning and tailor-made of guidelines. For example, blood pressure response to sodium varies among ethnic groups with Asians having a much higher tolerance to salt. In addition, these guidelines should be reexamined and amended every 2 years as new evidence-based studies and statistics about demographics become available. In this respect, we believe that the country-specific associations of HTN can play a leading role in education the public and the policy-makers [45].

Lastly, as it has been recently suggested the use of biomarkers can be a promising approach to improving detection and management of disease progression while optimizing health care expenditures. Currently, the potential of biomarkers to improve decision making, facilitate diagnosis and reduce health care costs is under investigation [46].

References

1. Kearney PM, et al. Global burden of hypertension: analysis of worldwide data. Lancet. 2005;365:217–23.
2. Perkovic V, et al. The burden of blood pressure-related disease a neglected priority for global health. Hypertension. 2007;50:991–7.
3. World Health Organization. A global brief on hypertension: silent killer, global public health crisis. Geneva: WHO; 2013 (WHO/DCO/WHD/2013.2).
4. Chockalingam A, Campbell NR, Fodor JG. Worldwide epidemic of hypertension. Can J Cardiol. 2006;22:553–5.
5. Nwankwo T, et al. Hypertension among adults in the United States: National Health and Nutrition Examination Survey, 2011-2012. NCHS Data Brief. 2013;133:1–8.
6. Redwood H. Hypertension, society, and public policy. Eur Heart J Suppl. 2007;9(suppl B):B13–8.
7. Fields LE, Burt VL, Cutler JA, Hughes J, Roccella EJ, Sorlie P. The burden of adult hypertension in the United States 1999 to 2000: a rising tide. Hypertension. 2004;44:398–404.
8. Ostchega Y, Yoon SS, Hughes J, Louis T. Hypertension awareness, treatment, and control – continued disparities in adults: United States, 2005-2006. NCHS Data Brief. 2008:1–8.
9. Wang G, Fang J, Ayala C. Hypertension-associated hospitalizations and costs in the United States, 1979–2006. Blood Press. 2014;23:126–33.
10. Ayala C, et al. Trends in hypertension-related death in the United States: 1980–1998. J Clin Hypertens (Greenwich). 2004;6:675–81.
11. Wang G, Zhang Z, Ayala C. Hospitalization costs associated with hypertension as a secondary diagnosis among insured patients aged 18–64 years. Am J Hypertens. 2010;23:275–81.
12. Wolff JL, Starfield B, Anderson G. Prevalence, expenditures, and complications of multiple chronic conditions in the elderly. Arch Intern Med. 2002;162:2269–76.
13. Hodgson TA, Cai L. Medical care expenditures for hypertension, its complications, and its comorbidities. Med Care. 2001;39:599–615.
14. Balu S, Thomas J. Incremental expenditure of treating hypertension in the United States. Am J Hypertens. 2006;19:810–6.
15. Fischer MA, Avorn J. Economic implications of evidence-based prescribing for hypertension: can better care cost less? JAMA. 2004;291:1850–6.
16. Moran AE, et al. Cost-effectiveness of hypertension therapy according to 2014 guidelines. N Engl J Med. 2015;372:447–55.
17. Goetzel RZ, et al. Health, absence, disability, and presenteeism cost estimates of certain physical and mental health conditions affecting US employers. J Occup Environ Med. 2004;46:398–412.
18. Tarride J-E, et al. A review of the cost of cardiovascular disease. Can J Cardiol. 2009;25:e195–202.
19. Weaver CG, et al. Healthcare costs attributable to hypertension Canadian Population-Based Cohort Study. Hypertension. 2015;66(3):502–8.
20. Campbell NRC, Chen G. Canadian efforts to prevent and control hypertension. Can J Cardiol. 2010;26:14C–7.
21. Prince MJ, et al. Hypertension prevalence, awareness, treatment and control among older people in Latin America, India and China: a 10/66 cross-sectional population-based survey. J Hypertens. 2012;30(1):177–87.
22. Dib MW, Riera R, Ferraz MB. Estimated annual cost of arterial hypertension treatment in Brazil. Rev Panam Salud Publica. 2010;27:125–31.
23. Arredondo A, Zuñiga A. Epidemiological changes and financial consequences of hypertension in Latin America: implications for the health system and patients in Mexico. Cad Saude Publica. 2012;28:497–502.
24. Eurostat. Eurostat statistics. Luxembourg: Statistical Office of the European Commission [Eurostat]; 2012.

25. Mennini FS, et al. Cost of poor adherence to anti-hypertensive therapy in Europe. CEIS Working Paper No. 299. 2013.
26. Degli Esposti E, et al. The PANDORA project: results of the cost of illness analysis. J Hum Hypertens. 2001;15:329–34.
27. Athanasakis K, et al. A short-term cost-effectiveness analysis of hypertension treatment in Greece. Hellenic J Cardiol. 2014;55:197–203.
28. Skroumpelos A, et al. The impact of economic crisis on chronic patients' self-rated health, health expenditures and health services utilization. Diseases. 2014;2:93–105.
29. Shin J-H, et al. Effects of the 2008 Global Economic Crisis on National Health Indicators: results from the Korean National Health and Nutrition Examination Survey. Korean J Fam Med. 2015;36:162–7.
30. Ngo AD, Rao C, Hoa NP, Adair T, Chuc NT. Mortality patterns in Vietnam, 2006: findings from a national verbal autopsy survey. BMC Res Notes. 2010;3:78.
31. Son PT, Quang NN, Viet NL, Khai PG, Wall S, Weinehall L, Bonita R, Byass P. Prevalence, awareness, treatment and control of hypertension in Vietnam-results from a national survey. J Hum Hypertens. 2012;26:268–80.
32. Ibrahim MM, Damasceno A. Hypertension in developing countries. Lancet. 2012;380:611–9.
33. Strategy H, Institute P. Cost effectiveness of hypertensive interventions in Vietnam. Research report. 2011.
34. Nguyen TP, et al. Direct costs of hypertensive patients admitted to hospital in Vietnam–a bottom-up micro-costing analysis. BMC Health Serv Res. 2014;14:514.
35. Wagner AK, et al. Costs of hospital care for hypertension in an insured population without an outpatient medicines benefit: an observational study in the Philippines. BMC Health Serv Res. 2008;8:1.
36. Dhitali SM, Arjun K. Dealing with the burden of hypertension in Nepal: current status, challenges and health system issues. Regional Health Forum. 2013;17:1.
37. Le C, et al. The economic burden of hypertension in rural south-west China. Trop Med Int Health. 2012;17:1544–51.
38. Nakamura K, et al. Treated and untreated hypertension, hospitalization, and medical expenditure: an epidemiological study in 314 622 beneficiaries of the medical insurance system in Japan. J Hypertens. 2013;31:1032–42.
39. Murray CJ, Lopez AD. Alternative projections of mortality and disability by cause 1990-2020. Global Burden of Disease Study. Lancet. 1997;349:1498–504.
40. Williams B, Poulter NR, Brown MJ, Davis M, McInnes GT, Potter JF, Sever PS, Thom SM, British Hypertension Society. Guidelines for management of hypertension: report of the fourth working party of the British Hypertension Society, 2004-BHS IV. J Hum Hypertens. 2004;18:139–85.
41. National Health Committee. Guidelines for the management of mildly raised blood pressure in New Zealand. Wellington: Ministry of Health; 1995.
42. Chobanian AV, Bakris GL, Black HR, Cushman WC, Green LA, Izzo JLJ, Jones DW, Materson BJ, Oparil S, Wright JTJ, Roccella EJ. The seventh report of the Joint National Committee on prevention, detection, evaluation, and treatment of high blood pressure: the JNC 7 report. JAMA. 2003;289:2560–72.
43. Gaziano TA, et al. Cost-effectiveness analysis of hypertension guidelines in South Africa absolute risk versus blood pressure level. Circulation. 2005;112:3569–76.
44. Constant AF, et al. Micro and macro determinants of health: older immigrants in Europe. IZA Discussion Paper No. 8754. 2014.
45. Frieden TR, King SM, Wright JS. Protocol-based treatment of hypertension: a critical step on the pathway to progress. JAMA. 2014;311:21–2.
46. Cohen JD. Hypertension epidemiology and economic burden: refining risk assessment to lower costs. Manag Care. 2009;18:51–8.

Chapter 22
Hypertension; Grey Zones, Future Perspectives

Emmanuel A. Andreadis

Abbreviations

ABP	Ambulatory Blood Pressure
ACC	American College of Cardiology
ACCORD BP	Action to Control Cardiovascular Risk in Diabetes Blood Pressure
ACEI	Angiotensin Converting Enzyme Inhibitor
AF	Atrial Fibrillation
AHA	American Heart Association
AOBP	Automated Office Blood Pressure
ARB	Angiotensin Receptor Blocker
ASH	American Society of Hypertension
BB	B-blocking agent
BHS	British Hypertension Society
BP	Blood pressure
CAD	Coronary Artery Disease
CBP	Central Blood Pressure
CCB	Calcium Channel Blocker
CDC	Centers for Disease Control
CHD	Coronary Heart Disease
CHEP	Canadian Hypertension Education Program
CKD	Chronic Kidney Disease
CVD	Cardiovascular Disease

E.A. Andreadis, M.D., Ph.D. (✉)
4th Department of Internal Medicine, "Evangelismos" State General Hospital,
AHEPA Building, Room 528, Ipsilantou 45-47, Athens, ATT 13122, Greece

Hypertension and Cardiovascular Disease Prevention Outpatient Clinic, "Evangelismos"
State General Hospital, Athens, Greece
e-mail: andreadise@usa.net

E.A. Andreadis (ed.), *Hypertension and Cardiovascular Disease*,
DOI 10.1007/978-3-319-39599-9_22

DBP	Diastolic Blood Pressure
DM	Diabetes Mellitus
ESH	European Society of Hypertension
GFR	Glomerular Filtration Rate
HBP	Home Blood Pressure
HTN	Hypertension
INVEST	International Verapamil-Trandolapril Study
ISH	International Society of Hypertension
JAMA	*Journal of the American Medical Association*
JNC 7	Seventh Joint National Committee
JNC 8	Eighth Joint National Committee
JSH	Japanese Society of Hypertension
LVMI	Left Ventricular Mass Index
MH	Masked Hypertension
NEJM	*New England Journal of Medicine*
NH	Nocturnal Hypertension
NHANES	National Health and Nutrition Examination Survey
NICE	National Institute of Health and Care Excellence
NIH	National Institute of Health
OBP	Office Blood Pressure
PCNA	Preventive Cardiovascular Nurses Association
SBP	Systolic Blood Pressure
SPRINT	Systolic Blood Pressure Intervention Trial
TIA	Transient Ischemic Attack
TOD	Target Organ Damage
VALUE	Valsartan Antihypertensive Long-term Use Evaluation Study
WCE	White Coat Effect
WCH	White Coat Hypertension

The Burden of Hypertension

Hypertension (HTN) is the leading cause of cardiovascular morbidity and mortality, and the single most important risk factor for cerebrovascular stroke [1]. Affecting 972 million people worldwide, its prevalence is estimated to increase from 26.4 % in 2000 to 29.2 % in 2025 [2]. Data from the National Health and Nutrition Examination Survey (NHANES) 2011–2012 support that the age-adjusted prevalence of HTN among U.S. adults aged 18 and over is 29.1 % [3]. This represents nearly one-third of the U.S. adult population [4]. Interestingly, high blood pressure (BP) is under control in only about half of these people while the rest of the population remains undertreated, untreated or even unaware of their condition [4]. Undoubtedly, HTN poses a major public health problem throughout the world which places an increasing economic burden on health resources [5].

Accurate Blood Pressure Measurements and Appropriate Use of Available Methods Are Essential to Hypertension Management

Early detection and accurate diagnosis of HTN are crucial steps in providing optimal care to afflicted patients. It has been demonstrated that uncontrolled HTN among adults is associated with increased mortality [6]. However, the diagnosis and management of HTN depends on accurate BP measurements. Consequently, trained (and regularly retrained) staff in standardized measurement techniques and BP devices validated in accordance with a recognized protocol, such as that of the European Society of Hypertension (ESH), are needed in order to obtain accurate BP measurements in clinical practice [6–8]. It is essential that these devices are checked regularly to ensure that their calibration remains within the European standard specification of ±3 mmHg [9] since calibration errors could result in one in five hypertensive patients not being diagnosed and, conversely, almost one third of patients being wrongly diagnosed with HTN [10]. Apart from obtaining a reliable BP measurement and making an accurate diagnosis of HTN through the use of properly validated and maintained BP equipment, we could also reach a more rational decision regarding treatment initiation and titration. Long-term follow-up of hypertensive patients is also based on proper evaluation of BP levels [10].

It is recommended that clinicians should adhere to published recommendations concerning the acquisition of BP measurement. It has been proposed that arm-cuff devices for BP measurement are preferable to wrist-cuff or finger-cuff devices since the latter have questionable accuracy and international guidelines do not support their use [11–13]. However, the use of wrist-cuff devices should be considered in cases of morbid obesity where an extremely large arm circumference is encountered [13]. Furthermore, it has been shown that the method used for BP assessment (auscultatory versus oscillometric), the patient's posture and body position, also play a crucial role in obtaining accurate BP measurements and have been extensively discussed several times in the international literature [14].

More than 100 years have passed since the legendary development of the sphygmomanometer by von Basch and the first non-invasive BP measurements. Subsequently, Scipione Riva-Rocci became the first to further develop the mercury sphygmomanometer in 1896, almost as we know it today, whereas it was Nikolai Korotkoff who first observed the sounds made by the constriction of the artery in 1905 [15]. Nowadays, the auscultatory method of BP measurement has been established worldwide as the standard for non-invasive BP measurement since it is out of the question that the mercury sphygmomanometer has higher accuracy [16]. However, its use is gradually being limited due to environmental concerns and practical reasons [17]. Technological advances have steadily increased the popularity of the oscillometric method of BP measurement [18]. Automatic home monitors that use the oscillometric technique are being used more and more by patients and health care workers [18]. Nonetheless, the reliability of home monitors has been questioned [19] because a few patients cannot overcome their anxiety when measuring their BP at home inducing thus higher BP levels compared to those taken by 24 h ambulatory blood pressure monitoring (24 h ABPM) [20].

Office or clinic measurement of blood pressure (OBP) remains the most common method for determining BP in everyday practice. In the majority of cases, conventional manual OBP readings are often inadequate for determining the status of an individual patient, mainly because readings are usually poorly performed and their variability is hard to control [21, 22]. In particular, casual OBP measurements may result in readings that are 10/5 mmHg higher, rendering the cut-off point as 150/95, and not the research-based 140/90, for defining HTN in routine clinical practice with devices such as the mercury sphygmomanometer [23]. To improve the accuracy of office measurements, three visits should be performed in order to diagnose HTN, and at least two readings should be taken at each visit [13, 23]. Notably, the European Society of Hypertension and Cardiology (ESH/ESC) guidelines acknowledge the importance of using oscillometric methods to evaluate the patient in clinical practice, rather than the mercury, aneroid or LED hybrid techniques [13]. Moreover, oscillometric measurements appear to be inaccurate and their value diminishes in cases of arrhythmias, as in atrial fibrillation (AF), whereas it has been paradoxically shown that manual BP measurements are still considered somewhat more reliable for patients with AF [23, 24]. OBP measurements cannot further indicate the patient's BP status and have been reported to be inaccurate and misleading, particularly in diagnosing white-coat hypertension (WCH) and masked hypertension (MH) [25, 26]. However, efforts aimed at improving the quality of routine manual OBP measurement have met with limited success.

The automated office BP (AOBP) technique that entails the use of a fully automated device with the patient resting alone in the examining room improves the accuracy of readings and correlates closely with the awake ambulatory BP technique [27–29]. Furthermore, it is a better predictor of target organ damage (TOD) than common office measurements, and seems to correlate well with 24-h ABP monitoring [30, 31]. Myers proposes using the same cut-off point of 135/85 mmHg for home and awake ambulatory BP, suggesting a lower BP threshold for HTN diagnosis [22]. Despite the potential of the AOBP technique for eliminating the white coat effect (WCE), it could be characterized as both time- and space-consuming [22, 28]. Although AOBP readings have many shortcomings if readings are elevated, they should at least serve as an indication for further assessment. As Myers stated "the days of a health professional diagnosing HTN by manually recording a patient's BP with a mercury sphygmomanometer may soon be over" [22]. The AOBP technique has currently been recognized by the 2015 Canadian Hypertension Education Program (CHEP) recommendations as a valuable tool in diagnosing HTN Table 22.1 [32].

Out-of-office BP techniques, such as home BP (HBP) and ambulatory BP (ABP) have evolved in the last 30 years. It is now acknowledged that these are superior to office readings in predicting clinical outcomes and subclinical organ damage and also in providing information on BP behavior out-of-office and in diagnosing various phenotypes of HTN such as WCH and MH [33, 34]. WCH, also known as "isolated office or clinic HTN", is defined as the occurrence of BP values greater

Table 22.1 Comparison between in-office blood pressure measurement methods

	OBP	AOBP
Indications	Basis for HTN screening	Accurate and unbiased observer evaluation of BP
Pros	Physician obtains multiple measurements	Physicians obtain multiple standardized automated measurements White coat phenomenon is lessened Correlates more closely with awake ABPM and TOD Gives similar levels with awake ABPM
Cons	Observer errors and bias Affected by the white coat phenomenon Annual service and recalibration is needed	Diastolic BP is overestimated in the presence of arrhythmia, such as AF Annual service and recalibration is needed

OBP office blood pressure, *HTN* hypertension, *AOBP* automated office blood pressure, *ABPM* ambulatory blood pressure monitoring, *TOD* target organ damage, *BP* blood pressure, *AF* atrial fibrillation

than 140/90 mmHg when measured in the office, but less than 135 mmHg systolic and 85 mmHg diastolic during daily life when measured using the 24-h ABP or HBP measurement technique [35]. Available data indicate that the prevalence of WCH ranges from ≈10 to ≈50 % and depends on the definition of normal for ambulatory BPs and/or the studied population [35]. MH is defined as normal OBP (<140/90 mmHg) but elevated out of the office readings (≥135/85 mmHg). This condition has a prevalence rate of 10–17 % [35] and in some studies as 50 % [35].

When the decision to start treatment is uncertain on the basis of OBP readings, the American Heart Association (AHA), American Society of Hypertension (ASH) and Preventive Cardiovascular Nurses Association (PCNA) propose home measurements in conjunction with ABP monitoring to facilitate the diagnosis. Current guidelines of both the ESH/ESC and those of the Japanese Society of Hypertension (JSH) 2014 highly recommend the use of HBP in clinical practice [14, 36]. To assist in the diagnosis and assessment of treatment, HBP measurements should be performed in strict accordance with the guidelines: "twice in the morning and evening and normally over 6 days" in order to provide accurate information [13]. In this way, BP readings approach mean daytime BP. Automated HBP devices can also monitor sleep BP. These readings approximate ABP measurements and have been correlated with TODs, including left ventricular mass index (LVMI) as evaluated by echocardiograph, and urine albumin excretion [37–39]. However, the HBP technique is not without its disadvantages, such as user misreporting, the over- or under-reporting of measurements taken in unrepresentative conditions, or risk of self-change treatment by the patient [39, 40].

ABP monitoring is the gold standard technique that has been available in clinical practice since the 1980s. Up to now, a steadily growing number of studies have been conducted with over 700 research articles being published annually. Regarded as the technique of choice for the diagnosis of WCH, MH and nocturnal hypertension

(NH), its prognostic ability is also greater than that of office or HBP measuring techniques [41]. Though prices are falling, there are several limitations when applying the technique in clinical practice, including restricted availability and imperfect reproducibility when the procedure is not standardized in terms of activity [41]. Various scientific organizations recommend the use of ABP measurements but this technique is not endorsed in clinical practice by the entire medical community. The National Institute of Clinical Excellence (NICE) has made strong recommendations for its use, stating that "if the clinic BP is ≥140/90 mmHg, offer ABPM to confirm the diagnosis of HTN" [42]. The guidelines issued in 2013 by ESH/ESC consider ABP monitoring as the "gold standard" for diagnosis and management of HTN [13]. They concluded that "ABP monitoring should be performed in subjects with suspected HTN in whom it is necessary to confirm the diagnosis of sustained HTN" [13]. The Australian consensus statement recommends clinic BP for screening and a combination of clinic, home and ambulatory measurements for diagnosis of HTN [43]. On the other hand, neither the eighth Joint National Committee (JNC 8) nor the AHA/ACC/CDC advisory publications mention ABP monitoring [13, 44, 45]. Furthermore, the higher cost of ABP monitoring in comparison to office and home techniques has restricted its use in the States as third party payers cannot cover its expense [45].

Despite new developments in the diagnosis of HTN, scientific communities are yet to be convinced of the use of out-of-office BP monitoring in decision-making in hypertensive patients. An unanswered question or a grey zone is that of how doctors should manage WCH patients. As the risk of cardiovascular disease (CVD) is higher in such patients compared with normotensive subjects, but lower than those with sustained HTN, prospective studies should be conducted in order to investigate the drug-related reduction of CVD risk in WCH subjects [46]. It should also be clarified whether the risk differs when WCH is diagnosed by ABP or HBP monitoring. Data are now available from the Ohasama Study on the long-term stroke risk as hypertensives with partial WCH, partial MH, defined as hypertensives only with home measurements or only with ambulatory technique, had a significant higher stroke risk than normotensives and comparable to those with complete masked or sustained hypertension [47]. Thus, they concluded that both home and 24 h ABPM measurements are needed to evaluate stroke risk accurately [47].

In the meantime, debate over the benefits of drug(s) in treated patients continues and there is no convincing evidence whether benefits are associated with clinical, 24-h or nighttime BP [13]. Furthermore, the usefulness of treating MH patients with increasing doses has not been completely documented. In subjects with MH, the 2013 ESH/ESC guidelines consider antihypertensive drug therapy since MH carries a cardiovascular risk very close to that of in- and out-of-office BP [13]. There is a lack of evidence regarding masked treated uncontrolled HTN in which the increase in therapy remains an unanswered question.

The estimation of central BP (c-BP) in clinical practice by non-invasive techniques has developed over the last decades. It is well known that the application of c-BP reflects the cardiac load and aortic hemodynamics more accurately than brachial BP [48]. However, a number of practical problems are encountered when

Table 22.2 Comparison between out-of-office blood pressure measurement methods

	HBP	ABP	CBP
Indications	Mandatory for accurate HNT diagnosis	Mandatory for accurate HNT diagnosis	Available with recent technological advancements
Pros	Improves patient compliance to treatment Improves HTN control rates Avoids white coat and masked HTN phenomena Avoids observer errors and bias Measurements are highly reproducible It is cheaper than ABP More widely available and more easy repeatable	It is the gold standard for HTN diagnosis It offers multiple measurements in a 24-h period Identifies white coat and masked HTN More reliable predictor of cardiovascular events than OBP	Office central pulse pressure is associated with cardiovascular events and TODs better than peripheral pulse pressure
Cons	Measurements need to be taken systematically at the same time of day and with respect to the dosing of patients' medications It does not provide BP data during routine day-to-day activities and during sleep	High cost of devices Results are often misinterpreted by physicians Time consuming Lack of reimbursement in most countries	Amplification is significantly influenced by CVD risk factors, gender and height

HTN hypertension, *HBP* home blood pressure, *ABP* ambulatory blood pressure, *CBP* central blood pressure, *OBP* office blood pressure, *AF* atrial fibrillation

using c-BP regarding office or ambulatory conditions. Similar central systolic BP (SBP) was found in subjects with normal BP, as well as in those with HTN and vice versa. This phenomenon is mainly unexplored in terms of potential risk stratification and needs to be addressed in future research Table 22.2 [48, 49].

The Development of Several Hypertension Guidelines Aids in Clinical Decision Making

Several HTN societies worldwide have proposed guidelines for achieving the ideal BP target and aim to help clinicians in clinical decision-making. However, these guidelines do not all concur. Hence, physicians are confused as to which recommendations should be followed and how to proceed with individual patients. Furthermore, ongoing research in the field of HTN is constantly changing and reforming current evidence. As a consequence, professional societies update HTN management guidelines from time to time in order to adapt to fresh emerging evidence. It is important to note that the role of these guidelines is not to substitute good clinical judgment but to offer recommendations for HTN management to HTN specialists. Careful use of available guidelines and good clinical judgment are central to optimal HTN management.

All current guidelines recommend antihypertensive drug therapy for patients with BP ≥140/90 mmHg [13, 44]. Recommendations concerning the threshold for initiating treatment advocate a somewhat more relaxed approach of <140/90 mmHg target in patients with diabetes mellitus (DM) or chronic kidney disease (CKD). However, some of the guidelines given by both ASH/ISH (International Society of Hypertension) and JNC 8 are so protracted as to become vague and others differ between them, thus creating confusion for internists, cardiologists and primary care physicians [12, 44].

The recommendations of the Seventh Joint National Committee (JNC-7) were released in 2003 [50] and remained in place until the publication of the work of the JNC-8 in JAMA in 2014 [44]. In contrast with the JNC-7 guidelines, which suggest a BP value of less than 140/90 mmHg as the treatment goal of BP for the general population, including the elderly [50], the JNC-8 recommends a BP goal for the general population of less than 140/90 mmHg, whereas it suggests a BP of less than 150/90 mmHg for the elderly [44]. Furthermore, for patients of all ages diagnosed with diabetes mellitus (DM) or chronic kidney disease (CKD), JNC-8 increased the BP goal from 130/80 to 140/90 mmHg [44]. CKD is defined as a glomerular filtration rate (GFR) of less than 60 mL/min per 1.73 m^2 for 3 or more months [51]. Regarding antihypertensive treatment, JNC-7 proposed a selection of pharmacological therapies based on the presence of comorbid conditions, such as the use of b-blocking agents (BBs) in patients suffering from coronary artery disease (CAD) [50]. Updated JNC-8 guidelines recommend the use of thiazide diuretics, calcium channel blockers (CCBs), and angiotensin-converting enzymes (ACEs) or angiotensin receptor blockers (ARBs) as first-line antihypertensive therapy for the general population [44]. ARBs and BBs, previously proposed as first-line treatment for black people according to JNC-7 [50], have now been eliminated, with thiazides and CCBs being considered as the appropriate selection for this group of patients. Another difference regarding HTN treatment is that patients with non-diabetic CKD need to be treated with ACEIs or ARBs, independently of the presence of proteinuria [44]. As well as ACEIs or ARBs for the treatment of diabetic hypertensives, thiazides and CCBs are now added as first-line treatment for this population [44].

Similar to JNC-7 and JNC-8, the ESH/ESC guidelines recommend a BP value of 140/90 mmHg as the favorable target for the general population [13]. European scientists suggest an SBP target of 140–150 mmHg for elderly patients beyond the age of 80 years, whereas they propose an SBP goal of less than 140 mmHg for fit elderly individuals under the age of 80 years [13]. Interestingly, the decision regarding the optimal BP target among frail, elderly individuals is left to the discretion of the clinician [13]. The term "frail" is used loosely to describe elderly people with a wide range of comorbid conditions, including general debility and cognitive impairment [52]. ESH/ESC, as opposed to the most recent published recommendations of the JAMA, sets a goal BP of less than 140/85 mmHg for diabetic patients with HTN, whereas both agree that an SBP of less than 140 mmHg should be the ideal target for hypertensives diagnosed with CKD [13, 44]. However, they recommend an SBP target of 130 mmHg if proteinuria is present. ESH/ESC recommend all drug classes as first-line agents for the treatment of systolic and diastolic HTN in the general population, as well as for the treatment of diabetics without evidence of proteinuria, whereas they propose the use of ACEIs or ARBs for diabetics with elevated 24-h urine albumin excretion [13]. This also applies to non-diabetic patients with CKD. Finally, European guidelines have no specific recommendations for black hypertensives [13].

Much the same as JNC-8, the ASH/ISH and CHEP guidelines propose a value of less than 140/90 mmHg as the ideal BP target for the general population [32, 44, 50]. Both the ASH/ISH and CHEP give instructions for BP less than 150/90 mmHg for elderly individuals beyond their 80s [12, 32]. Importantly, Canadian specialists recommend that pharmaceutical therapy be commenced when SBP values greater than 160 mmHg are encountered in the elderly over 80 years of age [32]. Similar to ESC/ESH guidelines, CHEP also leave the decision for optimal BP target among the frail, elderly population to the discretion of the clinician [32]. As in JNC-8, ASH/ISH suggest a goal BP of less than 140/90 mmHg for hypertensive patients with DM or CKD of all ages, whereas they underline that the cut-off point should drop to 130/80 mmHg for patients with nephropathy and concurrent proteinuria [12]. Additionally, CHEP sets a goal BP of less than 130/80 mmHg for diabetics and a goal of less than 140/90 mmHg for hypertensive patients with CKD of all ages [32].

Regarding treatment, the ASH/ISH guidelines recommend the selection of first-line antihypertensive therapy based on the comorbidities of individual patients (i.e. BBs in CAD) and their age. This instruction applies to the general hypertensive population [12]. The same guidelines consider the use of ACEIs or ARBs as first-line therapy for diabetic patients and non-diabetics with CKD. Furthermore, thiazide diuretics and CCBs are considered the appropriate drug classes for management of HTN in black individuals [12]. Importantly, for patients with BP ≥160/100 mmHg the ASH/ISH recommends that treatment be commenced with a combination of two drugs [12].

Similar to ESH/ESC recommendations, the CHEP urges physicians to use all classes of antihypertensive drugs as first-line HTN treatment for the general population, but discourages them against prescribing BBs for patients older than 60 years of age [13, 32]. Another similarity between them is that no recommendation is offered for HTN management in black people. For diabetic and non-diabetic patients with CKD, the use of ACEIs or ARBs is proposed by CHEP. In addition, thiazide diuretics, CCBs, ACEIs or ARBs, are suggested by the Canadian Organization as first-line treatment for diabetics without CKD [32].

The Australian guidelines for the management of HTN recommend a goal BP value of less than 140/90 mmHg (or lower if well-tolerated) for all adults [53]. For patients with associated conditions or end-organ damage, such as those with coronary heart disease (CHD), DM, CKD, proteinuria (24-h urine albumin excretion >300 mg) and a history of previous stroke or transient ischemic attack (TIA), the ideal BP target is set at values lower than 130 mmHg systolic and 80 mmHg diastolic [53]. Finally, for diabetic and non-diabetic patients with proteinuria exceeding the cut-off point of 1 g/day, values lower than 125/75 mmHg are considered as the favorable BP goal. Regarding HTN management, Australian physicians recommend treatment initiation with ACEIs or ARBS for patients with uncomplicated HTN, and CCBs and thiazide diuretics for patients aged 65 years or older, as monotherapy [53]. The Australian guidelines emphasize that antihypertensive therapy should be initiated with the lowest recommended dose. Moreover, for patients with associated conditions or comorbidities, it is recommended that clinicians should consider the benefits and contraindications of each drug class before initiating treatment, and that potential drug-drug interactions should also be taken into account. Interestingly, the Australian consensus statement recommends using clinic BP for screening and a combination of clinic, home and ambulatory measurements for diagnosis of HTN [53].

The British Hypertension Society (BHS) has published its recommendations along with the NICE [54]. BSH/NICE guidelines set a BP goal of lower than 140/90 mmHg in the general population, based on OBP measurements. This goal drops to less than 135/85 mmHg with ABP or HBP monitoring, which should always be confirmed by OBP measurements [54]. The same guidelines instruct clinicians to initiate drug therapy in low-risk patients after lifestyle modification to achieve goal BP lower than 160/100 mmHg OBP, or daytime ABP monitoring values less than 150/95 mmHg [54]. In cases with stage 1 HTN, drug treatment has been reserved for those with CV disease, diabetes, chronic kidney disease (CKD), target organ damage (TODs) or an estimated 10-year CV risk of ≥20 %. BBs are not recommended as first-line therapy in the BHS/NICE guidelines, whereas chlorthalidone and indapamide are considered the preferable diuretics for use in hypertensive patients [54]. Moreover, for patients aged 80 years or older, the cut-off point of 150/90 mmHg is set as the ideal target BP Tables 22.3, 22.4, 22.5, and 22.6 [54].

Such differences as those that emerge between the guidelines can lead to confusion for the practicing physician, thus establishing a grey zone in the treatment of HTN [55]. To explain the discrepancies between the two documents, the ASH/ISH authors stated "Because of the major differences in resources among points of care, it is not possible to create a uniform set of guidelines. For this reason, we have written a broad statement…and we expect that experts who are familiar with local circumstances will feel free to use their own judgment" [12].

Clearly, meta-analyses could help to answer other questions of equal practical medical importance that arise beyond the guidelines, such as whether cardiovascular risk reduction at different levels of baseline untreated BP or various outcomes is similar or different. In other words, the question is that of whether BP-lowering treatment should be applied to patients in different risk categories promising larger absolute treatment benefits [56]. To date, meta-analyses have concluded that a lower BP reduces cardiovascular risk and the benefits are proportional to the reduction of BP [57]. It is considered that the greater success of BP-lowering is achieved in grade 1 hypertension and in low-to-moderate risk patients. Furthermore, BP-lowering treatment induces greater absolute risk reduction in those with higher CVD risk levels [58, 59]. Although BP levels less than 130/80 mmHg appear safe, these levels add further reduction in CVD risk only in protecting against stroke. Interestingly,

Table 22.3 Comparison between hypertension guidelines in the adult general population and the elderly without comorbidities

	JNC 7	JNC 8	CHEP	ESH/ESC	ASH/ISH	Australian	BHS/NICE
	2003	2014	2015	2013	2014	2008 (updated 2010)	2011
BP target in the adult general population (mmHg)	<140/90	<140/90	<140/90	<140/90	<140/90	<140/90 or lower if well-tolerated	<140/90 (OBP) <135/85 (ABP/HBP)
BP target in the elderly (mmHg)	<140/90	<150/90 (>60 years of age)	SBP of < than 150 (>80 years of age) SBP of < 140/90 (<80 years of age) Initiate treatment when SBP is > than 160 Treatment initiation is based on clinician's discretion for frail elderlies	SBP of 140–150 (>80 years of age) SBP of < than 140 (<80 years of age) Treatment initiation is based on clinician's discretion for frail elderlies	<150/90 (>80 years of age)		<150/90 (>80 years of age)

BP blood pressure, *JNC-7* Seventh Joint National Committee, *JNC-8* Eighth Joint National Committee, *CHEP* Canadian Hypertension Education Program, *ESH/ESC* European Society of Hypertension/European Society of Cardiology, *ASH/ISH* American Society of Hypertension/International Society of Hypertension, *BHS/NICE* British Hypertension Society/National Institute for Health and Care Excellence, *SBP* systolic blood pressure, *OBP* office blood pressure, *ABP* ambulatory blood pressure, *HBP* home blood pressure

Table 22.4 Comparison between hypertension guidelines in patients with comorbidities

	JNC 7	JNC 8	CHEP	ESH/ESC	ASH/ISH	Australian	BHS/NICE
	2003	2014	2015	2013	2014	2008 (updated 2010)	2011
Goal BP in patients with DM	<130/80	<140/90	<130/80	<140/85	<140/90	<130/80	<140/90
Goal BP in patients with CKD	<130/80	<140/90	<140/90	SBP of < than 140 SBP of < than 130, if proteinuria is present	<140/90 <130/80, if proteinuria is present	<130/80, if proteinuria exceeds 300 mg/day <125/75, if proteinuria exceeds 1 g/day (± DM)	<140/90

BP blood pressure, *DM* diabetes mellitus, *CKD* chronic kidney disease, *JNC-7* Seventh Joint National Committee, *JNC-8* Eighth Joint National Committee, *CHEP* Canadian Hypertension Education Program, *ESH/ESC* European Society of Hypertension/European Society of Cardiology, *ASH/ISH* American Society of Hypertension/International Society of Hypertension, *BHS/NICE* British Hypertension Society/National Institute for Health and Care Excellence, *SBP* systolic blood pressure

Table 22.5 Comparison between hypertension guidelines regarding first-line therapy for systolic and diastolic hypertension in whites and blacks

	JNC 7	JNC 8	CHEP	ESH/ESC	ASH/ISH	Australian	BHS/NICE
	2003	2014	2015	2013	2014	2008 (updated 2010)	2011
Whites	Treatment selection is based on the presence of comorbid conditions (e.g. BBs in patients with CAD)	Thiazide diuretics, CCBs, ACEIs/ARBs	All drug classes (BBs are contraindicated in those >60 years of age)	All drug classes	Treatment selection is based on the presence of comorbidities and the age of patients	ACEIs, ARBs, CCBs Prescribe thiazide diuretics only if patients are >65 years of age	ACEIs or ARBs for those < than 55 years of age CCBs for those > than 55 years of age
Blacks	Thiazide diuretics, CCBs, ARBs, BBs	Thiazide diuretics, CCBs	No recommendation ACEIs are contraindicated for black people	No recommendation	Thiazide diuretics, CCBs	No recommendation?	CCBs for blacks

JNC-7 Seventh Joint National Committee, *JNC-8* Eighth Joint National Committee, *CHEP* Canadian Hypertension Education Program, *ESH/ESC* European Society of Hypertension/European Society of Cardiology, *ASH/ISH* American Society of Hypertension/International Society of Hypertension, *BHS/NICE* British Hypertension Society/National Institute for Health and Care Excellence, *BBs* beta blockers, *CAD* coronary artery disease, *CCBs* calcium channel blockers, *ARBs* angiotensin receptor blockers, *ACEIs* angiotensin converting enzyme inhibitors

Table 22.6 Comparison between hypertension guidelines regarding first-line therapy for patients with comorbidities

	JNC 7	JNC 8	CHEP	ESH/ESC	ASH/ISH	Australian	BHS/NICE
	2003	2014	2015	2013	2014	2008 (updated 2010)	2011
Non diabetic CKD	Initiate treatment with an ACEI or ARB in patients with proteinuria	Start treatment with an ACEI or an ARB, independently of the presence of proteinuria	ACEIs (use ARBs if ACE inhibitor-intolerant) if there is proteinuria, diuretics as additive therapy	Initiate treatment with an ACEI or ARB if proteinuria is present	Initiate treatment with an ACEI or ARB	For treatment selection, take into account: The benefits and contraindications of each drug class Potential drug-drug interactions	Offer a low-cost renin-angiotensin system antagonist If eGFR change is ≥25 % , or change in creatinine is ≥30 % : investigate other causes of a deterioration in renal function and if not, stop the or reduce the dose of the drug , and add an alternative if required
DM	Start treatment with an ACEI or an ARB	Thiazide diuretics, CCBs, ACEIs/ARBs	Concurrent CKD: Start treatment with an ACEI or an ARB CKD not present: Thiazide diuretics, CCBs, ACEIs/ARBs	Proteinuria present: Start treatment with an ACEI or an ARB Proteinuria absent: All drug classes are indicated	Start treatment with an ACEI or an ARB	For treatment selection, take into account: The benefits and contraindications of each drug class Potential drug-drug interactions	Once -daily ACE inhibitor Addition of a calcium-channel blocker or a diuretic

JNC-7 Seventh Joint National Committee, *JNC-8* Eighth Joint National Committee, *CHEP* Canadian Hypertension Education Program, *ESH/ESC* European Society of Hypertension/European Society of Cardiology, *ASH/ISH* American Society of Hypertension/International Society of Hypertension, *BHS/NICE* British Hypertension Society/National Institute for Health and Care Excellence, *CCBs* calcium channel blockers, *ARBs* angiotensin receptor blockers, *ACEIs* angiotensin converting enzyme inhibitors, *DM* diabetes mellitus, *CKD* chronic kidney disease hypertensive subjects with higher CVD risk level are associated with greater absolute residual risk [58–60]. The aforementioned data can help scientific societies and health services alike to provide recommendations that could facilitate decision-making for doctors.

In the future, scientific communities need to inform the population at large so as to protect it against the development of hypertension. Prevention could be achieved with lifestyle modification and regular measurements of HBP performed strictly according to the guidelines. Accurate information concerning BP status could serve to establish whether a person is hypertensive.

What Is the Optimal Blood Pressure Target?

Recently, the release of the results of the Systolic Blood Pressure Intervention Trial (SPRINT, ClinicalTrials.gov number, NCT01206062) at Scientific Sessions of the AHA on 9 November 2015 and online publication of the main results in the *New England Journal of Medicine* (*NEJM*) have intensified the debate as to what should be the optimal systolic BP goal [61]. SPRINT was a well-designed, large randomized clinical trial funded by the National Institutes of Health (NIH). It was conducted at 102 clinical sites in the United States (organized into five clinical center networks), including Puerto Rico. A total of 9361 persons participated in the study with an average systolic BP of 130–180 mmHg and an increased cardiovascular risk, but without diabetes [61]. Subjects considered as eligible for enrollment in the study included hypertensive individuals in the United States who were older than 50 years of age, had never had a stroke and were not diabetic, but were either older than 75 years of age (28 % of subjects), had chronic kidney disease, with an estimated GFR 20 ml/min/1.73 m^2 of body surface (28 % of subjects), or had clinical or subclinical cardiovascular disease or a Framingham score indicating a 10-year risk of >15 % of cardiovascular disease [61]. Individuals with difficult-to-control BP were excluded from the study [61]. More specifically, SPRINT compared the effects of antihypertensive treatment with participants being randomly allocated into two groups: intensive treatment with an SBP target of <120 mmHg and standard treatment with an SBP target of <140 mmHg [61]. The main finding of SPRINT was that a primary composite outcome of myocardial infarction, non-myocardial infarction, acute coronary syndrome, stroke, acute decompensated heart failure, and CVD death was reduced by 25 % in the intensive treatment group compared with the standard treatment group [61]. Similarly, all-cause mortality was reduced by ~27 % in the intensive treatment group. By 1-year post-randomization, the mean SBP was 121.5 mmHg in the intensive treatment group and 134.6 mmHg in the standard treatment group. Importantly, the mean numbers of antihypertensive medications were 2.8 and 1.8 in the intensive treatment and standard treatment groups, respectively [61]. Interestingly, several other trials have indicated benefits in individuals at increased CVD risk without HTN once lower SBP levels are reached [56].

It is noteworthy that the SPRINT trial was designed to identify any serious adverse events related to the more intensive treatment of HTN, such as orthostatic hypotension, syncope, bradycardia, electrolyte abnormalities, injurious falls and acute kidney injury or failure [62]. Whereas the hospital reports of acute kidney injury or failure and electrolyte abnormalities were significantly more common in the intensive than in the standard arm (4.1 and 3.1 % in the intensive arm versus 2.5 and 2.3 % in the standard arm, respectively), there was no significant difference between the two treatment groups in orthostatic hypotension with dizziness during standing BP measurement, injurious falls, or bradycardia [61]. However, the higher rates of some serious adverse events (such as hypotension, kidney failure and electrolyte abnormalities) observed in the intensive treatment group appear unlikely to outweigh the benefits overall [61]. Indeed, the estimation regarding the frequency of the aforementioned adverse events may be biased since the lack of blinding is inevitable in trials involving BP targets. In addition, the fact that individuals assigned to the intensive treatment group were examined more often than those in the standard arm, provided the former with the opportunity to report any adverse events more frequently [63]. Since individuals with diabetes mellitus, prior stroke and polycystic kidney disease were excluded from the SPRINT trial, it is not clear whether the trial results apply to them as well. To our knowledge, in The Action to Control Cardiovascular Risk in Diabetes Blood Pressure Trial (ACCORD BP), a total of 4733 participants with type 2 diabetes were randomly assigned to intensive therapy targeting a systolic BP of less than 120 mmHg, or standard therapy targeting an SBP of less than 140 mmHg [64]. The primary composite outcome was non-fatal myocardial infarction, non-fatal stroke, or death from cardiovascular causes, and the mean follow-up was 4.7 years. Researchers concluded that in patients with type 2 diabetes at high risk of cardiovascular events, targeting an SBP of less than 120 mmHg, as compared with less than 140 mmHg, did not reduce the rate of a composite outcome of fatal and non-fatal major cardiovascular events [64]. Although the ACCORD BP and the SPRINT trials used the same SBP target to determine the effects of intensive antihypertensive therapy in hypertensive individuals, the two trials had important differences. First of all, the ACCORD BP trial was about half the size of SPRINT [64, 65]. Secondly, the participants in the ACCORD BP trial were younger than those in SPRINT (mean age, 62 versus 68 years, respectively). Thirdly, SPRINT included a cohort with chronic kidney disease, whereas levels of serum creatinine >1.5 mg/dL constituted an exclusion criterion in ACCORD BP due to the use of metformin in the treatment of diabetes mellitus [65]. Finally, the main diuretic used in ACCORD BP trial for the treatment of HTN was hydrochlorothiazide whereas chorthalidone was the main diuretic used for the treatment of HTN in SPRINT trial [65]. Yet, the recent ACCORD-BP trial underscores that the risk of left ventricular hypertrophy was reduced in the intensive target arm when compared with the standard arm. This finding generally supports the SPRINT findings, where a lower CVD risk is achieved with tighter SBP control [66]. Other large, randomized controlled clinical trials are needed in the future to establish whether intensive BP-lowering treatment in diabetics leads to CVD risk reduction.

Clearly, the SPRINT trial results change the landscape on how we define and manage HTN [67]. Furthermore, there is no doubt that its results should be considered by the writing committee for the upcoming American College of Cardiology (ACC)/AHA BP guidelines. However, there are still some questions about SPRINT that remain unanswered. For example, what is the optimal SBP target for patients with preserved ejection fraction heart failure and those with low ejection fraction heart failure? [67]. Furthermore, intensive antihypertensive treatment regimen in SPRINT not only reduced SBP but also diastolic BP (DBP). The effects of reduced DBP on total CVD risk remain unclear [67]. In 2006, Messerli et al. demonstrated a J-shaped relationship between DBP and increased risk for CVD, and underlined the need for caution when DBP is reduced to <70 mmHg [68]. Similarly, the INVEST Study (Interventional Verapamil-Trandolapril Study) reported a higher risk for all-cause mortality and cardiovascular events in hypertensive patients with coronary artery disease when DBP drops to 70–80 mmHg [69]. On the other hand, results from the VALUE (Valsartan Antihypertensive Treatment Long-Term Use Evaluation) trial indicate no J-shaped relationship between DBP and increased CVD risk when the former goes down to levels below 70 mmHg [67, 70, 71].

Moreover, it should be mentioned that the SPRINT trial was based on automated office BP measurements and not on 24-h ambulatory BP measurements, which are considered as the gold standard for HTN diagnosis [61]. This issue should be carefully considered since under such conditions, overestimation and consequent overtreatment of HTN is possible [72].

Recently, Ettehad et al. conducted a systematic review and meta-analysis that indicated similar results to those of the SPRINT trial, where SBP lowering to levels <130 mmHg significantly reduced vascular risk across various baseline BP levels and comorbidities such as coronary heart disease, stroke, diabetes, heart failure and chronic kidney disease [73]. Likewise, Xu et al. showed that an SBP higher than 150 mmHg, as well as delays of greater than 1.4 months before medication intensification after systolic blood pressure elevation, and delays of greater than 2.7 months before blood pressure follow-up after antihypertensive medication intensification were associated with an increased risk of an acute cardiovascular event or death [74]. These findings support the importance of timely medical management and follow-up in the treatment of patients with HTN [74].

It is undeniable that all these important findings should be taken into consideration by writing committees when outlining the upcoming BP guidelines, in order to provide the safest and highest quality health care to patients who are always our first priority.

Interestingly, on the other side of the Atlantic Ocean, European researchers are conducting another large randomized clinical trial "The Stroke in Hypertension Optimal Treatment Trial (ESH-CHL-SHOT)" which is designed to test the hypothesis whether antihypertensive treatment programs aimed at reducing SBP to the usually recommended values (<145–135 mmHg), to a lower goal (<135–125 mmHg) or to even lower values (<125 mmHg) in elderly patients at high risk of recurrent stroke (previous recent stroke or transient ischemic attack) will result in progressively greater reductions in recurrent stroke, incidence of cardiovascular outcomes and cognitive decline [75, 76]. Parallely, the preventive efficacy of more and less intense LDL-C reductions is tested on the same outcomes [75]. However, this study is ongoing and researchers estimate that it will be completed in the following years [75]. Definitely, the results of this study will have a major impact on the international BP management guidelines.

Moreover, it was clearly demonstrated from a recent review and meta-analysis, published in Lancet by Xie et al. recently, that intensive BP reduction below currently recommended targets provides greater vascular protection, particularly for people at high risk for cardiovascular outcomes [77]. More specifically, the review, of 19 trials involving nearly 45,000 participants, showed that intensive BP lowering achieved in the trials significantly reduced major cardiovascular events, such as stroke, myocardial infarction (MI), albuminuria, and retinopathy progression, but had no impact on heart failure, cardiovascular death, total mortality, or end-stage kidney disease compared with less intensive regimens [77]. Thus, the authors strongly recommend the need for careful revision of existing clinical guidelines, to recommend more intensive blood-pressure–lowering treatment in high-risk patient groups [77].

Future Perspectives

BP is a potent determinant of CVD risk. However, further large, randomized controlled trials are needed to draw safe conclusions regarding what should be the optimal systolic and diastolic BP target in patients at increased CVD risk, in diabetics, or in the elderly (fit and frail) [78]. As Chobanian states: "Achieving stricter blood-pressure goals will probably require more careful titration of medications, greater use of combination drug preparations, more monitoring for adverse effects, and more frequent patient visits than currently occur". Moreover, technological advancement of available measurement BP techniques is imperative for optimal BP diagnosis and management. Undoubtedly, a high level of clinical suspicion and knowledge are required from the clinician for the early identification and treatment of HTN.

References

1. Chockalingam A, Campbell NR, Fodor JG. Worldwide epidemic of hypertension. Can J Cardiol. 2006;22:553–5.
2. Kearney PM, Whelton M, Reynolds K, Muntner P, Whelton PK, He J. Global burden of hypertension: analysis of worldwide data. Lancet. 2005;365:217–23.
3. Nwankwo T, Yoon SS, Burt V, Gu V. Hypertension among adults in the United States: National Health and Nutrition Examination Survey, 2011–2012. NCHC Data Brief. 2013;133:1–8.
4. Ong KL, Tso AW, Lam KS, Cheung BM. Gender difference in blood pressure control and cardiovascular risk factors in Americans with diagnosed hypertension. Hypertension. 2008; 51:1142–8.

5. Cohen JD. Hypertension epidemiology and economic burden: refining risk assessment to lower costs. Manag Care. 2009;18:51–8.
6. O'Brien E, Atkins N, Stergiou G, Karpettas N, Parati G, Asmar R, et al. European Society of Hypertension International Protocol revision 2010 for the validation of blood pressure measuring devices in adults. Blood Press Monit. 2010;15:23–38.
7. Stergiou GS, Karpettas N, Atkins N, O'Brien E. European Society of Hypertension International Protocol for the validation of blood pressure monitors: a critical review of its application and rationale for revision. Blood Press Monit. 2010;15:39–48.
8. de Greeff A, Lorde I, Wilton A, Seed P, Coleman AJ, Shennan AH. Calibration accuracy of hospital-based non-invasive blood pressure measuring devices. J Hum Hypertens. 2010;24:58–63.
9. Turner MJ, Irwig L, Bune AJ, Kam PC, Baker AB. Lack of sphygmomanometer calibration causes over- and under-detection of hypertension: a computer simulation study. J Hypertens. 2006;24:1931–8.
10. O'Brien E, Asmar R, Beilin L, Imai Y, Mallion JM, Mancia G, et al. European Society of Hypertension recommendations for conventional, ambulatory and home blood pressure measurement. J Hypertens. 2003;21:821–48.
11. Mourad A, Gillies A, Carney S. Inaccuracy of wrist-cuff oscillometric blood pressure devices: an arm position artefact? Blood Press Monit. 2005;10:67–71.
12. Weber MA, Schiffrin EL, White WB, Mann S, Lindholm LH, Kenerson JG, et al. Clinical practice guidelines for the management of hypertension in the community: a statement by the American Society of Hypertension and the International Society of Hypertension. J Clin Hypertens (Greenwich). 2014;16:14–26.
13. Mancia G, Fagard R, Narkiewicz K, Redon J, Zanchetti A, Böhm M, et al. 2013 ESH/ESC guidelines for the management of arterial hypertension. Task Force for the management of arterial hypertension of the European Society of Hypertension; Task Force for the management of arterial hypertension of the European Society of Cardiology. Blood Press. 2013;22:193–278.
14. Ogedegbe G, Pickering T. Principles and techniques of blood pressure measurement. Cardiol Clin. 2010;28:571–86.
15. Roguin A. Scipione Riva-Rocci and the men behind the mercury sphygmomanometer. Int J Clin Pract. 2006;60:73–9.
16. Tholl U, Forstner K, Anlauf M. Measuring blood pressure: pitfalls and recommendations. Nephrol Dial Transplant. 2004;19:766–70.
17. Pickering TG. What will replace the mercury sphygmomanometer? Blood Press Monit. 2003;8:23–5.
18. van Montfrans GA. Oscillometric blood pressure measurement: progress and problems. Blood Press Monit. 2001;6:287–90.
19. Pickering TG, Gerin W, Schwartz JE, Spruill TM, Davidson KW. Franz Volhard lecture: should doctors still measure blood pressure? The missing patients with masked hypertension. J Hypertens. 2008;26:2259–67.
20. Possidente Kaufman J, Ongaro Roberts S. The role of home blood pressure monitoring in hypertension control. J Clin Hypertens. 2001;3:171–3.
21. Reeves RA. The rational clinical examination. Does this patient have hypertension? How to measure blood pressure. JAMA. 1995;273:1211–8.
22. Myers MG, Godwin M, Dawes M, Kiss A, Tobe SW, Kaczorowski J. Measurement of blood pressure in the office: recognizing the problem and proposing the solution. Hypertension. 2010;55:195–200.
23. Stergiou GS, Parati G, Asmar R, O'Brien E, European Society of Hypertension Working Group on Blood Pressure Monitoring. Requirements for professional blood pressure monitors. J Hypertens. 2012;30:537–42.
24. Myers MG, Stergiou GS. Should oscillometric blood pressure monitors be used in patients with atrial fibrillation? J Clin Hypertens (Greenwich). 2015;17:565–6.

25. Myers MG, Godwin M, Dawes M, Kiss A, Tobe SW, Kaczorowski J. The conventional versus automated measurement of blood pressure in the office (CAMBO) trial: masked hypertension sub-study. J Hypertens. 2012;30:1937–41.
26. Myers MG, Godwin M, Dawes M, Kiss A, Tobe SW, Grant FC, et al. Conventional versus automated measurement of blood pressure in primary care patients with systolic hypertension: randomised parallel design controlled trial. BMJ. 2011;342:d286.
27. Myers MG. The great myth of office blood pressure measurement. J Hypertens. 2012;39: 1894–8.
28. Myers MG. Eliminating the human factor in office blood pressure measurement. J Clin Hypertens (Greenwich). 2014;16:83–6.
29. Andreadis EA, Angelopoulos ET, Tsakanikas AP, Agaliotis GD, Kravvariti SD, Mousoulis GP. Automated office versus home measurement of blood pressure in the assessment of morning hypertension. Blood Press Monit. 2012;17:24–34.
30. Andreadis EA, Agaliotis GD, Angelopoulos ET, Tsakanikas AP, Chaveless IA, Mousoulis GP. Automated office blood pressure and 24-h ambulatory measurements are equally associated with left ventricular mass index. Am J Hypertens. 2011;24:661–6.
31. Andreadis EA, Agaliotis GD, Angelopoulos ET, Tsakanikas AP, Kolyvas GN, Mousoulis GP. Automated office blood pressure is associated with urine albumin excretion in hypertensive subjects. Am J Hypertens. 2012;25:969–73.
32. Daskalopoulou SS, Rabi DM, Zarnke KB, Dasgupta K, Nerenberg K, Cloutier L, et al. The 2015 Canadian Hypertension Education Program Recommendations for blood pressure measurement, diagnosis, assessment of risk, prevention and treatment of hypertension. Can J Cardiol. 2015;31:549–68.
33. Baguet JP. Out-of-office blood pressure: from measurement to control. Integr Blood Press Control. 2012;5:27–34.
34. Mancia G, Parati G. Ambulatory blood pressure monitoring and organ damage. Hypertension. 2000;36:894–900.
35. Gorostidi M, Vinyoles E, Banegas JR, de la Sierra A. Prevalence of white-coat and masked hypertension in national and international registries. Hypertens Res. 2015;38:1–7.
36. Shimamoto K, Ando K, Fujita T, Hasebe N, Higaki J, Horiuchi M, et al. The Japanese Society of Hypertension Guidelines for the Management of Hypertension (JSH 2014). Hypertens Res. 2014;37:253–390.
37. O'Brien E, PARATI G, Stergiou G, et al. European Society of Hypertension position paper on ambulatory bold pressure monitoring. J Hypertens. 2013;31:1731–68.
38. Ishikawa J, Hoshide S, Eguchi K, Ishikawa S, Shimada K, Kario K, Japan Morning Surge-Home Blood Pressure Study Investigators Group. Nighttime home blood pressure and the risk of hypertensive target organ damage. Hypertension. 2012;60:921–8.
39. Stergiou GS, Jaenecke B, Giovas PP, Chang A, Chung-Yueh Y, Tan TM. A tool for reliable self-home blood pressure monitoring designed according to the European Society of Hypertension recommendations: the Microlife WatchBP Home monitor. Blood Press Monit. 2007;12:127–31.
40. Myers MG, Stergiou GS. Reporting bias: Achilles' heel of home blood pressure monitoring. J Am Soc Hypertens. 2014;8:350–7.
41. O'Brien E, Parati G, Stergiou G. Ambulatory blood pressure measurement what is the international consensus? Hypertension. 2013;62:988–94.
42. National Institute for Health and Clinical Excellence. Hypertension: clinical management of primary hypertension in adults [clinical guideline 127]. London: NICE; 2011.
43. Head GA, McGrath BP, Mihailidou AS, Nelson MR, Schlaich MP, Stowasser M, et al. Ambulatory blood pressure monitoring in Australia: 2011 consensus position statement. J Hypertens. 2012;30:253–66.
44. James PA, Oparil S, Carter BL, et al. 2014 evidence-based guideline for the management of high blood pressure in adults: Report from the panel members appointed to the Eighth Joint National Committee (JNC8). JAMA. 2014;311:507–20.

45. Go AS, Bauman MA, Coleman King SM, Fonarow GC, Lawrence W, Williams KA, Sanchez E, American Heart Association; American College of Cardiology; Centers for Disease Control and Prevention. An effective approach to high blood pressure control: a science advisory from the American Heart Association, the American College of Cardiology, and the Centers for Disease Control and Prevention. Hypertension. 2014;63:878–85.
46. Franklin SS, et al. White-coat hypertension new insights from recent studies. Hypertension. 2013;62:982–7.
47. Satoh M, Asayama K, Kikuya M, Inoue R, Metoki H, Tsubota-Utsugi M, et al. Long-term stroke risk due to partial white-coat or masked hypertension based on home and ambulatory blood pressure measurements. Hypertension. 2016;67:48–55.
48. McEniery CM, Cockcroft JR, Roman MJ, Franklin SS, Wilkinson IB. Central blood pressure: current evidence and clinical importance. Eur Heart J. 2014;35:1719–25.
49. Agabiti-Rosei E, Mancia G, O'Rourke MF, Roman MJ, Safar ME, Smulyan H, et al. Central blood pressure measurements and antihypertensive therapy a consensus document. Hypertension. 2007;50:154–60.
50. Chobanian AV, Bakris GL, Black HR, Cushman WC, Green LA, Izzo Jr JL, et al. Seventh report of the joint national committee on prevention, detection, evaluation, and treatment of high blood pressure. Hypertension. 2003;42:1206–52.
51. Johnson D. Diagnosis, classification and staging of chronic kidney disease. Kidney Health Australia. 2012:5–7.
52. Lally F, Crome P. Understanding frailty. Postgrad Med J. 2007;83:16–20.
53. National Heart Foundation of Australia (National Blood Pressure and Vascular Disease Advisory Committee).
54. National Clinical Guideline Centre (NCGC). Hypertension: the clinical management of primary hypertension in adults. Clinical Guideline 127. Methods, evidence and recommendations. Commissioned by the National Institute for Health and Clinical Excellence. London: NCGC; 2011.
55. Griffin BR, Schinstock CA. Thinking beyond new clinical guidelines: update in hypertension. Mayo Clinic Proc. 2015;90(2):273–9. Elsevier.
56. Law MR, Morris JK, Wald NJ. Use of blood pressure lowering drugs in the prevention of cardiovascular disease: meta-analysis of 147 randomised trials in the context of expectations from prospective epidemiological studies. BMJ. 2009;338:b1665.
57. Thomopoulos C, Parati G, Zanchetti A. Effects of blood pressure lowering on outcome incidence of hypertension. 1. Overview, meta-analyzes, and meta-regression analyses of randomized trials. J Hypertens. 2014;32:2285–95.
58. Celis H, Fagard RH. White-coat hypertension: a clinical review. Eur J Intern Med. 2004; 15:348–57.
59. Thomopoulos C, Parati G, Zanchetti A. Effects of blood pressure lowering on outcome incidence of hypertension. 2. Effects at different baseline and achieved blood pressure levels-overview and meta-analyzes of randomized trials. J Hypertens. 2014;32: 2296–304.
60. Thomopoulos C, Parati G, Zanchetti A. Effects of blood pressure lowering on outcome incidence of hypertension. 3. Effects in patients at different levels of cardiovascular risk-overview and meta-analyzes of randomized trials. J Hypertens. 2014;32:2305–14.
61. SPRINT Study Research Group. Wright JT Jr, Williamson JD, Whelton PK, Snyder JK, Sink KM, Rocco MV, et al. A randomized trial of intensive versus standard blood pressure control. N Engl J Med. 2015;373:2103–16.
62. Ambrosius WT, Sink KM, Foy CG, Berlowitz DR, Cheung AK, Cushman WC, et al. The design and rationale of a multicenter clinical trial comparing two strategies for control of systolic blood pressure: the Systolic Blood Pressure Intervention Trial (SPRINT). Clin Trials. 2014;11:532–46.
63. Cushman WC, Whelton PK, Fine LJ, Wright Jr JT, Reboussin DM, Johnson KC, et al. SPRINT trial results: latest news in hypertension management. Hypertension. 2016;67:263–5.

64. ACCORD Study Group. Cushman WC, Evans GW, Byington RP, Goff DC Jr, Grimm RH Jr, Cutler JA, et al. Effects of intensive blood-pressure control in type 2 diabetes mellitus. N Engl J Med. 2010;362:1575–85.
65. Jones DW, Weatherly L, Hall JE. SPRINT: what remains unanswered and where do we go from here? Hypertension. 2016;67:261–2.
66. Soliman EZ, Byington RP, Bigger JT, Evans G, Okin PM, Goff Jr DC, et al. Effect of intensive blood pressure lowering on left ventricular hypertrophy in patients with diabetes mellitus: action to control cardiovascular risk in diabetes blood pressure trial. Hypertension. 2015; 66:1123–9.
67. Touyz RM, Dominiczak AF. Successes of SPRINT, but still some hurdles to cross. Hypertension. 2016;67:268–9.
68. Messerli FH, Mancia G, Conti CR, Hewkin AC, Kupfer S, Champion A, et al. Dogma disputed: can aggressively lowering blood pressure in hypertensive patients with coronary artery disease be dangerous? Ann Intern Med. 2006;144:884–93.
69. Cooper-DeHoff RM, Handberg EM, Mancia G, Zhou Q, Champion A, Legler UF, et al. INVEST revisited: review of findings from the International Verapamil SR-Trandolapril Study. Expert Rev Cardiovasc Ther. 2009;7:1329–40.
70. Kjeldsen SE, Berge E, Bangalore S, Messerli FH, Mancia G, Holzhauer B, et al. No evidence for a J-shaped curve in treated hypertensive patients with increased cardiovascular risk: the VALUE trial. Blood Press. 2015;29:1–10.
71. Kjeldsen SE, Oparil S, Narkiewicz K, Hedner T. The J-curve phenomenon revisited again: SPRINT outcomes favor target systolic blood pressure below 120mmHg. Blood Press. 2016;25:1–3.
72. Esler M. SPRINT, or false start, toward a lower universal-treated blood pressure target in hypertension. Hypertension. 2016;67:261–2.
73. Ettehad D, Emdin CA, Kiran A, Anderson SG, Callender T, Emberson J, et al. Blood pressure lowering for prevention of cardiovascular disease and death: a systematic review and meta-analysis. Lancet. 2016;387:957–67.
74. Xu W, Goldberg SI, Shubina M, Turchin A. Optimal systolic blood pressure target, time to intensification, and time to follow-up in treatment of hypertension: population based retrospective cohort study. BMJ. 2015;350:h158.
75. Zanchetti A, et al. Continuation of the ESH-CHL-SHOT trial after publication of the SPRINT: rationale for further study on blood pressure targets of antihypertensive treatment after stroke. J Hypertens. 2016.
76. Zanchetti A, et al. Blood pressure and LDL-cholesterol targets for prevention of recurrent strokes and cognitive decline in the hypertensive patient: design of the European Society of Hypertension–Chinese Hypertension League Stroke in Hypertension Optimal Treatment randomized trial. J Hypertens. 2014;32:1888–97.
77. Xie X, Atkins E, Lv J, Bennett A, Neal B, Nikomiya T, et al. Effects of intensive blood pressure lowering on cardiovascular and renal outcomes: updated systematic review and meta-analysis. Lancet. 2016;387:435–43.
78. Chobanian AV. Time to reassess blood-pressure goals. N Engl J Med. 2015;373:2093–5.

Index

E.A. Andreadis (ed.), *Hypertension and Cardiovascular Disease*,
DOI 10.1007/978-3-319-39599-9_13

L

M

N

O

P

R

S

T

V

W

Printed by Printforce, the Netherlands